IMMUNOLOGY
&
SEROLOGY
IN LABORATORY MEDICINE

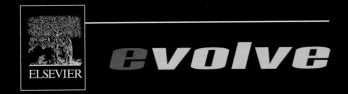

ELSEVIER

IMMUNOLOGY & SEROLOGY
IN LABORATORY MEDICINE

THIRD EDITION

Mary Louise Turgeon, EdD, MT(ASCP), CLS(NCA)

Acting Department Chair
Graduate and Post-Baccalaureate Program Director
Department of Medical Laboratory Science
Northeastern University
Boston, Massachusetts

Clinical Adjunct Assistant Professor
School of Medicine
Tufts University
Boston, Massachusetts

with 169 illustrations

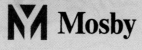

Mosby
An Affiliate of Elsevier

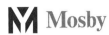

An Affiliate of Elsevier

11830 Westline Industrial Drive
St. Louis, Missouri 63146

IMMUNOLOGY & SEROLOGY IN LABORATORY MEDICINE, THIRD EDITION
Copyright © 2003, Mosby, Inc. All rights reserved.

Permissions may be sought directly from Elsevier's Health Sciences Rights
Department in Philadelphia, PA, USA: phone: (+1) 215 239 3804, fax: (+1) 215 239 3805,
e-mail: healthpermissions@elsevier.com. You may also complete your request on-line
via the Elsevier homepage (http://www.elsevier.com), by selecting 'Customer Support'
and then 'Obtaining Permissions'.

Notice

Pharmacology is an ever-changing field. Standard safety precautions must be followed, but as new research and clinical experience broaden our knowledge, changes in treatment and drug therapy may become necessary or appropriate. Readers are advised to check the most current product information provided by the manufacturer of each drug to be administered to verify the recommended dose, the method and duration of administration, and contraindications. It is the responsibility of the licensed prescriber, relying on experience and knowledge of the patient, to determine dosages and the best treatment for each individual patient. Neither the publisher nor the author assumes any liability for any injury and/or damage to persons or property arising from this publication.

Previous editions copyrighted 1990, 1996

Library of Congress Cataloging-in-Publication Data

Turgeon, Mary Louise.
 Immunology & serology in laboratory medicine / Mary Louise Turgeon.—3rd ed.
  p. ; cm.
 Includes bibliographical references and index.
 ISBN-13: 978 0-323-02371-9   ISBN-10: 0-323-02371-1
  1. Immunodiagnosis. 2. Serodiagnosis. I. Title: Immunology and serology in laboratory
medicine. II. Title.
  [DNLM: 1. Allergy and Immunology—Laboratory Manuals. 2. Serology—Laboratory
Manuals. 3. Immunologic Techniques—Laboratory Manuals. 4. Immunologic
Tests—Laboratory Manuals. QW 525 T936i 2003]
 RB46.5.T87 2003
 616.07'56—dc21
                                                    2002045243

  ISBN-13: 978 0-323-02371-9
  ISBN-10: 0-323-02371-1

Acquisitions Editor: Karen Fabiano
Developmental Editor: Ellen Wurm
Publishing Services Manager: Deborah Vogel
Project Manager: Mary E. Drone
Design Manager: Bill Drone

Printed in the United States of America

Last digit is the print number: 9 8 7 6 5 4 3

To my family and friends for their love and unending support

Contributor

Martin L. Caron, MT(ASCP), CLS(NCA)
Massachusetts General Hospital
Bone Marrow Transplant Program
Boston, Massachusetts

Preface

The intention of this third edition of *Immunology & Serology in Laboratory Medicine* is to continue to fulfill the needs of medical laboratory technology (clinical laboratory technician— CLT) and medical technology (clinical laboratory science— CLS) students and their instructors for a text that encompasses theory, practice, and clinical applications in the fields of immunology and serology. Practicing medical technologists and practitioners in other allied health disciplines can use this text as a reference.

The purpose of this edition continues to be to describe the basic concepts of immunology, to elucidate the underlying theory of procedures performed in clinical immunology and serology laboratories, to summarize clinical features and present case studies of selected infectious diseases and autoimmune disorders, and to discuss concepts of transplantation and tumor immunology. The major topical areas are organized into four primary sections. The initial two sections provide foundation knowledge and skills that progress from basic immunologic mechanisms and serologic concepts to the theory of laboratory procedures, including molecular techniques. The latter two sections emphasize medical applications of importance to clinical laboratory science. In addition, the latter two sections contain representative disorders of infectious and immunologic origin, as well as topics such as transplantation and tumor immunology. The sequence of the sections is designed to accommodate the core needs of clinical laboratory students in basic concepts, the underlying theory of procedures, and immunologic manifestations of infectious diseases. Because the needs of some students are more advanced in immunopathology, these topics are presented later in the book to allow students to analyze and evaluate abnormalities based on their knowledge of the preceding sections. Students may study specific components of the book, depending on the length and objectives of the course.

This third edition of *Immunology & Serology in Laboratory Medicine* capitalizes on the strengths of previous editions and presents additional or revised current information in each chapter. A topical outline is presented at the beginning of each chapter. These outlines should be of value to students in the organization of the material and may be of convenience to instructors in preparing lectures. Illustrations, photographs, and summary tables are used to visually clarify various conceptual themes and arrange detailed information. Chapter highlights and additional test questions are provided at the conclusion of each chapter. Twenty additional clinical case studies and more than 500 additional review questions have been added to this edition.

As in the previous editions, representative procedures are organized according to the format suggested by the NCCLS. This format introduces students to the typical procedural write-up encountered in a working clinical laboratory.

What's significantly new in the third edition? The knowledge base in the field of immunology continues to expand logarithmically. In Part One information related to lymphocyte development has been expanded. Knowledge related to soluble mediators of inflammation (e.g., cytokines) of importance to clinical laboratory scientists has been updated and expanded. Part Two, The Theory of Immunologic and Serologic Procedures, has been reorganized. Some methods have been replaced by more modern technology. A new chapter, Molecular Techniques, has been added to this section. Infrequently used but classic procedures, with the exception of the VDRL procedures, have been organized into a separate chapter to serve as a reference for students. Safety information has been updated to reflect the latest information required by laboratory staff. Part Three, Immunologic Manifestations of Infectious Diseases, has been revised to reflect new knowledge of each disease. Chapter 16 now includes presentations related to Ehrlichiosis and Borreliosis in addition to Lyme Disease. Chapter 20, Viral Hepatitis, includes a discussion of several new viral agents. Representative case studies have been added to the chapters in this section. Part Four, Immunologically and Serologically Related Disorders, has an expanded chapter on Transplantation with an additional chapter on Bone Marrow Transplantation. In addition, knowledge related to tumor immunology has been significantly expanded and presented in a separate chapter. Case studies have been added to chapters in this section.

Although the content of immunology continues to expand, *Immunology & Serology in Laboratory Medicine* is written for beginning students in immunology who need an emphasis on the medical aspects of the discipline and the practical aspects of serology. No attempt has been made to replace books written at more sophisticated reference levels. The third edition should provide students with a basic foundation in the theory and practice of clinical immunology and practical serology in a one- or two-term course. The text is appropriate for immunopathology or pathophysiology courses.

Mary L. Turgeon

Acknowledgments

My objective in writing *Immunology & Serology in Laboratory Medicine* continues to be to integrate basic science concepts and procedural theory in immunology and serology with relevant medical applications. Because the body of knowledge in immunology continues to expand, writing and revising a book that addresses the holistic needs of those in the clinical sciences continues to be a challenge. In addition, this book continues to provide me with the opportunity to share my experience and insight as a medical educator with others.

Special thanks to the following Northeastern University Medical Laboratory Science graduate students for their extensive research assistance: Esther Kumar (Chapter 16, Lyme Disease, and Appendix C, Chronic Fatigue Syndrome), Sara Fuller (Chapter 18, Cytomegalovirus, and Chapter 20, Viral Hepatitis), and Martin Caron (Chapter 29, Bone Marrow Transplantation). I am most appreciative of the efforts extended on my behalf by Karen Fabiano and Ellen Wurm at Elsevier.

Contents

Part One

Basic Immunologic Mechanisms

Chapter 1

An Overview of Immunology

LEARNING OBJECTIVES

At the conclusion of this chapter, the reader should be able to:
- Define the term immunology.
- Explain the function of the immune system.

- Describe the first line of defense, natural immunity, and adaptive immunity as body defense systems against microbial diseases.

Immunology is defined as the study of the molecules, cells, organs, and systems responsible for the recognition and disposal of foreign (nonself) material; how body components respond and interact; the desirable and undesirable consequences of immune interactions; and the ways in which the immune system can be advantageously manipulated to protect against or treat diseases. Immunologists in the Western Hemisphere generally exclude from the study of immunology the relationship between cells during embryonic development.

The immune system is composed of a large and complex set of widely distributed elements. Distinctive characteristics of the immune system include specificity, memory, mobility, replicability, and cooperativity. Specificity and memory are characteristics of lymphocytes (see Chapter 4). Various specific and nonspecific elements of the immune system demonstrate mobility; these include T and B lymphocytes, immunoglobulins, complement, and hematopoietic cells. For this reason, local sensitization (e.g., an insect bite) can result in systemic sensitization. In addition, specific and nonspecific cellular components of the immune system can replicate. Cooperativity is a required feature if optimal function of the immune system is to occur. Cooperative interaction involves specific cellular elements, cell products, and nonlymphoid elements.

The function of the immune system is to recognize self from nonself and to defend the body against nonself. Such a system is necessary for survival in all living organisms. The distinction of self from nonself is made by an elaborate, specific recognition system. Specific elements of the immune system are the lymphocytes. The immune system also has nonspecific effector mechanisms that usually amplify the specific functions. Nonspecific components of the immune system include mononuclear phagocytes, polymorphonuclear leukocytes, and soluble factors (e.g., complement).

Nonself substances can be as diverse as life-threatening infectious microorganisms or a lifesaving organ transplant. The desirable consequences of immunity include natural resistance, recovery, and acquired resistance to infectious diseases. A deficiency or dysfunction of the immune system can cause many disorders. Undesirable consequences of immunity include allergy, rejection of a transplanted organ, or an autoimmune disorder (a condition in which the body's own tissues are attacked as if they were foreign).

BODY DEFENSES: RESISTANCE TO MICROBIAL DISEASE

Before a pathogen can invade the human body, it must overcome the resistance provided by the body's immune system, which consists of nonspecific and specific defense mechanisms (Figure 1-1).

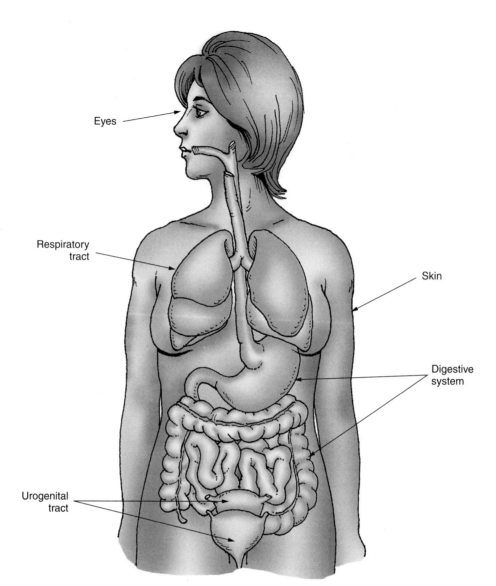

Figure 1-1   Natural body defenses. Body fluids, specialized cells, fluids, and resident bacteria (normal flora) allow systems such as the respiratory, digestive, urogenital, and integumentary to naturally defend the body against microbial infection.

First Line of Defense

The first line of defense or first barrier to infection is unbroken skin and mucosal membrane surfaces. These surfaces are of utmost importance in forming a physical barrier to many microorganisms because this is where foreign materials usually first contact the host. Keratinization of the upper layer of the skin and the constant renewal of the skin's epithelial cells, which repairs breaks in the skin, assist in the protective function of skin and mucosal membranes. In addition, the normal flora (microorganisms normally inhabiting the skin and membranes) deter penetration or facilitate elimination of foreign microorganisms from the body.

Secretions are also an important component in the first line of defense against microbial invasion. Mucus adhering to the membranes of the nose and nasopharynx traps microorganisms, which can be expelled by coughing or sneezing. Sebum (oil) produced by the sebaceous glands of the skin and lactic acid contained in sweat both possess antimi-

crobial properties. The production of ear wax is another example of a process that guards the auditory canals of the ear from infectious disease. Secretions produced in the process of eliminating liquid and solid wastes (e.g., the urinary and gastrointestinal processes) are important in physically removing potential pathogens from the body. The acidity and alkalinity of the fluids of the stomach and intestinal tract, as well as the acidity of the vagina, can destroy many potentially infectious microorganisms. Additional protection is provided to the respiratory tract by the constant motion of the cilia of the tubules.

In addition to the physical ability to wash away potential pathogens, tears and saliva also have chemical properties of value in defending the body. The enzyme lysozyme, which is found in tears and saliva, attacks and destroys the cell wall of susceptible bacteria, particularly certain gram-positive bacteria. Immunoglobulin A (IgA) antibody is another protective substance of importance in tears and saliva.

Thus the body has a wide variety of barrier-assisting defenses that protect against disease as the first line of defense. Although these barriers vary between individuals, they do assist in the general resistance to infectious organisms.

Natural Immunity

Natural (innate or inborn) resistance is one of the two ways that the body resists infection after microorganisms have penetrated the first line of resistance. The second form, acquired resistance, which specifically recognizes and selectively eliminates exogenous (or endogenous) agents, is discussed later in this chapter.

Natural immunity is characterized as a nonspecific mechanism. If a microorganism penetrates the skin or mucosal membranes, a second line of cellular and humoral defense mechanisms (Box 1-1) becomes operational. The elements of natural resistance include phagocytic cells, complement, and acute inflammatory reaction. Despite their relative lack of specificity, these components are essential because they are largely responsible for natural immunity to many environmental microorganisms. Phagocytic cells (see Chapter 3), which engulf invading foreign material, constitute the major cellular component. Complement proteins (see Chapter 5) are the major humoral (fluid) component of natural immunity. Other substances of the humoral component are lysozymes and interferon, which are sometimes described as natural antibiotics. Interferon is a family of proteins produced rapidly by many cells in response to viral infection; it blocks the replication of virus in other cells.

Tissue damage produced by infectious or other agents results in inflammation, a series of biochemical and cellular changes that facilitate the phagocytosis (the engulfing and destruction) of microorganisms or damaged cells. If the degree of inflammation is sufficiently extensive, it is accompanied by an increase in the plasma concentration of acute-phase proteins or reactants, a group of glycoproteins. Acute-phase proteins (see Chapter 5) are sensitive indicators of the presence of inflammatory disease and are especially useful in monitoring such conditions.

Adaptive Immunity

If a microorganism overwhelms the body's natural resistance, a third line of defensive resistance exists. Acquired or adaptive immunity is a more recently evolved mechanism. It allows the body to recognize, remember, and respond to a specific stimulus, an antigen. Adaptive immunity can result in the elimination of microorganisms and in the recovery from disease, and it frequently leaves the host with specific immunologic memory. This condition of memory or recall, acquired resistance, allows the host to respond more effectively if reinfection with the same microorganism occurs.

Adaptive immunity, like natural immunity, is composed of cellular and humoral components (Box 1-2). The major cellular component of this mechanism is the lymphocyte (see Chapter 4); the major humoral component is the antibody (see Chapter 2). Lymphocytes selectively respond to nonself materials, antigens, which leads to immune memory and a permanently altered pattern of response or adaptation to the environment. The majority of the actions of the two categories of the adaptive response, humoral-mediated and cell-

Box 1-1	Components of the Natural Immune System

CELLULAR

Mast cells
Neutrophils
Macrophages

HUMORAL

Complement
Lysozyme
Interferon

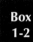

Box 1-2	Components of the Adaptive Immune System

CELLULAR

T Lymphocytes
B Lymphocytes
Plasma cells

HUMORAL

Antibodies
Cytokines

mediated immunity (Table 1-1), are exerted by the interaction of antibody with complement and the phagocytic cells of natural immunity, and of T cells with macrophages.

Humoral-Mediated Immunity

If specific antibodies have been formed to antigenic stimulation, they are available to protect the body against foreign substances. The recognition of foreign substances and subsequent production of antibodies to these substances are the specific meaning of immunity. Antibody-mediated immunity to infection is acquired if the antibodies are formed by the host or received from another source. These two types of acquired immunity (Table 1-2) are called active and passive immunity, respectively.

Active immunity can be acquired by natural exposure in response to an infection or natural series of infections, or it may be acquired by an intentional injection of an antigen. This intentional injection of antigen, vaccination, is an effective method of stimulating antibody production and memory (acquired resistance) without suffering from the disease. Suspensions of antigenic materials used for immunization are varied and may be of animal or plant origin. These products may be composed of living suspensions of weak or attenuated cells or viruses, killed cells or viruses, or extracted bacterial products such as the altered and no-longer-poisonous toxoids used to immunize against diphtheria and tetanus. The selected agents should stimulate the production of antibodies without clinical signs and symptoms of disease in an immunocompetent (a host that is able

---

TABLE 1-1   Characteristics of Humoral- and Cell-Mediated Immunity

	Humoral-Mediated Immunity	Cell-Mediated Immunity
Mechanism	Antibody-mediated	Cell-mediated
Cell type	B lymphocytes	T lymphocytes
Mode of action	Antibodies in serum	Direct cell-to-cell contact or soluble products secreted by cells
Purpose	Primary defense against bacterial infection	Defense against viral and fungal infections, intracellular organisms, tumor antigens, and graft rejection

---

TABLE 1-2   Comparison of Types of Acquired Immunity

	Type	Mode of Acquisition	Antibody Produced by Host	Duration of Immune Response
Active	Natural	Infection	Yes	Long
	Artificial	Vaccination	Yes	Long*
Passive	Natural	Transfer in vivo or colostrum	No	Short
	Artificial	Infusion of serum/plasma	No	Short

*Immunocompetent host.

---

to recognize a foreign antigen and build specific antigen-directed antibodies) and cause permanent antigenic memory. Booster vaccinations may be needed in some cases to expand the pool of memory cells. The mechanism of antigen recognition and antibody production is discussed in Chapter 2.

Artificial passive immunity is achieved by infusion of serum or plasma containing high concentrations of antibody. This form of passive immunity provides immediate antibody protection against microorganisms such as hepatitis A by administering preformed antibodies. These antibodies have been produced by another person or animal that has been actively immunized, but the ultimate recipient has not produced them. The recipient will only temporarily benefit from passive immunity for as long as the antibodies persist in their circulation.

In addition, passive immunity can be acquired naturally by the fetus because of the transfer of antibodies by the maternal circulation in utero. Maternal antibodies are also transferred to the newborn after parturition in the prelactation fluid, colostrum. For the newborn to have lasting protection, active immunity must occur.

Immediate hypersensitivity comprises a subset of the body's antibody-mediated mechanisms. This subset consists of the reactions primarily mediated by IgE, a class of immunoglobulins with unique biologic properties. Expression of immediate hypersensitivity results from:

1. Exposure to antigen (allergens)
2. Development of an IgE antibody response to the antigen
3. Binding of the IgE to mast cells
4. Reexposure to the antigen
5. Antigen interaction with antigen-specific IgE bound to the surface membrane of mast cells
6. Release of potent chemical mediators from sensitized mast cells
7. Action of these mediators on various organs

Atopic diseases are processes mediated by or related to IgE-immediate hypersensitivity. The most dramatic and devastating systemic manifestation of immediate hypersensitivity is anaphylaxis. Anaphylaxis is an immediate (type I) hypersensitivity reaction characterized by local reactions such as urticaria (hives) and angioedema (redness and swelling), or by systemic reactions in the respiratory tract, cardiovascular system, gastrointestinal tract, or skin. This type of reaction can be fatal. Other types of atopic diseases include allergic rhinoconjunctivitis, urticaria, angioedema, asthma, gastrointestinal allergy, and atopic dermatitis, an eczematous skin eruption.

In addition to IgE-dependent hypersensitivity, two other immunoglobulin-dependent (antibody-dependent) mechanisms and a fourth, cell-mediated, delayed-hypersensitivity mechanism exist. These clinical reactions are discussed in detail in Chapter 23. An alternate system of classification for hypersensitivity was developed by Gell and Coombs more than 2 decades ago. Characteristics of this classification of hypersensitivity are presented in Table 1-3.

Cell-Mediated Immunity

Cell-mediated immunity consists of immune activities that differ from antibody-mediated immunity (Table 1-1). Lymphocytes are the unique bearers of immunologic specificity, which depends on their antigen receptors. The full development and expression of immune responses, however, require that nonlymphoid cells and molecules primarily act as amplifiers and modifiers.

Cell-mediated immunity is moderated by the link between T lymphocytes and phagocytic cells (i.e., monocytes-macrophages).

A B type of lymphocyte can probably respond to a native antigenic determinant of the appropriate "fit"; a T type of lymphocyte responds to antigens presented by other cells in the context of major histocompatibility complex (MHC) proteins.

TABLE 1-3   Classification of Hypersensitivity Reactions

	Type I	Type II	Type III	Type IV
	Anaphylactic	**Cytotoxic**	**Immune Complex**	**T-Cell Dependent**
Antibody	IgE	IgG Possibly other	IgG IgM	None
Complement involved	No	Yes	Yes	No
Cells involved	Mast cells Basophils	Red cells White cells Platelets	Host tissue cells	T cells Macrophages
Examples	Anaphylaxis Hay fever Food allergy	Transfusion reactions Hemolytic disease of newborn Thrombocytopenia	Arthus reaction Serum sickness Pneumonitis	Allergy of infection Contact dermatitis

A T type of lymphocyte does not directly recognize the antigens of microorganisms or other living cells such as allografts (a graft of tissue from a genetically different member of the same species, e.g., a human kidney), but rather when the antigen is present on the surface of an antigen-presenting cell, the macrophage. Antigen-presenting cells (APCs) were at first thought to be limited to cells of the mononuclear phagocyte system. Recently, other kinds of cells (e.g., endothelial and glial), have been shown to have the ability to "present" antigens.

Lymphocytes are immunologically active through various types of direct cell-to-cell contact and by the production of soluble factors. The roles of various types of lymphocytes are discussed in Chapter 4. Nonspecific soluble factors (see Chapter 5) are made by or act on various elements of the immune system. These molecules are collectively called cytokines. Some mediators that act between leukocytes are called interleukins.

The term *delayed hypersensitivity* is often used synonymously with the term *cell-mediated immunity*. Delayed hypersensitivity, however, refers to the slow appearance of a secondary response in the skin; it dates back to the time when antibody responses were detected by immediate hypersensitivity and reflected the subtle difference in the length of time that it took for a delayed response to occur (e.g., tuberculin skin test). Cell-mediated immunity is responsible for the following immunologic events:

1. Contact sensitivity (e.g., poison-ivy dermatitis caused by binding of substance to the skin)
2. Delayed hypersensitivity (e.g., contact dermatitis)
3. Immunity to viral and fungal antigens
4. Immunity to intracellular organisms
5. Rejection of foreign-tissue grafts
6. Elimination of tumor cells bearing neoantigens
7. Formation of chronic granulomas (undegradable material such as tubercle bacilli, streptococcal cell walls, asbestos, or talc, sequestered in a focus of concentric macrophages that also contains some lymphocytes and eosinophils)

Under some conditions, the activities of cell-mediated immunity may not be beneficial. Suppression of the normal adaptive immune response (immunosuppression) by drugs or other means is necessary in conditions such as organ transplantation, hypersensitivity, and autoimmune disorders.

FACTORS ASSOCIATED WITH IMMUNOLOGIC DISEASE

Many of the same factors such as general health and the age of an individual are important in the development of immunologic and infectious disease; however, in the case of noninfectious diseases or disorders, additional factors may be important. These factors can include genetic predisposition to many disorders, nutritional status, and the individual's method of coping with stress.

Effect of Age on Immunity

Although nonspecific and specific body defenses are present in the unborn and newborn infant, many of these defenses are not completely developed in this group. Therefore young children are at greater risk for diseases, particularly infectious diseases.

A loss of immune defenses, not disease itself, may cause death in at least 30% of people more than 85 years old. In older adults certain natural barriers to infection break down. Changes in the skin resulting from the normal aging process allow it to be breached more readily. In the lung many of the specialized defenses against foreign invasion are weakened, including the cough reflex and bronchotracheal ciliary action. Other age-related changes include incomplete emptying of the bladder, which can lead to infection and alteration in the normal flora of the intestine; this is caused by immobilization or drug therapy. In addition, some age-associated diseases exert detrimental effects on the immune system. Diabetes, which is increasing in incidence in older adults, results in greater susceptibility to diseases such as septicemia and gangrene.

The ability to respond immunologically to disease is age related. It has been suggested that faulty immunologic reactions are involved in the aging process; however, the effect of aging on the immune response is highly variable. In studies of the cells of the immune system, a general decline in the quantity of some types of lymphocytes in the blood has been observed in some older adults. A decrease in lymphocyte subset types and aberrant functioning of immunoregulatory cells have been implicated as potential causes of many age-related immunologic dysfunctions that contribute to poor immunity in the elderly. It is not known whether enhancement of the immune response with methods such as tissue removal, dietary manipulation, cell grafting, and chemical intervention in older adults will be associated with clinical benefits; but immunomodulation may be a formidable tool to combat aging of the immune system in the future.

Role of Nutrition in Immunity

The importance of good nutrition to good health has always been emphasized. Good nutrition is known to be important to growth and development, and it is now suggested that a healthy diet is important in the aging process and in the triad of nutrition, immunity, and infection. The consequences of diet in many aspects of the immune response have been documented in multiple disorders. Every constituent of body defenses, including phagocytosis and humoral and cellular immunity, appears to be influenced by nutritional intake. Deficient or excessive intake of some dietary components such as vitamins and minerals can exert negative effects on the immune response (Table 1-4). Therefore a healthy diet is important for maximum functioning of the immune system.

Effects of a Proper Diet

The study of the relationship of nutrition to immunity is complex because of factors such as the diversity of the food we eat and the influence of environment on specific nutritional needs. Some nutritional associations hold true for the risk of malignancy and immune function, but others do not. The role of nutrition in the risk and treatment of malignancy has been studied. For example, low intake of vitamin A and high intake of fats have been associated with an increased risk of malignancy in humans. Both constituents also have a marked effect on the immune response. It has been suggested that the balance and absolute intake of multiple nutrients have an influence on susceptibility to infection, to host immune response, and possibly on susceptibility to and treatment of autoimmune disorders.

Food is a complex mixture of organic and inorganic substances and metals in varying proportions. Within each group of nutrients, each chemical can have a different effect on various physiologic functions. Specific components of food may impair or cause an abnormality in immune function by the following mechanisms:

1. Deficiency of a nutrient
2. Excess of a nutrient
3. An error of metabolism
4. Direct toxic effect and/or an allergic reaction

Deficiency of a Nutrient

Malnutrition caused by extremely reduced caloric intake or a deficiency, complete or partial, of a specific nutrient can pro-

---

TABLE 1-4 Examples of Suggested Effects of Increased or Decreased Levels of Vitamins and Minerals

Constituent	Effect
Water-Soluble Vitamins	
Folic acid	Deficiency has a profound effect on cell-mediated immunity.
Pantothenic acid	A deficiency in conjunction with pyridoxine deficiency is associated with the absence of antibodies.
Vitamin B_1 (thiamine)	Deficiency can produce abnormal phagocytosis.
Vitamin B_2 (riboflavin)	No disease is associated with deficiency. Specific role in human malignancy is unclear but believed to play a role in tumorgenesis.
Vitamin B_6 (pyridoxal, pyridoxine)	Deficiency during prenatal and postnatal development affects organs of the immune system, spleen, and thymus, respectively.
	Deficiency in children and adults can cause mild impairment (e.g., decreased lymphocytes), decreased hormones produced by immune organs (e.g., thymus), inability to produce antibodies to various antigens, and depression of delayed hypersensitivity.
	If there is simultaneous deficiency in pantothenic acid, complete absence of antibody production will occur.
Vitamin B_{12} (cobalamin)	Congenital deficiency of transcobalamin II,* associated with decreased white cells; the absence of immunoglobulins; impaired phagocytosis.
Vitamin C (ascorbic acid)	Increased or decreased amounts may negatively affect phagocytosis.
Fat-Soluble Vitamins and Congeners	
Vitamin A	Decreased intake of vitamin A and a high intake of fats are associated with an increased risk of malignancy.
Vitamin E	Increased intake of vitamin E improves cellular immune function.
Cadmium	Excess but subtoxic amounts have a negative effect on normal immune function.
Lead	Deficiency is associated with increase in severity of inflammatory lesion and antibody-forming cell response.
Copper	In excess, it has a dose-dependent immunosuppressive effect.
Iodine	Deficiency probably increases susceptibility to infection because iron is an integral part of microbicidal process.
Iron	Deficiency impairs T-cell–dependent antibody responses, particularly in association with vitamin E deficiency.
Selenium	

*Proteins that deliver vitamin B_{12} to the tissues.

duce abnormal immune function. Malnutrition has also been implicated in cancer risk and in abnormalities of immune function.

Protein deficiency is an example of a disorder that compromises the immune system. Patients with such deficiency have altered immune defenses such as decreased levels of IgA in secretions and decreased total levels and abnormal ratios of lymphocytic white cells. Abnormalities of immune function and increased susceptibility to infection are seen in alcoholics as a result of improper diet, but it is unclear to what degree dietary imbalance influences these abnormalities. These patients do have increased zinc and B-complex vitamin requirements.

Imbalanced intake of minerals can also cause immunologic abnormalities. For example, the amount of molybdenum in the diet influences the effect of copper intake. If molybdenum is deficient, the quantity of copper ingested can result in death if copper is deficient, death from toxicity if copper is excessive, or maintenance of good health if normal levels of copper are ingested.

Excess of a Nutrient

An excess of total calories or the increase of a specific nutrient can have immunologic consequence. Obesity, for example, has been implicated in cancer risk and in abnormalities of immune function. Obesity has been associated with a high incidence of infections, and infection-related mortality is higher in obese patients than in normal persons. Obese children have alterations in cell-mediated immune functions and white cell (neutrophil) function.

An example of the dire effects of an excess of a specific nutrient is seen in cases of rapid repletion of iron in malnourished children. If iron is replaced rapidly before resolution of their malnourished state, death or other serious complications from overwhelming sepsis can result. Although iron appears to be important for immune competence, the effect of iron on any specific individual depends on a balance between the host's iron-dependent immunocompetence and microbial need for iron.

Errors of Metabolism

Innate or acquired errors of metabolism that result in the inability to degrade or synthesize intermediate metabolites of a nutrient can lead to immune dysfunction or deficiency. The best examples are patients with the syndrome associated with the abnormal metabolism of purines.

In some cases a deficiency of adenosine deaminase has been associated with severe combined (cellular and humoral) deficiency caused by abnormal lymphocyte function. Children with a deficiency of adenosine deaminase have markedly depressed cellular and humoral immunity and are considered to have a defect at the level of the stem cell from which T and B cells are derived. At the present time, treatment to replace this enzyme involves red blood cell transfusion, which restores immunocompetence in most patients.

Another example of metabolic insufficiency that affects the immune system is the absence of the enzyme purine nucleoside phosphorylase in the purine salvage pathway. This absence is associated with the loss of cellular immunity only; patients with this disorder have normal humoral immunity.

Direct Toxic Effect or Allergic Reaction

Besides contaminants that can be present in food, naturally occurring toxins of plant or animal origin such as food additives

(nitrates, nitrites, and dyes) and chemicals produced during food processing or cooking (e.g., nitrosamines) can produce adverse effects. Although many natural toxins have medicinal properties, some types are associated with immunologic abnormalities or precipitate the manifestation of signs and symptoms of immune disorders, or both (Table 1-5). Food allergies are common and are believed to represent (type I) hypersensitivity reactions. Manufactured chemical food additives are particularly hazardous to asthmatics. When exposed to agents such as sulfites, asthmatics and others may manifest such signs as itching and hives, anaphylactic shock, or even death. Denatured rapeseed oil causes toxic oil syndrome. From ingestion of this toxin, an autoimmune disorder can develop.

Role of Proteins, Carbohydrates, and Lipids in Immunity

Proteins

Protein deficiency can have serious effects on the immune response and the ability of tumors and infections to prosper in a host. Malnutrition caused by lack of protein in children before 7 months old produces decreased levels of antibody production. Children suffering from malnutrition secrete and produce low levels of IgA in response to viral vaccines. Production of substances such as lysozyme and interferon is also decreased. These children fail to develop an inflammatory reaction in response to infection, and the degree of suppression of cell-mediated immunity correlates with the severity of the protein deficiency. Changes in phagocytosis are also noticed.

In patients with anorexia nervosa, an eating disorder prevalent in adolescent females, the consequences of protein depletion express themselves in immunologic terms. Anorexia nervosa causes depressed levels of proteins synthesized by the body, such as IgM and IgG antibodies, transferrin, and various complement components. Defects in phagocytosis are also observable. In adults chronic malnourishment causes higher incidences of postoperative wound infection, bacteremia, and/or pneumonia. Fasting, however, can be beneficial in certain conditions associated with autoimmune disorders.

Amino acids, the building blocks of proteins, are important to body defenses. Excess or decreased concentrations of

TABLE 1-5	Examples of Naturally Occurring Toxins
Type of Toxin	**Effect on Humans**
Allergens	Target organs may be skin, lungs, gastrointestinal tract, nervous system, or musculoskeletal system.
Carcinogens and mutagens	Aflatoxins are suspected in the pathogenesis of some malignancies.
Nonphysiologic amino acids	L-Canavine can induce or exacerbate the lupus syndrome.
Protease inhibitors	IgE antibodies to the Kunitz soybean inhibitor produce anaphylaxis and angioedema.

specific amino acids in the diet appear to affect immunity. For example, tryptophan and phenylalanine appear to be necessary for optimal production of antibodies. Depressed serum levels of the amino acid histidine in patients with disorders such as rheumatoid arthritis have been found to correlate with disease activity.

Lectins are also important to immunity. These proteins, many of which are glycoproteins, are immunologically important because of their ability to bind specific sugars on cell membranes. This binding thereby triggers cellular events such as mitosis.

Carbohydrates

Studies of carbohydrates support the concept that sugars such as glucose play a role in immunity. In humans the increased susceptibility of diabetics to infection has long been known. In diabetics, impaired phagocytosis has been demonstrated. Children with galactosemia are also at increased risk of bacterial infection. Increased levels of sugar, however, may not be the exclusive reason for these manifestations. Ketoacidosis, rather than hyperglycemia, may be important in susceptibility to infection.

Lipids

Both the total intake of specific fats and the relative balance of various dietary fats appear to play a major role in immunologic functions. In the skin, for example, long-chain saturated lipids and waxes provide a barrier to the outside environment. Essential fatty acid deficiency symptoms cause changes in the skin and impair wound healing.

Fish oils have been suggested as having a possible antiinflammatory role; however, high-fat diets have been correlated with promoting the action of carcinogens.

Role of Vitamins and Minerals in Immunity

Multiple vitamin deficiencies occurring alone or in combination are particularly prevalent among older adults and the sick. Vitamin deficiencies can compromise body defenses in various ways. For example, vitamin A is of major importance in maintaining the integrity of anatomic barriers (i.e., skin and mucosal membranes). Through their role in cell differentiation, vitamin A congeners and naturally occurring provitamins may play a significant role in susceptibility to cancer.

In the early 1970s the relationship between vitamin deficiencies and antibody formation was noted. A deficiency of vitamins such as pyridoxine, pantothenic acid, and folate profoundly impair antibody response. Moderate impairment is noted in deficiencies of riboflavin, thiamine, biotin, niacin-tryptophan, and vitamin A. Antibody response has not been observed as being defective in the presence of deficiencies of either vitamin B_{12} or vitamin D. Cellular immunity is affected profoundly by decreased levels of pyridoxine, folic acid, and vitamin A. Phagocytosis, however, may be specifically affected by the availability of vitamins such as vitamin C.

Excessive quantities of most of the heavy metals, even essential trace elements such as zinc, depress immunity and increase susceptibility to infections. Mineral deficiencies also produce markedly impaired cell-mediated immunity. Minerals such as calcium are important in the activation of complement. Calcium also has a regulatory effect on lymphocyte and phagocytic cell function. It is likely that calcium may indirectly affect critical sites of immune processes. Calcium intake and supplementation, however, do not appear to play a role in immune function. The role of fiber in immune function is not defined.

Relationship Between Brain and Immune System

Increasing scientific evidence supports age-old observations that psychosocial factors are closely associated with the development of certain physical and mental illnesses. The interlocking mechanisms of the nervous, endocrine, and immune systems have been shown to be significantly influenced by behavior, especially psychic and/or psychologic stress.

The relationship between psychologic stress (e.g., bereavement) and the occurrence of illness is illustrated by the fact that rates of illness and death tend to be higher among those who have recently lost a spouse. Abnormalities of immune functions have been found in bereavement, major affective disorders, and schizophrenia. In particular, psychopathologic populations and populations challenged by significant life events have been shown to have high levels of anxiety and depression that are associated with impaired cellular immunity. In contrast, a positive mental state may favorably influence health and longevity.

Psychoneuroimmunology

During the last 10 to 20 years, research findings have begun to confirm that the mind and body interact in remarkable ways. Studies show that stressful emotions can be translated into altered responses in the cells, glands, and organs of the immune system. The scientific discipline of psychoneuroimmunology is the study of interactions among behavior, the brain, and the immune system. It combines research in basic science with psychologic and psychosocial investigations to study the complex relationship of mind and body. This relationship may explain the correlation between increased susceptibility to certain diseases and psychologic events.

Stress and Disease

The ability of an individual to control stress both psychologically and neurochemically appears to be as critical a factor as the nature of stress itself. A patient's personality and coping style, the meaning of the stress, the presence of social supports, and other environmental factors determine how an individual will respond to any life event. Psychosocial factors are believed to influence susceptibility to infectious diseases as part of the response each organism has to a pathogenic microorganism. For example, biologic pathways exist that could allow psychologic factors to alter immune status in individuals positive for human immunodeficiency virus (HIV). It remains to be determined whether such factors can, in fact, act as cofactors in HIV progression.

In experimental observations, secretions of IgA were observed to be lower in high-stress times and higher in low-stress periods. A higher incidence of respiratory disease was also noted after a period of stress.

Studies support the concept that stress alone is not oncogenic; however, the inability to cope with stress may allow for the development and proliferation of tumor cells. The immune system appears to play a primary mediating role. Acute stress may initiate a transient, immunologically protective response, but prolonged or poorly controlled pychosocial stresses may result in depression of different components of the immune system. In addition, chronic stressors may persist well beyond the cessation of the actual stressor.

Hormonal Regulators of Stress and Immunity

Stress has a direct effect on hormone production. For example, deprivation of sleep causes elevations of stress-related hormones. Sleep disturbances correlate with a reduction of natural killer (NK) cell activity in major depression. Under these conditions the average lytic activity of these cells is reduced significantly. Sleep is important in the modulation of natural immunity, and even modest disturbances of sleep produce a reduction of NK cell activity.

In addition, several scientific observations support a hormonally mediated link between psychosocial stressors and impaired immune function. Hormones and catecholamines are also known to be mediating mechanisms regulated by the central nervous system (CNS) and have an influence on immune suppression and the pathogenesis of disease. Stimulation of the cortical-hypothalamic-pituitary axis leads to alteration in immune function, either indirectly by changes in secretion of hormones or neurotransmitters, or directly by the less well-documented bidirectional neuronal stimulation of lymphoid tissue.

Indirect endocrine system responses to stress include stimulation of the hypothalamus, which then initiates a response in the adrenal medulla with the subsequent release of catecholamines. The catecholamines, in turn, stimulate the release of a variety of other stress-related hormones. Alterations in concentrations of hormones (e.g., aldosterone, calcitonin, growth hormone, adrenocorticotropin, melanocyte-stimulating hormone, prolactin, thyrotropin, vasopressin, parathyroid hormone, thyroxine, glucagon, renin, erythropoietin, and gastrin) have also been documented in association with stress.

The autonomic nervous system, which is highly responsive to stress, in conjunction with corticosteroids, generally has an inhibitory effect on cell-mediated immunity. The impact on the immune system of other hormones released in response to stress is less clear. These responses, however, may be related to, or independent of, changes in the neuroendocrine system.

Immunologic Consequences of Stress

Numerous links between the brain, immune system, and nervous system have been shown to have an effect on the lymphoid elements of the immune system. Lymphocyte metabolism and proliferation are inhibited by increased production of the hormone corticosteroid. Lymphocytes have been observed to be elevated transiently with alterations of lymphocyte functions during periods of stress. Lymphoid organs are known to atrophy as a result of chronic stress, resulting in a decreased number of lymphocytes.

In addition, certain kinds of lymphocytes, NK cells, are affected by corticosteroids and catecholamines. These cells make up a subpopulation of lymphocytes functionally defined by their ability to spontaneously lyse select tumor and virally infected cells. NK cell lytic function is sensitive to modulation by cytokines, substances secreted by lymphocytes, and neuroendocrine mediators.

CNS modulation of NK cell activity and the presence of an interplay between cytokine activation and responsiveness to CNS immunoregulatory signals have been demonstrated. Recently, alterations in NK cell activity have been found in patients with major depression. The major depression-related reduction in NK cells was not related to alterations in peripheral NK cells.

Attention has also been given to the suggestion that a brain-immune system–nervous system link exists for mononuclear phagocytes. Phagocytosis, for example, is decreased by stress reactions. The fundamental biology and physiology of phagocytic cells are clearly consistent with such a role. Mononuclear phagocytes bear receptors on their surface for numerous ligands, including neuroendocrine peptides and hormones. In addition, macrophages can be modulated by a variety of lifestyle choices such as smoking and ingestion of alcohol and dietary lipids. Mononuclear phagocytes are key cells in the development of atherosclerosis and play significant roles in host protection against neoplasia and in the development of certain autoimmune diseases. In regard to atherogenesis, stress can potentiate the effects of a high-lipid diet in initiating formation of the macrophage-laden lesions of early atherosclerosis. In addition, oxidized lipids and catecholamines induce a macrophage phenotype that probably can promote development of atherosclerosis and lower host resistance to neoplasia.

In a study of self-reported life stress, immune reactivity was defined as changes in the numbers of monocytes, T lymphocytes and lymphocyte subsets, human leukocyte antigen (locus) DR (HLA-DR+) cells, and NK cells, as well as changes in in vitro proliferative responses of peripheral blood lymphocytes to antigens (e.g., pokeweed). Life stress influences reactivity of the immunologic parameters to the stressor. A high number of daily hassles was associated with a stressor-induced decrease in the number of T cells and NK cells in the peripheral blood. On the other hand, the number of HLA-DR+ cells in high life stress scorers decreased only slightly during the stressor, but increased in the control condition.

Immunologic Alterations in Mental Disorders

Specific mental illnesses have been shown to alter the immune system. Major depression may be accompanied by systemic immune activation or an inflammatory response with involvement of phagocytic cells, T-cell activation, and B-cell proliferation. In addition, an acute phase response with increased plasma levels of certain acute phase proteins, higher autoantibody (antinuclear, antiphospholipid) titers, increased prostaglandin secretion, and increased production of interleukin (IL)-1 beta and IL-6 by peripheral blood mononuclear cells have been observed. It is hypothesized that increased monocytic production of interleukins (IL-1 beta and IL-6) in severe depression may constitute key phenomena underlying the various aspects of the immune and acute phase response, while contributing to hypothalamic-pituitary-adrenal axis hyperactivity, disorder in serotonin metabolism, and vegetative symptoms (i.e., the sickness behavior of severe depression).

Some schizophrenic subjects also have evidence of immune activation. One marker that has been consistently elevated in schizophrenic patients is the serum-soluble IL-2 receptor (sIL-2R). Patients with obsessive-compulsive disorder have shown a positive relationship between sIL-2R and concentrations of transferrin receptors (TfR).

An increased risk of infection, autoimmune disease, and cancer has been noted in depressed patients. In these patients, inhibition of phagocytosis can be shown. Because patients with major depressive disorders have decreased lymphocytic mitotic activity, an altered immune response is suspected. Elevated levels of corticosteroids may also play a medicating role.

CHAPTER HIGHLIGHTS

Immunology is defined as the study of the molecules, cells, organs, and systems responsible for the recognition and disposal of nonself material; of how body components respond and interact; of the desirable or undesirable consequences of immune interactions; and of the ways in which the immune system can be advantageously manipulated to protect against or treat diseases.

The function of the immune system is to recognize self from nonself and to defend the body against nonself. The first line of defense against infection is unbroken skin and mucosal membrane surfaces. Secretions are also an important component in this first line of defense. Natural resistance is one of the two ways that the body resists infection if microorganisms penetrate the first line of resistance. Acquired resistance specifically recognizes and selectively eliminates exogenous or endogenous agents. Tissue damage produced by infectious or other agents results in inflammation, a series of biochemical and cellular changes that facilitates the phagocytosis of microorganisms or damaged cells. If the degree of inflammation is sufficiently extensive, it is accompanied by an increase in the plasma concentration of acute-phase proteins, a group of glycoproteins.

If a microorganism overwhelms the body's natural resistance, a third line of defensive resistance exists. Acquired or adaptive immunity is a more recently evolved mechanism; it allows the body to recognize, remember, and respond to a specific stimulus, an antigen. Antibody-mediated immunity to infection is acquired if the antibodies are formed by the host or received from another source. These two types of acquired immunity are called active and passive immunity, respectively.

Immediate hypersensitivity makes up a subset of the body's antibody-mediated effector mechanisms. This subset consists of the reactions primarily mediated by IgE. Cell-mediated immunity consists of immune activities that differ from antibody-mediated immunity. Lymphocytes are immunologically active through various types of direct cell-to-cell contact and by the production of cytokines for specific immunologic functions such as the recruitment of phagocytic cells to the site of inflammation. The term *delayed hypersensitivity* is often used synonymously with the term *cell-mediated immunity*. Delayed hypersensitivity, however, refers to the slow appearance of a secondary response in the skin.

Many of the same factors, such as general health and the age of an individual, are important considerations in the development of immunologic and infectious disease. These factors can include genetic predisposition to many disorders, nutritional status, and the individual's method of coping with stress. Psychoneuroimmunology shows that stressful emotions can be translated into altered responses in the cells, glands, and organs of the immune system. This relationship may explain the correlation between increased susceptibility to certain diseases and psychologic events.

REVIEW QUESTIONS

Questions 1-5. Match the following terms to their appropriate definitions or descriptions. (Use each answer only once.)

1. _____ immune system

2. _____ lymphocytes

3. _____ cooperative interaction

4. _____ nonspecific immune elements

5. _____ autoimmune disorder

    A. T and B types
    B. specific cellular elements, cell products, and nonlymphoid elements
    C. mononuclear phagocytes
    D. a condition in which the body's own tissues are attacked as if they were foreign
    E. can protect against or be manipulated to treat disease

Questions 6-10. On the following figure, identify each of the labeled body parts that constitute part of the body's natural defenses. Choose from the following answers:

    A. eyes
    B. digestive system
    C. skin
    D. respiratory tract
    E. urogenital tract

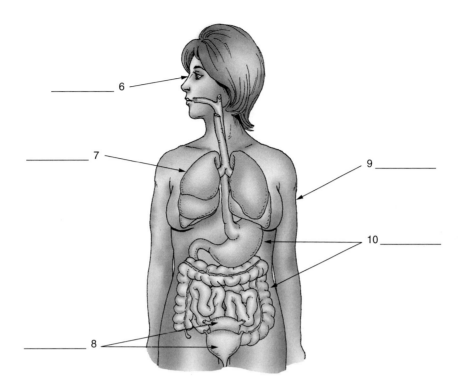

11. The first line of defense in protecting the body from infection includes all of the following components except:
   A. unbroken skin
   B. normal microbial flora
   C. phagocytic leukocytes
   D. secretions such as mucus

12. Natural immunity is characterized as being:
   A. innate or inborn
   B. able to specifically recognize exogenous or endogenous agents
   C. able to selectively eliminate exogenous or endogenous agents
   D. part of the first line of body defenses against microbial organisms

Questions 13 and 14. Complete the chart below from the following list of choices:
   A. lymphocytes
   B. macrophages
   C. mucus
   D. interferons

Components of the Natural Immune System

Cellular   Mast cells
             Neutrophils

             13. _____

Humoral   Complement
             Lysozyme

             14. _____

15. Another term for adaptive immunity is:
   A. antigenic immunity
   B. acquired immunity
   C. lymphocyte reactive immunity
   D. phagocytosis

16. Humoral components of the adaptive immune system include(s):
   A. T lymphocytes
   B. B lymphocytes
   C. antibodies
   D. saliva

Questions 17-28. Complete the table below, choosing from the following answers:

Possible answers for questions 17-20.
   A. infusion of serum of plasma
   B. transfer in vivo or colostrum
   C. vaccination
   D. infection

Possible answers for questions 21-24
   A. yes
   B. no

Possible answers for questions 25-28.
   A. short
   B. long

Comparison of the Types of Adaptive Immunity

Type	Mode of Acquisition	Antibody Produced by Host	Duration of Response
Active natural	17. _____	21. _____	25. _____
artificial	18. _____	22. _____	26. _____
Passive natural	19. _____	23. _____	27. _____
artificial	20. _____	24. _____	28. _____

29. Immediate hypersensitivity consists of the reactions primarily mediated by the _____ class of immunoglobulins.
    A. IgM
    B. IgG
    C. IgE
    D. IgA

30. The most immediate and severe manifestation of immediate hypersensitivity reaction is:
    A. anaphylaxis
    B. anaphylactoid
    C. itching
    D. sneezing

31. Delayed hypersensitivity is also referred to as:
    A. humoral
    B. cell mediated
    C. B cell
    D. cytotoxic

32. Older adults have _____ immunity than younger adults.
    A. better
    B. more active
    C. more passive
    D. poorer

BIBLIOGRAPHY

Adams DO: Molecular biology of macrophage activation: a pathway whereby psychosocial factors can potentially affect health, *Psychosom Med* 56(4):316-327, 1994.

Barrett JT: *Textbook of immunology,* ed 5, St Louis, 1988, Mosby.

Bergsma J: Illness, the mind, and the body. Cancer and immunology: an introduction, *Theor Med* 15(4):337-347, 1994.

Biondi M et al: Personality, endocrine and immune changes after eight months in healthy individuals under normal daily stress, *Psychother Psychosom* 62(3-4):176-184, 1994.

Brosschot JF et al: Influence of life stress on immunological reactivity to mild psychological stress, *Psychosoc Med* 56(3):216-224, 1994.

Claman HN: The biology of the immune system, *JAMA* 268(20): 2888-2892, 1992.

Corman LC: Effects of specific nutrients on the immune response, *Med Clin North Am* 69(4):759, 1985.

Cover H, Irwin M: Immunity and depression: insomnia, retardation, and reduction of natural killer cell activity, *J Behav Med* 17(2):217-223, 1994.

Edwards NL: Immunodeficiencies associated with errors in purine metabolism, *Med Clin North Am* 69(3):505, 1985.

Esterling BA et al: Chronic stress, social support, and persistent alterations in the natural killer cell response to cytokines in older adults, *Health Psychol* 13(4):291-298, 1994.

Gee A, Thiele GM, Johnson DR: Behaviorally conditioned modulation of natural killer cell activity: enhancement of baseline and activated natural killer cell activity, *Int J Neurosci* 77(1-2):139-152, 1994.

Irwin M et al: Partial sleep deprivation reduces natural killer cell activity in humans, *Fed Am Soc Exp Biol* 10:643-653, 1996.

Kemeny ME: Psychoneuroimmunology of HIV infection, *Psychiatr Clin North Am* 17(1):55-68, 1994.

Maes M et al: Natural killer cell activity in major depression: relation to circulating natural killer cells, cellular indices of the immune response, and depressive phenomenology, *Prog Neuropsycholpharmacol Biol Psychiatry* 18(4):717-730, 1994.

Maier SF, Watkins LR, Fleshner M: Psychoneuroimmunology: the interface between behavior, brain, and immunity, *Am Psychol* 49(12):1004-1017, 1994.

Rapaport JH, Lohr JB: Serum-soluble interleukin-2 receptors in neuroleptic-naive schizophrenic subjects and in medicated schizophrenic subjects with and without tardive dyskinesia, *Acta Psychiatr Scand* 90(5):311-315, 1994.

Rudbach JA, editor: *How aging affects immunity: Infectious Disease and Immunology Forum,* Chicago, 1984, Abbott Laboratories.

Schindler BA: Stress, affective disorders, and immune function, *Med Clin North Am* 69(3):585, 1985.

Ursin H: Stress, distress, and immunity, *Ann NY Acad Sci* 741(25):204-211, 1994.

Zorrilla EP, Redei E, DeRubeis RJ: Reduced cytokine levels and T-cell function in healthy males: relation to individual differences in subclinical anxiety, *Brain Behav Immun* 8(4):293-312, 1994.

Chapter 2

Antigens and Antibodies

LEARNING OBJECTIVES

At the conclusion of this chapter, the reader should be able to:
- Define the terms *antigen* and *antibody*.
- Name and describe the characteristics of each of the five immunoglobulin classes.
- Draw and describe a typical immunoglobulin G (IgG) molecular structure.

- Name the four phases of an antibody response.
- Describe the characteristics of a primary and secondary (anamnestic) response.
- Describe the method of production of a monoclonal antibody.

ANTIGEN CHARACTERISTICS

General Characteristics of Antigens

An antigen is a substance that stimulates antibody formation and has the ability to bind to an antibody. Foreign substances can be immunogenic or antigenic (capable of provoking an immune response) if their membrane or molecular components contain structures recognized as foreign by the immune system. These structures are called antigenic determinants, or epitopes. An epitope, as part of an antigen, reacts specifically with an antibody or T-cell receptor.

Not all surfaces act as antigenic determinants. Only prominent determinants on the surface of a protein are normally recognized by the immune system, and some of these are much more immunogenic than others. An immune response is directed against specific determinants, and resultant antibodies will bind to them with much of the remainder of the molecule being immunogenic.

The cellular membrane of mammalian cells chemically consists of proteins, phospholipids, cholesterol, and traces of polysaccharide. Polysaccharides (carbohydrates) in the form of either glycoproteins or glycolipids can be found attached to the lipid and protein molecules of the membrane. Most of these proteins are immunogenic when a different individual of the same species, such as erythrocytes and body tissues, is exposed to cells or tissues containing them. Outer surfaces of bacteria, such as a capsule or the cell wall, as well as the surface structures of other microorganisms, are immunogenic.

Cellular antigens of importance to immunologists include histocompatibility antigens, autoantigens, and blood group antigens. The normal immune system responds to foreignness by producing antibodies. For this reason, microbial antigens are also important to immunologists in the study of the immunologic manifestation of infectious diseases.

Histocompatibility Antigens

Nucleated cells such as leukocytes and tissues possess many cell-surface-protein antigens that readily provoke an immune response if transferred into a genetically different (allogenic) individual of the same species. Some of these antigens, which constitute the major histocompatibility complex (MHC), are much more potent than others in provoking an immune response. The MHC is referred to as the human leukocyte antigen (HLA) system in humans because its gene products were originally identified on white blood cells (human leukocytes). These antigens are second only to the ABO antigens in influencing the survival or graft rejection of transplanted organs. HLAs are the subject of numerous scientific investigations because of the strong association between individual HLAs and immunologic disorders. The HLA system is discussed in further detail in Chapter 28.

Autoantigens

The evolution of a recognition system that can recognize and destroy nonself material must also have safeguards to prevent damage to self-antigens. The body's immune system usually exercises tolerance to self-antigens, but in some situations antibodies may be produced in response to normal self-antigens. This failure to recognize self-antigens can result in autoantibodies directed at hormones, such as thyroglobulin. Specific autoantibodies are discussed in detail in Chapter 25.

Blood Group Antigens

Blood group substances are widely distributed throughout the tissues, blood cells, and body fluids. When foreign red cell antigens are introduced to a host, a transfusion reaction or hemolytic disease of the newborn can result. A brief description of these disorders is presented in Chapter 23. In addition, certain antigens, especially those of the Rh system, are integral structural components of the erythrocyte membrane. If these antigens are missing, the erythrocyte membrane is defective and results in hemolytic anemia. When antigens do not form part of the essential membrane structure (e.g., A, B, and H antigens), the absence of antigen has no effect on membrane integrity.

CHEMICAL NATURE OF ANTIGENS

Antigens, or immunogens, are usually large organic molecules that are either proteins or large polysaccharides and rarely, if ever, lipids. Antigens, especially cell-surface or membrane-bound antigens, can be composed of combinations of the biochemical classes (e.g., glycoproteins or glycolipids). For example, histocompatibility HLAs are glycoprotein in nature and are found on the surface membranes of nucleated body cells composed of both solid tissue and most circulating blood cells (e.g., granulocytes, monocytes, lymphocytes, and thrombocytes).

Proteins are excellent antigens because of their high molecular weight (MW) and structural complexity; lipids are considered inferior antigens because of their relative simplicity and lack of structural stability. However, when lipids are linked to proteins or polysaccharides, they may function as antigens. Nucleic acids are poor antigens because of relative simplicity, molecular flexibility, and rapid degradation. Antinucleic acid antibodies can be produced by artificially stabilizing them and linking them to an immunogenic carrier. Carbohydrates (polysaccharides) by themselves are considered too small to function as antigens. However, in the case of erythrocyte blood group antigens, protein or lipid carriers may contribute to the necessary size, and the polysaccharides present in the form of side chains confer immunologic specificity.

PHYSICAL NATURE OF ANTIGENS

For antigens to function effectively, several factors are important: foreignness, degradability, MW, structural stability, and complexity.

Foreignness

Foreignness is the degree to which antigenic determinants are recognized as nonself by an individual's immune system. The immunogenicity of a molecule depends to a great extent on its degree of foreignness. Normally an individual's immune system does not respond to self-antigens.

Degradability

For an antigen to be recognized as foreign by an individual's immune system, sufficient antigens to stimulate an immune response must be present. Foreign molecules, which are rapidly destroyed, will not be present long enough to provide adequate antigenic exposure.

Molecular Weight

The higher the MW, the better the molecule will function as an antigen. The number of antigenic determinants on a molecule is directly related to its size. Although large foreign molecules (MW >10,000) are better antigens, haptens, which are very small molecules, can bind to a larger carrier molecule and behave as antigens. If a hapten is chemically linked to a large molecule, a new surface structure is formed on the large molecule, which may function as an antigenic determinant.

Structural Stability

If a molecule is an effective antigen, structural stability is mandatory. If a structure is unstable (e.g., gelatin), the molecule will be a very poor antigen. Similarly, totally inert molecules are poor antigens.

Complexity

The more complex an antigen is, the greater its effectiveness. Complex proteins are better antigens than large, repeating polymers such as lipids, carbohydrates, and nucleic acids, which are relatively poor antigens.

GENERAL CHARACTERISTICS OF ANTIBODIES

Antibodies are specific glycoproteins referred to as immunoglobulins. Many antibodies can be isolated in the gamma globulin fraction of protein by electrophoresis separation (Figure 2-1). However, the term *immunoglobulin* (Ig)

has replaced gamma globulin because not all antibodies have gamma electrophoretic mobility. Antibodies can be found in blood plasma and in many body fluids such as tears, saliva, and colostrum.

The primary function of an antibody in body defenses is to combine with antigen, which may be enough to neutralize bacterial toxins or some viruses. A secondary interaction of an antibody molecule with another effector agent such as complement is usually required to dispose of larger antigens such as bacteria.

Determining the concentration of Ig can be of diagnostic significance in infectious and autoimmune diseases. Test methods to detect the presence and concentration of Igs are discussed in Chapters 7 to 11 and in chapters relating to specific diseases.

IMMUNOGLOBULIN CLASSES

Five distinct classes of Ig molecules are recognized in most higher mammals: IgM, IgG, IgA, IgD, and IgE. These Ig classes differ from each other in characteristics such as molecular weight (MW), sedimentation coefficients, and carbohydrate content (Table 2-1). In addition to the differences between classes, they vary within each class as well.

IgG

The major Ig in normal serum is IgG. This Ig diffuses more readily than others into the extravascular spaces, and it neutralizes toxins or binds to microorganisms in extravascular spaces. It is capable of crossing the placenta. In addition, when IgG complexes are formed, complement can be activated. IgG accounts for 70% to 75% of the total Ig pool. It is a 7S molecule, with a MW of approximately 150,000. One of the subclasses, IgG$_3$, is slightly larger (MW = 170,000) than the other subclasses.

Normal human adult serum values of IgG are 800 to 1800 mg/dL (90 to 210 IU/mL). In infants 3 to 4 months old, the level of IgG is approximately 350 to 400 mg/dL (40 to 45

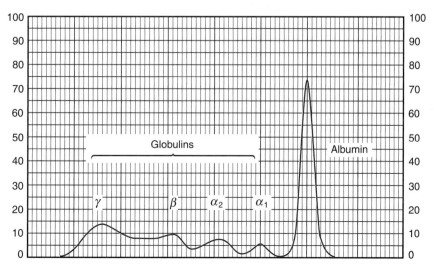

Figure 2-1 A tracing of the electrophoretic pattern of normal serum. (Redrawn from Barrett JT: *Textbook of immunology,* ed 5, St Louis, 1988, Mosby.)

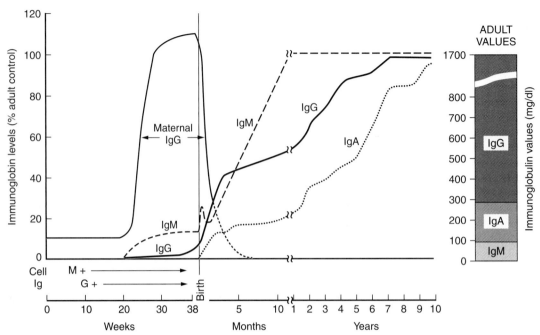

Figure 2-2   Immunoglobulin concentration in newborns, infants, and children. (Redrawn from Bauer JD: Clinical laboratory methods, ed 9, St. Louis, 1982, Mosby.)

TABLE 2-1	Characteristics of Immunoglobulin Classes				
	IgM	**IgG**	**IgA**	**IgE**	**IgD**
Molecular weight	900,000	160,000	360,000	200,000	160,000
Sedimentation coefficient	19S	7S	11S	8S	7S
Percent carbohydrate	12	8	7	12	12
Subclasses	None	IgG$_{1-4}$	Alpha 1,2	None	None
Serum concentration mg/dL*; adults	50-200	800-1600	150-400	0.002-0.05	1.5-40
Half-life (days)	5	21	6	2	

*Conversion factors: IgG 1 mg = 11.5 IU; IgA 1 mg = 57.7 IU; IgM 1 mg = 117 IU; IgD 1 mg = 709 IU.

IU/mL), and it gradually increases to 700 to 800 mg/dL (80 to 90 IU/mL) by the end of the first year of life (Figure 2-2). The average adult level is achieved before the age of 16 years (Figure 2-3). Other body fluids containing IgG include cord blood and cerebrospinal fluid (CSF). Cord blood contains 800 to 1800 mg/dL, and CSF contains 2 to 4 mg/dL of IgG.

Decreased levels of IgG can be manifested in primary (genetically determined) or secondary (acquired disorders associated with certain diseases) Ig deficiencies. Significant increases of IgG can be shown in a variety of diseases and disorders. These include:

1. Infectious diseases (e.g., hepatitis, rubella, infectious mononucleosis)
2. Collagen disorders (e.g., rheumatoid arthritis, systemic lupus erythematosus)
3. Hematologic disorders (e.g., polyclonal gammopathies, monoclonal gammopathies, monocytic leukemia, Hodgkin's disease)

Subclasses of Immunoglobulin

Within the major Ig classes are variants known as subclasses and subtypes. These subclasses differ in their heavy-chain com-

position and in some of their characteristics such as biologic activities (Table 2-2). Four IgG subclasses (IgG$_1$, IgG$_2$, IgG$_3$, IgG$_4$) exist. The subclasses occur in the approximate proportions of 66%, 23%, 7%, and 4%, respectively, in humans.

IgM

IgM accounts for about 10% of the Ig pool, and it is largely confined to the intravascular pool because of its large size. This antibody is produced early in an immune response and is largely confined to the blood. IgM is effective in agglutination and cytolytic reactions. In humans it is found in smaller concentrations than either IgG or IgA. The molecule has five individual heavy chains, with a MW of 65,000; the whole molecule has a MW of 900,000 and a sedimentation coefficient of 19S.

Normal values of IgM are 60 to 250 mg/dL (70 to 290 IU/mL) for males and 70 to 280 mg/dL (80 to 320 IU/mL) for females. Fifty percent of the adult levels are present at 4 months of age, and adult levels are obtained between 8 to 15 years. Cord blood contains >20 mg/dL. IgM is usually undetectable in CSF.

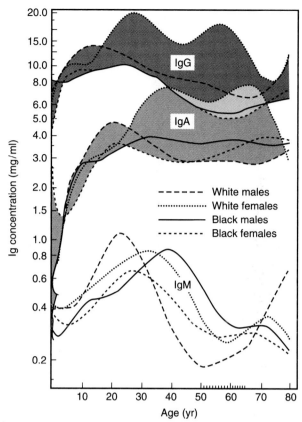

Figure 2-3 Serum immunoglobulins in 800 apparently healthy patients. (Redrawn from Bauer JD: *Clinical laboratory methods,* ed 9, St Louis, 1982, Mosby.)

| TABLE 2-2 | Characteristics of IgG Subclasses |

	IgG₁	IgG₂	IgG₃	IgG₄
Percentage of serum	65	24	7	4
Complement fixation	4+	2+	4+	+
Half-life (days)	23	23	8	23
Placental passage	+	?	+	+

IgM is decreased in primary (genetically determined) or secondary (acquired) Ig disorders. It can be increased in a wide variety of diseases and disorders. These conditions include:

1. Infectious diseases (e.g., subacute bacterial endocarditis, infectious mononucleosis, leprosy, trypanosomiasis, malaria, actinomycosis)
2. Collagen disorders (e.g., scleroderma)
3. Hematologic disorders (e.g., polyclonal gammopathies, monocytic leukemia, and monoclonal gammopathies such as Waldenström's macroglobulinemia)

IgA

IgA represents 15% to 20% of the total circulatory Ig pool. It is the predominant Ig in secretions such as tears, saliva, colostrum, milk, and intestinal secretions. IgA is synthesized largely by plasma cells located on body surfaces. If the IgA is produced by cells in the intestinal wall, it may pass directly into the intestinal lumen or diffuse into the blood circulation. As IgA is transported through intestinal epithelial cells or hepatocytes, it binds to a glycoprotein called the secretory piece. The secretory piece protects IgA from digestion by gastrointestinal proteolytic enzymes and forms a complex molecule named secretory IgA (SIgA).

SIgA is of critical importance in protecting body surfaces against invading microorganisms. It provides external surfaces of the body with protection from microorganisms because of its presence in seromucous secretions such as tears, saliva, nasal fluids, and colostrum.

IgA monomer is present in relatively high concentrations in human serum, including a concentration of 90 to 450 mg/dL (55 to 270 IU/mL) in normal adult humans. Twenty-five percent of the adult IgA level is reached at the end of the first year of life, and 50% at 3½ years. The average adult level is attained by age 16 years. IgA concentration in cord blood is >1 mg/dL, and CSF contains 0.1 to 0.6 mg/dL.

This Ig is decreased in primary (genetically determined) or secondary (acquired) Ig deficiencies. Significant increases in the concentration of serum IgA are associated with:

1. Infectious diseases (e.g., tuberculosis and actinomycosis)
2. Collagen disorders (e.g., rheumatoid arthritis)
3. Hematologic disorders (e.g., polyclonal gammopathies, monocytic leukemia, and the monoclonal gammopathy [IgA myeloma])
4. Liver disease (e.g., Laennec's cirrhosis and chronic active hepatitis)

IgD

IgD is found in very low concentrations in plasma, accounting for less than 1% of the total Ig pool. It is very susceptible to proteolysis and is primarily a cell membrane Ig found on the surface of B lymphocytes in association with IgM.

IgE

IgE is a trace plasma protein found in the blood plasma of unparasitized individuals. It has a MW of 188,000. IgE is of major importance because it mediates some types of hypersensitivity (allergic) reactions, allergies, and anaphylaxis and is generally responsible for an individual's immunity to invading parasites. The IgE molecule is unique in that it binds strongly to a receptor on mast cells and basophils and, together with antigen, mediates the release of histamines and heparin from these cells.

ANTIBODY STRUCTURE

Antibodies exhibit diversity among the different classes, which suggests that they perform different functions in addition to their primary function of antigen binding. Essentially each Ig molecule is bifunctional; one region of the molecule is concerned with binding to antigen, and a different region mediates binding of the Ig to host tissues, including cells of the immune system and the first component (C1q) of the classic complement system.

The primary core of an antibody consists of the sequence of amino acid residues linked by the peptide bond. All antibodies have a common basic polypeptide structure with a three-dimensional configuration. The polypeptide chains are linked by covalent and noncovalent bonds, which produce a unit composed of a four-chain structure based on pairs of identical heavy and light chains. The Igs IgG, IgD, and IgE occur only as monomers of the four-chain unit; IgA occurs in both monomeric and polymeric forms; IgM occurs as a pentamer with five four-chain subunits linked together.

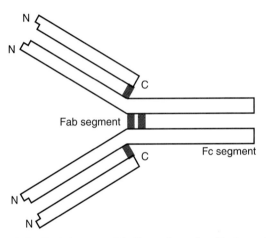

Figure 2-4   Basic immunoglobulin configuration. (Redrawn from Turgeon ML: *Fundamentals of immunohematology,* ed 2, Baltimore, 1995, Williams & Wilkins.)

Typical Immunoglobulin Molecule

The basic unit of an antibody structure is the homology unit or domain, of which a typical molecule has 12, arranged in two heavy and two light (H and L) chains, linked through cysteine residues by disulphide bonds so that the domains lie in pairs (Figure 2-4). The antigen-binding portion of the molecule (N-terminal end) shows such heterogeneity that it is known as the variable (V) region; the remainder is composed of relatively constant amino acid sequences, the constant (C) region. Short segments of about 10 amino acid residues within the variable regions of antibodies (or T cell receptor [TCR] proteins) form loop structures called complementary-determining regions (CDRs). Three hypervariable loops, also called CDRs, are present in each antibody heavy chain and light chain. Most of the variability between different antibodies or TCRs is located within these loops.

A classic model of antibody structure is displayed by the IgG molecule. Under electron microscopy, it appears Y-shaped (Figure 2-5). If the molecule is chemically treated to break interchain disulphide bonds, the molecule separates into four polypeptide chains. Light chains are small chains (MW = 25,000) common to all classes of Igs. The light chains are of two subtypes, kappa and lambda, which have different amino acid sequences and are antigenically different. In humans about 65% of Ig molecules have kappa chains, whereas 35% have lambda chains. The larger heavy chains (MW = 50,000 to 77,000) extend the full length of the molecule.

A general feature of the Ig chains is their amino acid sequence. The first 110 to 120 amino acids of both the light and heavy chains have a variable sequence and form the variable (V) region; the remainder of the light chains represents a constant (C) region with a similar amino acid sequence for each type and subtype. The remaining portion of the heavy chain is also constant for each type and has a hinge region. The class and subclass of an Ig molecule are determined by its heavy-chain type.

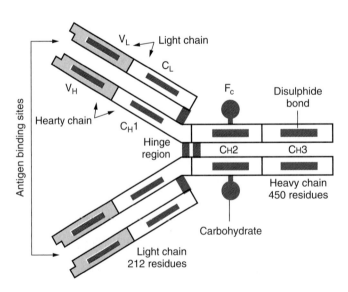

V_L and V_H = Variable regions
C_L and C_H = Constant regions

Figure 2-5   Redrawn from basic structure of IgG. (Redrawn from Turgeon ML: *Fundamentals of immunohematology,* ed 2, Baltimore, 1995, Williams & Wilkins.)

Fab, Fc, and Hinge Molecular Components

A typical monomeric IgG molecule consists of three globular regions (two Fab regions and an Fc portion) linked by a flexible hinge region. If the molecule is digested with a proteolytic enzyme such as papain (Figure 2-6), it splits into three approximately equal-size fragments. Two of these fragments retain the ability to bind antigen and are called the antigen-binding fragments (Fab fragments). The third fragment, which is relatively homogeneous and is sometimes crystallizable, is called the Fc portion. If IgG is treated with another proteolytic enzyme, pepsin, the molecule separates in a somewhat different manner. The Fc fragment is split into very small peptides and thus completely destroyed. The two Fab fragments remain joined to produce a fragment called F(ab)'2. This fragment possesses two antigen binding sites. If F(ab)'2 is treated to reduce its disulphide bonds, it breaks into two Fab fragments, each of which has only one antigen-binding site. Further disruption of the interchain disulphide bonds in the Fab fragments shows that each contains a light chain and half of a heavy chain, which is called the Fd fragment.

Electron microscopy studies of IgG reveal that the Fab regions of the molecule are mobile and can swing freely around the center of the molecule as if it were hinged. This hinge consists of a group of about 15 amino acids located between the CH1 and CH2 regions. The exact sequence of amino acids in the hinge is variable and unique for each Ig class and subclass. Because amino acids can rotate freely around peptide bonds, the effect of closely spaced proline amino acid residues is production of a universal joint, around which the Ig chains can swing freely. A remarkable feature of the hinge region is the presence of a large number of hydrophilic and proline residues. The hydrophilic residues tend to open up this region and thus make it accessible to proteolytic cleavage with enzymes such as pepsin and papain. This region also contains all of the interchain disulphide bonds except for IgD, which has no interchain links.

Structure of Other Igs

IgM

The IgM molecule is structurally composed of five basic subunits. Each basic subunit consists of two kappa or two lambda light chains and two mu heavy chains. The individual monomers of IgM are linked together by disulphide bonds in a circular fashion (Figure 2-7). A small cysteine-rich polypeptide, the J chain, must be considered an integral part of the molecule. IgM has carbohydrate residues attached to the C_{H3} and C_{H4} domains. The site for complement activation by IgM is located on this C_{H4} region. IgM is more efficient than IgG in activities such as the activation of complement cascade and agglutination.

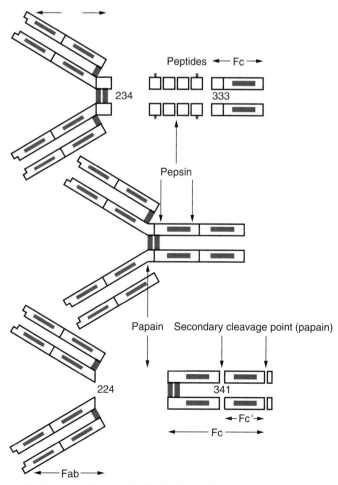

Figure 2-6 Enzymatic cleavage of human IgG1. (Redrawn from Turgeon ML: *Fundamentals of immunohematology,* ed 2, 1995, Williams & Wilkins.)

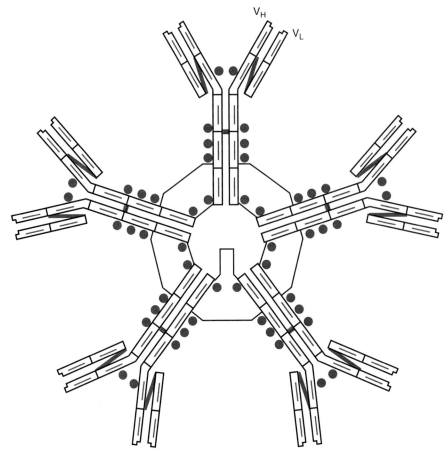

Figure 2-7 Pentameric polypeptide chain structure of human IgM. (Redrawn From Turgeon ML: *Fundamentals of immunohematology,* ed 2, Baltimore, 1995, Williams & Wilkins.)

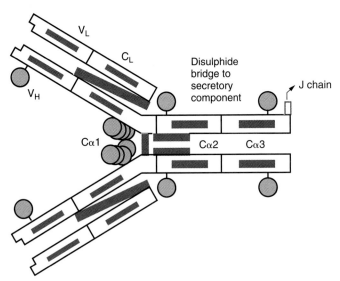

Figure 2-8 A molecule of IgA.

IgA

In humans more than 80% of IgA occurs as a typical four-chain structure consisting of paired kappa or lambda chains and two heavy chains (Figure 2-8). The basic four-chain monomer has a MW of 160,000; however, in most mammals plasma IgA occurs mostly as a dimer. In dimeric IgA the molecules are joined by a J chain linked to the Fc regions. Secretory IgA exists mainly in the 11S dimeric form and has a MW of 385,000 (Figure 2-9). This form of IgA is present in fluids and is stabilized against proteolysis when combined with another protein called the secretory component. In humans, variations in the heavy chains account for the subclasses IgA$_1$ and IgA$_2$.

IgD

The IgD molecule has a MW of 184,000 and consists of two kappa or lambda light chains and two delta heavy chains (Figure 2-10). It has no interchain disulphide bonds between its heavy chains and an exposed hinge region.

IgE

The IgE molecule is composed of paired kappa or lambda light chains and two epsilon heavy chains (Figure 2-11). It is unique in that its Fc region binds strongly to a receptor on mast cells and basophils and, together with antigen, mediates the release of histamines and heparin from these cells.

IMMUNOGLOBULIN VARIANTS

An antigenic determinant is the specific chemical determinant group or molecular configuration against which the immune response is directed. Because they are proteins, Igs themselves can function as very effective antigens when used to immunize mammals of a different species. When the resulting antiimmunoglobulins or antiglobulins are analyzed,

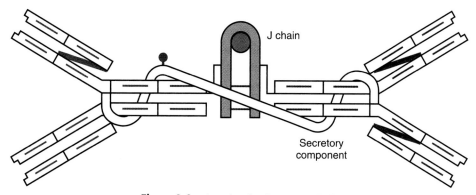

Figure 2-9   A molecule of secretory IgA.

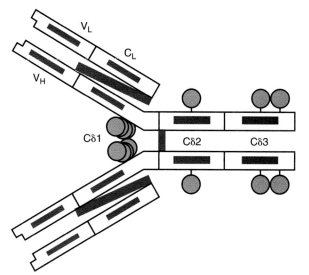

Figure 2-10   A molecule of IgD.

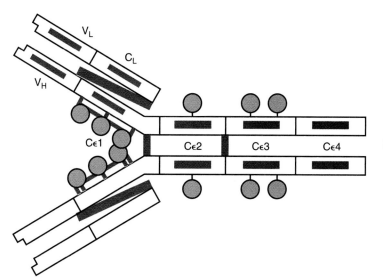

Figure 2-11   A molecule of IgE.

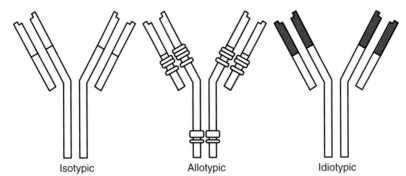

Figure 2-12   Variants of antibodies. (Redrawn from Turgeon ML: *Fundamentals of immunohematology*, ed 2, Baltimore, 1995, Williams & Wilkins.)

TABLE 2-3	**Immunoglobulin Variants**			
Variant	**Distribution**	**Variant**	**Location**	**Examples**
Isotypic	All variants in normal persons	Classes	C_H	IgM, IgE
		Subclasses	C_H	IgA$_1$, IgA$_2$
		Types	C_L	Kappa
				Lambda
Allotypic	Genetically controlled alternate forms—not present in all persons	Allotypes	Mainly C_H/C_L Sometimes V_H/V_2	Gm groups in humans
Idiotypic	Individually specific to each immunoglobulin molecule	Idiotypes	Variable regions	Probably one or more hypervariable regions forming the antigen-combining site

Modified from Roitt IM: *Essential immunology*, ed 5, Oxford, England, 1984, Blackwell Scientific.

three principal categories (Table 2-3) of antigenic determinants can be recognized: isotype, allotype, and idiotype (Figure 2-12).

Isotype Determinants

This class of antigenic determinants is the dominant type found on the Igs of all animals of a species. The heavy-chain, constant-region structures associated with the different classes and subclasses are termed *isotypic variants*. Genes for isotypic variants are present in all healthy members of a species. Determinants in this category include those specific for each Ig class such, as gamma for IgG, mu for IgM, and alpha for IgA, as well as the subclass-specific determinants kappa and lambda.

Allotype Determinants

The second principal group of determinants is found on the Igs of some, but not all, animals of a species. Antibodies to these allotypes (alloantibodies) may be produced by injecting the Igs of one animal into another member of the same species. The allotypic determinants are genetically determined variations representing the presence of allelic genes at a single locus within a species. Typical allotypes in humans are the Gm specificities on IgG (Gm is a marker on

IgG). In humans five sets of allotypic markers have been found: Gm, Km, Mm, Am, and Hv.

Idiotype Determinants

Idiotypes exist as a result of the unique structures on light and heavy chains. These individual determinants characteristic of each antibody are called the idiotypes. The idiotypic determinants are located in the variable part of the antibody associated with the hypervariable regions that form the antigen-combining site.

ANTIBODY SYNTHESIS

Production of antibodies is induced when the host's immune system comes into contact with a foreign antigenic substance and reacts to this antigenic stimulation. When an antigen is initially encountered, the cells of the immune system (see Chapters 3 and 4) recognize the antigen as nonself and either elicit an immune response or become tolerant to it, depending on the circumstances. An immune reaction can take the form of cell-mediated immunity (immunity dependent on T cells and macrophages) or involve the production of antibodies directed against the antigen. Whether a cell-mediated response or an antibody response takes place depends on the way in which the antigen is presented to the

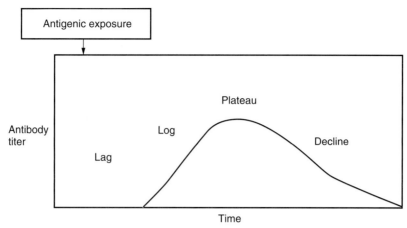

Figure 2-13   The four phases of an antibody response. (Redrawn from Turgeon ML: *Fundamentals of immunohematology,* ed 2, Baltimore, 1995, Williams & Wilkins.)

lymphocytes; many immune reactions display both kinds of responses. The antigenicity of a foreign substance is also related to the route of entry. Intravenous and intraperitoneal routes are stronger stimuli than subcutaneous and intramuscular routes. Subsequent exposure to the same antigen produces a memory response, or anamnestic response, and reflects the outcome of the initial challenge. In the case of antibody production, both the quantity and class of Igs produced vary.

Primary Antibody Response

After a foreign antigen challenge, an IgM antibody response proceeds in four phases (Figure 2-13), but the actual time period and levels of antibody (titer) depend on the characteristics of the antigen and the individual. The four phases are:
1. A lag phase when no antibody is detectable
2. A log phase in which the antibody titer increases logarithmically
3. A plateau phase during which the antibody titer stabilizes
4. A decline phase in which the antibody is catabolized

Secondary (Anamnestic) Response

Subsequent exposure to the same antigenic stimulus produces an antibody response that exhibits the same four phases as the primary responses (Figure 2-14). Repeated exposure to an antigen can take place many years after the initial exposure, but clones of the T memory cells will be stimulated to proliferate with subsequent production of antibody by the individual. However, an anamnestic response differs from a primary response in several important aspects:
1. Time. A secondary response has a shorter lag phase, a longer plateau, and a more gradual decline.
2. Type of antibody. IgM-type antibodies are the principal class formed in the primary response. Although some IgM antibody is formed in a secondary response, the IgG class is the predominant type formed.
3. Antibody titer. In a secondary response, antibody levels attain a higher titer. The plateau levels in a secondary response are typically 10-fold or more than the plateau levels in the primary response.

FUNCTIONS OF ANTIBODIES

The principal function of an antibody is to bind antigen. However, antibodies may exhibit secondary effector functions as well as behave like antigens. The significant secondary effector functions of antibodies (Table 2-4) are complement fixation and placental transfer. The activation of complement (see Chapter 5) is one of most important effector mechanisms of IgG_1 and IgG_3 molecules. IgG_2 seems to be less effective in activating complement; IgG_4, IgA, IgD, and IgE are ineffective in terms of complement activation. In humans most of the IgG subclass molecules are capable of crossing the placental barrier. It is not universally agreed whether IgG_2 crosses the placenta. Passage of antibodies across the placental barrier is important in the etiology of hemolytic disease of the newborn (see Chapter 23) and in conferring passive immunity to the newborn during the first few months of life.

ANTIGEN-ANTIBODY INTERACTION AND IMMUNE COMPLEXES

The ability of a particular antibody to combine with one antigen instead of another is referred to as its specificity. This property resides in the portion of the Fab molecule called the combining site, a cleft formed largely by the hypervariable regions of heavy and light chains. There is evidence, however, that an antigen may bind to larger, or even separate, parts of the variable region. The closer the fit between this site and the antigen determinant, the stronger the noncovalent forces such as hydrophobic or electrostatic bonds between them, and the higher the affinity between the antigen and antibody. Binding depends on a close three-dimensional fit, allowing weak intermolecular forces to overcome the normal repulsion between molecules. When more than one combining site interacts with the same antigen, the bond has greatly increased strength.

ANTIBODY SPECIFICITY AND CROSS-REACTIVITY

Antigen-antibody reactions can show a high level of specificity. Specificity exists when the binding sites of antibodies directed against determinants of one antigen are not

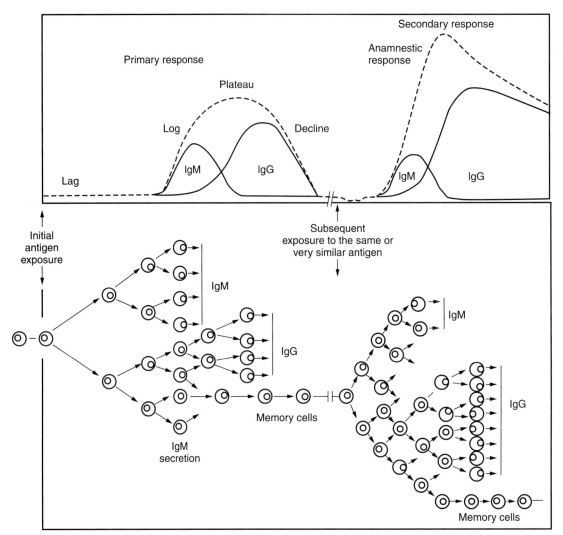

Figure 2-14   Primary and secondary antibody response. (Redrawn from Turgeon ML: *Fundamentals of immunohematology,* ed 2, Baltimore, 1995, Williams & Wilkins.)

TABLE 2-4	Comparison of Properties of Immunoglobulins							
	IgG$_1$	IgG$_2$	IgG$_3$	IgG$_4$	IgM	IgA	IgD	IgE
Complement fixation	2+	1+	3+	0	3+	0	0	0
Placental transfer	1+	+/−	+	1+	0	0	0	0

complementary to determinants of another, dissimilar antigen. When some of the determinants of an antigen are shared by similar antigenic determinants on the surface of apparently unrelated molecules, a proportion of the antibodies directed against one kind of antigen will also react with the other kind of antigen. This is called cross-reactivity. Antibodies directed against a protein in one species may also react in a detectable manner with the homologous protein in another species, which is another example of cross-reactivity.

Examples of cross-reactivity occur between bacteria that possess cell wall polysaccharides in common with mammalian erythrocytes. Intestinal bacteria, as well as other sub-

stances found in the environment, possess A-like or B-like antigens similar to the A and B erythrocyte antigens. If A or B antigens are foreign to an individual, production of anti-A or anti-B occurs, despite lack of previous exposure to these erythrocytic antigens. Cross-reacting antibodies of this type are heterophile antibodies.

Antibody Avidity

Each four-polypeptide-chain antibody unit has two antigen-binding sites, which allows them to be potentially multivalent in their reaction with an antigen. The strength with which a multivalent antibody binds a multivalent antigen is called avidity, in contrast to affinity (the bond between a single antigenic determinant and an individual combining site). When a multivalent antigen combines with more than one of an antibody's combining sites, the strength of the bonding is significantly increased. For the antigen and antibody to dissociate, all of the antigen-antibody bonds must be broken simultaneously.

Decreased avidity can result when an antigen has only one antigenic determinant (monovalent). In addition, a hapten is monovalent; therefore it can react with only one antigen-combining site.

Immune Complexes

The noncovalent combination of antigen with its respective, specific antibody is called an immune complex. An immune complex may be of the small (soluble) or large (precipitating) type, depending on the nature and proportion of antigen and antibody. Under conditions of antigen or antibody excess, small soluble complexes tend to predominate. If equivalent amounts of antigen and antibody are present, a precipitate may form. All antigen-antibody complexes, however, will not precipitate, even at equivalence.

Antibody can react with antigen that is fixed or localized in tissues or with antigen that is released or present in the circulation. Once formed in the circulation, the immune complex is usually removed by phagocytic cells of the body through the interaction of the Fc portion of the antibody with complement and with cell-surface receptors. Under normal circumstances this process does not lead to pathologic consequence, and it may be viewed as a major host defense against the invasion of foreign antigens. It is only in unusual circumstances that the immune complex persists as a soluble complex in the circulation, escapes phagocytosis, and is deposited in endothelial or vascular structures, where it causes inflammatory damage, the principal characteristic of immune complex disease; is deposited in organs such as the kidney; or inhibits useful immunity, such as to tumors or parasites. The level of circulating immune complex is determined by factors such as the rate of formation, the rate of clearance, and, most important, the nature of the complex formed (Box 2-1). Detection of immune complexes and the identification of the associated antigens are important to the clinical diagnosis of immune complex disorders.

MOLECULAR BASIS OF ANTIGEN-ANTIBODY REACTIONS

The basic Y-shaped Ig molecule is a bifunctional structure. The V regions are primarily concerned with antigen binding. When an antigenic determinant and its specific antibody combine, they interact through the chemical groups found on the surface of the antigenic determinant and on the surface of the hypervariable regions of the Ig molecule. Although the C regions do not form the antigen-binding sites, the arrangement of the C regions and hinge region give the molecule segmental flexibility, which allows it to combine with separated antigenic determinants.

Types of Bonding

Bonding of an antigen to an antibody takes place because of the formation of multiple, reversible, intermolecular attrac-

---

Box 2-1	**Factors Determining Immune Complex Level**

Nature of the antigen
  Quantity of available antigen
  Number of determinants (epitopes) per molecule
  Size
Nature of the antibody
  Quantity
  Affinity
  Class
    Valence
    Complement-fixing properties
    Reactivity with cellular receptors
Degree of lattice formation*
  Size of the complex
  Solubility properties
  Complement-fixing properties
  Clearance and distribution properties
Rate of formation
  Antigen availability
  Antibody synthesis rate
Rate of clearance
  Degree of lattice formation*
  Nature of the antigen
  Ability of the complex to react with complement or cellular receptors
  Condition of the mononuclear phagocytic system

Modified from McDougal JS, McDuffie FC: Detection and significance of immune complexes. In Spiefel HE, editor: *Advances in clinical chemistry,* New York, 1985, Academic Press.
*Lattice formation is the cross-linking between sensitized particles and antibodies resulting in aggregation (clumping).

---

tions between an antigen and amino acids of the binding site. These forces require proximity of the interacting groups. The optimum distance separating the interacting groups varies for different types of bond; however, all of these bonds act only across a very short distance and weaken rapidly as that distance increases.

The bonding of antigen to antibody is exclusively noncovalent. The attractive force of noncovalent bonds is weak when compared to covalent bonds, but the formation of multiple noncovalent bonds produces considerable total-binding energy. The strength of a single antigen-antibody bond is termed antibody affinity, and it is produced by the summation of the attractive and repulsive forces. The types of noncovalent bonds involved in antigen-antibody reactions are:

1. Hydrophobic bonds
2. Hydrogen bonding
3. Van der Waals forces
4. Electrostatic forces

Hydrophobic Bonds

The major bonds formed between antigens and antibodies are hydrophobic. Many of the nonpolar side chains of proteins are hydrophobic. When antigen and antibody molecules come together, these side chains interact and exclude water molecules from the area of the interaction. The exclusion of water frees some of the constraints imposed by the proteins, which results in a gain in energy and forms an energetically stable complex.

Hydrogen Bonds

Hydrogen bonding results from the formation of hydrogen bridges between appropriate atoms. Major hydrogen bonds in antigen-antibody interactions are O–H–O, N–H–N, and O–H–N.

Van der Waals Forces

Van der Waals forces are nonspecific, attractive forces generated by the interaction between electron clouds and hydrophobic bonds. These bonds occur because of a minor asymmetry in the charge of an atom as a result of the position of its electrons. They rely on the association of nonpolar, hydrophobic groups so that contact with water molecules is minimized. Although Van der Waals forces are very weak, they may become collectively important in an antigen-antibody reaction.

Electrostatic Forces

Electrostatic forces result from the attraction of oppositely charged amino acids located on the side chains of two amino acid residues. The relative importance of electrostatic bonds is unclear.

Goodness of Fit

The strongest bonding develops when antigens and antibodies are close to each other and when the shapes of both the antigenic determinants and the antigen-binding site conform to each other. This complementary matching of determinants and binding sites is referred to as goodness of fit (Figure 2-15).

A good fit will create ample opportunities for the simultaneous formation of several noncovalent bonds and few opportunities for disruption of the bond. If a poor fit exists, repulsive forces can overpower any small forces of attraction. Variations from the ideal complementary shape will produce a decrease in the total binding energy because of increased repulsive forces and decreased attractive forces. Therefore goodness of fit is important in determining the binding of an antibody molecule for a particular antigen.

Detection of Antigen-Antibody Reactions

In vitro tests detect the combination of antigens and antibodies. Agglutination tests are widely used in immunology to detect and measure the consequences of antigen-antibody in-

teraction. Other test types include precipitation reactions, hemolysis testing, and inhibition of agglutination. Tests such as the radioimmunoassay (RIA) and enzyme-linked immunosorbent assay (ELISA) measure immune complexes formed in an in vitro system. The principles of immunologic methods are discussed in Part Two.

Detection and quantitation of Igs is important in the laboratory investigation of infectious diseases and immunologic disorders (Table 2-5).

Influence of Antibody Types on Agglutination

Igs are relatively positively charged, and after sensitization or coating of particles, they reduce the zeta potential (the difference in electrostatic potential between the net charge at the cell membrane and the charge at the surface of shear). Antibodies can bridge charged particles by extending beyond the effective range of the zeta potential, which results in the erythrocytes closely approaching each other, binding, and agglutinating.

Antibodies differ in their ability to agglutinate. IgM-type antibodies, sometimes referred to as complete antibodies, are considerably more efficient than IgG or IgA antibodies in exhibiting in vitro agglutination when the antigen-bearing erythrocytes are suspended in physiologic (0.85%) sodium chloride (saline). Antibodies that do not exhibit visible agglutination of saline-suspended erythrocytes, even when bound to the cell's surface membrane, are considered to be nonagglutinating antibodies and may be called incomplete antibodies. Incomplete antibodies may fail to exhibit agglutination because the antigenic determinants are located deep within the surface membrane or may show restricted movement in their hinge region, causing them to be functionally monovalent.

TABLE 2-5	Role of Specific Immunoglobulins in Diagnostic Tests		
	IgG	**IgM**	**IgA**
Agglutination	1+	3+	Neg
Complement fixation	1+	3+	1+
Time of appearance after exposure to antigen (days)	3-7	2.5	3-7
Time to reach peak titer (days)	7-21	5-14	7-21

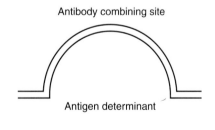

Good fit　　　　　　**Poor fit**

Figure 2-15　Goodness of fit.

MONOCLONAL ANTIBODIES

Monoclonal antibodies (MAbs) are purified antibodies cloned from a single cell. These antibodies exhibit exceptional purity and specificity and are able to recognize and bind to a specific antigen.

Discovery of the Technique

In 1975 Kohler and Miser first fused lymphocytes to produce a cell line that was both immortal and a producer of specific antibodies. The two scientists were awarded the Nobel Prize for Medicine in 1984 for the development of this hybridoma or cell hybrids made between different lines of cultured myeloma cells (plasma cells derived from malignant tumor strains) by using Sendai virus to induce the cells to fuse. Sendai virus is an influenza virus that characteristically causes cell fusion.

Initially Kohler immunized donors with sheep erythrocytes to provide a marker for the normal cells. After making the hybrids, he tested them to see if they still produced antibodies against the sheep erythrocytes. He discovered that some of the hybrids were manufacturing large quantities of specific antisheep erythrocyte antibodies.

This technique is referred to as somatic cell hybridization. The resulting hybrid cells secrete the antibody that is characteristic of the parent cell (e.g., antisheep erythrocyte antibodies). The multiplying hybrid cell culture is called a hybridoma. Hybridoma cells can be cloned (the process in which single cells are selected and grown). The Igs derived from a single clone of cells are termed monoclonal antibodies.

Monoclonal Antibody Production

Modern methods (Figure 2-16) for producing MAbs are refinements of the original technique developed by Kohler. Basically, hybridoma technique enables scientists to inoculate crude antigen mixtures into mice and then select clones producing specific antibodies against a single cell-surface antigen. The process of producing MAbs takes 3 to 6 months.

Mice are immunized with a specific antigen. Several doses of the antigen are given to ensure a vigorous immune response. After 2 to 4 days spleen cells are mixed with cultured mouse myeloma cells. Myeloma parent cells that lack the enzyme hypoxanthine phosphoribosyl transferase are selected because these cells cannot use hypoxanthine derived from the culture medium to manufacture purines and pyrimidines and, if unfused, will not survive in the culture medium. In addition, the mouse myeloma cell lines usually do not secrete Igs, thus simplifying the purification process.

Polyethylene glycol rather than Sendai virus is added to the cell mixture to promote cell membrane fusion. Only 1 in every 200,000 spleen cells actually forms a viable hybrid with a myeloma cell. Normal spleen cells do not survive in culture. The fused-cell mixture is placed in a medium containing *h*ypoxanthine, *a*minopterin, and *t*hymidine (HAT medium). Aminopterin is a drug that prevents myeloma cells from making their own purines and pyrimidines; because they cannot use hypoxanthine from the medium, they will die.

Hybrids resulting from the fusion of spleen cells and myeloma cells contain transferase provided by the normal spleen cells. Consequently, the hybridoma cells are able to use the hypoxanthine and thymidine in the culture medium and survive. They divide rapidly in HAT medium, doubling their numbers every 24 to 48 hours. About 300 to 500 hybrids can be generated from the cells of a single mouse spleen, although not all will be making the desired antibodies. After the hybridomas have been growing for 2 to 4 weeks, the supernatant is tested for specific antibody using methods such as ELISA or RIA. Clones that produce the desired antibody are grown in mass culture and recloned to eliminate non-antibody-producing cells.

Antibody-producing clones lose their ability to synthesize or secrete antibody after being cultured for several months. It is usual to freeze and store hybridoma cells in small aliquots. They may then be grown in mass culture or injected intraperitoneally into mice. Because hybridomas are tumor cells, they grow rapidly and induce the effusion of large quantities of fluid into the peritoneal cavity. This ascites fluid is rich in MAbs and can be easily harvested.

Uses of Monoclonal Antibodies

The greatest impact of MAbs in immunology has been on the analysis of cell membrane antigens. Because MAbs have a single specificity compared to the range of antibody molecules present in the serum, MAbs have multiple clinical applications including:

- Identifying and quantifying hormones
- Typing tissue and blood
- Identifying infectious agents
- Identifying clusters of differentiation for the classification and follow-up therapy of leukemias and lymphomas
- Identifying tumor antigens and autoantibodies
- Immunotherapy

Problems Related to Monoclonal Antibodies

MAb production has opened many possibilities in immunotherapy; however, ascites fluid of mice may yield commercially unsuitable antibody and the expansion of hybridomas in animals is becoming less acceptable because of humane and economic concerns. Several European countries have incorporated legislation limiting antibody production in mice. MAbs are extensively produced in vitro in Switzerland and Germany. Two popular alternative methods are bulk tissue culture in encapsulated or hollow fiber systems, and the expression of cloned antibody genes in high-producing eukaryotes using recombinant DNA technology.

Another problem is that MAbs, traditionally produced from mice, may be rejected by the human immune system. But human MAb production has proved to be quite complex. One current strategy involves transforming cells with Epstein-Barr virus and stabilizing them by extensive cloning. Another popular technique is the "humanization" of mouse MAbs. In this procedure, regions of the human myeloma protein are joined to the variable region of a mouse antibody. The production of true human antibodies is possible with the use of the polymerase chain reaction, but this procedure has limitations.

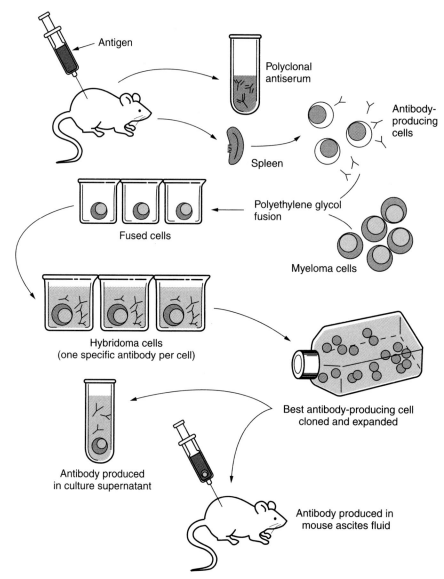

Figure 2-16 Production of monoclonal antibody. (Redrawn from Forbes BA, Sahm DF, Weissfeld AS: *Bailey & Scott's diagnostic microbiology,* ed 11, St Louis, Mosby, 2002.)

Hybridoma Data Bank

In 1983 the Committee on Data for Science and Technology and the International Union of Immunological Societies established an international Hybridoma Data Bank (HDB) to provide a comprehensive directory of information on hybridomas and other cloned cell lines and their immunoreactive products, such as MAbs. MAbs can be generated that react with specific epitopes. These molecules and their biologic origins are described in the database. The terminology used to describe the reactivity of MAbs covers the taxonomy of each genus, species, and strain of organism, as well as the cells, subcellular structures, organs, tissues, and biochemical substances and their components that were derived from these organisms.

HDB holds data on various aspects of hybridomas and their immunoreactive products. Information on the construction of the hybridoma and the reactivity and nonreactivity of its secreted product is included. Information on the availability of an individual hybridoma and its MAb product are included.

CHAPTER HIGHLIGHTS

Foreign substances can be immunogenic if their membrane or molecular components contain structures that are recognized as foreign by the immune system. These structures are called antigenic determinants or epitopes. Cellular antigens of importance to immunologists include HLAs, autoantigens, and blood group antigens. The normal immune system responds to foreignness by producing antibodies. For this reason, microbial antigens are also important in the study of the immunologic manifestation of infectious diseases.

Nucleated cells possess many cell-surface-protein antigens, which readily provoke an immune response if transferred into an (allogenic) individual of the same species. Some of these antigens (e.g., the MHC), are much more potent than others in provoking an immune response. This MHC is referred to as the HLA system. The body's immune system usually exercises tolerance to self-antigens, but in some situations antibodies may be produced in response to normal self-antigens. Antigens are usually large organic molecules that are either proteins or polysaccharides and rarely, if ever, lipids. For antigens to function effectively, several factors are important: foreignness, degradability, MW, structural stability, and complexity. Although large foreign molecules are better antigens, haptens, which are very small molecules, can bind to larger carrier molecules and behave as antigens.

Agglutination of particles to which soluble antigen has been absorbed produces a serum method of demonstrating precipitins. Examples of artificial carriers include latex particles and colloidal charcoal. Antibodies are specific glycoproteins referred to as immunoglobulins. Many antibodies can be isolated in the gamma globulin fraction of protein by electrophoresis separation. However, the term *immunoglobulin* (Ig) has replaced gamma globulin because not all antibodies have gamma electrophoretic mobility.

Antibodies can be found in blood plasma and many body fluids such as tears, saliva, and milk. The primary function of an antibody in body defenses is to combine with antigen, which may be enough to neutralize bacterial toxins or some viruses. A secondary interaction of an antibody molecule with another effector agent such as complement is usually required to dispose of larger antigens such as bacteria.

Five distinct classes of Ig molecules are recognized in most higher mammals: IgM, IgG, IgA, IgD, and IgE. These Ig classes differ from each other in characteristics such as MW, sedimentation, coefficient, and carbohydrate content. Antibodies exhibit diversity among the different classes, which suggests that they perform different functions in addition to their primary function of antigen binding. Each Ig molecule is essentially bifunctional: one region of the molecule is concerned with binding to antigen, while a different region mediates binding of the Ig to host tissues, including cells of the immune system and the first component (C1q) of the classic complement system.

The primary structure of a protein is based on the sequence of amino acid residues linked by the peptide bond. The basic unit of an antibody structure is the homology unit or domain, of which a typical molecule has 12, arranged in two heavy and two light (H and L) chains, linked through cysteine residues by disulphide bonds so that the domains lie in pairs.

Variations between the regions of different antibody molecules are responsible for differences in antigen binding and in biologic functioning. The antigen-binding portion of the molecule (N-terminal end) shows such heterogeneity that it is known as the variable region; the remainder is relatively constant, but some heterogeneity in form is observed in classes and subclasses.

A typical monomeric IgG molecule consists of three globular regions (two Fab regions and a Fc portion) linked by a flexible hinge region. If the molecule is digested with a proteolytic enzyme such as papain, it splits into three approximately equal-size fragments. Two of these fragments retain the ability to bind antigen and are called the antigen-binding (Fab) fragments. The third fragment, which is relatively homogeneous and sometimes crystallizable, is called the Fc portion.

An antigenic determinant is the specific chemical determinant group or molecular configuration against which the immune response is directed. Because they are proteins Igs themselves can function as effective antigens when used to immunize mammals of a different species. When the resulting antiimmunoglobulins or antiglobulins are analyzed, three principal categories of antigenic determinants can be recognized: isotype, allotype, and idiotype.

Production of antibodies is induced when the host's immune system comes into contact with a foreign antigenic substance and reacts to this antigenic stimulation. When an antigen is initially encountered, the cells of the immune system recognize the antigen as nonself and either elicit an immune response or become tolerant to it, depending on the circumstances. An immune reaction can take the form of cell-mediated immunity (immunity-dependent on T cells and macrophages) or involve the production of antibodies directed against the antigen.

After a foreign antigen challenge, an IgM antibody response proceeds in four phases, but the actual time period and titer depend on the characteristics of the antigen and the individual. The four phases are the lag, log, plateau, and decline. Subsequent exposure to the same antigenic stimulus produces an antibody response that exhibits the same four phases as the primary responses.

Repeated exposure to an antigen can take place many years after the initial exposure, but clones of the T memory cells will be stimulated to proliferate with subsequent production of antibody by the individual. An anamnestic response, however, differs from a primary response in several important aspects, namely, time, type of antibody produced, and the titer of antibody.

The ability of a particular antibody to combine with one antigen instead of another is referred to as its specificity. This property resides in the portion of the Fab molecule called the combining site, a cleft formed largely by the hypervariable regions of heavy and light chains. There is evidence, however, that an antigen may bind to larger, or even separate, parts of the variable region. The closer the fit between this site and the antigen determinant, the stronger the noncovalent forces—such as hydrophobic or electrostatic bonds—between them, and the higher the affinity between the antigen and antibody.

Binding depends on a close three-dimensional fit, allowing weak intermolecular forces to overcome the normal repulsion between molecules. When more than one combining site interacts with the same antigen, the bond has greatly increased strength. When some of the determinants of an antigen are shared by similar antigenic determinants on the surface of apparently unrelated molecules, a proportion of the antibodies directed against one kind of antigen will also react with the other kind of antigen. This is called cross-reactivity.

The strength with which a multivalent antibody binds a multivalent antigen is termed avidity, in contrast to affinity. When a multivalent antigen combines with more than one of an antibody's combining sites, the strength of the bonding is significantly increased. For the antigen and antibody to dissociate, all of the antigen-antibody bonds must be broken simultaneously. Decreased avidity can result from an antigen having only one antigenic determinant (monovalent). In addition, a hapten is monovalent; therefore it can react with only one antigen-combining site.

The noncovalent combination of antigen with its respective, specific antibody is called an immune complex. An immune complex may be of the small (soluble) or large (precipitating) type, depending on the nature and proportion of antigen and antibody. Bonding of antigen to antibody is exclusively noncovalent and may be of several types: hydrophobic bonds, hydrogen bonding, Van der Waals forces, or electrostatic forces.

In vitro tests detect the combination of antigens and antibodies. Tests such as agglutination tests are widely used in immunology to detect and measure the consequences of antigen-antibody interaction. Other test types include precipitation reactions, hemolysis testing, and inhibition of agglutination. Tests such as the RIA and ELISA measure immune complexes formed in an in vitro system.

Antibodies differ in their ability to agglutinate. IgM-type antibodies, sometimes referred to as complete antibodies, are considerably more efficient than IgG or IgA antibodies in exhibiting in vitro agglutination when the antigen-bearing erythrocytes are suspended in physiologic (0.85%) sodium chloride. Antibodies that do not exhibit visible agglutination of saline-suspended erythrocytes, even when bound to the cell's surface membrane, are considered to be nonagglutinating antibodies and may be called incomplete antibodies.

MAbs are purified antibodies cloned from a single cell. These antibodies are engineered to bind to a single specific antigen. MAbs bound to cell-surface antigens now provide a method for classifying and identifying specific cellular membrane characteristics, such as in the typing of erythrocyte and leukocyte antigens.

REVIEW QUESTIONS

1. A synonym for an antigenic determinant is:
   A. immunogen
   B. epitope
   C. binding site
   D. polysaccharide

2. Genetically different individuals are referred to as:
   A. allogenic
   B. heterogenic
   C. autogenic
   D. isogenic

3. Antigenic substances can be composed of:
   A. large polysaccharides
   B. proteins
   C. glycoproteins
   D. all of the above

4. Which of the following characteristics of an antigen is the least important?
   A. foreignness
   B. degradability
   C. molecular weight
   D. the presence of large, repeating polymers

5. The chemical composition of an antibody is:
   A. protein
   B. lipid
   C. carbohydrate
   D. glycoprotein

Questions 6-10. Match the following characteristics with the appropriate antibody subclass (use an answer only once).

6. _____ IgM

7. _____ IgG

8. _____ IgA

9. _____ IgE

10. _____ IgD

   A. the highest in plasma/serum concentration in normal individuals
   B. has the shortest half-life
   C. 19S
   D. can exist as a dimer
   E. has no known subclasses

Questions 11-15. Match the following characteristics with the appropriate antibody.

11. _____ IgG

12. _____ IgM

13. _____ IgA

14. _____ IgD

15. _____ IgE

   A. predominant Ig in secretions
   B. increased in infectious diseases, collagen disorders, and hematologic disorders
   C. mediates some types of hypersensitivity reactions
   D. primarily a cell membrane Ig
   E. produced early in an immune response

Questions 16-18. Match each of the following antigenic determinant terms with its appropriate definition.

16. _____ isotype

17. _____ allotype

18. _____ idiotype

   A. found on the Igs of some, but not all, animals of a species
   B. dominant type found on Igs of all animals of a species
   C. individual determinants characteristic of each antibody

Questions 19-22. Arrange the sequence of events of a typical antibody response.

19. _____

20. _____

21. _____

22. _____

    A. plateau
    B. lag phase
    C. log phase
    D. decline

23. Which of the following characteristics is not true of an anamnestic response compared to a primary response?
    A. has a shorter lag phase
    B. has a longer plateau
    C. antibodies decline more gradually
    D. IgM antibodies predominate

24. Which type of antibody is capable of placental transfer?
    A. IgM
    B. IgG
    C. IgA
    D. IgD

Questions 25-28. Match the following terms and their respective definitions.

25. _____ specificity

26. _____ affinity

27. _____ avidity

28. _____ immune complex

    A. the strength of bond between a single antigenic determinant and an individual combining site
    B. the noncovalent combination of an antigen with its respective specific antibody
    C. the ability of an antibody to combine with one antigen instead of another
    D. the strength with which a multivalent antibody binds to a multivalent antigen

29. Which of the following type(s) of bonding is (are) involved in antigen-antibody reactions?
    A. hydrophobic
    B. hydrogen
    C. Van der Waals
    D. all of the above

30. Monovalent antibodies may also be referred to as:
    A. complete antibodies
    B. incomplete antibodies

31. Which of the following is an accurate statement about monoclonal antibodies? Monoclonal antibodies are:
    A. antibodies engineered to bind to a single epitope
    B. purified antibodies cloned from a single cell
    C. used to classify and identify specific cellular membrane characteristics
    D. all of the above

32. Antigens are characterized by all of the following information except that they:
    A. are usually large organic molecules
    B. are usually lipids
    C. can be glycolipids or glycoproteins
    D. are also called immunogens

33. The immunogenicity of an antigen depends to a great extent on:
    A. its biochemical composition
    B. being structurally unstable
    C. its degree of foreignness
    D. having a low molecular weight

34. Antibodies are also referred to as:
    A. Igs
    B. haptens
    C. epitopes
    D. gamma globulins

Questions 35-39. Match each of the individual Igs to the appropriate lettered description.

35. _____ IgM

36. _____ IgG

37. _____ IgA

38. _____ IgE

39. _____ IgD

    A. accounts for 10% of Ig pool, largely confined to the intravascular space
    B. mediates some types of hypersensitivity
    C. found in tears, saliva, colostrum, milk, and intestinal secretions
    D. makes up less than 1% of total Igs
    E. diffuses more readily into extravascular spaces, neutralizes toxins, binds to microorganisms

Questions 40 and 41. Label the components of the basic immunoglobulin (Ig) configuration in the following figure.

Possible answers for question 40.
    A. Fc segment
    B. FAB segment
    C. hinge region
    D. disulphide bond

Possible answers for question 41.
    A. Fc segment
    B. FAB segment
    C. hinge region
    D. disulphide bond

42. It is not true that IgM is:
    A. composed of five basic subunits
    B. more efficient in the activation of the complement cascade and agglutination than IgG
    C. predominant in an initial antibody response
    D. predominant in a secondary (anamnestic) response

Questions 43-46. Label the four phases of an antibody response on the following figure, choosing from the following answers:
    A. log
    B. plateau
    C. lag
    D. decline

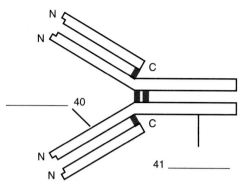

(Redrawn from Turgeon ML: *Fundamentals of immunohematology,* ed 2, Baltimore, 1995, Williams & Wilkins.)

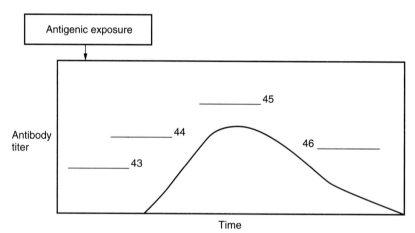

(Redrawn from Turgeon ML: *Fundamentals of immunohematology,* ed 2, Baltimore, 1995, Williams & Wilkins.)

47. In a secondary (anamnestic) response, all of the following characteristics are correct except:
    A. IgG is the predominant antibody type
    B. it has a shorter lag phase
    C. the antibody titer is lower
    D. it has a more gradual decline in antibody response

48. Bonding of antigen to antibody consists of:
    A. hydrogen bonding
    B. van der Waals forces
    C. electrostatic forces
    D. noncovalent bonding

49. The strongest bond of antigen and antibody chiefly results from the:
    A. type of bonding
    B. goodness of fit
    C. antibody type
    D. quantity of antibody

50. Monoclonal antibodies have all of the following characteristics except:
    A. purified antibodies
    B. having been cloned from a single cell
    C. having been engineered to bind to a single specific antigen
    D. frequent occurrence in nature

BIBLIOGRAPHY

Baron EJ, Peterson LR, Finegold SM: *Bailey and Scott's diagnostic microbiology,* ed 9, St Louis, 1994, Mosby.

Barrett JT: *Textbook of immunology,* ed 5, St Louis, 1988, Mosby.

Bellanti JA: *Immunology: basic processes,* Philadelphia, 1979, WB Saunders.

McDougal JS, McDuffie FC: Detection and significance of immune complexes, *Adv Clin Chem* 24:4, 1985.

Ritzmann SE, Daniels JC, editors: *Serum protein abnormalities,* Boston, 1985, Little, Brown.

Ritzmann SE, editor: *Physiology of immunoglobulins,* New York, 1982, Alan R Liss.

Roitt IM: *Essential immunology,* ed 5, Oxford, England, 1984, Blackwell Scientific Publications.

Turgeon ML: *Fundamentals of immunohematology,* ed 2, Baltimore, 1995, Williams & Wilkins.

Chapter 3

The Cells and Cellular Activities of the Immune System: Granulocytes and Mononuclear Cells

LEARNING OBJECTIVES

At the conclusion of this chapter, the reader should be able to:
- Describe the functions of granulocytes, monocytes-macrophages, and lymphocytes-plasma cells as components of the immune system.
- Name and describe the signs and symptoms of abnormal neutrophil function.
- Explain the process of phagocytosis.
- Discuss the role of monocytes-macrophages in cellular immunity.

The entire leukocytic cell system is designed to defend the body against disease. Each cell type, however, has a unique function and behaves both independently and, in many cases, in cooperation with other cell types. Leukocytes can be functionally divided into the general categories of granulocyte, monocyte-macrophage, and lymphocyte-plasma cell. The primary phagocytic cells are the polymorphonuclear neutrophilic (PMN) leukocytes and the mononuclear monocytes-macrophages. The lymphocytes participate in body defenses primarily through the recognition of foreign antigen and/or production of antibody. Plasma cells are antibody-synthesizing cells.

ORIGIN AND DEVELOPMENT OF BLOOD CELLS

Embryonic blood cells, excluding the lymphocyte type of white blood cell, originate from the mesenchymal tissue that arises from the embryonic germ layer, the mesoderm. The sites of blood cell development, hematopoiesis, follow a definite sequence in the embryo and fetus:

1. The first blood cells are primitive red blood cells (erythroblasts) formed in the islets of the yolk sac during the first 2 to 8 weeks of life.
2. Gradually the liver and spleen replace the yolk sac as the sites of blood cell development. By the second month of gestation, the liver becomes the major site of hematopoiesis, and granular types of leukocytes have made their initial appearance. The liver and spleen predominate from about 2 to 5 months of fetal life.
3. In the fourth month of gestation, the bone marrow begins to produce blood cells. After the fifth fetal month, the bone marrow begins to assume its ultimate role as the primary site of hematopoiesis.

The cellular elements of the blood are produced from a common, multipotential, hematopoietic (blood-producing) cell, the stem cell. After stem cell differentiation, blast cells arise for each of the major categories of cell types: erythrocytes, megakaryocytes, granulocytes, monocytes-macrophages, lymphocytes, and plasma cells. Subsequent maturation of these cells will produce the major cellular elements of the circulating blood, the erythrocytes, thrombocytes, and specific types of leukocytes. In normal peripheral or circulating blood, the following types of leukocytes can be found in order of frequency: neutrophils, lymphocytes, monocytes, eosinophils, and basophils.

GRANULOCYTIC CELLS

Granulocytic leukocytes can be further subdivided on the basis of morphology into neutrophils, eosinophils, and basophils. The neutrophil, basophil, and eosinophil each begin as the multipotential stem cell in the bone marrow. The major role of each of these cells in body defenses is unusual.

Neutrophils

The neutrophilic leukocyte, particularly the PMN type, provides an effective host defense against bacterial and fungal infections. Although the monocytes-macrophages and other granulocytes are also phagocytic cells, the neutrophil is the principal leukocyte associated with phagocytosis (Figure 3-1) and a localized inflammatory response. The formation of an inflammatory exudate (pus), which develops rapidly in an inflammatory response, is composed primarily of neutrophils and monocytes.

Mature neutrophils are found in two evenly divided pools, the circulating and marginating pools. The marginating granulocytes adhere to the vascular endothelium. In the peripheral blood, these cells are only in transit to their potential sites of action in the tissues. Movement of granulocytes from the circulating pool to the peripheral tissues occurs by a process called diapedesis (movement through the vessel wall). Once in the peripheral tissues, the neutrophils are able to carry out their function of phagocytosis.

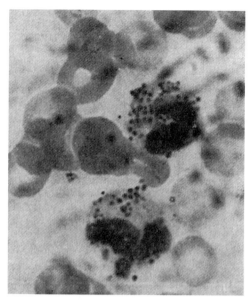

Figure 3-1   The two phagocytic cells have engulfed numerous *Staphylococcus aureus* cells. (From Barrett JT: *Textbook of immunology,* ed 5, St Louis, 1988, Mosby.)

The granules of segmented neutrophils contain various antibacterial substances including lysosomal hydrolases, lysozyme, and peroxidase. Some of these granules are typical lysosomes. During the phagocytic process, however, the powerful antimicrobial enzymes that are released also disrupt the integrity of the cell itself. Neutrophils are also steadily lost to the respiratory, gastrointestinal, and urinary systems, where they participate in generalized phagocytic activities. An alternate route for the removal of neutrophils from the circulation is phagocytosis by cells of the mononuclear-phagocytic system.

Signs and Symptoms of Abnormal Neutrophil Function

That patients with quantitative or qualitative defects of neutrophils have a high rate of infection illustrates the importance of the neutrophil to body defenses. Individuals with a marked decrease of neutrophils (neutropenia) or severe defects in neutrophil function frequently suffer from recurrent systemic bacterial infections such as pneumonia, disseminated cutaneous pyogenic lesions, and other types of life-threatening bacterial and fungal infections.

Leukocyte mobility may be impaired in diseases such as rheumatoid arthritis, cirrhosis of the liver, and chronic granulomatous disease. Defective locomotion or leukocyte immobility can also be seen in patients receiving steroids and in those with lazy leukocyte syndrome. A marked defect in the cellular response to chemotaxis, an important step in phagocytosis, can be seen in patients suffering from diabetes mellitus, Chédiak-Higashi anomaly, and sepsis, and in those with high levels of antibody immunoglobulin E (IgE) such as in Job's syndrome.

Congenital Abnormalities of Neutrophil Structure and Function

A small number of patients have congenital abnormalities (Box 3-1) of neutrophil structure and function.

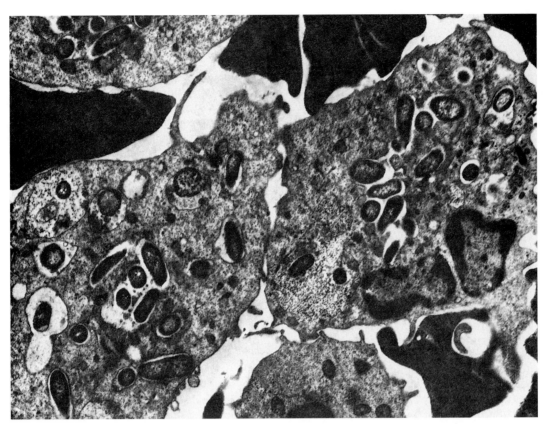

Figure 3-2 Undigested bacteria are numerous within the phagosomes of these phagocytes taken from a patient with chronic granulomatomous disease. (From Barrett JT: *Textbook of immunology,* ed 5, St Louis, 1988, Mosby.)

Box 3-1	Congenital Abnormalities of Neutrophil Structure or Function

Chédiak-Higashi syndrome
Chronic granulomatosus disease
CR3 deficiency
Myeloperoxidase deficiency
Specific granule deficiency

Chédiak-Higashi Syndrome

The Chédiak-Higashi syndrome represents a qualitative disorder of neutrophils. It is a rare familial disorder inherited as an autosomal recessive trait and expressed as an abnormal granulation of neutrophils. Neutrophils having giant granules display impaired chemotaxis and delayed killing of ingested bacteria.

Chronic Granulomatosus Disease

The chronic granulomatosus diseases (CGDs) are a genetically heterogeneous group of disorders of oxidative metabolism affecting the cascade of events required for hydrogen peroxide production by phagocytes. Multiple types of inheritance of the disorder have been described, including sex-linked (X-chromosome–linked) in 66% of cases, an autosomal-recessive in 34% of cases, and an autosomal-dominant in <1% of cases. Patients with the autosomal-recessive form may have a less severe clinical course than patients with the X-linked form.

The onset is during infancy, with one third of patients dying before age 7 years because of infections. In 1966 it was observed that in the presence of normal or elevated leukocyte counts, the neutrophilic granulocytes in vitro ingested (Figure 3-2) and destroyed only streptococci, not staphylococci. Subsequent testing revealed that the cells from patients with CGD can phagocytize non-hydrogen-peroxide–producing bacteria such as *Staphylococcus aureus* and gram-negative rods, the Enterobacteriaceae, but they cannot destroy them. In the X-linked form the defective leukocytes fail to exhibit increased anaerobic metabolism during phagocytosis because of a cytochrome b_{558} deficiency (which expresses itself as a defect in the 91,000-dalton glycoprotein membrane anchor of the cytochrome complex); or these defective leukocytes produce hydrogen peroxide as the result of a deficiency of the enzyme myeloperoxidase.

Patients with this abnormality suffer from infections with catalase-positive bacteria and fungi affecting the skin, lungs, liver, and bones. They also develop granuloma resulting from a lack of resolution of inflammatory foci, even after the infection has been eliminated. This leads to extensive granuloma formation and, in some circumstances, impairment of physiologic processes such as obstruction of the esophagus or urinary tract.

Complement Receptor 3 Deficiency

The complement receptor (CR3) deficiency is a rare condition inherited as an autosomal-recessive trait. A deficiency of CR3 on phagocytic cells presents as a leukocyte adhesion deficiency. Leukocyte adhesion deficiency type I (LAD-I) is due to a deficiency of CD18. LAD-II is due to absent Sialyl-Lewis X (SeLeX, CD15s).

A CR3 deficiency in neutrophils is associated with marked abnormalities of adherence-related functions, including decreased aggregation of neutrophils to each other after activation, decreased adherence of neutrophils to endothelial cells, poor adherence and phagocytosis of opsonized microorganisms, defective spreading, and decreased diapedesis and chemotaxis. Patients with this disorder may also lack an intravascular marginating pool of neutrophils. Defects in T lymphocytes are characterized by faulty lymphocyte-mediated cytotoxicity with poor adherence to target cells. Abnormalities of B lymphocytes have also been observed.

Clinically a deficiency can manifest itself by delayed separation of the umbilical cord. Other signs and symptoms include early onset of bacterial infections, including skin infections, mucositis, otitis, gingivitis, and periodontitis. A depressed inflammatory response and neutrophilia can be observed.

Myeloperoxidase Deficiency

A deficiency of myeloperoxidase is inherited as an autosomal recessive trait on chromosome 17. Myeloperoxidase is an iron-containing heme protein responsible for the peroxidase activity characteristic of azurophilic granules; it accounts for the greenish color of pus. Human neutrophils contain many granules of various sizes that are morphologically, biochemically, and functionally distinct. The azurophilic granules normally contain myeloperoxidase. In this disorder azurophilic granules are present, but myeloperoxidase is decreased or absent. If phagocytes are deficient in myeloperoxidase, the patient's phagocytes manifest a mild-to-moderate defect in bacterial killing and a marked defect in fungal killing in vitro.

Persons with a myeloperoxidase deficiency are generally healthy and do not have an increased frequency of infection. The absence of increased susceptibility to infection is probably because other microbicidal mechanisms compensate for the deficiency. Patients with diabetes and myeloperoxidase deficiency, however, may have deep fungal infections caused by *Candida* species.

Specific Granule Deficiency

Specific granule deficiency is believed to be an autosomal-recessive disease. It is caused by a failure to synthesize specific granules and some contents of other granules during differentiation of neutrophils in the bone marrow. Persons with specific granule deficiency suffer from recurrent, severe bacterial infections of the skin and deep tissues. A depressed inflammatory response is also manifested.

Eosinophils and Basophils

Although eosinophils and basophils are capable of participating in phagocytosis, they possess less phagocytic activity. The ineffectiveness of these cells results from both the small number of cells in the circulating blood and the lack of powerful digestive enzymes. Both the eosinophils and basophils, however, are functionally important in body defense.

Eosinophils

The eosinophil is considered to be a homeostatic regulator of inflammation. Functionally this means that the eosinophil attempts to suppress an inflammatory reaction to prevent the excessive spread of the inflammation. The eosinophil may also play a role in the host defense mechanism because of its ability to kill certain parasites.

A functional property related to the membrane receptors of the eosinophil is the ability of the cell to interact with the larval stages of some helminth parasites and to damage them by way of oxidative mechanisms. Certain proteins released from eosinophilic granules damage antibody-coated *Schistosoma* parasites and may account for damage to endothelial cells in hypereosinophilic syndromes.

Basophils

Basophils have high concentrations of heparin and histamine in their granules, which play an important role in acute, systemic, hypersensitivity reactions (see Chapter 23). Degranulation (Figure 3-3) occurs when an antigen such as pollen binds to two adjacent IgE antibody molecules located on the surface of mast cells. The events resulting from the release of the contents of these basophilic granules include increased vascular permeability, smooth muscle spasm, and vasodilation. If this reaction is severe, it can result in anaphylactic shock.

A newly identified class of compounds, the leukotrienes, mediate the inflammatory functions of leukocytes. The observed systemic reactions related to this compound were previously attributed to the slow-reacting substance of anaphylaxis.

Monocytes and Macrophages

In the past the mononuclear monocyte-macrophage was known only as a scavenger cell. Only recently has its role as a complex cell of the immune system in the host defense against infection been recognized.

The Mononuclear-Phagocyte System

The macrophage and its precursors are widely distributed throughout the body (Figure 3-4). These cells are considered to constitute a physiologic system, the mononuclear-phagocyte system, which includes promonocytes and their precursors in the bone marrow, monocytes in the circulating blood, and macrophages in tissues. This collection of cells is considered to be a system because of their common origin, similar morphology, and common functions, including rapid phagocytosis mediated by receptors for IgG and the major fragment of the third component of complement C3.

Macrophages and their known precursor, the monocytes, migrate freely into the tissues from the blood to replenish and reinforce the macrophage population (Figure 3-5). Macrophages exist as either fixed or wandering cells. Specialized macrophages such as the pulmonary alveolar macrophages are the dust phagocytes of the lung that function as the first line of defense against inhaled foreign particles and bacteria. Fixed macrophages line the endothelium of capillaries and the sinuses of organs such as the bone marrow, spleen, and lymph nodes. These cells, along with the network of reticular cells of the spleen, thymus, and other lymphoid tissues, make up the mononuclear-phagocyte system (Figure 3-6). The term *mononuclear-phagocyte system* has replaced the older term, *reticuloendothelial system*.

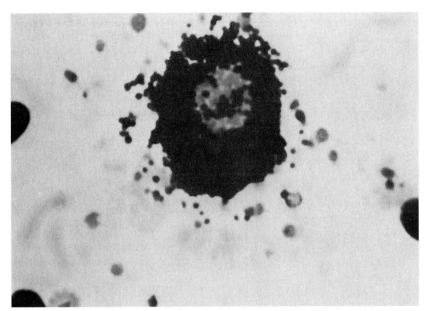

Figure 3-3 A mast cell that has begun to discharge its granules. The light area in the center of the cell, partially shielded by granules, is the nucleus. (From Barrett JT: *Textbook of immunology,* ed 5, St Louis, 1988, Mosby.)

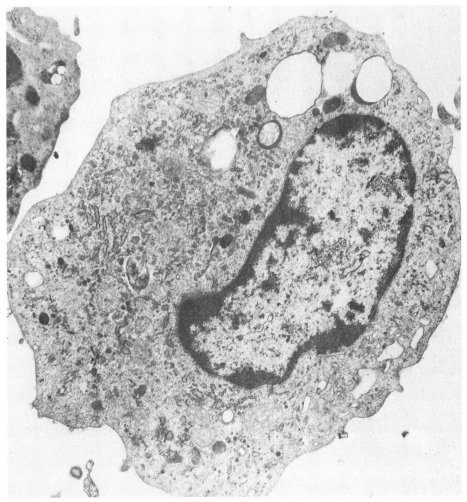

Figure 3-4 Electron micrograph of a macrophage. (From Barrett JT: *Textbook of immunology,* ed 5, St Louis, 1988, Mosby.)

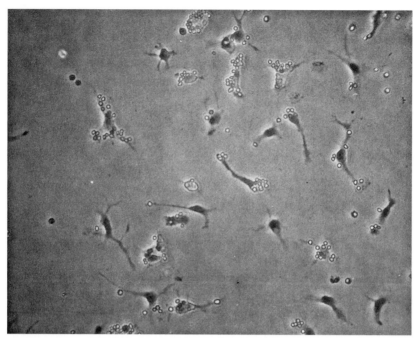

Figure 3-5 Macrophages in culture. Note their elongated form, indicative of their motility. The cellular refractile bodies are erythrocytes that the macrophages are phagocytosing. (From Barrett JT: *Textbook of immunology,* ed 5, St Louis, 1988, Mosby.)

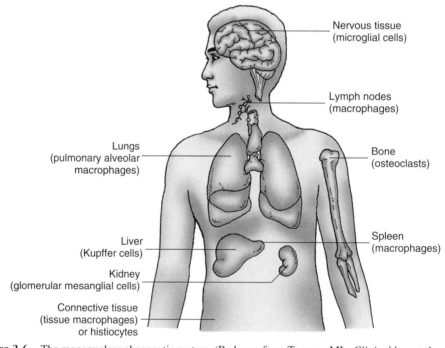

Nervous tissue
(microglial cells)

Lymph nodes
(macrophages)

Lungs
(pulmonary alveolar
macrophages)

Bone
(osteoclasts)

Liver
(Kupffer cells)

Spleen
(macrophages)

Kidney
(glomerular mesanglial cells)

Connective tissue
(tissue macrophages)
or histiocytes

Figure 3-6 The mononuclear phagocytic system. (Redrawn from Turgeon ML: *Clinical hematology: theory and procedures,* ed 3, Philadelphia, 1999, Lippincott-Williams & Wilkins.)

Development of Monocytes-Macrophages

Cells of the macrophage system originate in the bone marrow from the multipotential stem cell. This common, committed progenitor cell can differentiate into either the granulocyte or monocyte-macrophage pathway, depending on the microenvironment and chemical regulators. Maturation and differentiation of these cells may be in various directions.

Circulating monocytes may continue to have a multipotential and give rise to different types of macrophages.

Functionally the most important step in the maturation of macrophages is the cytokine-drive conversion of the normal resting macrophage to the activated macrophage. Macrophages can be activated during infection by the release of macrophage-activating cytokines such as interferon gamma and granulocyte-colony stimulating factor, from T lymphocytes specifically sensitized to antigens from the infecting microorganisms. This interaction constitutes the basis of cell-mediated immunity. In addition, macrophages exposed to an endotoxin release a hormone, tumor necrosis factor-alpha-cachectin, which can itself activate macrophages under certain in vitro conditions.

The terminal stage of development in the mononuclear-phagocyte cell line is the multinucleated giant cell, which characterizes granulomatous inflammatory diseases such as tuberculosis. Both monocytes and macrophages can be shown in the lesions in these diseases before the formation of giant cells; they are thought to be the precursors to the multinucleated cells.

FUNCTIONS OF MONOCYTES-MACROPHAGES IN HOST DEFENSE

Functionally, monocytes-macrophages have phagocytosis as their major role. However, these cells perform at least three distinct but interrelated functions in host defense. The categories of host defense functions of monocytes-macrophages include:

1. Phagocytosis
2. Antigen presentation and induction of the immune response
3. Secretion of biologically active molecules

The principal functions of mononuclear phagocytes in body defenses result from the changes that take place in these functions when the macrophage is activated. These changes are presented in Box 3-2.

Phagocytosis

Macrophages carry out the fundamental function of ingesting and killing invading microorganisms such as intracellular parasites, *Mycobacterium tuberculosis,* and some fungi. In addition, macrophages remove and eliminate such extracellular pathogens as pneumococci from the blood circulation. It is also known that the macrophage has the capacity to phagocytize particulate and aggregated soluble materials. This process is enhanced by the presence of receptors on the surface of the Fc portion of IgG and the C3 complement component. The ability to internalize soluble substances undoubtedly supports the increased microbicidal and tumoricidal ability of activated macrophages. Another important phagocytic function of macrophages is their ability to dispose of damaged or dying cells (Figure 3-7). Macrophages lining the sinusoids of the spleen are particularly important in ingesting aging erythrocytes. They are also involved in removing tissue debris, repairing wounds, and removing debris as embryonic tissues replace one another.

Phagocytic activity increases when there is tissue damage and inflammation, which releases substances that attract macrophages. Activated macrophages migrate more vigorously in response to chemotactic factors and should enter sites of inflammation (e.g., locations of infection or cancer) more efficiently than resting macrophages. Migration of monocytes into different body tissues appears to be a random phenomenon in the absence of localized inflammation. An essential factor in the protective function of monocytes is the capacity of the cell to move through the endothelial wall of blood vessels (diapedesis) to the site of microbial invasion in tissues.

Box 3-2	**Functions of Mononuclear Phagocytes**

INCREASED ACTIVITY IN ACTIVATED MACROPHAGES

Antigen presentation
Chemotaxis
Glucose transport and metabolism
Microbicidal activity
Phagocytosis (variable activity, depending on particle)
Phagocytosis-associated respiratory burst
Pinocytosis
Tumoricidal activity

INCREASED CONSTITUENTS IN ACTIVATED MACROPHAGES

Acid hydrolases
Angiogenesis factor
Arginase
Collagenase
Complement components*
Cytolytic proteinase
Fibronectin
Interleukin-1
Interferon (alpha and beta)
Plasminogen activator
Tumor necrosis factor—cachetin†

DECREASED CONSTITUENTS IN ACTIVATED MACROPHAGES

Apolipoprotein E and lipoprotein lipase
Elastase
Prostaglandins, leukotrienes

CONSTITUENT DEMONSTRATING NO CHANGE IN ACTIVATED MACROPHAGES

Lysoenzyme

Modified from Johnston RVB: Monocytes and macrophages, *N Engl J Med* 318(12):749, 1988.
*Increased or no change.
†When stimulated.

The attracting forces for monocytes—chemotactic factors—include complement products and chemoattractants derived from neutrophils, lymphocytes, or cancer cells.

The activity of mononuclear phagocytes against cancer cells in humans is less well understood than the phagocytosis of microorganisms. Phagocytes are thought to suppress the growth of spontaneously arising tumors. The ability of these cells to control malignant cells may not involve phagocytosis, but it may be related to secreted cellular products such as lysosomal enzymes, oxygen metabolites (e.g., hydrogen peroxide), proteinases, and tumor necrosis factor-alpha (TNF-α) (cachetin). The proteolytic enzymes present on the surface membrane of monocytes could also have a role in tumor rejection.

Antigen Presentation and Induction of the Immune Response

The phagocytic property of the macrophage is particularly important in the processing of antigens as part of the immune response. Macrophages are believed to process antigens and

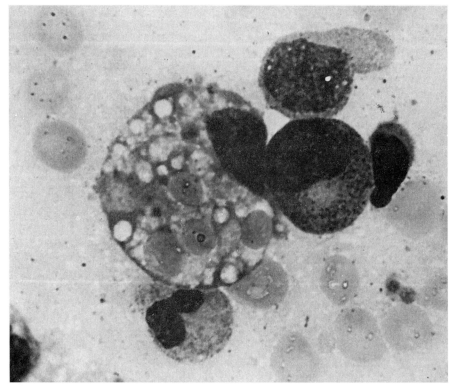

Figure 3-7 Bone marrow macrophage showing erythrophagocytosis. (From Bauer JD: *Clinical laboratory methods,* ed 9, St Louis, 1982, Mosby.)

physically present this biochemically modified and more reactive form of antigen to lymphocytes (particularly T-helper cells) as an initial step in the immune response. Recognition of antigen on the macrophage surface by T lymphocytes, however, requires an additional match of the surface class II gene product of the major histocompatibility complex (MHC). This gene product is the Ia product in the mouse and D gene region product in humans. With proper recognition, the macrophage secretes a lymphocyte-activating factor (interleukin-1 [IL-1]), lymphocyte proliferation ensues, and the immune response (T- and/or B-cell response) is facilitated.

Secretion of Biologically Active Molecules

It has been discovered that monocytes-macrophages release many factors associated with host defense and inflammation. In this role these cells serve as supportive "accessory" cells to lymphocytes, at least partly by releasing soluble factors. In cellular immunity, monocytes assume a "killer role" in that they are activated by sensitized lymphocytes to phagocytize offending cells or antigen particles. This is important in fields such as tumor immunology.

In addition to their phagocytic properties, monocytes-macrophages are able to synthesize a number of biologically important compounds, including transferrin, complement, interferon, pyrogens, and certain growth factors. Approximately 100 distinct substances have been identified as being secreted by monocytes-macrophages.

Blood monocytes and tissue macrophages are primary sources of the polypeptide hormones called IL-1, which have a particularly potent effect on the inflammatory response. IL-1 also supports B-lymphocyte proliferation and antibody production, as well as T-lymphocyte production of lymphokines. The increased synthesis of IL-1 by activated macrophages could contribute to enhancement of the immune response. Endotoxin also induces the synthesis of IL-1. This effect is achieved at least partly by stimulation of the macrophages to release TNF-α, which then stimulates the production of IL-1 by endothelial cells and macrophages. Activated macrophages release much more TNF-α than do resting macrophages that are exposed to endotoxin. Both TNF-α and IL-1 can induce the fever and synthesis of acute-phase reactants (discussed later in this chapter) that characterize inflammation.

Monocyte-Macrophage Disorders

Monocyte-macrophage has been shown to be abnormal in a variety of diseases (Table 3-1). The abnormality is partial, and no related association with increased susceptibility to infection has been established. In cases of severely depressed migration of monocytes, however, it is likely that this dysfunction predisposes a patient to infection because other defects of host defense coexist in these disorders.

The signs and symptoms of abnormalities of monocyte-macrophage function are extremely evident in some conditions. The profound defect of phagocytic killing exhibited by patients with CGD results in the formation of subcutaneous abscesses and abscesses in the liver, lungs, spleen, and lymph nodes. Cancer patients with a defective monocyte cytotoxicity may develop this defect because tumors have the ability to release factors that suppress the generation of toxic oxygen metabolites by macrophages. In newborn infants depressed chemotaxis, killing, and decreased synthesis of the phagocytosis-promoting factors fibronectin, C3, and complement factor B have been observed. In addition, the new-

TABLE 3-1	Primary and Secondary Abnormalities of Monocyte-Macrophage Function
Abnormality	**Condition**
Defect in phagocyte killing	Chronic granulomatosus disease, corticosteroid therapy, newborn infants, viral infections
Defective monocyte cytotoxicity	Cancer, Wiskott-Aldrich syndrome
Defective release of macrophage-activating factors	Acquired immunodeficiency syndrome (AIDS), intracellular infections (e.g., lepromatous leprosy, tuberculosis, visceral leishmaniasis)
Depressed migration	AIDS, burns, diabetes, immunosuppressive therapy, newborn infants
Impaired phagocytosis	Congenital deficiency of CD11-CD18, monocytic leukemia, systemic lupus erythematosus

born infant's macrophages may not respond effectively to infection because his or her lymphocytes have impaired the production of the macrophage activator interferon gamma.

Qualitative disorders of monocytes-macrophages reflect themselves as lipid storage diseases including a number of rare autosomal-recessive disorders. In these conditions the expression in macrophages of a systemic enzymatic defect permits the accumulation of cell debris normally cleared by macrophages. The macrophages are particularly prone to accumulate undegraded lipid products. Resistance to infection can be impaired, at least partially, because of an impairment in macrophage function. Disorders of this type include Gaucher's disease and Niemann-Pick disease.

Gaucher's Disease. Gaucher's disease is an inherited disease caused by a disturbance in cellular lipid metabolism. It is most frequently discovered in children, and the prognosis varies from patient to patient. If the disease is mild, the patient may live a relatively normal life. If the disease is severe, the patient may die prematurely.

The disorder represents a deficiency of beta glucocerebrosidase, the enzyme that normally splits glucose from its parent sphingolipid, glucosylceramide. As the result of this enzyme deficiency, cerebroside accumulates in histiocytes (macrophages). Gaucher's cells are rarely found in the circulating blood. The typical Gaucher cell is large, with one to three eccentric nuclei and a characteristically wrinkled cytoplasm. These cells are found in the bone marrow, spleen, and other organs of the mononuclear-phagocyte system. Production of erythrocytes and leukocytes decreases as these abnormal cells infiltrate the bone marrow.

Niemann-Pick Disease. Niemann-Pick disease is similar to Gaucher's disease in being an inherited abnormality of lipid metabolism. Niemann-Pick disease afflicts infants and children, with the average patient's life expectancy being 5 years.

This disorder represents a rare autosomal-recessive deficiency of the enzyme sphingomyelinase. It is characterized by massive accumulation of sphingomyelin in the mononuclear phagocytes. The characteristic cell in this disorder, Pick's cell, is similar in appearance to Gaucher's cell; however, the cytoplasm of the cell is foamy in appearance.

Phagocytosis and Acute Inflammation

Tissue damage results in inflammation, a series of biochemical and cellular changes that facilitate the phagocytosis of invading microorganisms or damaged cells. If inflammation is sufficiently extensive, it is accompanied by an increase in the plasma concentration of acute-phase reactants (see Chapter 5).

Phagocytosis is mediated by macrophages and neutrophils. Phagocytosis involves the ingestion and digestion of microorganisms, insoluble particles, damaged or dead host cells, cell debris, or activated clotting factors.

Inflammation is characterized by redness, heat, swelling, and pain. The primary objective of inflammation is to localize and eradicate the irritant and repair the surrounding tissue. The inflammatory response involves three major stages:
1. Dilation of capillaries to increase blood flow
2. Microvascular structural changes and escape of plasma proteins from the bloodstream
3. Leukocyte transmigration through endothelium and accumulation at the site of injury

The Process of Phagocytosis

Phagocytosis can be divided into several stages (Figure 3-8): chemotaxis, adherence, engulfment, phagosome formation and fusion, and digestion and destruction. The physical occurrence of damage to tissues, either by trauma or microbial multiplication, releases substances such as activated complement components and/or the products of infection to initiate phagocytosis.

Chemotaxis. Various phagocytic cells continually circulate throughout the blood, lymph, gastrointestinal system, and respiratory tract. When trauma occurs, the neutrophils arrive at the site of injury and can be found in the beginning exudate in less than 1 hour. Monocytes are slower in moving to the inflammatory site. Macrophages resident in the tissues of the body are already in place to deal with an intruding agent. Additional macrophages from the bone marrow and other tissues can occur in severe infections.

Segmented neutrophils are able to gather quickly at the site of injury because they are actively motile. The marginating pool of neutrophils, adhering to the endothelial lining of nearby blood vessels, migrates through the vessel wall to the interstitial tissues. This ameboid movement is called extravasation or diapedesis. Several mediators produced both by microorganisms and by the cells participating in the inflammatory process (e.g., IL-1), which is released by macrophages as a result of infection or tissue injury. Another is histamine, released by circulating basophils, tissue mast cells, and blood platelets. Mediators cause capillary and venular dilation.

Cells are guided to the site of injury by the chemoattractant substances. This event is termed chemotaxis. A chemotactic response is defined as a change in the direction of movement of a motile cell in response to a concentration gradient of a specific chemical, chemotaxin. Chemotaxins can induce both a positive movement toward and a negative

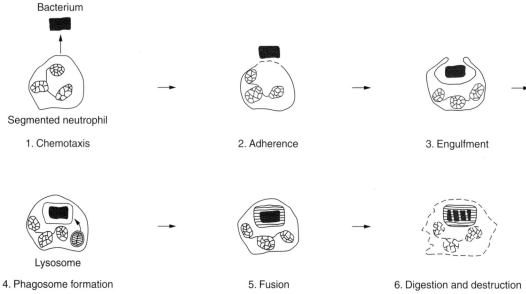

Figure 3-8   The process of phagocytosis. (Redrawn from Turgeon ML: *Clinical hematology: theory and procedures,* ed 3, Philadelphia, 1999, Lippincott-Williams & Wilkins.)

movement away from a chemotactic response. Antigens function as chemoattractants and when antigenic material is present in the body, phagocytes are attracted to its source by moving up its concentration gradient.

Phagocytes detect antigens using various cell-surface receptors. The speed of phagocytosis can be increased markedly by bringing into action two attachment devices present on the surface of phagocytic cells:

- Fc receptor: binds the Fc portion of antibody molecules, chiefly IgG. The IgG will have attached the organism via its Fab site
- Complement receptor: the third component of complement (C3) also binds to organisms and then attaches to the complement receptor

This coating of the organisms by molecules that speed up phagocytosis is termed opsonization, and the Fc portion of antibody and C3 are called opsonins.

Adherence. The leukocyte adhesion cascade is a sequence of adhesion and activation events that ends with the cell exerting its effects on the inflamed site. At least five steps of the adhesion cascade are capture, rolling, slow rolling, firm adhesion, and transmigration. All of these five steps appear to be necessary for effective leukocyte recruitment to the site of injury. These steps are not phases of inflammation but represent the sequence of events involving different leukocytes in the same microvessel.

The process known as capture or tethering represents the first contact of a leukocyte with the activated endothelium. Capture occurs after margination, which allows phagocytes to move in a position close to the endothelium. P-selectin on endothelial cells is the primary adhesion molecule for capture and the initiation of rolling. In addition, many studies suggest that L-selectin also exhibits an important role in capture. A number of other adhesion molecules have been implicated in capture, although the level of actual involvement varies—PECAM-1, ICAM-1, VE-cadherin, CD11a/CD18 (LFA-1), IAP (CD47), and VLA-4 (4β1 integrin).

The inflammatory response begins with a release of inflammatory chemicals into the extracellular fluid. Sources of these inflammatory mediators, the most important of which are histamine, prostaglandins, and cytokines, are injured tissue cells, lymphocytes, mast cells, and blood proteins. The presence of these chemicals promotes and furthers the reactions to inflammation, which are redness, heat, swelling, and pain.

The transit time through the microcirculation and, more specifically, the contact time during which the leukocyte is in close proximity with the endothelium, appears to be a key parameter in determining the success of the recruitment process as reflected in firm adhesion.

Engulfment. On reaching the site of infection, phagocytes engulf the foreign matter and destroy it. Eosinophils can also undergo this process, except that they kill parasites. After the phagocytic cells have arrived at the site of injury, the bacteria can be engulfed through active membrane invagination. Pseudopodia are extended around the pathogen, pulled by interactions between the Fc receptors and Fc antibody portions on the opsonized bacterium. Pseudopodia meet and fuse, thereby internalizing the bacterium and enclosing it in a phagocytic vacuole or phagosome.

The principal factor in determining whether phagocytosis can occur is the physical nature of the surface of both the bacteria and the phagocytic cell. The bacteria must be more hydrophobic than the phagocyte. Some bacteria such as *Diplococcus pneumoniae* possess a hydrophilic capsule and are not normally phagocytized. Most nonpathogenic bacteria are easily phagocytized because they are very hydrophobic. The presence of certain soluble factors such as complement, a plasma protein, coupled with antibodies, and chemicals such as acetylcholine enhance the phagocytic process. Enhancement of phagocytosis through the process of opsonization, the coating of a particle with certain plasma factors, can speed up the ingestion of particles. If the surface tensions are conducive to engulfment, the phagocytic cell

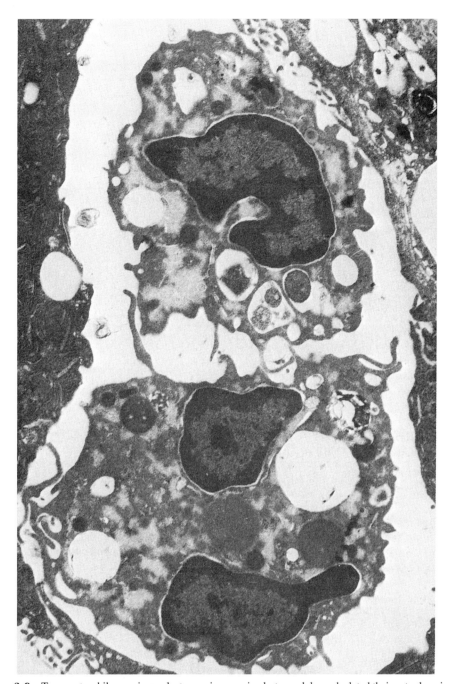

Figure 3-9   Two neutrophils seen in an electron-microscopic photograph have depleted their cytoplasmic granules during phagocytosis. The upper cell contains bacteria at different levels of destruction in the phagolysosomes just below its nucleus. (From Barret JT: *Textbook of immunology,* ed 5, St. Louis, 1988, Mosby.)

membrane invaginates. This invagination leads to the formation of an isolated vacuole, a phagosome, within the cell.

Digestion. Digestion follows ingestion of particles, with the required energy being primarily provided by anaerobic glycolysis. Granules in the phagocyte cytosol then migrate to and fuse with the phagosome to form the phagolysosome. These granules contain degradatory enzymes and are of three types:

1. Primary or azurophilic granules containing enzymes (e.g., lysozyme, myeloperoxidase)
2. Secondary or specific granules containing substances (e.g., lactoferrin)
3. Tertiary granules containing, for example, caspases

Degranulation of the neutrophil (Figure 3-9) releases substances from the granules of neutrophils with antibacterial substances such as lactoferrin, lysozyme, defensin, and bactericidal permeability in increasing protein. Elastase, which is one of several substances that can damage host tissues, is also released. The myeloperoxidase granules are responsible for the action of the oxygen-dependent, myeloperoxidase-mediated system. Hydrogen peroxide and an oxidizable cofactor serve as major factors in the actual killing of bacteria within the vacuole. Other oxygen-independent systems such as alterations in pH, lysozymes, lactoferrin, and the granular cationic proteins also participate in the bactericidal process.

Monocytes are particularly effective as phagocytic cells because of the large amounts of lipase in their cytoplasm. Lipase is able to attack those bacteria such as *M. tuberculosis* with a lipid capsule. Monocytes are further able to bind and destroy cells coated with onocomplement-fixing antibodies because of the presence of membrane receptors for specific components or types of immunoglobulin.

As the result of the release of lytic enzymes, the neutrophils die and are in turn phagocytized by macrophages. Macrophage digestion proceeds without risk to the cell unless the ingested material is toxic. However, if the ingested material damages the lysosomal membrane, the macrophage will also be destroyed because of the release of lysosomal enzymes.

During phagocytosis, cells demonstrate increased metabolic activity, referred to as "respiratory burst." This results in the production by the phagocyte of large quantities of reactive oxygen species (ROS), which are released into the phagocytic vesicle. This phenomenon is achieved by the activity of the enzyme NADPH oxidase. Together, the granule-mediated and NADPH oxidase-mediated effects elicit microbicidal results. NADPH oxidase forms the centerpiece of the phagocyte-killing mechanism and is activated in about 2 seconds. The NADPH oxidase generates ROS by generating the superoxide radical; the associated cyanide-insensitive increase in oxygen consumption is called the respiratory burst.

The importance of the oxygen-dependent microbicidal mechanism is dramatically illustrated by patients with a severe congenital deficit in bacterial killing that results from the inability to produce superoxide. This syndrome is CGD. CGD results from defects in the genes encoding individual components of the enzyme system responsible for oxidant production. Acquisition of oxidase activity occurs in the course of myeloid cell maturation, and the genes for several of its components have been identified. This system also lends itself to analysis of the transcriptional and translational events that occur during cellular differentiation and under the influence of specific cytokines.

Rather than being discarded by exocytosis, some peptides undergo an important separate process at this stage. Instead of being eliminated, they attach to a host molecule called MHC class II and end up being expressed on the surface of the cell within a groove on the MHC molecule (antigen presentation).

Subsequent Phagocytic Activity. If invading bacteria are not phagocytized at entry into the body, they may establish themselves in secondary sites such as the lymph nodes or various body organs. These undigested bacteria produce a secondary inflammation, where neutrophils and macrophages again congregate. If bacteria escape from secondary tissue sites, a bacteremia will develop. In patients who are unresponsive to antibiotic intervention, this situation can prove fatal.

Neutrophils As Mediators of Noninfectious Inflammatory Diseases

Although neutrophils provide the major means of defense against bacterial and fungal infections, they can also be destructive to host tissues. The same oxidative and nonoxidative processes that destroy microorganisms can affect adjacent host tissues. A number of disease states correspond to

Box 3-3	Noninfectious Diseases in Which Signs, Symptoms, and Injury May Be Partly Mediated by Neutrophils

Autoimmune arthritides
Autoimmune vasculitis
Dermatophytic disorders
   Autoimmune bullous dermatoses
   Behçet's disease
   Psoriasiform dermatoses
   Pyoderma gangrenosum
   Sweet's syndrome
Glomerulonephritis
Gout
Inflammatory bowel disease
Malignant neoplasms at the site of chronic inflammation
Myocardial infarction
Respiratory disorders
   Adult respiratory distress syndrome
   Asthma and allergic asthma
   Emphysema

inappropriate phagocytosis (Box 3-3). Inappropriate prolonged activation of the NADPH oxidase is one example. This process occurs when the phagocytes attempt to engulf particles that are too large. The phagocyte releases oxygen radicals and granule contents onto the particle, but these escape into the surrounding tissues, generating tissue damage. This is often observed in response to dust inhalation and smoking (e.g., nicotine) and in persistent infections such as cystic fibrosis. In addition, many autoimmune diseases are thought to be due to inappropriate activation of the process of phagocytosis, whereby the body attacks its own cells and tissues. Examples include rheumatoid arthritis, multiple sclerosis, and Graves' disease.

CELL-SURFACE RECEPTORS

Cellular communication is essential to development, tissue organization, and function of all multicellular organisms. Cells communicate with each other and with their environment via soluble mediators and during direct contact (e.g., phagocytosis). An immunologic response is a result of the interactions of various leukocytes with each other and with other cells in the body. These interactions occur through cell-surface receptors that mediate cell-cell binding or "adhesion" of leukocytes.

Discovery of several cell surface receptors involved in cellular communication has been a key factor in understanding the mechanisms underlying inflammatory and immune phenomena. Three protein families—the Ig family, the integrin family, and the recently designated selectin family—are associated in a network of cellular interactions in the immune system.

Members of the Ig superfamily include antigen-specific receptors, such as the T-cell receptor and surface immunoglobulin (Ig), as well as antigen-independent receptors and their counterreceptors such as CD2 and lymphocyte function associated molecule-3. Ig superfamily members function in cell activation, differentiation, and cell-cell interaction. In some cases, both an adhesion receptor and the counterreceptor to which it binds are members of the Ig superfamily.

Three selectin family molecules—endothelial cell adhesion molecule-1, leukocyte adhesion molecule (LAM-1, Mel-14), and CD62, also known as platelet activation-dependent granule-external membrane protein and granule membrane protein of 140 KD (GMP-140)—have been implicated in a number of leukocyte adhesion phenomena, including leukocyte homing to lymphoid tissue. Selectins are expressed on both leukocytes and endothelial cells. Mel-14 functions early in neutrophil-endothelium adhesion.

The integrin family consists of at least 14 alpha/beta heterodimers divided into subfamilies with distinct structural and functional characteristics. The subfamily of leukocyte integrins contains three members (LFA-1, Mac-1, and p150,95). These molecules are glycoproteins composed of noncovalently associated alpha and beta subunits. LFA-1 is expressed on all leukocytes, whereas Mac-1 and p150,95 are found primarily on granulocytes and monocytes.

The integrin family is phylogenetically ancient. Integrin family members engage in interactions with cell-surface ligands and extracellular matrix components (EMC). ECM components, including fibronectin, collagen, and laminin, have been shown to be ligands for members of the beta 1 and beta 3 subfamilies. Members of these subfamilies are of great significance in embryogenesis, growth and repair, and hemostasis. The leukocyte integrins—or beta 2 subfamily—have been shown to be involved in a diverse number of leukocyte adhesion-dependent phenomena, giving them a critical role in inflammatory and immune responses. The term *integrin* was initially used to emphasize that these receptors integrate signals from the extracellular environment with the intracellular cytoskeleton. A signal is transduced from outside to inside the cell.

In addition to the involvement of these receptors in a variety of immune functions, integrin molecules play a role in the spread of malignant cells. The major cause of death in malignant disease is not the primary tumor but rather the metastasis of tumor cells to distant sites within the body. Metastasis is a complex, multistep process that begins with the detachment of a few tumor cells from the primary tumor. The tumor cells then move into the circulatory system, where they can be transported to other organs. While in the circulatory system, the tumor cells must survive the natural defense system of the body before attaching to and invading the tissues of another organ. A better understanding of the metastatic process could provide the basis for diagnostic and therapeutic strategies.

Disease States Involving the Leukocyte Integrins

Leukocyte adhesion deficiency (see p. 40) is characterized by impaired leukocyte adhesion that ultimately leads to recurrent and often fatal bacterial and fungal infections. Patients with this clinical syndrome suffer from chronic granulocytosis, recurrent gingivitis, and lack of pus formation. Leukocytes from LADI patients are deficient in the leukocyte beta$_2$-integrin subunit. Patients are categorized as severely and moderately deficient. Moderately deficient patients may survive to adulthood with treatment of recurrent infections, but severely deficient patients will die early in

childhood because of overwhelming infection unless they receive a bone marrow transplant.

Screening Test For Phagocytic Engulfment

Principle

A mixture of bacteria and phagocytes is incubated and examined for the presence of engulfed bacteria. This simple procedure may be useful in supporting the diagnosis of impaired neutrophilic function in conjunction with clinical signs and symptoms (Figure 3-10).

Specimen Collection and Preparation

No special preparation of the patient is required before specimen collection. The patient must be positively identified when the specimen is collected. The specimen label should be completed at the bedside and include the patient's full name, date, patient's hospital identification number, and phlebotomist's initials.

Blood should be drawn by an aseptic technique. A minimum of 2 mL of heparin blood (green-top evacuated tube) or 15 to 20 heparinized capillary tubes are required. The specimen should be centrifuged, and the test should be performed promptly.

Reagents, Supplies, and Equipment

1. Broth culture of *Bacillus subtilis* or *Staphylococcus* coagulase-negative species
2. Microscope slides
3. Pasteur pipettes and rubber bulb
4. 12- × 75-mm test tubes
5. Wright's stain

Quality Control

A fresh, heparinized sample of blood from a healthy volunteer should be tested simultaneously.

Procedure

1. Label two 12- × 75-mm-test tubes: "patient" and "control."
2. Add 4 to 8 drops of the buffer coat from either the patient's heparinized blood or from the normal control to the respectively labeled test tubes.
3. Add 2 to 3 drops of the bacterial broth culture to each tube.
4. Incubate both tubes at room temperature or 37° C for 30 minutes.
5. Place 1 drop of the incubated specimen on a glass slide and prepare a smear.
6. Air-dry the slides and stain with Wright's stain.

Wright's Stain Procedure

a. Cover each smear generously with filtered Wright's stain and allow the stain to remain on the slide for at least 5 minutes.

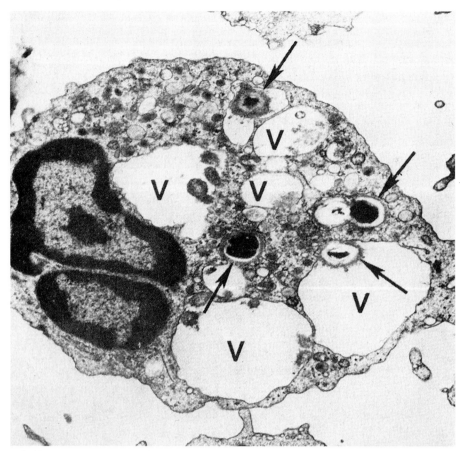

Figure 3-10   An electron photomicrograph from a polymorphonuclear leukocyte from a normal control patient incubated with staphylococci for 30 minutes. Many bacteria (*see arrows*) in various stages of destruction are evident within the cell. Note the cytoplasmic vacuoles (V) around and adjacent to degenerating bacteria. (From Bauer JD: *Clinical laboratory methods,* ed 9, St Louis, 1982, Mosby.)

b. Slowly add distilled water or buffer to the stain until the buffer begins to overflow the stain. Watch for the appearance of a metallic luster.

c. Gently blow on the slide to mix the stain and buffer.

d. Allow the buffer to remain on the slide for at least 5 minutes.

e. Gently wash the stain and buffer off the slide with distilled water.

f. Air-dry or carefully blot the slide between two sheets of bibulous paper.

7. Place a drop of immersion oil on each smear and examine microscopically with the oil (×100) immersion objective.

Reporting Results

Positive—demonstration of the engulfment of bacteria
Negative—no engulfment of bacteria

Procedure Notes

Sources of Error

This procedure may produce false-negative results if the blood specimen is not fresh or if a coagulase-positive *Staphylococcus* specimen is used. It is important to distinguish between granules and cocci. In addition, the bacteria must be intracellular and not extracellular for the test to be positive.

Clinical Applications

The failure of phagocytes to engulf bacteria can support the diagnosis of neutrophilic dysfunction; however, these results must be used in conjunction with patient signs and symptoms.

Limitations

This is a simple screening procedure for engulfment. The presence of engulfed bacteria does not demonstrate that the bacteria have been destroyed.

CHAPTER HIGHLIGHTS

The entire leukocytic cell system is designed to defend the body against disease. However, each cell type has a unique function and behaves both independently and, in many cases, in cooperation with other cell types. The primary phagocytic cells are the neutrophilic leukocytes and the mononuclear monocytes-macrophages. The cellular elements of the blood are produced from a common, multipotential, hematopoietic cell, the stem cell. After stem cell differentiation, blast cells arise for each of the major categories of cell types: erythrocytes, megakaryocytes, granulocytes, monocytes-macrophages, lymphocytes, and plasma cells. Subsequent maturation of these cells produce the major cellular elements of the circulating blood, the erythrocytes, thrombocytes, and specific types of leukocytes. In normal peripheral or circulating blood, the following types of leukocytes can be found in order of frequency: neutrophils, lymphocytes, monocytes, eosinophils, and basophils.

That patients with quantitative or qualitative defects of neutrophils have a high rate of infection illustrates the importance of the neutrophil to body defenses. The neutrophilic leukocyte provides an effective host defense against bacterial and fungal infections. Although the monocytes-macrophages and other granulocytes are also phagocytic cells, the neutrophil is the principal leukocyte associated with phagocytosis and a localized inflammatory response.

In the past the mononuclear monocyte-macrophage was known only as a scavenger cell. Recently its role as a complex cell of the immune system in the host defense against infection has been recognized. Qualitative disorders of monocytes-macrophages reflect themselves as lipid storage diseases, including a number of rare autosomal-recessive disorders.

Tissue damage results in inflammation, a series of biochemical and cellular changes that facilitate the phagocytosis of invading microorganisms or damaged cells. If inflammation is sufficiently extensive, it is accompanied by an increase in the plasma concentration of acute-phase reactants.

Phagocytosis can be divided into several stages: movement of cells, engulfment, and digestion. If bacteria are not effectively immobilized, subsequent phagocytic activity may take place. Although neutrophils provide the major means of defense against bacterial and fungal infections, they can also be destructive to host tissues. The accumulation of neutrophilic infiltrates and the side effects of phagocytosis can be important as the cause of tissue destruction in a number of noninfectious disease processes.

Cells communicate with each other and with their environment via soluble mediators and during direct contact (e.g., phagocytosis). These interactions occur through cell surface receptors that mediate cell-cell binding or "adhesion" of leukocytes.

Three protein families—the Ig family, the integrin family, and the recently designated selectin family—are associated in a network of cellular interactions in the immune system. Leukocyte adhesion deficiency is characterized by impaired leukocyte adhesion that ultimately leads to recurrent and often fatal bacterial and fungal infections.

REVIEW QUESTIONS

1. The major site of hematopoiesis in the second month of gestation is the:
   A. yolk sac
   B. spleen
   C. liver
   D. bone marrow

2. The principal type of leukocyte in the process of phagocytosis is the:
   A. eosinophil
   B. basophil
   C. monocyte
   D. neutrophil

3. Chronic granulomatosus disease represents a defect of:
   A. oxidative metabolism
   B. abnormal granulation of neutrophils
   C. diapedesis
   D. chemotaxis

4. A primary function of the eosinophil is:
   A. phagocytosis
   B. suppression of the inflammatory response
   C. reacting in acute, systemic hypersensitivity reactions
   D. antigen recognition

5. The cells of the mononuclear phagocytic system include:
   A. monocytes and promonocytes
   B. monocytes and macrophages
   C. lymphocytes and monocytes
   D. Both A and B

6. The host defense function(s) of monocytes-macrophages include(s):
   A. antigen presentation
   B. phagocytosis
   C. secretion of biologically active molecules
   D. all of the above

7. The surface MHC class II gene product is important in:
   A. antigen recognition by T lymphocytes
   B. antigen recognition by B lymphocytes
   C. synthesis of antibody by plasma cells
   D. phagocytosis

Questions 8-12. Match the appropriate monocyte-macrophage abnormality with its respective condition.

8. _____ defect in phagocytic killing

9. _____ defective monocyte cytotoxicity

10. _____ defective release of macrophage-activating factors

11. _____ depressed migration

12. _____ impaired phagocytosis

   A. Wiskott-Aldrich syndrome
   B. burns or diabetes
   C. systemic lupus erythematosus
   D. corticosteroid therapy
   E. intracellular infections

Questions 13-16. Arrange the steps of phagocytosis in the proper sequence.

13. _____

14. _____

15. _____

16. _____

    A. digestion of bacteria
    B. increase in chemoattractants at site of tissue damage
    C. ingestion of bacteria
    D. movement of phagocytic cells

Questions 17-20. Match the following cell types to their respective functions. (An answer can be used more than once.)

17. _____ polymorphonuclear neutrophilic (PMN) leukocytes

18. _____ lymphocytes

19. _____ mononuclear monocytes-macrophages

20. _____ plasma cells

    A. primary phagocytic cells
    B. antibody-synthesizing cells
    C. recognition of foreign antigen and/or production of antibody

Questions 21-23. Arrange the sites of blood cell development (hematopoiesis) in the embryo and fetus in the correct sequence.

21. _____ site of initial red blood cell production

22. _____ predominant site from 2 to 5 months of fetal life

23. _____ ultimate site of primary hematopoiesis

    A. liver and spleen
    B. yolk sac
    C. bone marrow

24. Patients with a marked decrease in neutrophils or severe defects in neutrophil function:
    A. have a high rate of infection
    B. suffer from recurrent systemic bacterial infections
    C. suffer from recurrent life-threatening fungal infections
    D. all of the above

Questions 25-28. Match each disorder/deficiency to its characteristics.

25. _____ chronic granulomatosus disease

26. _____ lazy leukocyte syndrome

27. _____ Chédiak-Higashi anomaly

28. _____ myeloperoxidase deficiency

    A. marked defect in cellular response to chemotaxis
    B. fail to exhibit increased anaerobic metabolism during phagocytosis
    C. mild to marked defect in bacteria-killing ability of neutrophils
    D. defective leukocyte locomotion

29. Which statement about eosinophils is not correct?
    A. they are homeostatic regulators of inflammation
    B. they attempt to suppress an inflammatory reaction
    C. they are able to kill most parasites
    D. they interact with the larval stages of some helminth parasites

30. Which statement about basophils is not true?
    A. they have a high concentration of heparin in the granules
    B. they have a high concentration of histamine in the granules
    C. they react with two adjacent IgA molecules on mast cells
    D. they are associated with anaphylactic shock

31. The cells that constitute the physiologic, mononuclear-phagocytic system, do not include:
    A. promonocytes and their precursors
    B. monocytes in circulating blood
    C. macrophages in tissues
    D. polymorphonuclear neutrophils

Questions 32-36. Identify the types of mononuclear phagocytic cells found in the various locations indicated in the illustration. Choose from the following answers:
  A. Kupffer cells
  B. macrophages
  C. microglial cells
  D. histiocytes

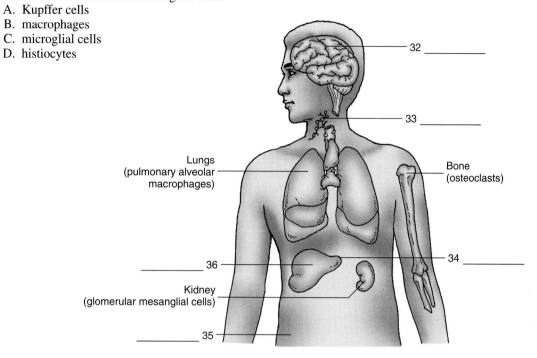

(From Turgeon ML: *Clinical hematology: theory and procedures,* ed 3, Philadelphia, 2000, Lippincott-Williams & Wilkins.

Questions 37-40. Name the steps in the process of phagocytosis as illustrated in the illustration. Choose from the following answers:
  A. engulfment
  B. chemotaxis
  C. phagosome formation
  D. adherence

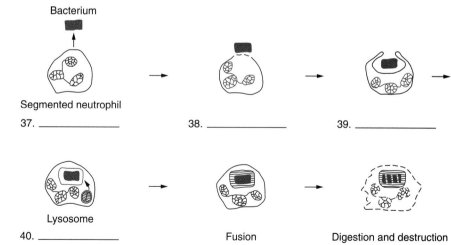

(From Turgeon ML: *Clinical hematology: theory and procedures,* ed 3, Philadelphia, 2000, Lippincott-Williams & Wilkins.)

BIBLIOGRAPHY

Barrett J: *Textbook of immunology,* ed 5, St Louis, 1988, Mosby.

Busby J, Caranasos GJ: Immune function, autoimmunity, and selective immunoprophylaxis, *Med Clin North Am* 71(1), 1987.

Etzion: A: Integrins: the molecular glue of life, *Hosp Pract* 35(3): 102, 2000.

Gee GK et al: *Body defenses—Part A, Integrated science for the health professions laboratory manual,* Corning, New York, 1985, Corning College Press.

Jandl JH: *Blood,* Boston, 1987, Little, Brown.

Johnston RB: Monocytes and macrophages, *N Engl J Med* 318(12): 747-752, 1988.

Katz P: Clinical and laboratory evaluation of the immune system, *Med Clin North Am* 69(3):453-459, 1985.

Larson RS, Springer TA: *Structure and function of leukocyte integrins. Immunological reviews,* No 114, pp 181-217, Copenhagen, Denmark, 1990, Munksgaard.

Ledue TB et al: The relationship between serum levels of lipoprotein (a) and proteins associated with the acute-phase response, *Clin Chim Acta* 223(1-2):73-82, 1993.

Malech HL, Malech JI: Neutrophils in human diseases, *N Engl J Med* 317(11):687-692, 1987.

Noti JD: Laboratory of molecular biology, *Guthrie J* 63(2):51-53, 1994.

Roitt IM: *Immunology,* London, 1985, Gower Medical Publishing.

Rotrosen D: The respiratory burst oxidase. In Gallin JI, Goldstein IM, Snyuderman R, editors: *Inflammation: basic principles and clinical correlates,* ed 2, New York, 1992, Raven Press.

Turgeon ML: *Clinical hematology,* ed 3, Philadelphia, 1999, Lippincott-Williams & Wilkins.

Turgeon ML: *Fundamentals of immunohematology,* ed 2, Baltimore, 1995, Williams & Wilkins.

Chapter 4

The Cells and Cellular Activities of the Immune System: Lymphocytes and Plasma Cells

LEARNING OBJECTIVES

At the conclusion of this chapter, the reader should be able to:
- Name and describe the function of primary and secondary lymphoid tissue.
- Explain the function of T lymphocytes in immunity.
- Explain the function of B lymphocytes in immunity.
- Describe the evaluation of suspected lymphocytic or plasma cell defects.
- Name and compare disorders with immunologic (lymphocytic or plasma cell) origin.

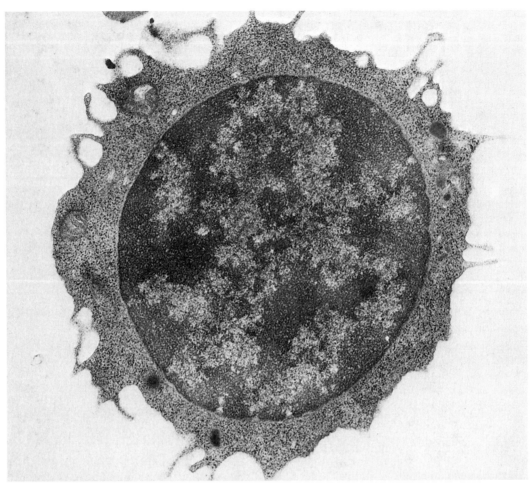

Figure 4-1   Electron photomicrograph of a lymphocyte. (From Barrett JT: *Textbook of immunology,* ed 5, St Louis, 1988, Mosby.)

LYMPHOCYTES AND PLASMA CELLS

Lymphocytes (Figure 4-1) represent the only immunologically specific cellular components of the immune system. Any immune response involves the interaction of many different cell types, and it is not possible to consider cell-mediated responses and antibody-mediated responses entirely separately. T cells play an important role in the regulation of virtually all immune responses by providing help for antibody production by B lymphocytes (B cells) and by providing growth factors for B cells, T cells, and several other cell types. The cytotoxic subset of lymphocytes carry out important effector functions; it is one of the cell types that is responsible for destroying virally infected cells, tumor cells, and allogeneic transplant cells.

Anatomic Origin and Development of Lymphocytes

In addition to the activities of the granulocytes and monocytes-macrophages, the lymphocytes and plasma cells are the cornerstone of the immune system. Lymphocytes recognize foreign antigens, directly destroy some cells, and produce antibodies as plasma cells.

Sites of Lymphocytic Development

In mammalian immunologic development (Figure 4-2), the precursors of lymphocytes arise from progenitor cells of the yolk sac and liver. Later in fetal development and throughout the life cycle, the bone marrow becomes the sole provider of undifferentiated progenitor cells, which can further develop into lymphoblasts. Continued cellular development and proliferation of lymphoid precursors occur as the cells travel to the primary and secondary lymphoid tissues.

Primary Lymphoid Tissue

The primary lymphoid organs are the thymus and the bursa of Fabricius in birds (Figure 4-3). In mammals both the bone marrow (and/or fetal liver) and thymus are classified as primary or central lymphoid organs (Figure 4-4). Mammals have no bursa of Fabricius, but the bone marrow and other sites are considered to be the bursal equivalent.

   The Thymus. Early in embryonic development, the stroma and nonlymphoid epithelium of the thymus are derived from the third and fourth pharyngeal pouches. This structure, located in the mediastinum, exercises control over the entire immune system. It is believed that the development of diversity occurs mainly in the thymus and bone marrow,

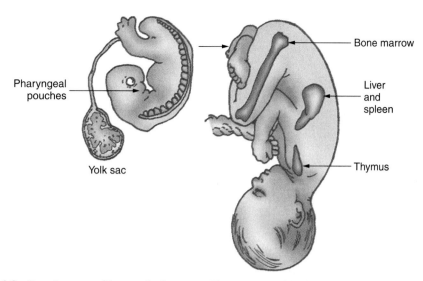

Figure 4-2   Development of immunologic organs. The anatomy of the human fetus illustrates the development of the mammalian immune system. Cells of the pharyngeal pouches migrate into the chest and form the thymus. Precursors of lymphocytes originate early in embryonic life in the yolk sac and eventually migrate to the bone marrow via the spleen and liver.

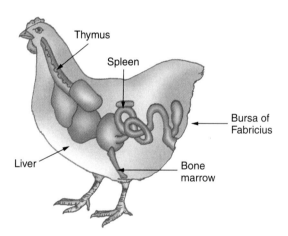

Figure 4-3   Avian immunologic organs. The immune system in birds is focused in two organs, the thymus and the bursa of Fabricius.

although clonal expansion can occur anywhere in the peripheral lymphoid tissue.

Progenitor cells that migrate to the thymus proliferate and differentiate under the influence of the humoral factor, thymosin. These lymphocyte precursors with acquired surface membrane antigens are referred to as thymocytes. The reticular structure of the thymus allows a significant number of lymphocytes to pass through it to become fully immunocompetent (able to function in the immune response), thymus-derived T cells. The thymus also regulates immune function by secretion of multiple soluble hormones.

Many cells die in the thymus and are apparently phagocytized, a mechanism to eliminate lymphocyte clones reactive against self-antigens. Viable cells migrate to the secondary tissues. The absence or abnormal development of the thymus results in a T-lymphocyte deficiency. Involution of the thymus is the first age-related change occurring in the immune system of humans. The thymus gradually loses up to 95% of its mass (Figures 4-5 and 4-6) during the first 50

years of life. The accompanying functional changes of decreased synthesis of thymic hormones and the loss of ability to differentiate immature lymphocytes are reflected in an increased number of immature lymphocytes both within the thymus and as circulating peripheral blood T cells. Most of the changes in immune function, such as dysfunction of T and B lymphocytes, elevated levels of circulating immune complexes, increases in autoantibodies, and monoclonal gammopathies (see Chapter 24 for a complete discussion of representative examples of these disorders), are correlated to involution of the thymus. Immune senescence may account for the increased susceptibility of older adults to infections, autoimmune disease, and neoplasms.

Bone Marrow.   The bone marrow is the source of progenitor cells. These cells can differentiate into lymphocytes and other hematopoietic cells (e.g., granulocytes, erythrocytes, and megakaryocyte populations). In mammals the bone marrow also supports eventual differentiation of mature T and B lymphocytes, probably from a common lymphoid cell

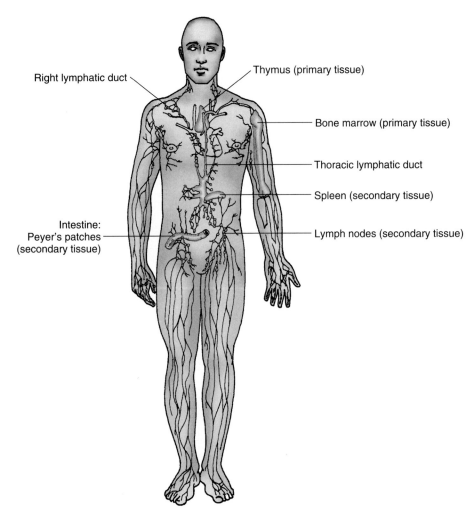

Figure 4-4   Human primary and secondary tissues. (Redrawn from Turgeon ML: *Clinical hematology: theory and procedures,* ed 3, Philadelphia, 1999, Lippincott, Williams & Wilkins.)

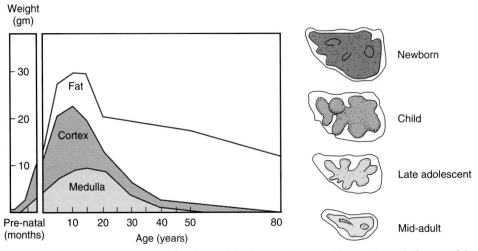

Figure 4-5   Thymic development. The histology of the thymus changes with age. The main feature of these changes is a loss of cellularity with increasing age.

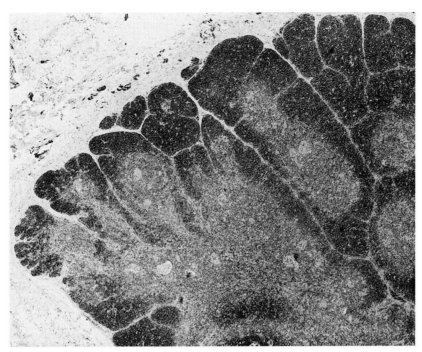

Figure 4-6   Normal thymus gland from infant, showing lobulated structure, distinct corticomedullary junction, and prominent Hassall's corpuscles of medulla (×25). (From Kissane JM: *Anderson's pathology,* ed 9, St Louis, 1990, Mosby.)

progenitor. It is believed that the bone marrow and gut-associated lymphoid tissue (GALT) may also play a role in the differentiation of progenitor cells into B lymphocytes. These structures function as the bursal equivalent in humans. It is from the term, *bursa,* that the B lymphocytes derive their name.

Secondary Lymphoid Tissues

The secondary lymphoid tissues include lymph nodes (Figure 4-7), spleen, gut-associated lymphoid tissue, thoracic duct, bronchus-associated lymphoid tissue, skin-associated lymphoid tissue, and blood. Mature lymphocytes and accessory cells (antigen-presenting cells, APCs)) are found throughout the body, although the relative percentages of T and B cells are different in different locations. The approximate percentage of lymphocytes in lymphoid organs is described in Table 4-1.

Proliferation of the T and B lymphocytes in the secondary or peripheral lymphoid tissues is primarily dependent on antigenic stimulation.

The T lymphocytes or T cells (Figure 4-8) populate the following:

1. Perifollicular and paracortical regions of the lymph nodes
2. Medullary cords of the lymph nodes
3. Periarteriolar regions of the spleen
4. Thoracic duct of the circulatory system

The B lymphocytes or B cells multiply and populate:

1. Follicular and medullary (germinal centers) of the lymph nodes
2. Primary follicles and red pulp of the spleen
3. Follicular regions of GALT
4. Medullary cords of the lymph nodes

Lymph Nodes. Lymph nodes act like lymphoid filters in the lymphatic system. Lymph nodes respond to antigens introduced distally and routed to them by afferent lymphatics. Generalized lymph node reactivity can occur after systemic antigen challenge (e.g., serum sickness).

Spleen. The spleen acts like a lymphatic filter within the blood vascular tree. It is an important site of antibody production in response to intravenous particulate antigens (e.g., bacteria). The spleen is also a major organ for the clearance particles.

Gut-Associated Lymphoid Tissue. GALT includes lymphoid tissue in the intestines (Peyer's patches) and the liver. GALT features immunoglobulin A (IgA) production and involves a unique pattern of lymphocyte recirculation. Pre-B cells develop in Peyer's patches and, after meeting antigen from the gut, many enter the general circulation and then return back to the gut. GALT is also important for the development of tolerance to ingested antigens.

Thoracic Duct. Thoracic duct lymph is a rich source of mature T cells. Chronic thoracic duct drainage can cause T-cell depletion and has been used as a method of immunosuppression.

Bronchus-Associated Lymphoid Tissue. Bronchus-associated lymphoid tissue includes lymphoid tissue in the lower respiratory tract and in the hilar lymph nodes. It is mainly associated with IgA production to inhaled antigens.

Skin-Associated Lymphoid Tissue. Antigens introduced via the skin are presented via epidermal Langerhans cells, which are bone marrow-derived accessory cells. These epidermal cells then interact with lymphocytes in the skin and/or in draining lymph nodes.

Blood. The blood is an important lymphoid organ and immunologic effector tissue. Circulating blood has enough

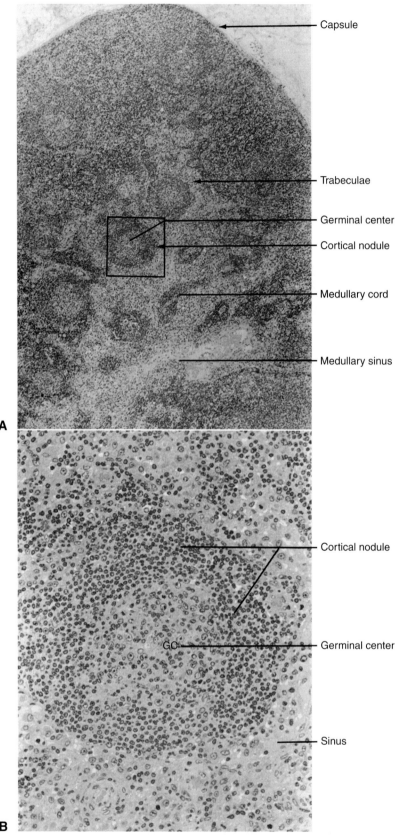

Figure 4-7   A, Lymph node (×90). Cortical nodule (enclosed by triangle; is enlarged in *B*). **B,** Lymph node (×450). Enlargement of cortical nodule seen in *A*. (From Anthony CP, Thibodeau GA: *Textbook of anatomy and physiology,* ed 12, St Louis, 1987, Mosby.)

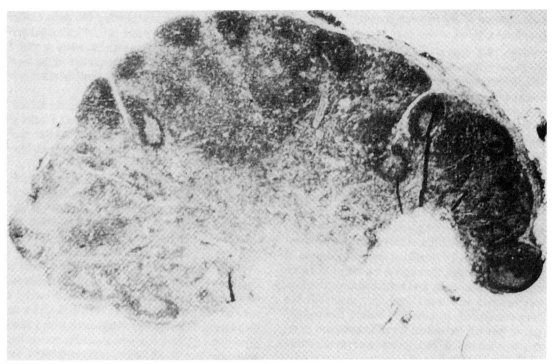

Figure 4-8 Normal lymph node of a child, showing germinal centers, deep cortical areas, and medullary cords. T cells are located in the deep cortical areas, whereas B cells are located in germinal centers and medullary cords. (Courtesy Dr. Richard O'Reilly, New York.)

TABLE 4-1	Approximate Percentage of Lymphocytes in Lymphoid Organs	
Lymphoid Organ	T Lymphocytes (%)	B Lymphocytes (%)
Thymus	100	0
Blood	80	20
Lymph nodes	60	40
Spleen	45	55
Bone marrow	10	90

Modified from Claman HN: Biology of the immune response, *JAMA* 268(20):2792, 1992.

mature T cells to produce a graft-versus-host reaction. In addition, blood transfusions have been responsible for inducing acquired immunologic tolerance in kidney allograft patients.

Blood is the most frequently sampled lymphoid organ. It is assumed that what is found in blood samples represents what is present in other lymphoid tissues. Although this may be a true representation, it is not always accurate.

Circulation of Lymphocytes

The mature T lymphocyte survives for several months or years, whereas the average life span of the B lymphocytes is only a few days. Lymphocytes move freely between the blood and lymphoid tissues. This activity, referred to as lymphocyte recirculation, enables lymphocytes to come in contact with

processed foreign antigens and to disseminate antigen-sensitized memory cells throughout the lymphoid system. Clonal expansion may occur regionally, as in lymph nodes draining a contact allergic reaction, and then the whole body becomes susceptible to rechallenge because T cells recirculate (but generally are excluded from returning to the thymus). Research has shown that a pool of T-cell clonal elements is developed by a combination of positive selection of those clones able to recognize and react to foreign antigens, and negative selection (purging) of those clones able to interact with self-antigens in a damaging way.

Recirculation of lymphocytes back to the blood is via the major lymphatic ducts. Lymphocytes enter the lymph node (Figure 4-9) from the blood circulation via arterioles and capillaries to reach the specialized postcapillary venules. From the venule the lymphocytes enter the node and will either remain in the node or pass through the node and return to the circulating blood. Lymphatic fluid, lymphocytes, and antigens from certain body sites enter the lymph node through the afferent lymphatic duct and exit the lymph node through the efferent lymphatic duct.

LYMPHOID AND NONLYMPHOID SURFACE MEMBRANE MARKERS

Before 1979 human lymphocytes could be classified as T or B cells. Observation of these cells with an electron microscope (Figure 4-10) revealed that T lymphocytes have a relatively smooth surface compared with the rough pattern of the B lymphocytes.

The introduction of monoclonal antibody testing led to the present identification of surface membrane markers on

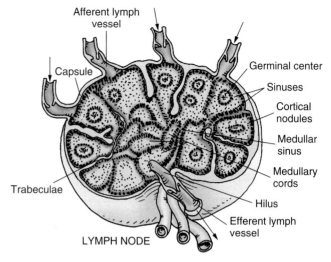

Figure 4-9 Structure of a lymph node. Several afferent valved lymphatics bring lymph to the node. An efferent lymphatic leaves the node at the hilus. Note that the artery and vein enter and leave at the hilus. (Redrawn from Anthony CP, Thibodeau GA: *Textbook of anatomy and physiology,* ed 12, St Louis, 1987, Mosby.)

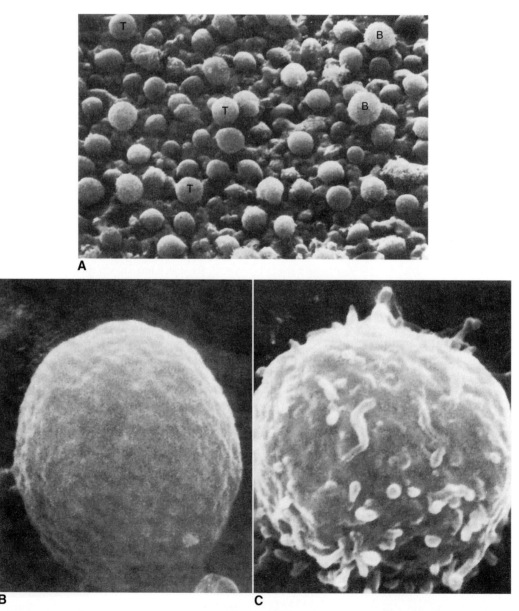

Figure 4-10 Scanning electron photomicrograph of T- and B-lymphocyte cell surface membranes. **A,** T = T lymphocytes, B = B lymphocytes; **B,** T lymphocytes; **C,** B lymphocyte. (From Polliack A et al: Identification of human B and T lymphocytes by scanning electron microscope, *J Exp Med* 138:607-624, 1973.)

lymphocytes and other cells. In practical terms, surface markers are used to identify and enumerate various lymphocyte subsets, establish lymphocyte maturity, classify leukemias, and monitor patients on immunosuppressive therapy.

Cell surface molecules recognized by monoclonal antibodies are called antigens (because antibodies can be produced against them) or markers (because they identify and discriminate between or mark different cell populations). Originally surface markers were named according to the antibodies that reacted with them, but a uniform nomenclature system has now been adopted. In this system a surface marker that identifies a particular lineage or differentiation stage with a defined structure and that can be identified with a group or cluster of monoclonal antibodies is called a member of a cluster of differentiation (CD) (see Table 4-2 for some of the most commonly used cluster designations).

Markers can be grouped into several categories:
- Some are specific for cells of a particular lineage or maturational pathway.
- Some vary in expression, depending on the state of activation or differentiation of the same cells. For example, when CD antigen identification is used to classify lymphocyte subsets, most helper T lymphocytes are CD3+, CD4+, CD8-; most cytotoxic lymphocytes are CD3+, CD4-, CD8+. In addition to using CD classification for the identification and separation of lymphocytes, CD antigens are involved in various lymphocyte functions. The two most frequent functions are:
1. Promotion of cell-to-cell interactions and adhesion
2. Transduction of signals that lead to lymphocyte activation

TABLE 4-2 Cell Differentiation Antigens

Antigen	Earlier Designations	Distribution
CD1a	Leu-6	<1% T cells
CD2	T-11, Leu-5b	78%-88% T cells, NK cells
CD3	T3, Leu-4	68%-82% mature T cells (T-cell receptor complex)
CD3+CD2	Leu-4+5b	83% ± 5% T cells, NK cells
CD4	T4, Leu-3a	35%-55% mature T cells, monocytes
CD4	Leu-3a+3b	29%-55% mature T cells
CD5	Leu-1	65%-79% T cells, B-cell subset
CD7	Leu-9	75% T cells and NK cells
CD8	T8, Leu-2a	20%-36% mature T cells
	Leu-2b	19%-37% mature T cells
CD10	CALLA	>90% of common ALLs, common acute lymphoblastic leukemia antigen, granulocytes, immature B cells
CD11b	Leu-M15	Monocytes, NK cells, granulocytes 25%-35% some T cells
CD11c	Leu- M5 (Anti-CR3)	100% monocytes, macrophages, histiocytic lymphomas, NK cells, hairy-cell and acute myeloid leukemia
CD14	Leu- M3	>85% monocytes/macrophages, granulocytes
CD15	Leu- M1	80%-100% monocytes, >95% mature granulocytes
CD16	Leu-11a	8%-22% NK cells, granulocytic neutrophils
	Leu-11b	
	Leu-11c	
CD19	Leu-12	5%-15% B cells
CD20	B4, B1	5%-15% B cells
	Leu-16	
CD21	B2	5%-15% mature B cells, dendritic cells
CD22	Leu-14	5%-15% B cells
CD23	Leu-20	<10% B cells, activated B cells
CD25	Tac	15%-40% activated T cells, some B cells
	IL-2 receptor	
CD29	4B4	Some CD4+ and CD8+ cells
CD32	2EI	B monocytes, granulocytes, platelets
CD33	Leu-M9	>95% monocytes, granulocytes, acute myeloid leukemia
CD34	JPCA-1	Bone marrow progenitor cells, TdT+ cells, some acute leukemias
CD35	CR$_1$	5%-15% B cells, a few T cells, monocytes, granulocytes
CD38	Leu-17	24%-44% T cells, NK cells, activated T cells, B cell subset
CD43	Leu-22	80%-90% reactive T cells, CD5+ B cells, monocytes, granulocytes, NK cells
CD45 RA	2H4	Some CD4+ and CD8+ cells, some B cells, monocytes
CD45 RO	UCH-1	Some CD4+ and CE 8+ cells
CD57	Leu-a7	13%-27% T-cell and NK-cell subsets
CD69	Leu-23	<10% activated T cells, B cells, and NK cells
CD71	Transferrin receptor	100% of lymphoblasts and monocytes, tumor cell lines, nucleated red blood cells

Lymphocyte Characteristics

Type	Function(s)	Phenotypic Marker	Peripheral Blood (% of Total)
Helper T(T$_H$)	Stimulate B cell growth and differentiation *(humoral immunity)*, macrophage activation by secreted cytokines *(cell-mediated immunity)*	CD3+, CD4+, CD8-	50-60
Cytolytic T(T$_c$)	Lysis of virus-infected cells, tumor cells, allografts *(cell-mediated immunity)*, Macrophage activation by secreted cytokines *(cell-mediated immunity)*	CD3+, CD4-, CD8+	20-25
Natural killer cells	Lysis of virus-infected cells, *(antibody-dependent cellular cytotoxicity)*	Fc receptor for IgG or cells CD16	~10
B cells	Antibody production *(humoral immunity)*	Fc receptors, MHC class II, CD19, CD 21	10-15

T LYMPHOCYTES

Most total circulating lymphocytes (Table 4-3) are T cells derived from bone marrow progenitor cells that mature in the thymus gland. These cells are responsible for cellular immune responses and are involved in the regulation of antibody reactions in conjunction with B lymphocytes.

During cellular development, T-lymphocyte-associated antigens vary (Figure 4-11). Some antigens appear early in cellular development and remain on mature T cells. Others appear at an early or intermediate stage of cellular maturation and are lost before maturity. When mature T cells leave the thymus, their T-cell receptors (TCRs) are either CD4+ or CD8+, and the cells gain functional maturity with their entry into the peripheral blood circulation.

T cells develop into a variety of clones, each bearing a different CD3 molecule specific for a particular antigen-major histocompatibility complex (MHC). Markers present on all T cells are used to evaluate total T-cell numbers. The cells that react strongly with self-antigen are generally deleted during maturation.

T-Lymphocyte Subsets

The CD4+ subset was initially described as representing the helper-inducer T cell; the CD8+ subset was initially described as representing the suppressor-cytotoxic T cells. The complexity of the T cells has increased with recent reports describing subpopulations of the cells. T cells can be subdivided into several populations using various operational and phenotypic parameters.

Helper T Lymphocytes

Helper T lymphocytes can be assigned to one of several subsets, including:
- T$_H$1 (responsible for cell-mediated effector mechanisms)
- T$_H$2 (play a greater role in the regulation of antibody production)
- T$_H$0 (an intermediate category)

These divisions are not absolute and there is considerable overlap or redundancy in function between the different subsets. This classification is based according to the in vitro blends of cytokines they produce. T$_H$1 and T$_H$2 (Figure 4-12)

cells can promote development of cytotoxic cells and are believed to develop from T$_H$0 cells. T$_H$1 cells interact most effectively with mononuclear phagocytes; T$_H$2 release cytokines that are required for B cell differentiation.

T$_H$1 (Figure 4-13, *A*) responses are characterized by high interferon-gamma (IFN-gamma) production and promote elimination of intracellular pathogens. T$_H$2 (Figure 4-13, *B*) responses, characterized by interleukin-4 (IL-4) and IL-5, promote a different type of effector response that involves immunoglobulin E production and eosinophils capable of elimination of larger extracellular pathogens (e.g., helminths). In situations of repeated pathogen exposure or persistent infections, the polarization of T-cell responses serves to focus the antigen-specific response on a specific effector pathway.

Many factors can influence the terminal differentiation of lymphocytes:
- The type of APC
- The affinity of the specific antigenic peptide
- The kinds of costimulatory molecules expressed by APCs
- The cytokines acting on the T cell during primary activation through the TCR

A hierarchy is apparent among these factors and is determined by the mechanism by which they influence T-cell differentiation. Certain cytokines acting directly on T cells during primary activation appear the most proximal or direct mediators of CD4+ T-cell differentiation. The presence of IL-12 during primary T-cell activation leads to strong development of Th1 responses, and IL-4 promotes Th2 development. Activation through the TCR is a requirement for initiating terminal differentiation, but the signals from the TCR appear to be *phenotype neutral*.

Certain T cells carry out delayed hypersensitivity reactions. These T cells react with antigen class II MHC on APCs and create their effects mainly via cytokine production. These cells generally are of the CD4+ phenotype.

T cells can also be differentiated into two populations depending on whether they use an alpha-beta (TCR2) or a gamma-delta (TCR1) antigen receptor. The TCR consists of a heterodimer and a number of associated polypeptides that form the CD3 complex. The dimer recognizes processed anti-

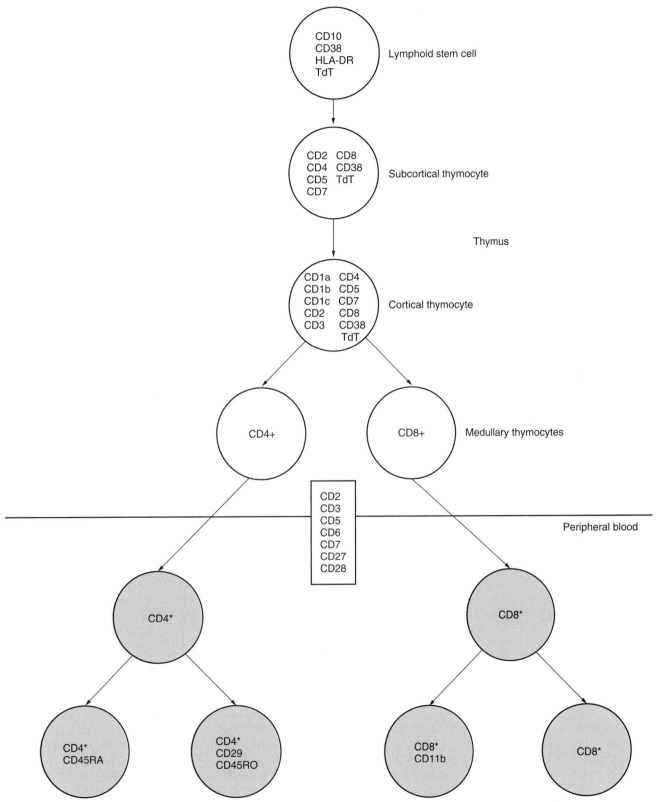

Figure 4-11   Lymphoid CD antigen expression in T lymphocytes. *Also includes CD2, CD3, CD5, CD6 (subset), CD7, CD11c (subset), CD27 (subset), CD28 (subset), CD45RB (subset), CDW49d, CDW49f, CD57 (subset), CDW60 (subset), CDW70, CD73 (subset), CDW75 (subset), CD76 (subset). Note: Activated T cells express CD2R, CD25, CD26, CD30, CD38, CDW49b, CD69, CDW70, CD71.

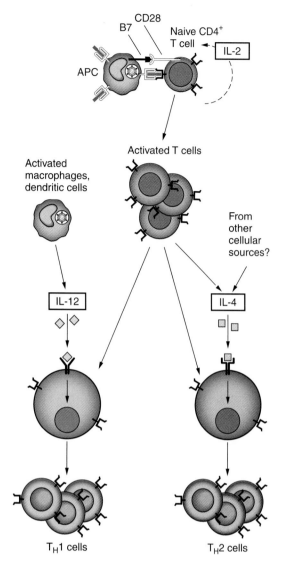

Figure 4-12   The differentiation of naïve CD4+ helper T cells into T$_H$1 and T$_H$2 effector cells. After their activation by antigen and co-stimulators, naïve helper T cells may differentiate into T$_H$1 and T$_H$2 cells under the influence of cytokines. IL-12 produced by microbe-activated macrophages and dendritic cells stimulates differentiation of CD4+ T cells into T$_H$1 effectors. In the absence of IL-12, the T cells themselves (and perhaps other cells) produce IL-4, which stimulates their differentiation into T$_H$2 effectors. (Redrawn from Abbas AK, Lichtman AH: *Basic immunology: functions and disorders of the immune system,* Philadelphia, 2001, WB Saunders.)

gen associated with an MHC molecule. The CD3 complex is required for receptor expression and is involved in signal transduction. TCR1 cells constitute less than 5% of total lymphocytes, but appear in greater proportions in some sites (e.g., skin and vagina). These cells appear to recognize different antigens than TCR2 cells, including carbohydrate and intact protein antigens. In addition, some TCR1 cells do not require antigen to be processed or to be presented by MHC molecules.

Cytotoxic Lymphocytes

Cytotoxic lymphocytes (T$_c$) are effector cells found in the peripheral blood that are capable of directly destroying virally infected target cells. Most T$_c$ are CD8+ and recognize anti-

gen on the target cell surface associated with MHC class I molecules (HLA-A, -B, -C) or class I MHC alone. This process is demonstrated by the immune response to virus-infected cells or tumor cells (Figure 4-14). In addition to destruction of virally infected class I–bearing targets, T$_c$ are major effectors in allograft organ rejection. Cytotoxic T cells express either CD4 or CD8, depending on the major histocompatibility antigen restriction (MHC) that governs their antigen recognition (i.e., class I or class II antigens) (Figure 4-15).

T suppressor (T$_s$) cells are functionally defined T cells that downregulate the actions of other T and B cells. These cells have no unique markers. Although antigen-specific suppression was described in 1970, and many investigators believe that T suppressor cells are critical in various phases of immunoregulation, peripheral tolerance, and autoimmunity, their mode of action is unclear. Many are CD8+ and may operate via secretion of free TCRs.

Antigen Processing and Antigen Presentation to T Cells

Antigen-presenting cells are a group of functionally defined cells capable of taking up antigens and presenting them to lymphocytes in a form that they can recognize. Antigens are taken up by antigen-presenting cells (e.g., dendritic cells, macrophages, B cells, and sometimes even tissue cells) in various ways. Some antigens are taken up by APCs in the periphery and transported to the secondary lymphoid tissues; other APCs normally resident in lymphoid tissues intercept antigen as it arrives. B cells recognize antigen in a native form.

There are two major pathways of antigen processing within the APC and target cell.

1. The endogenous pathway processes proteins that have been internalized, processed into fragments, and reexpressed at the cell surface membrane in association with MHC molecules. In this pathway, proteins in the cytoplasm are cleaved into peptide fragments of ~20 amino acids in length. These fragments are then transported into the lumen of the endoplasmic reticulum via the transporter associated with antigen processing complex, where they encounter newly formed heavy-chain molecules of MHC class I and their associated beta$_2$ microglobulin (beta$_2$m) light chains. The heavy chain, light chain, and peptide form a trimeric complex, which is then transported to and expressed on the cell surface. T cells that express the CD8+ cell-surface marker recognize antigens that are presented by MHC class I molecules. CD8+ functions as a coreceptor in this process, binding to an invariant region of the MHC class I molecule.

2. In the exogenous pathway soluble proteins are taken up from the extracellular environment, generally by specialized or "professional" APCs. The antigens are then processed in a series of intracellular acidic vesicles called endosomes. During this process, the endosomes intersect with vesicles that are transporting MHC class II molecules to the cell surface. CD4+ T cells recognize antigens that are presented by MHC class II molecules. As with CD8, the CD4 molecule functions as a coreceptor, increasing the strength of the interaction between the T cell and the APC.

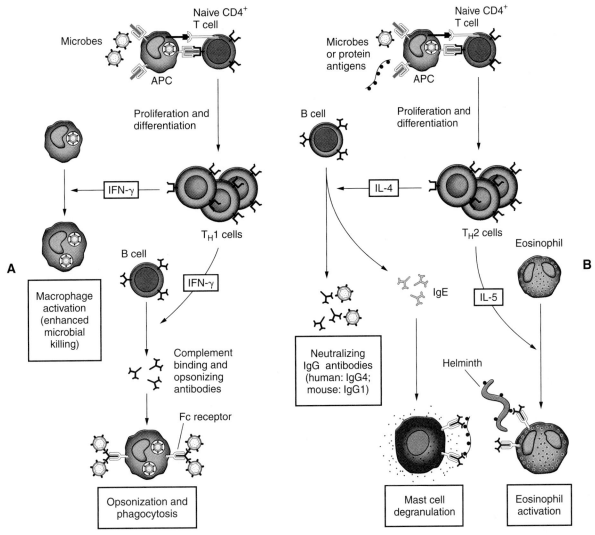

Figure 4-13   The functions of T_H1 and T_H2 subsets of CD4+ helper T lymphocytes. **A,** T_H1 cells produce the cytokine IFN-gamma, which activates phagocytes to kill ingested microbes and stimulates the production of antibodies that promote the ingestion of microbes by the phagocytes. **B,** T_H2 cells specific for microbial or nonmicrobial protein antigens produce the cytokines IL-4, which stimulates the production of IgE antibody, and IL-5, which activates eosinophils. IgE participates in the activation of mast cells by protein antigens and coats helminths for destruction by eosinophils. T_H2 cells also stimulate the production of other antibodies (IgG4 in humans) that neutralize microbes and toxins but do not bind to Fc receptors or activate complement efficiently. (Redrawn from Abbas AK, Lichtman AH: *Basic immunology: functions and disorders of the immune system,* Philadelphia, 2001, WB Saunders.)

For both systems of antigen presentation, recognition of the antigen by the T cells is described as being MHC restricted; that is, the T cells recognize only antigen presented by self-MHC molecules.

Antigen Recognition by T Cells

T cells are clonally restricted so that each T cell expresses a receptor able to interact with a given peptide. Each lymphocyte makes only one type of antigen receptor and can recognize only a very limited number of antigens. As receptors differ on each clone of cells, the entire lymphocyte population has an enormous number of different, specific antigen receptors.

The TCR of most T lymphocytes is composed of an alpha and beta polypeptide chain, with constant regions located close to the cell surface and the part that binds to the antigenic peptide of appropriate fit located away from the cell surface. It is the difference in the structure of the distal regions of the alpha and beta chains that allows the development of different clones of T cells. The TCR reacts with antigen in the context of class I or II MHC molecules on an APC (Figure 4-16).

T cells recognize protein antigens in the form of peptide fragments presented at the cell surface by MHC I or MHC II molecules. When the antigen-specific TCR on the T-cell surface (specifically the zeta-beta chains) of the CD3 complex interacts with the appropriate peptide–MHC complex, it triggers phosphorylation of the intracellular domains of the CD3 zeta chains. Subsequently, the zeta-associated protein 70 (ZAP-70) binds to the phosphorylated zeta chains, and is activated.

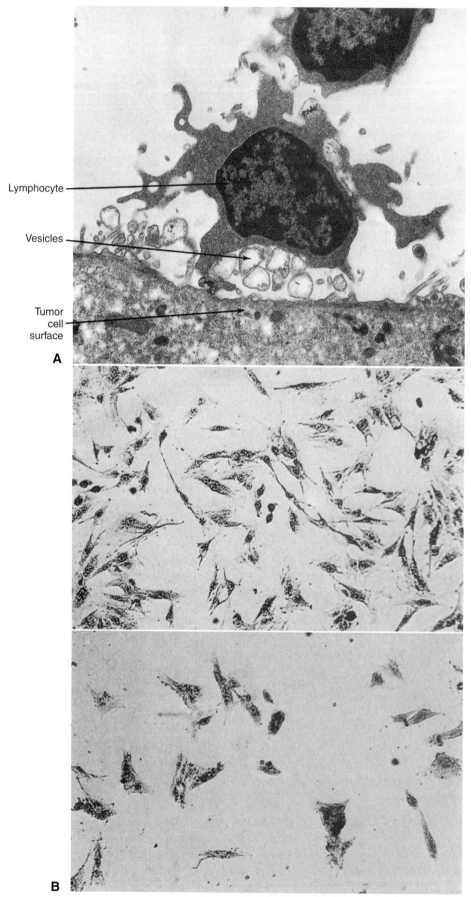

Lymphocyte

Vesicles

Tumor
cell
surface

A

B

Figure 4-14   **A,** Transmission electron photomicrograph demonstrating the initial stages of the attack of a cytotoxic lymphocyte on a tumor cell, only a portion of which is seen. Notice the vesicles and blebs of cytoplasm being shed by the lymphocyte. **B,** The effects of cytotoxic lymphocytes on tumor cells. 1. The tumor cells before contact with the immune lymphocytes. 2. The tumor cells after this contact. Note that many cells have detached from the surface, some cells are swollen, and few cells exhibit the morphology of normal cells. (From Barrett JT: *Textbook of immunology,* ed 5, St Louis, 1988, Mosby.)

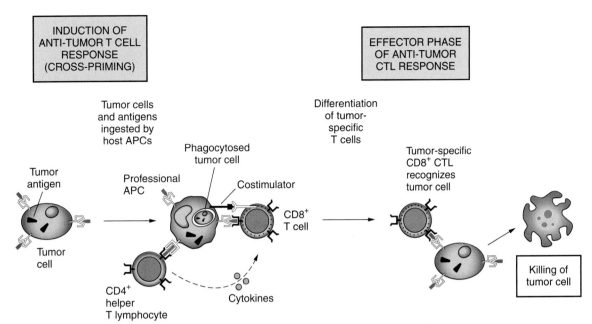

Figure 4-15   Induction of CD8+ T-cell responses against tumors. CD8+ T-cell responses to tumors may be induced by cross-priming (also called cross-presentation), in which the tumor cells and/or tumor antigens are taken up by professions APCs, processed, and presented to T cells. In some cases, B7 costimulators expressed by the APCs provide the second signals for the differentiation of the CD8+ T cells. The APCs may also stimulate CD4+ helper T cells, which provide the second signals for CTL development. Differentiated CTLs kill tumor cells without a requirement for costimulation or T-cell help. (From Abbas AK, Lichtman AH: *Basic immunology: functions and disorders of the immune system,* Philadelphia, 2001, WB Saunders.)

Simultaneous coligation of the cell marker CD4 (or CD8) with the MHC II (or class I) molecule results in the phosphorylation of particular kinases. These events stimulate the activation of at least three intracellular signaling cascades. T-cell activation also requires a second costimulatory signal (e.g., interaction between the cell markers CD28 on the T cell and CD80 on the APC). This interaction also triggers several intracellular signaling pathways. Activation of T cells can lead to:

- Cell division
- Cytokine secretion by the T cell
- Expression by the T cell of antigens associated with the activated state

Activated T cells frequently express "activation antigens" (Table 4-4). Expression of CD69 occurs within 12 hours of activation, followed by CD25 (IL-2 receptor) and CD71 (the transferring receptor) in 1 to 3 days.

Alternatively, in the case of T_c, interaction with antigen via the specific TCR leads to destruction of target cells.

If a cell does not receive a full set of signals, it will not divide, and may even become anergic. Peripheral T cells generally exist in a resting state (G_0 or G_1). T cell activation is a complex reaction involving transmembrane signaling and intracellular enzyme activation steps. It is through soluble cytokines that the T-cell regulation influences the action of other T cells, accessory cells, and nonimmune constituents. When activated by the proper signals, T cells may carry out one or more of the following functions: proliferation, differentiation, production of cytokines, and development of effector function.

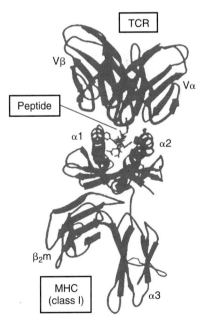

Figure 4-16   The recognition of a peptide-MHC complex by a T-cell antigen receptor. This ribbon diagram is drawn from the crystal structure of the extracellular portion of a peptide-MHC complex bound to a TCR that is specific for the peptide displayed by the MHC molecule. The peptide can be seen attached to the cleft at the top of the MHC molecule, and one residue of the peptide contacts the V region of a TCR. (Redrawn from Bjorkman PJ: MHC restriction in three dimensions: a view of T cell receptor/ligand interactions, *Cell* 89:167-170, 1997. © Cell Press; with permission.)

TABLE 4-4   T-Cell Activation Profile

Components	Reference Range (% positive)
CD2	75-92
CD3	63-84
CD69+ and CD3+	0-2
CD25+ and CD2+	0-5
CD71+ and CD2+	0-8
HLA-DR+ (Class II HLA) and CD3+	1-9
TCR alpha-beta	59-84
TCR gamma-delta	0-10

Source: ARUP: *Interpretive Data Guide,* ed 2, Spring, 1999. p. 473.

TABLE 4-5   Natural Killer Cell Profile

Components	Reference Interval (% positive)
CD2	75-92
CD3	63-84
CD5	61-88
CD7	73-94
CD8	14-39
CD16	1-12
CD56	7-27
CD57	1-26

Source: ARUP: *Interpretive data guide,* ed 2, Spring, 1999.

T-Independent Antigen Triggering

Some antigens, particularly polysaccharide polymers (e.g., dextran), can trigger B cells without help from T cells. These are called T-independent antigens. In general they are not strong, provoke mainly IgM responses, and induce little immunologic memory.

NATURAL KILLER AND K-TYPE LYMPHOCYTES

A subpopulation of circulating lymphocytes, the natural killer (NK) and K-type lymphocytes (~10%), lack conventional antigen receptors of T or B cells. These lymphocytes are classified as a population of effector lymphocytes that produce mediators (e.g., interferon and IL-2).

Although these cells were previously classified as null cells, monoclonal antibodies demonstrate that these cells express a variety of surface membrane markers (Table 4-5). Most of these cells lack CD3 but express CD2, CD16, CD56, CD57, and occasionally CD8.

Natural Killer Cells

A total of 70% to 80% of NK cells have the appearance of large granular lymphocytes (LGLs). Up to about 75% of LGLs function as NK cells, and LGLs appear to account fully for the NK activity in mixed cell populations.

NK cells destroy target cells through an extracellular, non-phagocytic mechanism referred to as a cytotoxic reaction, MHC-unrestricted cytolysis. Target cells include tumor cells, some cells of the embryo, cells of the normal bone marrow and thymus, and microbial agents. Increasing evidence suggests that a considerable number of NK cells may be present in other tissues, particularly in the lungs and liver, where they may play important roles in inflammatory reactions and in host defense, including defense against certain viruses such as cytomegalovirus and hepatitis virus. NK cells will actively kill virally infected target cells, and if this activity is completed before the virus has time to replicate, a viral infection can be combated.

Several cytokines affect NK-cell activation and proliferation. NK cells are highly responsive to IL-2, IL-7, and IL-12.

These cytokines generate high cytokine-activated killer activity in these cells. In addition, NK cells synthesize a number of cytokines involved in the modulation of hematopoiesis and immune responses, and in the regulation of their own activities.

Target cell recognition-molecular identification and analysis of NK cell receptor(s) involved in target cell recognition are currently being intensively researched. These molecules are mainly classified under the family of cell adhesion molecules (CAMs). The main class of effector CAMs that have been shown to mediate NK-cell functions is the leukocyte integrins, more specifically, the $beta_2$ class of integrins.

Several NK cell surface molecules involved in target cell recognition and binding have been identified. NK cells recognize targets using several cell surface molecular receptors (e.g., CD2, CD69, and NKR-P1) and a high density of the Fc receptor CD16 of IgG (FC-R III). They also receive inhibitory signals from MHC class I on potential target cells, transduced via killer inhibitory receptor on the NK cell. CD56 may mediate interactions between effector and target cells. NK cells are able to bind and lyse antibody-coated nucleated cells through a membrane Fc receptor that can recognize a part of the heavy chain of immunoglobulins. This enables NK cells to mediate antibody-dependent, cell-mediated cytotoxic (ADCC) activities. Some, if not all, of the activation of NK cells has been shown to be mediated by CD16. CD16 exerts a regulatory role in the cytolytic function of NK cells. NK cells respond to cross-linking of CD16 and CD69 as follows:

- Increasing the rate of proliferation of NK cells
- Elevating the levels of tumor necrosis factor production within 4 hours of stimulation
- Increasing the expression of CD69 on the cell surface of NK cells
- Increasing the cytotoxicity activity against a normally resistant cell line (P815)

K-Type Lymphocytes

K killer cells are mononuclear cells that can kill target cells sensitized with antibody, which they engage via their Fc receptors. Most K cells are non-T, non-B lymphocytes, but macrophages and eosinophils can also have K cell activity.

K-type cells exhibit a different kind of cytotoxic mechanism than NK cells. The target cell must be coated with low concentrations of IgG antibody; this is referred to as an ADCC reaction. An ADCC reaction may be exhibited both by K cells and by phagocytic and nonphagocytic myelogenous-type leukocytes. K cells are capable of lysing tumor cells. Although morphologically similar to a small lymphocyte, the precise lineage of the K cell is uncertain.

B LYMPHOCYTES

B cells represent a small proportion of the circulating peripheral blood lymphocytes. B-1 and B-2 cells are B cell subsets. B cells are distinguished by the CD5 marker, appear to form a self-renewing set, respond to a number of common microbial antigens, and occasionally generate autoantibodies. B-2 cells account for the majority of the B lymphocytes in adults. This subset generates a greater diversity of antigen receptors and responds effectively to T-dependent antigen.

B cells are derived from progenitor cells through an antigen-independent maturation process occurring in the bone marrow and GALT. Participation of B cells in the humoral immune response is accomplished by reacting to antigenic stimuli by dividing and differentiating into plasma cells. Plasma cells or antibody-forming cells are terminally differentiated B cells. These cells are entirely devoted to antibody production, a primary host defense against microorganisms.

The specific antibodies produced are able to bind to infected cells and free organisms bearing the antigen, then inactivate those cells or organisms and destroy them. The condition of hyperacute rejection of transplanted organs is also mediated by B cells. In addition, antigenic stimulation prompts B cells to multiply.

Cell Surface Markers

Primitive B-cell precursors have delta chains in their cytoplasm and no Ig on their surface. More differentiated (but still immature) B cells have intact cytoplasmic IgM and surface IgM. Mature B cells lose their cytoplasmic IgM and add surface IgD to the surface IgM. These changes appear to occur in the absence of antigen and depend on cytokines.

In humans there is evidence of the existence of four types of B cell markers. These include:

1. Ig receptor. The best studied B cell surface marker is the Ig receptor. This receptor is actually an antibody molecule with antigenic specificity. According to the clonal selection theory, B cells exist in the body with Ig receptors specific for antigen before exposure to the antigenic substances. When specific antigen exposure does occur, the antigen will select the B cell having an Ig receptor with the best fit.

   Following binding and cooperative interaction with T cells, B cells undergo transformation into plasma cells. The secreted antibody in turn has the same specificity as the Ig receptor on the B cell. Virtually all of the antibody produced by plasma cells is secreted (plasma cells have few Ig receptors), but 90% of the antibody produced by B cells is expressed as surface Ig receptors. Some antigens (e.g. lipopolysaccharides from some gram-negative organisms) can bind to the Ig receptor and also stimulate an antibody response independent of T- cell cooperation (T-independent antigens). This type of response, however, is generally of low intensity and is class-restricted to the production of IgM antibody.

   B cells have surface immunoglobulins (sIg) (except for very immature lymphocytes and mature plasma cells) that are normally polyclonal (i.e., kappa and lambda light chains are present on the cytoplasmic membrane of B cells). Mu and delta heavy chains are usually found with either the kappa or lambda chains on any one cell surface. Gamma and alpha are rarely found on the surface of properly prepared, normal lymphocytes.

2. An Fc receptor that specifically binds the Fc portion of IgG antibody. The function of this receptor may be to aid B cells in binding to antigen already bound to antibody.

3. Receptors that bind fragments of the cleaved complement component C3 have been reported on the surface of approximately 75% of B cells. This receptor binds C3b, iC3b (inactivated C3b), and C3d, but the function of these receptors is not totally understood.

4. B cell surface antigens coded by the class II genes of the MHC.

B-Cell Activation

B cells can be stimulated in their resting state to enlarge, develop synthetic machinery, divide, mature, and secrete antibody. The proper signals for this sequence depend on the type of triggers, which can be specific or nonspecific and polyclonal. Specific activation involves the antigen that is complementary to the particular Ig on the surface. Nonspecific activation occurs with B-cell mitogens.

Efficient antibody production to complex protein antigens requires T-cell help (which, in turn, develops from APC presentation of antigen to the T cell). Activated T cells secrete a variety of cytokines that, together with the specific antigen, trigger the B cell to develop into an antibody-secreting cell. This process also involves "IgG-class switching."

In the immune response to a foreign protein, the first antibodies to appear are of the IgM class (or isotype). As the response proceeds, other isotypes (IgG, IgA, and IgE) emerge as the result of immunoglobulin-class switching. The isotype switch has considerable clinical importance because each of the four major isotypes has specialized biologic properties. IgG is the principal class of antibody in interstitial fluids, and IgA is the protective antibody of mucosal surfaces. Isotype switching requires collaboration between antibody-synthesizing B cells and helper CD4+ T cells. In this collaboration, the B cell uses IgM molecules on its surface to capture the antigen and present the antigen to the T cell. Contact between the collaborating lymphocytes is enhanced by complementary pairs of adhesion molecules. Some of these molecules (e.g., CD4 and MHC class II antigens) are constitutively expressed on the surfaces of T and B cells. Others, by contrast, are induced. For instance, contact between B and T cells induces the T cell to express a ligand for the B cell surface molecule CD40. In turn, CD40 interacts with the newly expressed CD40 ligand on the T cell, and this leads to the expression of another B-cell surface molecule, B7. The latter's partner on the surface of the T lymphocyte is CD28. These cooperative and synergistic interactions between the T cell and B cell induce the secretion of cytokines such as IL-2 and IL-4.

Isotype switching requires two signals. The first is delivered by an interleukin, the second by the binding of CD40 to its ligand on the T cell. In the process of switching from IgM synthesis to IgE synthesis, IL-4 makes the IgE gene in the B cell accessible to the switch machinery that is set in motion when CD40 binds to its ligand. In this process, the gene that encodes the variable region (the part of the antibody molecule that contains the antigen binding site) moves from its position near the gene that encodes for IgM to a position near the gene that encodes for IgE.

OTHER KINDS OF LYMPHOCYTES

Virgin or naive lymphocytes are cells that have not encountered their specific antigen. These cells do express high molecular weight variants of leukocyte common antigen.

Memory cells are populations of long-lived T or B cells that have been stimulated by antigen. These cells can make a quick response to a previously encountered antigen. Memory B cells carry surface IgG as their antigen receptor; memory T cells express the CD45RO variant of the leukocyte common antigen and increased levels of adhesion molecules (e.g., LFA-3 and VLA-4).

PLASMA CELL BIOLOGY

The function of plasma cells is the synthesis and excretion of Igs. Plasma cells are not normally found in the circulating blood but are found in the bone marrow in concentrations that do not normally exceed 2%. Plasma cells arise as the end stage of B-cell differentiation into a large, activated plasma cell.

The pathway from the B lymphocyte to the antibody-synthesizing plasma cell (Figure 4-17) occurs when the B cell is antigenically stimulated and undergoes transformation as a result of the stimulation of various interleukins. The immune antibody response begins when individual B lymphocytes encounter an antigen that binds to their specific Ig surface receptors. After receiving an appropriate "second signal" provided by interaction with helper T cells, these antigen-binding B cells undergo transformation and proliferation to generate a clone of mature plasma cells that secrete a specific type of antibody.

An increase in plasma cells can be seen in a variety of nonmalignant disorders such as viral disorders (e.g., rubella and infectious mononucleosis), allergic conditions, chronic infections, and collagen diseases. In plasma cell dyscrasias, the plasma cells can be greatly increased or can completely infiltrate the bone marrow (e.g., multiple myeloma or Waldenström's macroglobulinemia).

Antibody molecules secreted by plasma cells consist of four chains (two light chains and two heavy chains, based on molecular weight) and can be enzymatically cleaved into Fab and Fc fragments. The Fab portion of the molecule binds antigen and contains the light chains and their antigenic markers (kappa, lambda). The Fc fragment (this fragment

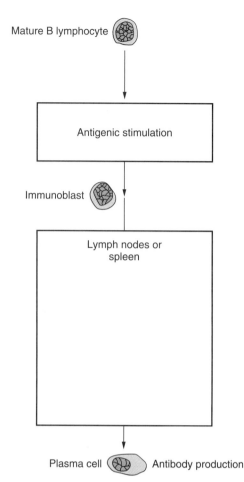

Figure 4-17   Plasma cell development from B lymphocytes. (Redrawn from Turgeon ML: *Clinical hematology: theory and procedures,* ed 3, Philadelphia, 1999, Lippincott-Williams & Wilkins.)

readily crystallizes after enzymation, and c represents crystallizably) contains the markers that distinguish the different classes of antibody (M, G, A, D, E) and sites that will bind and activate complement and bind to Fc receptors on cells. The amino acid sequence for most of the antibody protein is constant, except for the antigen-binding portion of the molecule that has a hypervariable region and accounts for the various antigenic specificities that the antibody is programmed to recognize.

ALTERATIONS IN LYMPHOCYTE SUBSETS

The normal functioning of helper cells and suppressor cells in the immune response can be reversed under certain conditions. For example, the target cell for human T-cell leukemia (HIV) is phenotypically a helper cell but functionally a suppressor cell. Functionally the helper-inducer subset cells signal B cells to generate antibodies, control production and switching of types of antibodies formed, and activate suppressor cells. The suppressor-cytotoxic lymphocytes control and inhibit antibody production either by suppressing helper cells or by turning off B cell differentiation. The normal ratio of helper cells and suppressor cells (approximately 2:1) can be reversed under certain conditions.

CHANGES IN LYMPHOCYTE SUBPOPULATIONS WITH AGING

Except for inconsistent values seen in extremely elderly persons, the total number of T cells in the peripheral blood is relatively stable throughout adult life; however, there is a change in the distribution of T-cell subpopulations. A decrease in the number of suppressor cells and an increase in the helper cell population are demonstrated in older adults.

The effect of aging on the immune response is highly variable, but the ability to respond immunologically to disease is age related. It has been suggested that faulty immunologic reactions such as aberrant functioning of immunoregulatory cells, effector T cells, and antibody-producing B cells contribute to poor immunity in older adults. Functional deficits of T lymphocytes with aging, causing impairment of cell-mediated immunity, have been identified. In addition, skin testing reveals decreases in the intensity of delayed hypersensitivity in older adults. The proliferative response of T lymphocytes to mitogens or antigens such as *Mycobacterium tuberculosis* or varicella zoster virus is impaired.

A decrease in T-helper cells is the primary cause of impaired humoral response seen in older adults. Although the total number of B cells and total concentration of Ig produced remains unchanged, the serum concentration of IgM is decreased. Concentrations of IgA and IgG have been shown to be increased.

EVALUATION OF SUSPECTED DEFECTS

Although more than 50 genetically determined immunodeficiency syndromes have been reported since 1952, defects in immunity were considered rare until acquired immunodeficiency syndrome (AIDS) emerged more than 20 years ago. This growing list of primary and secondary diseases (Table 4-6) now encompasses all major components of the immune system, including lymphocytes, phagocytic cells, and complement proteins. Clinical and laboratory tests for the evaluation of patients with suspected disorders must be informative, reliable, and cost-effective.

A complete blood cell count and erythrocyte sedimentation rate (ESR) are among the most cost-effective screening tests. If the ESR is normal, chronic bacterial infection is unlikely. If the absolute neutrophil count is normal, congenital and acquired neutropenias and severe chemotactic defects are eliminated. If the absolute lymphocyte count is normal, the patient is not likely to have a severe T-cell defect. The absolute lymphocyte count is the number of lymphocytes in the total white blood cell population (Box 4-1).

Evaluation of Suspected Defects: Cell-Mediated Immune System

Deficiencies of cell-mediated immunity (discussed in detail later in this chapter) are often suspected in individuals with recurrent viral, fungal, parasitic, and protozoan infections.

TABLE 4-6   Initial Evaluation of Suspected Immunodeficiency

Suspected Deficiency	Appropriate Laboratory Procedures
All suspected immunodeficiencies	Complete blood count with platelet evaluation
	Erythrocyte sedimentation rate
Antibody deficiency	Screen for anti-A and anti-B isoagglutinins
	Screen for antibodies to diphtheria or tetanus toxoids
T-cell deficiency	Absolute lymphocyte count
	Intradermal skin test to *Candida albicans* 1:1000 or 1:100
Phagocytic cell deficiency	Absolute neutrophil count
	Nitroblue tetrazolium test

Box 4-1   Absolute Lymphocyte Count

An example of a determination of the absolute number of lymphocytes:

Absolute Number = Total Leukocyte Count × % of Lymphocytes

Total Leukocyte Count = 25×10^9/L

Relative Number Percentage (%) of Lymphocytes = 76%

Absolute Number = 19×10^9/L

Patients with AIDS (see Chapter 22) exhibit some of the most severe manifestations of cell-mediated immunity.

One avenue of testing involves delayed hypersensitivity skin testing to determine the integrity of the patient's cell-mediated immune response. More than 90% of normal adults will react to one of the following antigens within 48 hours after antigen exposure: *Candida albicans,* trichophyton, tetanus toxoid, mumps, and streptokinase-streptodornase. Reactivity to histoplasmin or purified protein derivative (PPD) is positive in patients with active infection or previous exposure to histoplasmosis or tuberculosis, respectively; therefore they are not useful in the assessment of anergy.

The number of T lymphocytes, the primary effector cell in cell-mediated reactions, can be determined by a number of different techniques. The "gold standard" has previously been the E (erythrocyte rosette formation) technique. Development of monoclonal antibodies, however, has permitted a quick and specific method for determining the number of T cells. The method of testing is by use of immunofluorescent techniques in which the fluorescent microscope or fluorescence-activated cell sorter (FACS) is used. Additional testing can include functional testing or the measurement of biologic response modifiers such as IL-2 (T-cell growth factor).

Evaluation of Suspected Defects: Humoral System

The humoral system can be screened for abnormalities by quantitating the concentration of IgM, IgG, and IgA. An initial simple screening can be determined by the presence and titer of antibodies to type A and B red blood cell antigens.

Testing of Lymphocytes

In functional testing phenotypes are enumerated in proportional relationship to one another. Functional assays evaluate the response of lymphocytes to nonspecific mitogens. In the case of T lymphocytes, mitogens such as pokeweed mitogen or specific antigens such as PPD are used. Functional testing of B lymphocytes is confined to determining the response to pure B cell mitogen such as *Staphylococcus aureus*-Cowan strain and antibody production. These substances provoke DNA synthesis and mitosis or production of antibodies that can determine which cells are functioning abnormally. A patient may have a normal proportion of phenotypically defined suppressor cells, but functional tests might show that those cells are impaired.

Several tests were used before the introduction of highly specific fluorescent monoclonal antibody tests to distinguish T and B cells. T lymphocytes were defined by their ability to form rosettes with sheep erythrocytes (Figure 4-18); they were further subclassified by their ability to form rosettes with Ig or bovine erythrocytes coated with complement (a soluble blood protein consisting of nine components, C1-C9, which if activated can lead to rupture of the cellular membrane). This test demonstrates that the surface membrane of T cells had receptors for attachment to normal sheep erythrocytes. B cells had membrane-bound antibody and receptors including the complement (C3) receptor. The presence of the C3 receptor could be demonstrated by the ability of B cells to bind erythrocytes with complement to form the erythrocyte-antibody-complement rosettes. B lymphocytes were indisputably characterized by their surface membrane Ig markers. Using these techniques, a population of non-B, non-T cells could also be shown.

DISORDERS WITH IMMUNOLOGIC ORIGINS

A breakdown in any part of the immune mechanism can lead to disease. These disorders can involve progenitor cells, phagocytosis (see Chapter 3), T cells, B cells, or complement (see Chapter 5).

Immunologic disorders can be divided into primary (dysfunction in the immune organ itself) and acquired or secondary (disease or therapy causing an immune defect) processes. A third category, diseases mediated through immune mechanisms, can also be included. In this section, the general characteristics of immunodeficiency disorders and examples of immunodeficiency disorders are discussed. Because of its complexity and contemporary importance, AIDS is discussed in detail in a separate chapter (see Chapter 22). Other immune disorders such as immunoproliferative disorders and autoimmune disorders are presented in detail in Chapters 24 to 27.

Immune Disorders

Immune deficiency disorders may be caused by defects in the quality (defects) or quantity (deficiencies) of lymphocytes, and they may be congenital or acquired. These conditions may be combined disorders or either T or B cell disorders (Table 4-7).

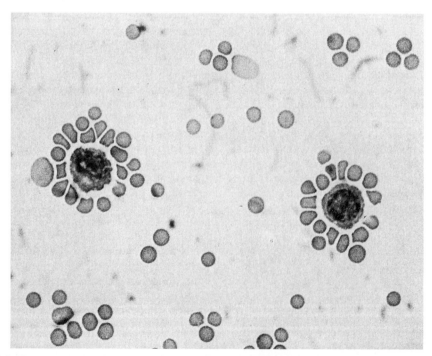

Figure 4-18 A rosette in Giemsa-stained cytocentrifuge preparation from a normal adult peripheral blood sample. (From Bauer JD: *Clinical laboratory methods,* ed 9, St Louis, 1982, Mosby.)

Primary Immune Disorders

Diseases associated with a primary defect (Box 4-2 and Table 4-8) in the immune response are composed of 40% T-cell disorders, 50% B-cell disorders, 6% phagocytic abnormalities, and 4% complement alterations (Figure 4-19). The most common T-cell deficiency states are those associated with a concurrent B-cell abnormality. Primary immunodeficiency disorders are predominantly seen (75%) in children under the age of 5 years.

T-Cell and Combined Immunodeficiency Disorders

DiGeorge's Syndrome

Etiology. This T-cell defect is a congenital anomaly that represents faulty embryogenesis of the endodermal derivation of third and fourth pharyngeal pouches, which results in aplasia of the parathyroid and thymus glands. At

TABLE 4-7   Examples of T- and B-Cell Disorders

T-Cell Disorder	B-Cell Disorder
Congenital	
Thymic hypoplasia (DiGeorge's syndrome)	Bruton's agammaglobulinemia
Acquired	
Acquired immune deficiency syndrome	Autoimmune disorders
Hodgkin's disease	Multiple myeloma
Chronic lymphocytic leukemia	
Systemic lupus erythematosus	

autopsy, parathyroid and a vestigial thymus may be found in ectopic locations. The newborn infant may exhibit an assortment of facial and vascular anomalies. These combined abnormalities are collectively referred to as pharyngeal pouch syndrome. In addition to the established embryonic cause of the disorder, a question of a nutrient (zinc) deficiency in utero has been suggested as a cause of this process.

Signs and Symptoms. DiGeorge's syndrome is present at birth. Initial manifestations can include hypocalcemic tetany, unusual facies, and congenital heart defects. An increased susceptibility to viral, fungal, and disseminated bacterial infections such as acid-fast bacilli, *Listeria* monocytogenes, and *Pneumocystis carinii* result from the defect of T cells normally controlled by cell-mediated immunity. Infants usually die of sepsis during the first year of life.

Immunologic Manifestations. Peripheral lymphoid tissue appears to be normal except for depletion of T cells in the thymus-dependent zones such as the subcortical region of the lymph nodes and the perifollicular and periarteriolar lymphoid sheaths of the spleen. Lymph node paracortical areas and thymus-dependent regions of the spleen show variable degrees of depletion.

In the circulating blood lymphopenia is generally present, although in some cases the concentration of lymphocytes is normal. However, an abnormally high CD4+ : CD8+ ratio is present due to a decrease in CD8+ cells. Most patients with DiGeorge's syndrome have a decreased percentage of cells expressing the CD3+ (mature T cell) antigen. Because patients do demonstrate lymphocytes capable of differentiating to the more mature surface markers such as CD4+, a small rudimentary thymus is believed to be present in these patients. Lymphocytic responsiveness to antigenic and mitogenic stimulation can be absent, reduced, or normal depending on the degree of thymic deficiency. Cell-mediated immune reactions such as delayed hypersensitivity and skin allograft rejections, however, are absent or feeble.

Box 4-2	**Primary Immunodeficiency Diseases**

T CELLS

Combined immunodeficiency
   Thymic alymphoplasia
   Swiss type
   Adenosine deaminase deficiency
   Nezelof syndrome
DiGeorge's syndrome (thymic hypoplasia)
Wiskott-Aldrich syndrome
Chronic mucocutaneous candidiasis
Immunodeficiency associated with nucleoside phosphorylase
   deficiency
Short-limbed dwarfism
Ataxia-telangiectasia
Thymoma
Leukocyte adhesions deficiency

B CELLS

Selected IgA deficiency associated with:
   Normal state
   Allergy
   Autoimmune disease
   Central nervous system disease
   Gastrointestinal disorders
   Malignancy
   Pulmonary infections
X-linked infantile agammaglobulinemia
X-linked immunodeficiency with hyper-IgM
Common variable hypogammaglobulinemia
Selective IgM deficiency
IgG subclass deficiency

Modified from Graziano FM, Bell CL: The normal immune response and what can go wrong. In Corman LC, Katz D, editors: *Symposium on clinical immunology I, Medical Clinics of North America,* Philadelphia, WB Saunders 69(3):445, 1985.

TABLE 4-8	Genetic Basis of Representative Immunodeficiency Diseases

Disorder	Chromosomal Map Location of Faulty Gene
DiGeorge's syndrome	22?
Nezelof syndrome (including PNP) deficiency	14q13.1
Severe combined immuno-deficiency syndrome	Xq13-21.1 (X-linked)
Wiskott-Aldrich syndrome	Xp11-11.3
Ataxia-telangiectasia	11q22.3
Hyperimmunoglobulinemia E	Unknown
LAD, CD-11-18 deficiency	21q22.3
Lymphocyte activation defects	Unknown
X-linked agammaglobulinemia	X q222
Transient hypogammaglobu-linemia of infancy	Unknown
CVID (acquired hypogamma-globulinemia)	6p21.3?
IgG subclass deficiencies	2p11; 14q32.3
Selective IgA deficiencies	6p21.3?
Immunodeficiency with hyper-M	Xq24-27
X-linked lymphoproliferative disease	Xq24-26

CVID, Common variable immunodeficiency; *LAD,* leukocyte adhesion disorder.

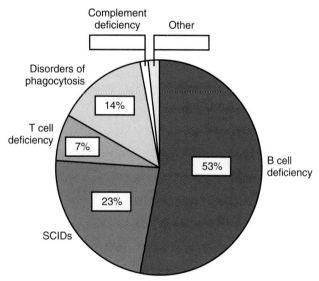

Figure 4-19   Distribution of immunodeficiencies.

Serum immunoglobulin concentrations are near normal. IgA may be diminished and IgE levels elevated. Antibody response to primary antigenic stimulation may be unimpaired.

Nezelof Syndrome (Cellular Immunodeficiency With Immunoglobulins)

Etiology. An autosomal-recessive pattern of inheritance is often seen. The defect appears to exist on chromosome 14q13.1.

Signs and Symptoms. Nezelof syndrome is the primary immunodeficiency disorder most likely to be confused with AIDS in the pediatric age group. Infants suffer from failure to thrive, recurrent or chronic pulmonary infections, oral or cutaneous candidiasis, chronic diarrhea, recurrent skin infections, gram-negative sepsis, urinary tract infections, and/or severe varicella.

Immunologic Manifestations. This syndrome is characterized by lymphopenia, neutropenia, and eosinophilia. In addition, diminished lymphoid tissue and abnormal thymus architecture are observed. Peripheral lymphoid tissues are hypoplastic and demonstrate paracortical lymphocyte depletion. Lymphocyte responses to mitogens, antigens, and allogeneic cells are profoundly depressed but not totally absent. Normal or increased serum levels of most of the five immunoglobulin classes are manifested. Antibody-forming capacity has been reported to be normal in one third of cases.

Severe Combined Immunodeficiency

Etiology. Severe combined immunodeficiency (SCID) is caused by inappropriate development of progenitor cells into lymphocyte precursors. This hereditary and invariably fatal disorder in infants results from the lack of both T and B cells and the consequent inability to synthesize antibody.

Recently mutations in the IL-2 receptor complex, a hematopoietic growth factor, have been shown to cause X-linked severe combined immunodeficiency in humans. Two modes of inheritance are known: autosomal recessive or X-linked recessive. X-linked recessive SCID is thought to be the most common form of SCID in this country, which accounts for the 3:1 ratio of males to females with the disorder.

Half the patients with autosomal SCID have a concomitant deficiency of adenosine deaminase, an aminohydrolase that converts adenosine to inosine. Analysis by cDNA probe has revealed that the deficiency results from a hereditable point mutation in the adenosine deaminase gene. Another variant with a severe deficiency in T-cell immunity but normal B-cell concentrations is associated with purine nucleotide phosphorylase deficiency.

There are two main forms of defective expression of MHC antigens. In a less common cause of SCID, "bare lymphocyte syndrome," an MHC class I antigen deficiency is present. In another form of defective expression, MHC class I antigen deficiency plus the absence of class II antigens is present. Patient lymphocytes cannot be typed by standard serologic cytotoxicity tests.

Signs and Symptoms. No important differences in signs and symptoms exist between the two major genetic types of SCID. Initial manifestations of SCID are repeated debilitating infections beginning within the first 6 months of life. These infections are dominated by bacterial, viral, and fungal infections of the respiratory and intestinal systems and skin. Infants with SCID usually die within 3 years of birth from lung abscesses, pneumocystis pneumonitis, or a common viral disorder such as chickenpox or measles.

Immunologic Manifestations. The thymus and other lymphoid organs are severely hypoplastic. The bone marrow is devoid of lymphoblasts, lymphocytes, and plasma cells. Lymphocytes are also absent from lymphoid tissues such as the spleen, tonsils, appendix, and intestinal tract. Variable hypogammaglobulinemia with decreased serum IgM and IgA levels and poor to absent antibody production are representative characteristics. Moderate lymphocytopenia is detectable early in infancy. T cell functions are decreased. The circulating blood contains no CD4+, CD8+, or CD3+ cells. The percentage of B cells is usually normal.

Patients with the X-linked form of SCID usually appear similar to those with the autosomal recessive form, except they generally tend to have an increased percentage of B cells. However, the defect affects B lineage cells as well as T lineage cells.

Chronic Mucocutaneous Candidiasis (CMC)

Etiology. This disorder results from a primary defect in cell-mediated immunity. T cells specifically fail to recognize only the *Candida* antigen.

Signs and Symptoms. Patients with CMC usually survive to adulthood. The manifestation of the disorder is candida infection of mucous membranes, the scalp, skin, and nails. Endocrine abnormalities, often polyendocrinopathies, are frequently associated with fungal manifestation. Sudden death from adrenal insufficiency has been reported in patients with CMC.

Immunologic Manifestations. Patients suffering from this disorder demonstrate normal skin reactions to testing to all antigens except *Candida*.

B Cell: Antibody Deficiency Disorders

Because the primary function of B cells is to produce antibody, the major clinical manifestation of a B-cell deficiency is an increased susceptibility to severe bacterial infections. Selective IgA deficiency is the most common B-cell disorder, occurring in 1 of every 400 to 800 persons. Because IgA is the primary Ig in secretions, a lack of it contributes to pulmonary infections, gastrointestinal disorders, and allergic respiratory disorders. The majority of cases (50% of reported cases are associated with Ig deficiencies) is autoimmune in nature, including rheumatoid arthritis, systemic lupus erythematosus, thyroiditis, and pernicious anemia.

Bruton's X-linked Agammaglobulinemia

Etiology. Although it has been questioned whether a functional T-cell defect may have been responsible for the lack of B-cell development in this B-cell immunodeficiency, the cause is generally believed to result from a maturation failure during early B-cell differentiation. The defective LSA gene has been mapped to the q22 region of the proximal part of the long arm of the X chromosome.

Signs and Symptoms. This disorder occurs primarily in young boys, but scattered cases have been identified in girls. Manifestations of this disorder begin in the first or second year of life. Hypersusceptibility to infection does not develop until 9 to 12 months after birth because of passive protection by residual maternal Ig. Thereafter patients repeatedly acquire infections with high-grade extracellular pyogenic organisms such as streptococci. This disorder is characterized by sinopulmonary and central nervous system infectious episodes and severe septicemia, but patients are not abnormally susceptible to common viral infection (excluding fulminant hepatitis) or to enterococci or most gram-negative organisms. Chronic fungal infections are not usually present.

An autoimmune phenomenon, especially a juvenile rheumatoid arthritis type of disease, has also been associated with X-linked agammaglobulinemia. In addition, patients are highly vulnerable to a malignant form of dermatomyositis that eventually involves destructive T-cell infiltration surrounding the small vessels of the central nervous system. In addition to infections and connective tissue disorders, agammaglobulinemic patients also suffer from hemolytic anemia, drug eruptions, atopic eczema, allergic rhinitis, and asthma.

Immunologic Manifestations. The diagnosis of X-linked agammaglobulinemia is suspected if serum concentrations of IgG, IgA, and IgM are notably below the appropriate level for the patient's age. Tests for natural antibodies to blood group substances and for antibodies to antigens given during standard courses of immunization (e.g., diphtheria) are useful in distinguishing this disorder from transient hypogammaglobulinemia of infancy.

B cells are virtually absent from bone marrow and lymphoid tissues. A deficiency or absence of peripheral blood B lymphocytes is usually noted in this disorder. If B cells are present, they are unresponsive to T cells and incapable of antibody synthesis or secretion. Surface Igs (SIgs) are absent. However, patients do have normal numbers of CD3+ and CD8+ cells, and many have normal CD+4 cells. Male children possess normal T-cell function; therefore homograft rejection mechanisms are intact, and delayed hypersensitivity reaction for both tuberculin and skin contact types can be elicited.

Common Variable Immunodeficiency

Etiology. Common variable immunodeficiency (CVID) is a form of primary acquired agammaglobulinemia. It occurs equally in males and females. The etiology of this disease seems to be heterogeneous, with abnormalities of B-cell maturation, antibody production, antibody secretion, or T-cell regulation. Family clusters have been reported in which first-degree relatives of patients with selective IgA deficiency have a high incidence of abnormal immunoglobulin concentration, autoantibodies, autoimmune disease, and malignant neoplasms. Recent findings of rare alleles or deletions of the class III MHC in patients with IgA deficiency of CVID suggest that the susceptibility gene(s) is (are) on chromosome 6.

Signs and Symptoms. This disorder usually manifests itself in the second or third decade of life. The signs and symptoms include frequent sinopulmonary infections, diarrhea, endocrine, and autoimmune disorders, and malabsorption difficulties such as malabsorption of vitamin B_{12}. Intestinal giardiasis is also prevalent.

Immunologic Manifestations. Both the concentration and/or near absence of serum and secretory IgA is thought to be the most common well-defined immunodeficiency disorder. The pattern of inheritance suggests an autosomal function of antibodies are usually compromised. The number of B cells is usually normal or mildly depressed. Despite a normal number of circulating immunoglobulin-bearing B lymphocytes and the presence of lymphoid cortical follicles, blood lymphocytes do not differentiate into immunoglobulin-producing cells. In most patients the defect appears to be intrinsic to the B cell. The primary defect in immunoglobulin synthesis may be caused by the absence or dysfunction of CD4+ cells or by increased CD8+ supressor cell activity. Therefore cellular immunity and immunoglobulin production are both impaired by the interaction between helper and suppressor T-cell subsets. Lymph nodes lack plasma cells, but they may show striking follicular hyperplasia.

The total IgG level may be normal, but a subclass of the Ig (usually IgG_2 or IgG_3) is deficient. Both IgA and IgM may be detectable, but IgM levels may be elevated.

In addition, some patients may suffer from thymoma and refractory anemia.

Immunoglobulin Subclass Deficiencies

Some patients have been reported to have deficiencies of one or more of the subclasses of IgG despite normal total IgG serum concentrations. Most of those with absent or very low concentrations of IgG_2 have been patients with selective IgA deficiency.

Selective IgA Deficiency

Etiology. An isolated absence mode. It is commonly seen in pedigrees containing individuals with CVID. IgA deficiency has been noted to evolve into CVID, and the recent find of rare alleles and deletions of MHC class III genes in both conditions suggests a common basis.

Signs and Symptoms. This condition is commonly associated with ill health. Infections occur predominantly in the respiratory, gastrointestinal, and urogenital tracts. There is no clear evidence that patients with this disorder have any increased susceptibility to viral agents. IgA deficiency has been noted in patients treated with phenytoin, sulfasalazine, penicillamine, or gold. This suggests that environmental factors may lead to expression of the defect.

Immunologic Manifestations. As many as 44% of patients with selective IgA deficiency demonstrate antibodies to IgA. Severe or fatal anaphylactic reactions after intravenous administration of blood products containing IgA and anti-IgA antibodies (particularly IgE anti-IgA antibodies) have occurred.

Immunodeficiency with Elevated IgM (Hyper-M)

Etiology. A sex-linked mode of inheritance has been noted in some pedigrees. The abnormal gene in the X-linked type has been localized to Xq24-Xq27. However, more than one genetic cause is suspected.

Signs and Symptoms. Patients with this defect become symptomatic during the first or second year of life, with recurrent pyogenic infections, including otitis media, sinusitis, pneumonia, and tonsillitis. Hemolytic anemia and thrombocytopenia have been observed. Transient, persistent, or cyclic neutropenia is a common feature.

Immunologic Manifestations. This disorder is characterized by extremely low concentrations of IgG and IgA and, most frequently, markedly elevated concentrations of polyclonal IgM. Normal or slightly reduced numbers of IgM and/or IgD B lymphocytes have been observed.

Transient Hypogammaglobulinemia of Infancy

Unlike patients with Bruton's X-linked agammaglobulinemia or CVID, patients with transient hypogammaglobulinemia of infancy can synthesize antibodies to A and B red blood cell antigens if they lack the antigen(s), and to diphtheria and tetanus toxoids. Antibody production usually occurs by 6 to 11 months of age. This antibody production occurs before Ig levels become normal.

X-Linked Lymphoproliferative Disease (Duncan's Disease)

Etiology. This disease is caused by a recessive trait. The defective gene has been localized to the Xq26-Xq27 region.

Signs and Symptoms. The disease is characterized by an inadequate immune reaction to infection with Epstein-Barr virus (EBV) (see Chapter 19 for a full discussion of infectious mononucleosis). Infected patients are apparently healthy until they experience infectious mononucleosis. Two thirds of more than 100 patients studied died of overwhelming EBV-induced B-cell proliferation during mononucleosis. A majority of patients surviving the primary infection developed hypogammaglobulinemia and/or B-cell lymphomas.

Immunologic Manifestations. A marked impairment in production of antibodies to the EBV nucleus has been noted in afflicted patients. In contrast, titers of antibodies to the viral capsid antigen range from zero to markedly elevated.

Antibody-dependent, cell-mediated cytotoxicity against EBV-infected cells has been low in many patients. NK cell function is also depressed. There is also a deficiency in long-lived T-cell immunity to EBV.

Partial Combined Immunodeficiency Disorders

Wiskott-Aldrich Syndrome (Immunodeficiency with Thrombocytopenia and Eczema)

Etiology. The primary defect in this uncommon X-linked recessive pediatric disease is caused by a specific inability to respond to polysaccharide antigens (e.g., pneumococci). An immunodeficiency and poor humoral immune response to bacterial polysaccharide antigen results.

Signs and Symptoms. Wiskott-Aldrich syndrome is characterized by the triad of thrombocytopenic purpura, increased susceptibility to infection, and eczema (atopic dermatitis). Afflicted boys rarely survive past 10 years. Thrombocytopenia and bleeding are common. Platelets are small and with an intrinsic defect. Patients usually die from sepsis, hemorrhage, or malignancy.

Immunologic Manifestations. In this disorder a progressive deterioration of the thymus takes place, leading to a defect in cellular immunity and the attrition of T-cell populations from the lymph nodes and spleen. Decreased numbers of T cells and alteration in the normal T4:T8 ratio of lymphocytes are manifested. Serum levels of IgM are low, but IgG concentrations are usually normal. IgA levels are normal or elevated, and IgE levels are usually elevated.

Hereditary Ataxia-Telangiectasia

Etiology. This autosomal-recessive disorder apparently results from the coexistence of a T-cell deficiency with a defect in DNA repair, which leads to extreme nonrandom chromosome instability. The sites of chromosomal breakage involve chromosomes 7 and 14 in more than 50% of cases.

Signs and Symptoms. Ataxia telangiectasia is characterized by ataxia and choreoathetosis in infancy. Multiple telangiectasia appears on exposed oculocutaneous surfaces during childhood. A high incidence of malignancy such as lymphoma is also displayed. Children with this disorder eventually die of respiratory insufficiency and sepsis.

Immunologic Manifestations. The thymus is hypoplastic or dysplastic, and the thymus-dependent zones of the lymph nodes are void of cells. About 80% of patients lack serum and secretory IgA, and some develop IgG antibodies to injections of IgA. The signs and symptoms of the disease appear to result from a concomitant T-cell deficiency, a deficiency of DNA repair, and disordered IgG synthesis.

Hyperimmunoglobulinemia E Syndrome

Etiology. This disorder has a presumed autosomal-dominant pattern of inheritance.

Signs and Symptoms. This is a relatively rare primary immunodeficiency syndrome characterized by recurrent severe staphylococcal abscesses. Patients have histories from infancy of staphylococcal abscesses involving the skin, lungs, joints, and other sites; persistent pneumatoceles develop as a result of the recurrent pneumonias. Pruritic dermatitis also occurs.

Immunologic Manifestations. Patients have elevated levels of serum IgE and IgD; usually normal concentrations of IgG, IgA, and IgM are present. Poor antibody and cell-mediated responses to neoantigens are demonstrated. In addition, a decreased percentage of T cells with the memory (CD45RO) has been noted.

Leukocyte Adhesion Deficiency or CD-11-CD-18 Deficiency

Etiology. This condition is due to mutations in the gene or chromosome 21q22.3.

Signs and Symptoms. Patients with this syndrome have histories of delayed separation of the umbilical cord, omphalitis, gingivitis, recurrent skin infections, repeated otitis media, pneumonia, peritonitis, perianal abscesses, and impaired wound healing. A lack of pus formation has also been noted. Patients frequently suffer from severe, life-threatening bacterial and fungal infections, although their blood neutrophil counts are usually elevated. Affected individuals do not have increased susceptibility to viral infections or malignant neoplasms.

Immunologic Manifestations. All cytotoxic lymphocyte functions are markedly impaired because of the lack of lymphocyte function antigen 1; deficiency of the lymphocyte function antigen also interferes with immune cell interaction and immune recognition. Patients also display an absence of abnormal phagocytic cell adherence and chemotaxis and a reduced respiratory burst with phagocytosis.

T-Cell Activation Defects

Some patients have experienced:
- Defective surface expression of the CD3-T cell antigen receptor complex caused by mutation in the gene encoding the CD3-gamma subunit
- Defective signal transduction from the T-cell antigen receptor to intracellular metabolic pathways
- Pretranslational defect in IL-2 and/or other cytokine production

These conditions are characterized by the presence of T cells that appear phenotypically normal but fail to proliferate or produce cytokines in response to stimulation with mitogens, antigens, or other signals delivered to the T-cell antigen receptor. Patient problems are similar to other T cell-deficient individuals, and some patients with severe T-cell activation defects may clinically resemble patients with SCID.

Other Primary Immunodeficiencies

In addition to hereditary or congenital disorders of lymphocytes, there are several primary immune defects involving the complement system and phagocytic cells.

Complement Deficiency

Deficiencies in all of the components of the complement system (see Chapter 5) have been described (Table 4-9). These deficiencies are genetic in origin. Unusual susceptibility to infection is characteristic of some of these components, particularly deficiencies involving C3, C5, C6, and C7.

A functional deficiency of the polymorphonuclear neutrophilic leukocytes is chronic granulomatous disease (CGD) (see Chapter 3). This fatal syndrome usually begins with the onset of symptoms during the first year of life.

Secondary Immunodeficiencies

A secondary immunodeficiency can result from a disease process that causes a defect in normal immune function (Box 4-3), which leads to a temporary or permanent impairment of one or multiple components of immunity in the host. Patients with secondary immunodeficiencies, which

TABLE 4-9	Complement Deficiencies
Deficient Component	**Common Types of Infections**
C1 (r/q)	Gram-positive, mainly respiratory
C2	Gram-positive, recurrent respiratory, meningitis, sepsis, tuberculosis
C3	Gram-positive, recurrent
C4	Gram-positive, sepsis, meningitis
C5	Meningitis (*Neisseria meningitidis*), disseminated gonococcal infection
C6	Meningitis (*N. meningitidis*), disseminated gonococcal infection
C7	Meningitis (*N. meningitidis*)
C8	Meningitis (*N. meningitidis*), disseminated gonococcal infection
C9	Meningitis (*N. meningitidis*)

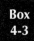

Box 4-3 Secondary Immunodeficiencies

HEMATOLOGIC LYMPHOPROLIFERATIVE DISORDERS

Hodgkin's disease and lymphoma
Leukemia
Myeloma, macroglobulinemia
Agranulocytosis and aplastic anemia
Sickle cell disease

OTHER SYSTEMIC PROCESSES AND METABOLIC DISORDERS

Nephrotic syndrome
Protein-losing enteropathy
Diabetes mellitus
Malnutrition
Hepatic disease
Uremia
Aging

VIRAL INFECTION

Acquired immunodeficiency syndrome

SURGICAL PROCEDURES AND TRAUMA

Splenectomy
Burns

IMMUNOSUPPRESSIVE AGENTS

Antimetabolites
Corticosteroids
Radiation

Modified from Graziano FM, Bell CL: The normal immune response and what can go wrong. In Corman LC, Katz D, editors: *Symposium on clinical immunology I, Medical Clinics of North America,* Philadelphia, WB Saunders 69(3):445, 1985.

TABLE 4-10	Immune-Mediated Disease
Allergic hypersensitivity	Foods, drugs, aeroallergens (dust, pollens, molds)
Contact hypersensitivity	Poison ivy, nickel, cosmetics
Transfusion Reactions	
Autoimmune disease	Systemic lupus erythematosus, rheumatoid arthritis, vasculitis syndromes, hemolytic anemia, idiopathic thrombocytopenia, pernicious anemia, Goodpasture's disease, myasthenia gravis, Graves' disease

are much more common than primary deficiencies, have an increased susceptibility to infections, as is seen in the primary immunodeficiencies.

Immunosuppressive agents and burns are major causes of secondary immunodeficiencies. Immunosuppressive agents have been demonstrated to affect, in varying degrees, every component of the immune response. In burn patients, septicemia is a common complication in those who survive the initial period of hemodynamic shock. The mechanism that seems most critical in thermal injury is disruption of the skin; however, interference with phagocytosis and deficiencies of serum Ig and complement levels have also been observed.

Immune-Mediated Disease

The immune system is normally efficient in eliminating foreign antigens. The nature of the antigen or the genetic makeup of the host, however, can cause alterations of the immune response that can be injurious and can lead to immune-mediated disease (Table 4-10). In these disorders, the immune response is normal but the reactivity is heightened, prolonged, or inappropriate.

Allergic reactions (see Chapter 23) are of major concern. These reactions are characterized by an immediate response on exposure to an offending antigen and the release of mediators (e.g., histamine, leukotrienes, and prostaglandins) that are capable of initiating signs and symptoms. Although allergic reactions are associated with IgE, not all allergic reactions are IgE-mediated. Complement activation by immune complexes or via the alternative complement pathway has been shown to release complements C3a and C5a anaphylatoxins capable of producing similar reactions.

Autoimmune disease (see Chapter 25) is thought to be caused by antibody or T-cell sensitization with autologous "self" antigens. Several of the postulated mechanisms of this process include:

- *Altered antigen or neoantigen.* Such antigens may be created by chemical, physical, or biologic processes. Hemolytic anemia caused by a drug interaction is an example of this process occurring in red blood cells.
- *Shared or cross-reactive antigens.* Evidence suggests that poststreptococcal disease occurs through this mechanism.

Case Study

History and Physical Examination

ML is a 38-year-old Caucasian female who came to the Emergency Department of her local hospital because of increasing difficulty breathing. She also reported that she has experienced chronic diarrhea for the last 18 months.

Her physical examination revealed a cachectic woman with bilateral rales and splenomegaly. After a chest x-ray confirmed the presence of pneumonia and bronchiectasis, the patient was admitted to the hospital.

The patient's condition worsened. Her respiratory insufficiency increased, and she developed renal failure and disseminated intravascular coagulation (DIC). She

Assay	Patient's Results	Reference Range
Complete blood count		
Hemoglobin	9.8 g/dL	11.5-13.5 g/dL
Hematocrit	24%	34%-42%
Total leukocyte count	9.0×10^9/L	$4.5-9.0 \times 10^9$/L
PMNs	87%	40%-60%
Lymphocytes	13%	20%-40%
Absolute lymphocytes	1.17×10^9/L	$>1.1 \times 10^9$/L
Stool culture	Normal biota (flora)	Normal biota (flora)
Ova and parasite examination	*Giardia lamblia*	Negative for all ova and parasites
Serum total protein	5.5 g/dL	
Serum electrophoresis	Hypogammaglobulinemia	
Immunoelectrophoresis		
IgM	0.7g/L	0.6-2.5g/l
IgG	2.2g/L	6.8-15.5 g/L
IgA	Undetectable	0.7-3.0g/L
Follow-Up		
CD4+	20%	35% to 55%
CD8+	26%	18% to 32%
Absolute CD4 count	0.26×10^9/L	$>0.43 \times 10^9$/L

was subsequently transferred to a tertiary care medical center.

Medical History

The patient had a childhood history of multiple episodes of bronchitis and middle ear infections (otitis media). In her late 20s she began to suffer from sinusitis, frequent diarrhea, and a chronic productive cough. She had two bouts of pneumonia, one of which required hospitalization. One year before the current episode the patient developed extreme difficulty breathing (dyspnea) when exercising. During the last year she lost almost 30 lbs and became so weak that she could no longer lead a normal life.

Family History

She had no family history of frequent infections, immunodeficiency, or autoimmune disorders.

Laboratory Data

On admission to the tertiary medical center, a blood count, serum protein, serum protein electrophore sis, immunoglobulin electrophoresis, stool culture, and ova and parasite examination were administered (see the chart above).

The patient was found to be anergic. Tetanus, rubella, and diphtheria titers were nonprotective despite previous immunizations.

The patient was diagnosed with common variable immunodeficiency. She was treated with intravenous immunoglobulin on a monthly basis. She also received metronidazole for her *Giardia lamblia* intestinal infection. After 1 year of immunoglobulin therapy, the patient gained weight and returned to a normal lifestyle.

Questions and Discussion

1. Does the patient's medical history suggest an immunodeficiency?

   A history of repeated infections in childhood is suggestive of an immunologic defect.
2. Which laboratory findings are significant?

   In common variable immunodeficiency, hypogammaglobulinemia is a hallmark of the disorder. The laboratory finding of a decreased number of CD4+ lymphocytes and decreased levels of immunoglobulins is important. *Giardia lamblia* is commonly detected in patients with this disorder.
3. How often is common variable immunodeficiency diagnosed in adults?

   Common variable immunodeficiency usually manifests itself in the second or third decade of life.

Diagnosis

Common variable immunodeficiency

CHAPTER HIGHLIGHTS

Lymphocytes represent the cellular components of the specific system of body defense. These cells function in either cell-mediated immunity or humoral immunity. Although cell-mediated and humoral immunity are not entirely independent and are frequently cooperative, they can be discussed as distinct systems.

The primary lymphoid organs in mammals are the bone marrow (and/or fetal liver) and thymus. Stem cells that migrate to the thymus proliferate and differentiate under the influence of the humoral factor, thymosin. These lymphocyte precursors with acquired surface membrane antigens are referred to as thymocytes. It is believed that the bone marrow and GALT may also play a role in the differentiation of stem cells into B lymphocyte functions as the bursal equivalent in humans. The secondary lymphoid tissues include the lymph nodes, spleen, and Peyer's patches in the intestine. Proliferation of the T and B lymphocytes in the secondary or peripheral lymphoid tissues is primarily dependent on antigenic stimulation. Lymphocytes display a great diversity of biologic and chemical properties such as size, density, charge, surface structure, and function. Several major categories of lymphocytes are recognized by the presence of cell surface membrane markers. These categories are the T cells and B cells, and the NK and K-type lymphocytes. Soluble mediators are secreted by monocytes, lymphocytes, or neutrophils, providing the language for cell-to-cell communication. Some of the most important soluble mediators are migration inhibition factor, IL-2 (T-cell growth factor), chemotactic factors, and IL-1. Except for inconsistent values seen in extremely elderly persons, the total number of T cells in the peripheral blood is relatively stable throughout adult life. There is, however, a change in the distribution of T-cell subpopulations. A decrease in the number of suppressor cells and an increase in the helper cell population are demonstrated in older adults. The effect of aging on the immune response is highly variable, but the ability to respond immunologically to disease is age related.

The function of plasma cells is the synthesis and excretion of immunoglobulins. Plasma cells are not normally found in the circulating blood but in the bone marrow in concentrations not normally exceeding 2%. Two well-established pathways of plasma cell development have been documented. Some plasma cells arise from immature plasma cells; others arise as the end stage of B cell differentiation into a large, activated plasma cell.

The introduction of monoclonal antibody testing led to the present identification of surface membrane markers. Relating monoclonal antibodies to cell surface antigens now provides a method for classifying and identifying specific cellular membrane characteristics. Separate subsets of T cells have been recognized with monoclonal antibodies. T cells are divided into two subsets: the suppressor/cytotoxic subset and the helper/inducer subset. During T-cell development, associated membrane antigens vary. In humans there is evidence of the existence of four types of B cell markers: Ig receptor, an Fc receptor, receptors that bind fragments of the cleaved complement component C3, and B cell surface antigens coded by the class II genes of the MHC. The best-studied B cell surface marker is the Ig receptor. This receptor is actually an antibody molecule with antigenic specificity. Although NK cells have long been classified as null cells, monoclonal antibodies demonstrate that NK cells share a variety of surface membrane markers with T cells. Some surface membrane markers associated with monocytes, granulocytes, or B cells are also demonstrable.

T cells respond to antigen by dividing, and they are responsible for delayed hypersensitivity, graft rejection, bacterial and viral killing, and elimination by direct cytotoxic effects or by release of soluble mediators. Deficiencies of cell-mediated immunity are often suspected in individuals with recurrent viral, fungal, parasitic, and protozoan infections. Patients with AIDS exhibit some of the most severe manifestations of cell-mediated immunity. The number of T lymphocytes, the primary effector cells in cell-mediated reactions, can be determined by a number of different techniques. The "gold standard" has previously been the E rosette technique. Development of monoclonal antibodies, however, has permitted a quick and specific method for determining the number of T cells. The method of testing is by use of immunofluorescent techniques in which the fluorescent microscope or FACS is used. Additional testing can include functional testing or the measurement of biologic response modifiers such as IL-2 using bioassay and radioimmunoassay.

The humoral system can be screened for abnormalities by quantitating the concentration of IgM, IgG, and IgA. However, serum protein electrophoresis may not be sensitive enough to detect selective Ig class deficiencies. IgD and IgE are not useful in the determination of a suspected humoral deficiency. The number of B lymphocytes in the peripheral blood and lymphoid organs can be determined by several different techniques. The most common procedure involves the detection of SIg.

A breakdown in any part of the immune mechanism can lead to disease. These disorders can involve stem cells, phagocytosis, T cells, B cells, or complement. Immunologic disorders can be divided into primary-acquired and those mediated through immune mechanisms. Immune deficiency disorders may be caused by defects in the quality or quantity of lymphocytes, and they may be congenital or acquired. These conditions may be combined disorders or either T- or B-cell disorders. Diseases associated with a primary defect in the immune response are composed of 40% T-cell disorders, 50% B-cell disorders, 6% phagocytic abnormalities, and 4% complement alterations. The most common T-cell deficiency states are those associated with a concurrent B-cell abnormality. Primary immunodeficiency disorders are predominantly seen in children under age 5 years. Primary immune disorders include severe combined immunodeficiency hereditary ataxia telangiectasia, chronic mucocutaneous candidiasis, Bruton's X-linked agammaglobulinemia, common variable hypogammaglobulinemia, and Wiskott-Aldrich syndrome.

REVIEW QUESTIONS

1. A function of the cell-mediated immune response not associated with humoral immunity is:
   A. defense against viral and bacterial infection
   B. initiation of rejection of foreign tissues and tumors
   C. defense against fungal and bacterial infection
   D. antibody production

2. The primary or central lymphoid organs in humans are the:
   A. bursa of Fabricius and thymus
   B. lymph nodes and thymus
   C. bone marrow and thymus
   D. lymph nodes and spleen

3. All of the following are a function of T cells except:
   A. mediation of delayed hypersensitivity reactions
   B. mediation of cytolytic reactions
   C. regulation of the immune response
   D. synthesis of antibody

Questions 4-7. Match the type of lymphocyte with its function (use an answer only once).

4. _____ T cells

5. _____ B cells

6. _____ K-type lymphocytes

7. _____ natural killer (NK)

   A. antibody-dependent, cell-mediated cytotoxicity reaction (ADCC)
   B. cellular immune response
   C. cytotoxic reaction
   D. humoral response
   E. phagocytosis

Questions 8-10. Match the surface membrane marker with the appropriate normal T-cell type.

8. _____ CD4

9. _____ CD8

10. _____ CD3

   A. all or most T lymphocytes
   B. helper-inducer T cells
   C. suppressor-cytotoxic T cells

Questions 11-14. Match the appropriate type of cell situation with a condition/disease.

11. _____ decreased helper cells

12. _____ increased helper cells

13. _____ decreased suppressor cells

14. _____ increased suppressor cells

   A. Kawasaki's disease
   B. infectious mononucleosis
   C. acquired immunodeficiency syndrome
   D. acute graft-versus-host disease

15. All of the following are B-cell surface membrane markers except:
   A. SIg
   B. F_C receptor
   C. C3 receptor
   D. CD4

Questions 16-21. Match the following congenital or acquired disorders with the major type of lymphocyte affected.

16. _____ thymic hypoplasia

17. _____ AIDS

18. _____ chronic lymphocytic leukemia

19. _____ systemic lupus erythematosus

20. _____ multiple myeloma

21. _____ Bruton's agammaglobulinemia

   A. congenital T-cell disorder
   B. congenital B-cell disorder
   C. acquired T-cell disorder
   D. acquired B-cell disorder

22. The majority of diseases associated with a primary defect are _____ disorders.

   A. T cell
   B. B cell
   C. complement
   D. phagocytic

23. Severe combined immunodeficiency is caused by:
   A. T-cell depletion
   B. B-cell depletion
   C. inappropriate development of stem cells
   D. phagocytic dysfunction

24. DiGeorge's syndrome is caused by:
   A. faulty embryogenesis
   B. deficiency of calcium in utero
   C. inappropriate stem cell development
   D. an autosomal-recessive disorder

25. The major clinical manifestation of a B-cell deficiency is:
   A. impaired phagocytosis
   B. diminished complement levels
   C. increased susceptibility to bacterial infections
   D. increased susceptibility to parasitic infections

26. Bruton's agammaglobulinemia is:
   A. an acquired disorder
   B. an autosomal genetic disorder
   C. a sex-linked genetic disorder
   D. a disorder occurring primarily in young females

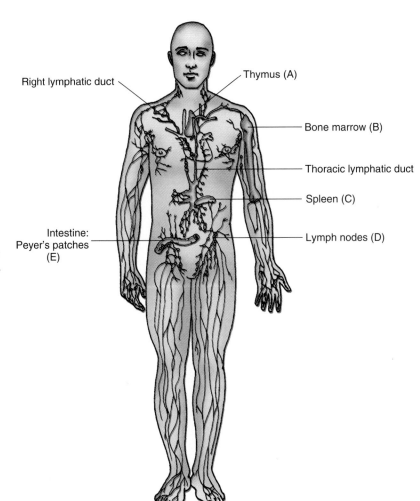

Right lymphatic duct

Thymus (A)

Bone marrow (B)

Thoracic lymphatic duct

Spleen (C)

Lymph nodes (D)

Intestine:
Peyer's patches
(E)

(Redrawn from Turgeon ML: *Clinical hematology: theory and procedures,* ed 3, Philadelphia, 1999, Lippincott Williams & Wilkins.)

27. Which of the following disorders does not result in a secondary immunodeficiency?
A. sickle cell disease
B. uremia
C. AIDS
D. poison ivy hypersensitivity

28. The primary lymphoid tissues in mammals are:
A. thymus and bursa of Fabricius
B. thymus and bone marrow
C. thymus and fetal liver
D. both B and C

29. In mammalian immunologic development, the precursors of lymphocytes arise from progenitor cells of the:
A. yolk sac
B. bone marrow
C. liver
D. both A and C

30. The thymus is embryologically derived from the:
A. yolk sac
B. pharyngeal pouches
C. lymphoblasts
D. bone marrow

31. Identify the sites of secondary tissue in the diagram above.
A. A, B, C
B. B, C, D
C. B, D, E
D. C, D, E

32. The process of aging causes the thymus to:
A. decrease in size
B. not change over time
C. lose cellularity
D. both A and C

33. T lymphocytes can also be referred to as:
A. mast cells
B. memory cells
C. phagocytic cells
D. short-lived cells

34. Which of the following characteristics is not true of T lymphocytes?
A. they can form a suppressor/cytotoxic subset
B. they can be helpers/inducers
C. they can be CD4+ or CD8+
D. they synthesize and secrete immunoglobulin

Questions 35 and 36. Match each to the appropriate function.

35. _____ T lymphocytes

36. _____ B lymphocytes

    A. cellular immune response
    B. humoral antibody response

Questions 37-39. Match each to the appropriate function.

37. _____ cytotoxic or effector T cells

38. _____ helper or regulator T cells

39. _____ suppressor T cells

    A. secrete a variety of cytokines
    B. recognize antigens associated with class I MHC
    C. inhibit response of helper T cells

40. Natural killer cells:
    A. produce interferon
    B. produce IL-2
    C. were previously called null cells
    D. all of the above

41. K type cells:
    A. synthesize antibody
    B. secrete antibody
    C. destroy by cytotoxic reaction
    D. phagocytize target cells

Questions 42-45. Complete the chart, choosing from the following answers:

    A. screening for anti-A and anti-B isoagglutinins
    B. erythrocyte sedimentation rate
    C. absolute neutrophil count
    D. absolute lymphocyte count

Initial Evaluation of Suspected Immunodeficiency

Suspected Deficiency	Appropriate Laboratory Procedures
All suspected deficiencies	42. _____ Complete CBC with platelet evaluation
Antibody deficiency	43. _____ Screening for antibodies to diphtheria or tetanus toxoids
T cell deficiency	44. _____ Intradermal skin test
Phagocytic cell deficiency	45. _____

46. Calculate the absolute lymphocyte count, when the following conditions exist:

    Total leukocyte count = 20×10^9/L
    Relative % of lymphocytes = 50%

    A. 5×10^9/L
    B. 10×10^9/L
    C. 15×10^9/L
    D. 20×10^9/L

Questions 47-49. Match.

    A. chronic lymphocytic leukemia
    B. Bruton's agammaglobulinemia
    C. multiple myeloma

T Cell Disorder	B Cell Disorder
Congenital	
DiGeorge's syndrome	47. _____
Acquired	
AIDS	48. _____
Hodgkin's disease	
Systemic lupus erythematosus	49. _____

Questions 50-53. Identify the distribution of immunodeficiencies, as shown in the following illustration.

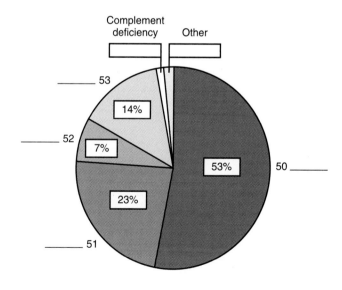

    A. T cell disorder
    B. B cell disorder
    C. severe combined immunodeficiency (SCID)
    D. disorders of phagocytosis

BIBLIOGRAPHY

Akella R: Laboratory of tumor immunology, *Guthrie J* 63(2):49-50, 1994.

Alberts B et al: *Molecular biology of the cell,* ed 2, New York, 1989, Garland Publications.

Arnaiz-Villena A et al: Primary immunodeficiency caused by mutation in the gene encoding the CD-3-(gamma) subunit of the T lymphocyte receptor, *N Engl J Med* 327(8):529-532, 1992.

Beezhold DH: Immune regulation, *Guthrie J* 59(1):3-8, 1990.

Buckley RH: Immunodeficiency diseases, *JAMA* 268(20):2797-2806, 1992.

Busby J, Caranasos GJ: Immune function, autoimmunity, and selective immunoprophylaxis, *Med Clin North Am* 69(3):465-470, 1985.

Claman HN: The biology of the immune response, *JAMA* 268(20):2790-2796, 1992.

Cooper MD, Lawton AR: The development of the immune system, *Scientific American,* 1974, pp 59-70.

D'Andrea AD: Cytokine receptors in congenital hematopoietic disease, *N Engl J Med* 330(12):839-846, 1994.

Denny T et al: Lymphocyte subsets in healthy children during the first 5 years of life, *JAMA* 267(11):1484-1488, 1992.

Geha RS, Rosen FS: The genetic basis of immunoglobulin-class switching, *N Engl J Med* 330(14):1008-1009, 1994.

Graziano FM, Bell CL: The normal immune response and what can go wrong. In Corman LC, Katz P, editors: *Med Clin North Am Symposium on Clinical Immunology I,* Philadelphia, 1985, WB Saunders.

Heinzel FP: Infections in patients with humoral immunodeficiency, *Hospital Practice,* 1989, pp 97-123.

Nightengale SL: New therapy for severe combined immunodeficiency disease, *JAMA* 263(22):2995, 1990.

Sneller MC: New insights into common variable immunodeficiency, *Ann Intern Med* 118(9):720-730, 1993.

Turgeon ML: *Clinical hematology,* ed 3, Philadelphia, 1999, Lippincott Williams & Wilkins.

Turgeon ML: *Fundamentals of immunohematology,* ed 2, Baltimore, 1995, Williams & Wilkins.

Yocum MW, Kelso JM: Common variable immunodeficiency: the disorder and treatment, *Mayo Clinic Proc* 66:83-96, 1991.

Chapter 5

Soluble Mediators of the Immune System

LEARNING OBJECTIVES

At the conclusion of this chapter, the reader should be able to:
- Name and compare the three complement activation pathways.
- Describe the mechanisms and consequences of complement activation.
- Explain the biologic functions of the complement system.
- Name and describe alterations in complement levels.

- Briefly describe the assessment of complement levels.
- Name and compare various other types of nonspecific mediators of the immune system (e.g., cytokines, interleukins, tumor necrosis factor, hematopoietic growth factors, and chemokines).
- Discuss the clinical applications of C-reactive protein.
- Compare acute-phase reactant methods.

TABLE 5-1　Three Main Physiologic Activities of the Complement System

Activity	Responsible Complement Protein
1. Host defense against infection	
Opsonization	Covalently bonded fragments of C3 and C4
Chemotaxis and leukocyte activation	C5a, C3a, and C4a; anaphylatoxin leukocyte receptors
Lysis of bacterial and mammalian cells	C5-C9 membrane attack complex
2. Interface between innate and adaptive immunity	
Augmentation of antibody	C3b and C4b bound to immune complexes and to antigen
Responses	C3 receptors on B cells and antigen-presenting cells
Enhancement of immunologic memory	C3b and C4b bound to immune complexes and to antigen; C3 receptors on follicular dendritic cells
3. Disposal of waste	
Clearance of immune complexes from tissues	C1q; covalently bonded fragments of C3 and C4
Clearance of apoptotic cells	C1q; covalently bonded fragments of C3 and C4

Source: Modified from Walport MJ: Complement, *N Engl J Med* 344(14):1058, 2001.

TABLE 5-2　Initiators of the Three Activation Pathways of Complement

Pathway	Initiators
Classic	Immune complexes
	Apoptotic cells
	Certain viruses and gram-negative bacteria
	C-reactive protein bound to ligand
Alternative	Various bacteria, fungi, viruses, or tumor cells
Mannose-binding lectin	Microbes with terminal mannose groups

Modified from Walport MJ: Complement, *N Engl J Med* 344(14): 1058, 2001.

The immune system is composed of the phylogenetically oldest and highly diversified innate immune system, and the adaptive immune system. Some of the components of the innate or natural immune system (e.g., phagocytosis) have been discussed in previous chapters. In this chapter the other components of the innate immune system—the complement system and other circulating effector proteins of innate immunity (e.g., cytokines and acute-phase reactants) are discussed).

THE COMPLEMENT SYSTEM

Complement is a heat-labile series of 18 plasma proteins, many of which are enzymes or proteinases. Collectively these proteins are a major fraction of the beta 1 and beta 2 globulins. The complement system displays three overarching physiologic activities, which are initiated in various ways (Tables 5-1 and 5-2):
1. Classic pathway
2. Alternative pathway
3. Mannose-binding lectin pathway
Proteins of the classic activation pathway and the terminal sequence are called components and are symbolized by the

letter C followed by a number (e.g., C4). Proteins of the alternative activation pathway are called factors and are symbolized by letters such as B. Control proteins include the inhibitor of C1 (C1 INH), the C4b/C3b inactivator (now called factor I), and (beta) 1H globulin (now called factor H).

Activation of Complement

Normally complement components are present in the circulation in an inactive form. In addition, the control proteins C1 INH, factor I, factor H, and C4-bp (C4-binding protein) are normally present to inhibit uncontrolled complement activation.

The classic pathway (Figure 5-1) is initiated by the complexing of antigen to its specific antibody, either IgG or IgM, and is the primary amplifier of the biologic effects of humoral immunity. The alternative pathway is activated by contact with a foreign surface such as the polysaccharide coating of a microorganism, and it amplifies nonimmune defense against microbial infection and other biologic alterations. It is probable that under normal physiologic conditions, the activation of one pathway also leads to the activation of the other. Either of the two routes leads to a common final pathway. Both pathways convert C3 to C3b, the central event of the common final pathway, which in turn leads to the activation of the lytic complement sequence, C5-C9, and cell destruction. A third set of plasma proteins that function as membrane attack complexes becomes assembled into the structures responsible for lytic lesions in the lipid bilayer of the cell membrane and disrupts membrane integrity.

After complement is initially activated, each enzyme precursor is activated by the previous complement component or complex, which is a highly specialized proteinase. This converts the enzyme precursor to its catalytically active form by limited proteolysis. During this activation process, a small peptide fragment is cleaved, a membrane-binding site is exposed, and the major fragment binds. As a consequence, the next active enzyme of the sequence is formed. Because each enzyme can activate many enzyme precursors, each step is amplified; therefore the whole system forms an amplifying cascade.

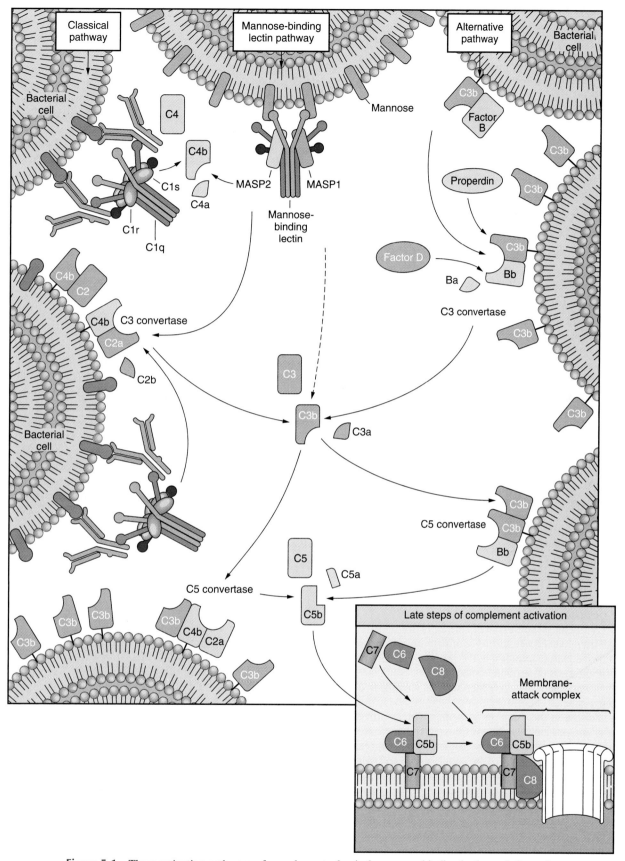

Figure 5-1 Three activation pathways of complement: classical, mannose-binding lectin, and alternative pathways. The three pathways converge at the point of cleavage of C3. The classical pathway is initiated by the binding of the C1 complex (which consists of C1q, two molecules of C1r, and two molecules of C1s) to antibodies bound to an antigen on the surface of a bacterial cell. The mannose-binding lectin pathway is initiated by binding of the complex of mannose-binding lectin and the serine proteases mannose-binding lectin—associated proteases 1 and 2 (MASP1 and MASP2, respectively) to arrays of mannose groups on the surface of a bacterial cell. The alternative pathway is initiated by the covalent binding of a small amount of C3b to hydroxyl groups on cell-surface carbohydrates and proteins and is activated by low-grade cleavage of C3 in plasma. (Redrawn from Walport MJ: Complement, *N Engl J Med* 344(14):1058-1066. 2001.)

TABLE 5-3	Receptors for C3 Fragments	
Receptor Name	Specificity	Cellular Distribution
CR1	C3b (1C3b)	Erythrocytes, granulocytes, monocytes, B cells, glomerular visceral epithelial cells, dendritic cells
CR2	C3dg (C3d)	B cells
CR3	1C3b	Monocytes, granulocytes, natural killer cells

From Stein J: *Internal medicine,* ed 2, Boston, 1987, Little, Brown.

Complement Receptors

Various cell types express surface membrane glycoproteins that react with one or more of the fragments of C3 produced during complement activation and degradation. The functions of these receptors depend on the type of cell manifesting them and are, in many instances, incompletely understood (Table 5-3). The complement receptor 1 (CR1) is important in enhancing phagocytosis. CR1 is the only receptor on human erythrocytes and serves as a cofactor in the cleavage of C3b to iC3b by factor I. CR2 may have an effect on lymphocytes in their response to mitogens or antigen stimulation. CR3 is known to be important in host defense mechanisms such as phagocytosis.

Effects of Complement Activation

The activation of complement and the products formed during the complement cascade have a variety of physiologic and cellular consequences. Physiologic consequences include blood vessel dilation and increased vascular permeability. The cellular consequences include the following:

1. Cell activation such as the production of inflammatory mediators.
2. Cytolysis or hemolysis, if the cells are erythrocytes. The most important biologic role of complement in blood group serology is the production of cell membrane lysis of antibody-coated targets.
3. Opsonization, which renders cells vulnerable to phagocytosis.

In addition to the function of complement as a major effector of antigen-antibody interaction, physiologic concentrations of complement have been found to induce profound alteration in the molecular weight, composition, and solubility of immune complexes. The activation of complement may also play a role in mediating hypersensitivity reactions. This process may occur either from direct alternative pathway activation by IgE-antigen complexes or through a sequence initiated by the activated Hageman coagulation factor that causes the generation of plasmin, which subsequently activates the classic pathway. In either case, activation of complement components from C3 onward leads to the generation of the anaphylatoxins in an immediate hypersensitivity reaction.

CLASSIC PATHWAY

The classic complement pathway is one of the major effector mechanisms of antibody-mediated immunity. The principal components of the classic pathway are C1 through C9. The sequence of component activation does not follow the expected numeric order. The sequence is C1, 4, 2, 3, 5, 6, 7, 8, and 9.

C3 is present in the plasma in the largest quantities; fixation of C3 is the major quantitative reaction of the complement cascade. Although the principal source of synthesis of complement in vivo is debatable, the majority of the plasma complement components are made in hepatic parenchymal cells, except for C1 (a calcium-dependent complex of the three glycoproteins C1q, C1r, and C1s), which is primarily synthesized in the epithelium of the gastrointestinal and urogenital tracts.

The classic pathway is composed of three stages:

1. Recognition
2. Enzymatic activation
3. Membrane attack leading to cellular destruction

Fixation of the C1 Complex

The recognition unit of the complement system is the C1 complex: C1q, C1r, and C1s, an interlocking enzyme system. The C1 complex is a unique feature of the classic pathway leading to C3 conversion. C1 fixation occurs when the C1q subcomponent binds directly to an immunoglobulin (Ig) molecule. The other two subcomponents, C1r and C1s, do not bind to the Ig but are involved in subsequent activation of the classic pathway. Whether C1 fixation occurs depends on a number of factors. These conditions include:

- *Subclass of Ig.* Only certain subclasses of Ig such as IgM and most of the IgG subclasses can fix C1 even under optimal conditions.
- *Spatial or configurational constraints.*

A single IgM molecule is potentially able to fix C1, but at least a pair of IgG molecules is required for this purpose. The amount of C1 fixed is directly proportional to the concentration of IgM antibodies; however, this is not true of IgG molecules.

The C1q molecule is potentially multivalent for attachment to the complement fixation sites of Ig. The structures of C1q peptide chains are formed into three subunits of six chains each. Each subunit consists of a Y-shaped pair of triple helices joined at the stem and ending in a globular head. The globular ends are assumed to be the sites for multivalent attachment to the complement-fixing sites in immune-complexed Igs. The sites on the IgG molecules are on the CH2 domains and probably on the CH4 domain of IgM. The complement-fixing site may become exposed after complexing of the Ig, or the sites may always be available but need multiple attachments by C1q with critical geometry to achieve the necessary avidity.

C1r and C1s are chemically similar; however, C1r forms dimers, whereas C1s binds monovalently to C1r. C1r and C1s form a tetrad complex that binds to C1q in the presence of Ca^{++} ion. The mechanism of C1r by C1q is unknown because C1q is not known to have enzymatic activity. However, it is known that C1r and C1s activate in sequence still attached to C1q and that both proteins become typical serine-histidine esterases on activation. C1s is the only substrate for C1r. C1s will activate C4 and C2, the next components in the classic complement sequence, but C1r will not.

Fixation and Activation of C4 by the C1qrs Complex

C1s splits a peptide C4a from the N-terminal part of the alpha chain of the C4 component, leaving a large fragment, C4b. This reaction occurs in the fluid phase of the plasma around the C1s catalytic site, and a reactive internal thioester bond is revealed on C4b. The stable binding of C4b molecules to membranes has less than 10% efficiency. Binding occurs in proximity to the site of activation, either to the C1qrs complex or to the adjacent erythrocyte membrane. C4b molecules that fail to bind become inactive and decay.

C1s is weakly proteolytic for free intact C2 but highly active against C2 that has complexed with C4b molecules in the presence of Mg^{++} ions. This reaction will occur only if the C4bC2 complex forms close to the C1s. The resultant C2b fragment joins with C4b to form the new C4b2a enzyme, the classic pathway C3 convertase. The catalytic site of the C4b2a complex is probably in the C2b peptide. A smaller C2a fragment from the C2 component is lost to the surrounding environment. The C4b2a enzyme is unstable and decays with a half-life of 5 minutes at 37° C because of the release and decay of C2b.

There are two chief constraints on the activities of C1s on C4 and C2 and on the stable formation of the C4b2a complex:

1. The action of the proteinase inhibitor, C1 esterase
2. The effect of C3b inactivator

C1 esterase inhibitor binds to C1s and C1r. This activity may not be important in restraining the action of C1s at a local membrane site, but it is extremely important in preventing the excessive action of free C1 on C4 and C2 in the fluid phase.

C3b inactivator has the ability to disintegrate membrane-bound C4b. This action destroys the acceptor site for C2, which prevents the formation of C4b2a convertase.

Action of C4b2a Complex on C3

The complement cascade reaches its full amplitude at the C3 stage, which represents the heart of the system. The C4b2a complex, referred to as classic pathway C3 convertase, activates C3 molecules by splitting the peptide, C3 anaphylatoxin, from the N-terminal end of the peptide of C3. This exposes a reactive-binding site on the larger fragment, C3b. Consequently, clusters of C3b molecules are activated and bound near the C4b2a complex. Each catalytic site can bind several hundred C3b molecules, even though the reaction is very inefficient because C3 is present in high concentration. Only one C3b molecule combines with C4b2a to form the final proteolytic complex of the complement cascade.

Action of C3b on C5

C3b splits C5a from the alpha chain of C5 to initiate C5b fixation and the beginning of the membrane attack complex. No further proteinases are generated in the classic complement sequence. Other bound C3b molecules not involved in the C4b2a3b complex form an opsonic macromolecular coat on the erythrocyte or other target, which renders it susceptible to immune adherence by C3b receptors on phagocytic cells.

C5-9 Membrane Attack Complex

Fixation of C5b to biologic membrane is followed by the sequential addition of C6, C7, C8, and C9. When fully assembled in the correct proportions, they form the membrane attack complex. The C5bC6 complex is hydrophilic, but with the addition of C7 to the C567 complex, the complex has additional detergent and phospholipid-binding properties as well. This occurrence of both hydrophobic and hydrophilic groups within the same complex may account for its tendency to polymerize and form small protein micelles (a packet of chain molecules in parallel arrangement). In free solution uncombined C567 has a half-life of about 0.1 second. It can attach to any lipid bilayer within its effective diffusion radius, which produces the phenomenon of reactive lysis on innocent "bystander" cells. Once membrane bound, C567 is relatively stable and can interact with C8 and C9.

C5-8 polymerizes C9 to form a tubule known as the membrane attack complex, which bridges the membrane. By complexing with C9, the osmotic cytolytic reaction is accelerated. This tubule is a hollow cylinder with one end inserted into the lipid bilayer and the other end projected from the membrane. Although the micellar arrangement of the membrane insertion region has not been positively established, a structure of this form can be assumed to disturb the lipid bilayer sufficiently to allow the free exchange of ions as well as water molecules across the membrane. The consequence in a living cell is that the influx of Na^+ and H_2O leads to disruption of osmotic balance, which produces cell lysis.

ALTERNATE PATHWAY

The alternate pathway shows points of similarity with the classic sequence. Both pathways generate a C3 convertase that activates C3 to provide the pivotal event in the final common pathway of both systems. However, in contrast to the classic pathway, which is initiated by the formation of antigen-antibody reactions, the alternate complement pathway is predominantly a nonantibody-initiated pathway.

Microbial and mammalian cell surfaces can activate the alternate pathway in the absence of specific antigen-antibody complexes. Factors capable of activating the alternate pathway include inulin, zymosan, a polysaccharide complex from the surface of yeast cells, bacterial polysaccharides and endotoxins, and the aggregated Igs IgG_2, IgA, and IgE. In paroxysmal nocturnal hemoglobinuria (PNH), the patient's erythrocytes act as an activator and result in the excessive lysis of these erythrocytes. This nonspecific activation is a major physiologic advantage because host protection can be generated before the induction of a humoral immune response.

A key feature of the alternate pathway is that the first three proteins of the classic activation pathway—C1, C4, and C2—do not participate in the cascade sequence. The C3A component is considered to be the counterpart of C2a in the classic pathway. C2 of the classic pathway structurally resembles factor B of the alternate pathway. The omission of C1, C4, and C2 is possible because activators of the alternate pathway catalyze the conversion of another series of normal serum proteins, which leads to the activation of C3. It was previously believed that properdin, a normal protein of human serum, was the first protein to function in the alternate pathway; thus the pathway was originally named after this protein.

The uptake of factor B onto C3b occurs when C3b is bound to an activator surface. However, C3b in the fluid phase or attached to a nonactivator surface will preferentially bind to factor H and so prevent C3b,B formation. C3b and factor B combine to form C3b,B, which is converted into an active C3 convertase, C3b,Bb. This results from the loss of a small fragment, Ba (a glycine-rich alpha$_2$ globulin believed to be physiologically inert), through the action of the enzyme, factor D. The C3b,Bb complex is able to convert more C3 to C3b, which binds more factor B. And so the feedback cycle continues.

The major controlling event of this pathway is factor H, which prevents the association between C3b and factor B. Factor H blocks the formation of C3b,Bb, the catalytically active C3 convertase of the feedback loop. Factor H (previously called beta$_1$H) competes with factor B for its combining site on C3b, eventually leading to C3 inactivations. Factors B and H apparently occupy a common site on C3b. The factor that is preferentially bound to C3b depends on the nature of the surface to which C3b is attached. Polysaccharides are called activator surfaces and favor the uptake of factor B on the chain of C3b, with the corresponding displacement of factor H. In this situation, binding of factor H is inhibited, and consequently factor B will replace H at the common binding site. When factor H is excluded, C3b is thought to be formed continuously in small amounts. Another controlling point in the amplification loop depends on the stability of the C3b,Bb convertase. Ordinarily C3b,Bb decays because of the loss of Bb with a half-life of approximately 5 minutes. However, if properdin (P) binds to C3b,Bb, forming C3b,BbP, the half-life is extended to 30 minutes.

The association of numerous C3b units, factor Bb, and properdin on the surface of an aggregate of protein or the surface of a microorganism has potent activity as a C5 convertase. With the cleavage of C5, the remainder of the complement cascade continues as in the classic pathway.

MANNOSE-BINDING LECTIN PATHWAY

Mannose-binding lectin is a member of a family of calcium-dependent lectins, the collectins (collagenous lectins), and is homologous in structure to C1q. Mannose-binding lectin, a pattern-recognition molecule of the innate immune system, binds to arrays of terminal mannose groups on a variety of bacteria.

A deficiency of mannose-binding lectin is caused by one of three point mutations in the gene for mannose-binding lectin, each of which reduces levels of the lectin. After the discovery that the binding of mannose-binding lectin to mannose residues can initiate complement activation, the mannose-binding lectin-associated serine protease (MASP) enzymes were discovered. MASP activates complement by interacting with two serine proteases called MASP1 and MASP2. These components comprise the mannose-binding lectin pathway.

BIOLOGIC FUNCTIONS OF COMPLEMENT PROTEINS

The biologic functions of the complement system (Table 5-4) fall into two general categories:
  1. Cell lysis by the membrane attack complex (MAC)

TABLE 5-4   Selected Complement Components and Functions

Complement Component(s)	Function
C5-C9	Lysis of cells
C3B, IC3B	Opsonization in phagocytosis
C5A>C3A>>C4A	Anaphylatoxins/inflammation (vascular responses)
C5A	Polymorphonuclear leukocytes activation
Classic complement Pathway, C3B, ?iC3b, C3dg	Immune complex removal B-lymphocyte activation

  2. Biologic effects of proteolytic fragments of complement

The first category is the situation in which the MAC leads to osmotic lysis of a cell.

The second category encompasses multiple other effects of complement in immunity and inflammation that are mediated by the proteolytic fragments generated during complement activation. These fragments may remain bound to the same cell surfaces where complement has been activated or may be released into the blood or extracellular fluid. In either situation, active fragments mediate their effects by binding to specific receptors expressed on various types of cells, including phagocytic leukocytes and the endothelium.

In contrast, the absence of an integral component of the classic, alternative, or terminal lytic pathways can lead to decreased complement activation and a lack of complement-mediated biologic functions.

Alterations in Complement Levels

The complement system can cause significant tissue damage in response to abnormal stimuli. Biologic effects of complement activation can occur as a reaction to persistent infection or an autoantibody response to self-antigens. In these infectious or autoimmune conditions, the inflammatory or lytic effects of complement may contribute significantly to the pathology of the disease.

Complement activation is also associated with intravascular thrombosis, which leads to ischemic injury to tissues. Complement levels may be abnormal in certain disease states (e.g., rheumatoid arthritis or systemic lupus erythematosus [SLE]) and in some genetic disorders.

Elevated Complement Levels

Complement can be elevated in many inflammatory conditions. Increased complement levels are often associated with inflammatory conditions, trauma, or acute illness such as myocardial infarction because separate complement components (e.g., C3) are acute-phase proteins. However, these elevations are common and nonspecific. Therefore increased levels are of limited clinical significance.

Decreased Complement Levels

Low levels of complement suggest one of the following biologic effects:

TABLE 5-5	Complement Deficiency in Humans
Complement Deficiency	**Associated Diseases**
C1q	SLE-like syndrome; decreased secondary to agammaglobulinemia
C1r	SLE-like syndrome; dermatomyositis, vasculitis, recurrent infections and chronic glomerulonephritis, necrotizing skin lesions, arthritis
C1s	SLE, SLE-like syndrome
C1 INH	Hereditary angioedema, lupus nephritis
C2	Recurrent pyogenic infections, SLE, SLE-like syndrome, discoid lupus, membranoproliferative glomerulonephritis, dermatomyositis, synovitis, purpura, Henoch-Schönlein purpura, hypertension, Hodgkin's disease, chronic lymphocytic leukemia, dermatitis herpetiformis, polymyositis
C3	Recurrent pyogenic infections, SLE-like syndrome, arthralgias, skin rash
C3 inactivator	Recurrent pyogenic infections, urticaria
C4	SLE-like syndrome, SLE, dermatomyositis-like syndrome, vasculitis
C5	*Neisseria* infections, SLE
C5 dysfunction	Leiner's disease, gram-negative skin and bowel infection
C6	*Neisseria* infections, SLE, Raynaud's phenomenon, scleroderma-like syndrome, vasculitis
C7	*Neisseria* infections, SLE, Raynaud's phenomenon, scleroderma-like syndrome, vasculitis
C8	*Neisseria* infections, xeroderma pigmentosa, SLE-like syndrome

Modified from Cassidy JT, Petty RE: Immunodeficiency and arthritis. In Cassidy JT, editor: *Textbook of pediatric rheumatology,* New York, 1982, John Wiley & Sons; Wedgewood RJ, Rosen FS, Paul HW: Primary immunodeficiency disease, *Birth Defects* 19:345, 1983; and Pahwa R et al: Treatment of the immunodeficiency diseases, *Springer Semin Immunopathol* 1:355, 1978.
SLE, Systemic lupus erythematosus.

- Complement has been excessively activated recently
- Complement is currently being consumed
- A single complement component is absent because of a genetic defect

Specific component deficiencies are associated with a variety of disorders (Table 5-5). Deficiencies of complement account for a small percentage of primary immunodeficiencies (<2%), but depression of complement levels frequently coexists with SLE and other disorders associated with an immunopathologic process (Figure 5-2 and Box 5-1).

Deficiencies in any of the protein components of complement are usually due to a genetic defect which leads to abnormal patterns of complement activation. If regulatory components are absent, excess activation may occur at the wrong time or at the wrong site. The potential consequences of increased activation are excess inflammation and cell lysis, and consumption of complement components.

Hypocomplementemia can result from the complexing of IgG or IgM antibodies capable of activating complement. Depressed values of complement are associated with diseases that give rise to circulating immune complexes. Because of the rapid normal turnover of the complement proteins—within 1 or 2 days of the cessation of complement activation by immune complexes—complement levels return to normal rapidly.

Three types of complement deficiency can cause increased susceptibility to pyogenic infections:
1. Deficiency of the opsonic activities of complement
2. Any deficiency that compromises the lytic activity of complement
3. Deficient function of the mannose-binding lectin pathway.

Increase susceptibility to pyogenic bacteria (e.g., *Haemophilus influenzae* and *Streptococcus pneumoniae*) occurs in patients with defects of antibody production, complement proteins of the classic pathway, or phagocyte function. The sole clinical association between inherited deficiency of components of the membrane-attack complex and infection is with neisserial disease, particularly *Neisseria meningitidis.* Low levels of mannose-binding lectin in young children with recurrent infections suggest that the mannose-binding lectin pathway is important during the interval between the loss of passively acquired maternal antibody and the acquisition of a mature immunologic repertoire of antigen exposure.

DIAGNOSTIC EVALUATION

During immune complex reactions, certain complement proteins become physically bound to the tissue in which the immunologic reaction is occurring. These proteins can be demonstrated in tissue by appropriate immunopathologic stains. The most frequent evaluation of complement, however, is by serum/plasma assay (Table 5-6). Complement components (e.g., C3 and C4) can be assessed nephelometry. These assays are useful in diagnosis and monitoring of patients.

Assessment of Complement

Procedures that can be used in diagnostic immunology include the following:

C1 Esterase Inhibitor (C1 Inhibitor)

C1 measures the activity and/or concentration of C1 inhibitor in serum. A deficiency of this protein is characteristic of

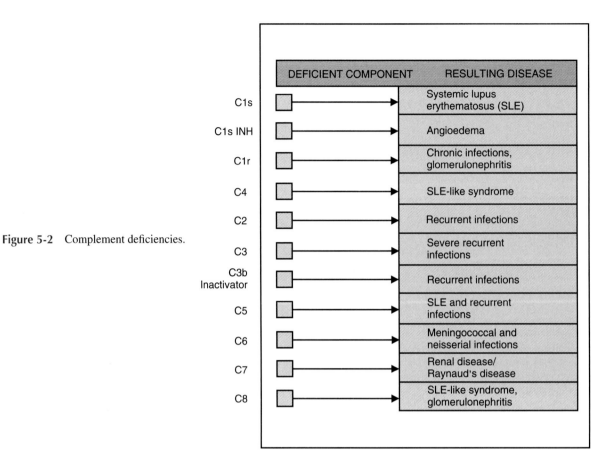

Figure 5-2   Complement deficiencies.

DEFICIENT COMPONENT	RESULTING DISEASE
C1s	Systemic lupus erythematosus (SLE)
C1s INH	Angioedema
C1r	Chronic infections, glomerulonephritis
C4	SLE-like syndrome
C2	Recurrent infections
C3	Severe recurrent infections
C3b Inactivator	Recurrent infections
C5	SLE and recurrent infections
C6	Meningococcal and neisserial infections
C7	Renal disease/ Raynaud's disease
C8	SLE-like syndrome, glomerulonephritis

> **Box 5-1**   **Diseases Associated With Hypocomplementemia**
>
> **RHEUMATIC DISEASES WITH IMMUNE COMPLEXES**
>
> Systemic lupus erythematosus
> Rheumatoid arthritis (with extraarticular disease)
> Systemic vasculitis
> Essential mixed cryoglobulinemia
>
> **GLOMERULONEPHRITIS**
>
> Poststreptococcal
> Membranoproliferative
>
> **INFECTIOUS DISEASES**
>
> Subacute bacterial endocarditis
> Infected atrioventricular shunts
> Pneumococcal sepsis
> Gram-negative sepsis
> Viremias (e.g., hepatitis B surface antigenemia, measles)
> Parasitic infections (e.g., malaria)
>
> **DEFICIENCY OF CONTROL PROTEINS**
>
> C1 inhibitor deficiency: hereditary angioedema
> Factor I deficiency
> Factor H deficiency

hereditary angioedema (HAE). Some patients demonstrate catalytically inactive protein.

C1r, C1s, C2, C3, C4, C5, C6, C7, C8

Homozygous deficiencies predispose a patient to autoimmune disease (especially SLE) and to arthritis, chronic glomerulonephritis, infections, and vasculitis.

C1q

The complement component C1q is evaluated in serum. Decreased levels can be demonstrated in patients suffering from hypocomplementemic urticarial vasculitis, severe combined immunodeficiency, or X-linked hypogammaglobulinemia.

C1q Binding

This procedure measures the binding of immune complexes containing IgG_1, IgG_2, or IgG_3, and/or IgM to the complement component C1q. High values of C1q binding are associated with the presence of circulating immune complexes of the type that interact with the classic pathway of complement activation. This test can be useful as a prognostic tool at diagnosis and during remission of acute myelogenous leukemia.

C2

C2 is the most common complement deficiency. It is an autosomal-recessive disorder (C2 gene is on chromosome 6 in the major histocompatibility complex [MHC]). The incidence rate is 1:28,000 to 1:40,000; the carrier state is 1.2% in the general population.

TABLE 5-6	Interpretation of Complement Activation by Individual Components				
Complement Determination	Classic Pathway	Alternative Pathway	Improper Specimen*	Inflammation
CH_{50}	Decreased	Decreased, normal	Decreased	Increased
C3	Decreased	Decreased	Normal	Increased
C4	Decreased	Normal	Decreased	Increased

*Results if specimen is improperly stored or too old.

One-half of patients with homozygous C2 deficiency have no symptoms; those with symptoms have infections with *S. pneumoniae, N. meningitidis,* and *H. influenzae.* Fifty percent of symptomatic patients exhibit a lupus-like disorder with photosensitivity and rash.

C3

C3 is also an acute phase protein. Elevated values can indicate an acute inflammatory disease. Although C3 lies at the junction of the two pathways, it is much more severely depressed when activation occurs via the alternative pathway. Extremely decreased levels are seen in patients with post-streptococcal glomerulonephritis and in patients with inherited (C3) complement deficiency. This component is also decreased in cases of severe liver disease and in SLE patients with renal disease.

C3b Inhibitor (C3b Inactivator)

The C3b component of complement causes low complement C3 levels, the absence of C3PA in serum, and high C3b levels. A deficiency of C3b inhibitor is associated with an increased predisposition to infection.

C3PA (C3 Proactivator, Properdin Factor B)

The factor B component is consumed by activation of the alternative complement pathway. Assessment of C3PA indicates whether a decreased level of C3 results from the classic or alternate pathways of complement activation. Decreased levels of C3 and C4 demonstrate activation of the classic pathway. Decreased levels of C3 and C3PA with a normal level of C4 indicate complement activation via the alternative pathway.

Activation of the classic pathway (and sometimes with accompanying alternative pathway activation) is associated with disorders such as immune complex diseases, various forms of vasculitis, and acute glomerulonephritis. Activation of the alternative pathway is associated with many disorders, including chronic hypocomplementemic glomerulonephritis, diffuse intravascular coagulation, septicemia, subacute bacterial endocarditis, PNH, and sickle cell anemia.

In SLE, both the classic and alternative pathways are activated.

C4

The C4 level often provides the most sensitive indicator of disease activity. C4 is also an acute phase reactant. Elevated C4 levels can indicate an acute inflammatory reaction or a malignant condition. Measurement of C4 may demonstrate inflammation or infection long before it is clinically evident by standard assessment methods (e.g., total white blood count and leukocyte differential, febrile response, or an elevated erythrocyte sedimentation rate [ESR]).

C4 is destroyed only when the classic pathway is activated. A decreased C4 level with elevated anti-n-DNA and antinuclear antibody titers confirm the diagnosis of SLE in a patient. In these cases of SLE, the periodic assessment of C4 can be useful in monitoring the progress of the disorder. Patients with extremely low C4 in the presence of normal levels of the C3 component may be demonstrating the effects of a genetic deficiency of either C1 inhibitor or C4. Reduction of C3 and C4 components implies that activation of the classic pathway has been initiated.

C4 Allotypes

The antigenically distinct forms of C4A and C4B are located on the sixth chromosome in the major histocompatibility complex. Identification of C4 allotypes in conjunction with specific human leukocyte antigens (HLAs) are markers for disease susceptibility.

C5

A genetic deficiency of the C5 component is associated with increased susceptibility to bacterial infection and is expressed as an autoimmune disorder (e.g., SLE). In the case of dysfunction of C5 (Leiner's disease), the patient is predisposed to infections of the skin and bowel characterized by eczema. In these patients the level of C5 is normal, but the C5 component fails to promote phagocytosis.

C6

A decreased quantity of C6 predisposes an individual to significant *Neisseria* (bacteria) infections.

C7

A decreased level of C7 is associated with Raynaud's phenomenon, sclerodactyly, telangiectasia, and severe bacterial infections caused by *Neisseria* species.

C8

A decreased quantity of C8 is associated with SLE. A C8 deficiency makes patients highly susceptible to *Neisseria* infections.

Properdin Deficiency

Properdin acts to stabilize the alternative pathway C3 converase (C3bBb). A deficiency leads to bacterial infections, often meningococcemia. This disorder is an X-linked recessive trait.

Hereditary Angioedema

This disorder is a deficiency in a complement protein. Infections are not usually a significant problem. This disorder is autosomal dominant, unlike other complement deficiencies. Two types exist: type 1 (low antigen level and low functional protein) and type 2 (normal antigen level with low function).

Familial Mediterranean Fever

This is a defect in protease in peritoneal and synovial fluid. This disorder is transmitted as an autosomal-recessive on chromosome 16. Patients with the defect experience recurrent episodes of fever and inflammation in the joints and pleural/peritoneal fluid.

OTHER SOLUBLE MEDIATORS OF THE IMMUNE RESPONSE

Cytokines

Migratory inhibitory factor (MIF) was the first cytokine activity to be described. MIF is a T-cell-derived activity that immobilizes macrophage migration. This may cause phagocytes to be retained and accumulate at sites of inflammation.

TABLE 5-7 Examples of Cytokines of Innate and Adaptive Immunity

Innate Immunity	Adaptive Immunity
Chemokines	Interferon-gamma (IFN-gamma)
Interferons type 1 (IFN-alpha, IFN-beta)	Interleukin-2 (Il-2)
Interleukin-1 (Il-1)	Interleukin-4 (Il-4)
Interleukin-6 (Il-6)	Interleukin-5 (Il-5)
Interleukin-10 (Il-10)	Interleukin-13 (Il-13)
Interleukin-12 (Il-12)	Lymphotoxin (Lt)
Interleukin-15 (Il-15)	Transforming growth factor-beta (TGF-beta)
Interleukin-18 (Il-18)	
Tumor necrosis factor (TNF)	

Cytokines are the focus of a great deal of current research, and the list of individual cytokines steadily increases. Cytokines are synthesized and secreted by the cells associated with innate and adaptive immunity (Tables 5-7 and 5-8) in response to microbial and other antigen exposure.

The generic term, *cytokines,* has become the preferred name for this class of mediators. Because many cytokines are made by leukocytes and act on other leukocytes, they are also referred to by the imperfect but descriptive term, interleukins (ILs). As cytokines are discovered and characterized, they are assigned a number using a standard nomenclature (e.g., IL-1).

Cytokines are polypeptide products of activated cells that control a variety of cellular responses and thereby regulate the immune response. Many cytokines are released in response to specific antigens; however, they are nonspecific in the sense that their chemical structure is not determined by the stimulating antigen. Most cytokines have multiple activities and act on numerous cell types (Tables 5-9 and 5-10). Hematopoietic and lymphoid cell compartments are regulated by a complex network of interacting cytokines. The colony-stimulating factors (CSFs) and the ILs have been shown to play important roles in normal proliferation, differentiation, and activation of several hematopoietic and lymphoid lineages.

Cytokines have a variety of roles in host defense. In innate immunity, cytokines mediate early inflammatory reactions to microbial organisms and stimulate adaptive immune responses. In contrast, in adaptive immunity, cytokines stimulate proliferation and differentiation of antigen-stimulated lymphocytes and activate specialized effector cells (e.g., macrophages).

Cytokines are very potent even in minute concentrations. Their action is usually limited to affecting cells in the local area of their production, but they can have systemic effects as well.

As a group, cytokines differ molecularly but they also have common properties. Common properties include the ability to:

- Secrete cytokines in rapid bursts that have been synthesized in response to cellular activation

TABLE 5-8 Some Comparative Features of Innate and Adaptive Immunity

Feature	Innate Immunity	Adaptive Immunity
Examples	TNF-alpha, IFN-beta, IL-1, IL-12	IFN-gamma, IL-2, IL-4, IL-5
Major cell source	Macrophages, NK cells	T lymphocytes
Major physiologic function	Mediators of innate immunity and inflammation (local and systemic)	Adaptive immunity: regulation of lymphocyte growth and differentiation, activation of effector cells (macrophages, eosinophils, mast cells)
Stimuli	LPS (endotoxin), bacterial peptidoglycans, viral RNA, T-cell–derived cytokines (IFN-gamma)	Protein antigens
Quantity produced	Possibly high, detectable in serum	Usually low, usually undetectable in serum
Effects on body	Local and systemic	Usually local
Roles in disease	Systemic diseases	Local tissue injury
Inhibitors	Corticosteroids	Cyclosporine, FK-506

Source: Modified from Abbas AK, Lichtman AH, Pober JS: *Cellular and molecular immunology,* ed 4, Philadelphia, 2000, WB Saunders.

TABLE 5-9	Origin and Immunoregulatory Activity of Cytokines	

Cytokines	Origin	Prominent Biologic Activities
Interleukins		
IL-1 alpha	Macrophages, epithelial cells	Fever, T-cell activation, macrophage activation
IL-1 beta	Macrophages, epithelial cells	Fever, T-cell activation, macrophage activation
IL-1 RA	Macrophages	Binds IL-1 receptor as natural antagonist of IL-1
IL-2 (T-cell growth factor)	T cells	Proliferation and clonal expansion of activated T cells; activates cytotoxic cells; induces other lymphokines
IL-3 (multicolony colony-stimulating factor)	Activated T cells	Promotes the growth of early hematopoietic cell lines
IL-4	T cells, mast cells	Growth factor for early activation of resting B cells; induces HLA-DR molecules on B cells and macrophages; governs B cell isotype switching to IgG$_1$ and IgE; growth and differentiation of T cells, mast cells, granulocytes, megakaryocytes, and erythrocytes
IL-5	T cells, mast cells, ? B cells	Growth and differentiation-inducing factor for activated T and B cells; eosinophil differentiation and proliferation; induces class specific B cell differentiation (IgA production)
IL-6	Macrophages, mitogen activated T cells, fibroblasts	Growth and final differentiation factor for B cells; induces acute phase response; growth factor for T and B cells; T cell activation; cytolytic T cell activation factor
IL-7	Bone marrow stroma	Early T and B cell differentiation and maturation
IL-8 (NAP-1)	Monocytes, keratinocytes, fibroblasts	Chemotaxis and activation of neutrophils
IL-9	T cells	Proliferation of T cells; thymocytes; mast cells
IL-10	T cells, mast cells, ? B cells	Inhibition of cytokine synthesis in various cells; proliferation of mast cells
IL-11	Bone marrow stroma	Regulator of hematopoiesis—stimulates the production of megakaryocyte and myeloid progenitors; increases the number of Ig-secreting B lymphocytes
IL-12 (NK stimulatory factor)	B cells, macrophages	Enhances the activity of cytotoxic effector T cells; acts as a growth factor for activated NK/lymphokine-activated killer cells and for activated T cells of both the CD4+ and CD8+ subsets
IL-13	T-cells	Possesses many biologic effects similar to IL-4, its receptor is a subunit of IL-4 receptor; inhibits the proliferation of leukemic pro-B cells; does not act on T-lymphocytes
IL-14	Acts as a B-cell growth factor	Hyperproduction of this interleukin enables the progression of B-cell type non-Hodgkin's lymphoma (NHL-B); its antibodies slow down the growth of NHL-B
IL-15	T-cells	Biologically similar to IL-2; acts in many ways as synergist, particularly in LAK-cells' induction process; increases the antitumoral activities of T-killer and NK cells, and can be a chemotractant for T lymphocytes; endogenous IL-15 is a key condition for IFN-gamma synthesis
IL-16	Monocytes, CD8+, and B lymphocytes	Acts as a T-cell chemoattractant; increases the mobility of CD4+ T cells and with IL-2 promotes their activation; found in high levels in patients with stage III and IV cancers; IFN-alpha, histamine, and serotonin increase the production of IL-16
IL-17	CD4+ lymphocytes	Induces granulopoiesis via G-CSF; can reinforce the antibody-dependent tumor cell destruction; takes part in the regulation of many cytokines IL-1, IL-4, IL-6, IL-10, IL-12, IFN-gamma; histamine and serotonin increase the production of IL-17
IL-18		Acts as a synergist with IL-12 in some of their effects, especially in the induction of IFN gamma production and inhibition of angiogenesis; a high IFN-gamma production under an integrated effect of IL-18 and IL-12 suppresses tumor growth

Continued

TABLE 5-9   Origin and Immunoregulatory Activity of Cytokines—cont'd

Cytokines	Origin	Prominent Biologic Activities
Interleukins—cont'd		
IL-19	Monocytes	Lipopolysaccharides and GM-CSF stimulates synthesis of IL-19; the biologic function is similar to that of IL-10; regulates the functions of macrophages, suppresses the activities of T_H1 and T_H2; increases the synthesis of bcl-2 protein, thereby influencing apoptosis of tumor and immune cells
IL-20	Keratinocytes	Plays an important role in skin inflammations with synthesis increased in psoriasis; biologic activities similar to those of IL-10 and can stimulate the tumor growth
IL-21		Regulates hematopoiesis and immune response, influences the development of lymphocytes; similar to IL-2 and IL-15 in antitumor defense system; promotes high production of T lymphocytes, fast growth and maturation of NK cells, and fast growth of B lymphocytes
IL-22	Activated T-cells	Similar to IL-10 but does not prohibit the production of proinflammatory cytokines through monocytes in response to LPS; IL-22 is somewhat similar to IFN-alpha, beta, and gamma
IL-23		Activator of the transcription factor STAT4 (signal transducer and activator of the transcription factor-4), which acts as a stimulant on particular populations of memory T cells
IL-25	T_H2 T cells	Supports proliferation of cells in the lymphoid lineage. IL-25 has been demonstrated to be capable of amplifying allergic type inflammatory responses by its actions on other cell types in mice
Interferons		
IFN-alpha	Leukocytes	Antiviral, increased MHC class I expression
IFN-beta	Fibroblasts, epithelial cells	Antiviral, increased MHC class I expression
IFN-gamma	T cells, NK cells	Major macrophage activator; induces MHC class II molecules on many cells and can synergize with tumor necrosis factor; augments NK cell activity; antagonist to IL-4

TABLE 5-10   Immunoregulatory Activity of Other Cytokines

Factor	Target Cells	Prominent Biologic Activities
Tumor Necrosis Factor (TNF)		
TNF-alpha (cachectin)	Macrophages, NK cells	Local inflammation, endothelial activation
TNF-beta (lymphotoxin)	T cells, B cells	Killing, endothelial activation
Tumor necrosis family		
CD40 ligand	T cells, mast cells	B-cell activation, class switching
TNF Family		
CD27 ligand	T cells	Stimulates T-cell proliferation
CD30 ligand	T cells	Stimulates T- and B-cell proliferation
Chemokines		
Membrane cofactor protein (MCP-1)	Macrophages, others	Chemotactic for monocytes

Modified from Claman HN: The biology of the immune response, *JAMA* 268(20):2791, 1992; Janeway C, Travers P, *Immunobiology*, ed 3, New York, 1997, Current Biology Ltd, Garland Publishing; and Abbas AK, Lichtman AH, Pober JS: *Cellular and molecular immunology*, ed 4, Philadelphia, 2000, WB Saunders.

TABLE 5-11	Cytokine Receptor Families
Family	**Members**
Type I (hemopoietin) receptors	IL-2, IL-3, IL-4, IL-5, IL-6, IL-7, IL-9, IL-11, IL-12, IL-13, IL-15, GM-CSF, G-CSF, growth hormone, prolactin
Type II receptors	IFN-alpha, IFN-beta, IFN-gamma
Tumor necrosis factor (TNF)	TNF-alpha, LT, CD40 ligand, Fas ligand, nerve growth factor
Immunoglobulin superfamily receptors	IL-1, M-CSF, stem cell factor
Seven transmembrane alpha-helical receptors	Chemokines

From Abbas AK, Lichtman AH, JS Pober: *Cellular and molecular immunology*, ed 4, Philadelphia, 2000 WB Saunders, p. 239.

- Bind to specific membrane receptors on target cells
- Regulate receptor expression in T and B cells, which drives positive amplification or negative feedback
- Act on different cell types (pleiotropism)
- Excite the same functional effects with multiple cytokines (redundancy)
- Act close to the site of synthesis either on the same cell (autocrine action) or on a nearby cell (paracrine action)
- Influence the synthesis and actions of other cytokines

Cytokines act on other cells by bonding to cytokine receptors on the surface of cells.

Individual cytokines have characteristic functions and differ in how they transduce signals as a consequence of the binding of the cytokines. All cytokine receptors (Table 5-11) consist of one or more transmembrane proteins whose extracellular portions are responsible for cytokine binding and whose cytoplasmic portions are responsible for initiating the intracellular signaling pathways. These six pathways are:

1. Janus kinase (JAK/STAT) pathway
2. Tumor-necrosis factor (TNF) receptor signaling by TRAFs (tumor necrosis receptor-associated factor)
3. TNF receptor signaling by death domains
4. Toll receptor signaling
5. Receptor-associated tyrosine kinases
6. G-protein signaling

Receptors for different cytokines are classified into families (see Table 5-11) on the basis of conserved extracellular domain structures. Once ligand binding occurs, these receptors activate associated intracellular proteins that induce apoptosis or stimulate gene expression, or both.

Interleukins

At least 25 different ILs have been identified. A characteristic of ILs is that secreted peptides and proteins mediate local interactions between leukocytes but do not bind antigen. ILs include molecules that are made by and that act on lymphocytes.

ILs have widely overlapping functions. These molecules modulate inflammation and immunity by regulating growth, mobility, and differentiation of lymphoid cells. Each of the ILs has been shown to be a distinct molecule by gene cloning and sequencing. In addition, each IL functions through a separate receptor system.

IL-1

IL-1, formerly called lymphocyte-activating factor, is found in two forms: IL-1 alpha and IL-1 beta. IL-1 stimulates IL-2–dependent T lymphocyte proliferation, increases the expression of IL-2 receptors, and enhances the proliferation and differentiation of B lymphocytes. IL-1 serves primarily as a cofactor by activating the resting T cell and inducing the synthesis of other lymphocytes.

The principal function of IL-1 is as a mediator of the host inflammatory response to infections and other inflammatory stimuli. Biologic effects of IL-1 are similar to TNF. In low concentrations, it acts as a mediator of local inflammation; in large concentrations, it enters the bloodstream and exerts endocrine effects. IL-1 is a potent mediator at the systemic level in the acute-phase response. This cytokine induces fever, increases the synthesis of acute-phase reactants by hepatocytes, stimulates prostaglandin release, and initiates metabolic wasting (cachexia).

In addition, IL-1 is a potent mediator of inflammation, and the overproduction or chronic release of IL-1 has been implicated in the pathogenesis of arthritis, fibrosis, and toxic shock syndrome. Research into understanding the regulatory mechanisms involved in controlling IL-1 release is ongoing. Acquisition of this knowledge is important to eventually controlling chronic inflammation. The IL-1 family consists of three structurally related polypeptides. The first two are IL-1 alpha and IL-1 beta, each of which has a broad spectrum of both beneficial and harmful biologic actions; the third is IL-1-receptor antagonist, which inhibits the activities of IL-1. Among the properties of the two forms of IL-1 is the ability to induce fever, sleep, anorexia, and hypotension. IL-1 stimulates the release of pituitary hormones; increases the synthesis of collagenases, resulting in the destruction of cartilage; and stimulates the production of prostaglandins, leading to a decrease in the pain threshold. IL-1 has also been implicated in the destruction of beta cells of the islets of Langerhans, the growth of myelogenous leukemia cells, inflammation associated with arthritis and colitis, and the development of atherosclerotic plaques. IL-1 also has host defense properties.

The third member of the IL-1 family, IL-1-receptor antagonist, provides some protection against the disease-provoking effects of IL-1. It is a specific inhibitor of IL-1 activity that acts by blocking the binding of IL-1 to its cell surface receptors. This receptor antagonist may be beneficial in patients with sepsis, arthritis, and some forms of chronic myelogenous leukemia.

IL-2

IL-2, formerly called T-cell growth factor, is best known for its ability to initiate proliferation or clonal expansion of antigen-stimulated T cells. Activation of T lymphocytes by IL-1 results in the rapid expression of IL-2 receptors.

The binding of IL-2 to its receptor results in the clonal expansion of antigen-activated T cells; removal of the antigen leads to a decrease in IL-2 receptor expression, which appears to limit the clonal expansion of the T cells. IL-2 receptor (IL-2R) consists of three noncovalently associated proteins: alpha, beta, and gamma. Because antigen stimulation enhances expression of the complete IL-2R, T cells that recognize antigen are also the cells that proliferate preferentially in response to physiologic levels of IL-2 produced during adaptive immune responses. IL-2 produced by T cells on antigen recognition is responsible for the proliferation of the antigen- specific cells, promotes proliferation and differentiation of other immune cells, and potentiates apoptotic death of antigen-activated T cells.

IL-2 also dramatically enhances the cytolytic activity of a population of natural killer (NK) cells against certain tumor cells. This property has led to the much-publicized use of IL-2 in clinical trials with cancer patients. These cells are known as lymphokine-activated killer cells (LAK).

IL-3

IL-3 has a wide spectrum of activities on hematopoietic cells. This cytokine was originally known as multicolony-stimulating factor because IL-3 promotes the expansion of cells that differentiate into all known mature cell types.

The therapeutic use of recombinant IL-3 may enable stimulation of dysfunctional bone marrow under a number of conditions. IL-3 may be useful in the treatment of the cytopenias associated with viral infections, certain anemias, or after bone marrow transplantation and chemotherapy.

IL-4

IL-4 was originally isolated as B cell-stimulating factor-1, a growth factor for the early activation of resting B cells. IL-4 is known to be the major stimulus for the production of IgE antibodies and for the development of T_H2 cells from naïve CD4+ helper T cells. IL-4 is also the principal cytokine that stimulates B cell Ig heavy chain class switching to the IgE isotype. IL-4 functions as autocrine growth factor for differentiated T_H2 cells. IL-4 also antagonizes the macrophage-activating effects of interferon (IFN)-gamma and thus inhibits cell-mediated immune reactions, which may be one of the mechanisms by which T_H2 cells function as inhibitors of immune inflammation. This cytokine has the potential therapeutic application of limiting allergic reactions.

IL-5

IL-5, originally called T-cell replacing factor or B-cell growth factor-2, shares many of the same activities as IL-4. IL-5 specifically stimulates the proliferation of B cells and production of IgA antibodies. The major function of IL-5 is to activate eosinophils and serve as the link between T-cell activation and eosinophilic inflammation. Therefore the major actions of IL-5 are to stimulate the growth and differentiation of eosinophils and to activate mature eosinophils.

Because of its development-promoting activity, IL-5 alone or in combination with other ILs could be considered for the treatment of immunodeficiencies.

IL-6

IL-6 functions in both innate and adaptive immunity. It was originally called interferon (IFN)-beta-2 and B-cell-stimulating factor 2. In adaptive immunity, IL-6 stimulates the growth of B cells that have differentiated into antibody producers. IL-6 functions to induce secretion of Ig as well.

IL-6 has potent systemic effects similar to those of IL-1 and TNF (e.g., fever-inducing activity and stimulating the release of acute-phase reactants). It appears that IL-1, TNF, and IL-6 are the major factors that induce the acute-phase response, and that their overproduction may result in chronic inflammation and/or death.

IL-7

IL-7 was originally called lymphopoietin-1. IL-7 stimulates survival and expansion of immature precursors committed to the T- and B-cell lineages. Early B-cell progenitor cells respond to IL-7 until they begin to display IgM on the surface. Once IgM appears on the cell membrane, B cells become unresponsive to IL-7. IL-7 also mimics IL-2 as a growth factor for mature T cells.

IL-8

IL-8 was originally described as a monocyte-derived neutrophil chemotactic factor. IL-8 appears to be an inflammatory cytokine that is chemotactic for both neutrophils and T cells. It is a potent stimulator of neutrophils, and it activates the respiratory burst and the release of both specific and azurophilic granular contents.

IL-9

IL-9 is a potent lymphocyte growth factor. It supports the growth of some T-cell lines and of bone marrow-derived mast cell progenitors. In addition, it has been demonstrated to support growth of erythroid blast-forming units. IL-9 may play a role in autocrine growth of tumors in large-cell anaplastic lymphomas and Hodgkin's disease. Hodgkin and Reed-Sternberg cells produce IL-9 transcripts and protein and express surface-binding sites for IL-9.

IL-10

IL-10 inhibits activated macrophages. This process includes inhibition of production of IL-12 and TNF by activated macrophages, and inhibition of the expression of costimulators and class II MHC molecules on macrophages. In vitro IL-10 stimulates the proliferation of human B cells.

IL-10 may contribute to the profound immunosuppression of TNF-gamma release that occurs during kala azar resulting from *Leishmania donovani*. The ability of IL-10 to turn down cytokine synthesis provides negative feedback.

In patients with intermediate or high-grade non-Hodgkin's lymphoma, the presence of detectable serum IL-10 at diagnosis has been correlated to a significantly shorter overall and progression-free survival. Patients with stage IV disease and detectable serum IL-10 have a particularly poor prognosis (less than 4 years of survival).

IL-11

IL-11 is a recently described bone marrow, stromal-derived cytokine that appears to be a multifunctional regulator of hematopoiesis. IL-11 has been shown to synergize with IL-3 to stimulate production of megakaryocyte and myeloid progenitors and to increase the number of Ig-secreting B lymphocytes both in vivo and in vitro.

IL-11 acts in a manner similar to IL-6 on hematopoietic progenitor cells. It is known to promote differentiation of normal human B cells. IL-11 does not result in significantly increased DNA synthesis or Ig secretion of B cell alone. IL-11 promotes differentiation of human B lymphocytes only in the presence of accessory T cells and monocytes. A minor component of this effect may be through stimulation of IL-6 production by CD4+/45RA–T cells and monocytes. IL-11 might regulate malignant cells of the megakaryocytic line.

IL-11 is in clinical use to treat patients with platelet deficiencies resulting from cancer chemotherapy.

IL-12

IL-12, also known as NK cell stimulatory factor or cytotoxic lymphocytic maturation factor, enhances the activity of cytotoxic effector cells. IL-12 is the principal mediator of the early innate immune response to intracellular microbial agents and is a key inducer of cell-mediated immunity, the adaptive immune response to these agents.

IL-12 is a critical component for initiating a sequence of responses involving macrophages, NK cells, and T cells that eradicate intracellular microbial agents.

This cytokine was first identified by its ability to synergize with IL-2 in augmenting cytotoxic lymphocyte responses. Although IL-12 shares the functional properties of enhancing the cytotoxic function of NK cells and activated T cells with IL-2, it appears to act via a distinct mechanism independent of IL-2.

In addition, IL-12 is a growth factor for activated NK/LAK cells and for activated T cells of both the CD4+ and CD8+ subsets.

The biologic actions of IL-12 include:
- Stimulates the production of IFN-gamma by NK cells and T cells
- Stimulates the differentiation of CD4+ helper T cells into IFN-gamma–producing T_H1 cells
- Enhances the cytolytic functions of activated NK cells and CD8+ cytologic T cells

IL-13

IL-13 possesses many biologic effects similar to IL-4; in fact, its receptor is a subunit of IL-4 receptor. IL-13 is structurally similar to IL-4 and mimics the effects of IL-4 on nonlymphoid cells (e.g., macrophages). It appears to have less of an effect on T or B cells than does IL-4. The major action of IL-13 on macrophages is to inhibit their activation and to antagonize IFN-gamma.

IL-14

IL-14 acts as a B-cell growth factor. Hyperproduction of this IL enables the progression of B-cell type non-Hodgkin's lymphoma (NHL-B); conversely, its antibodies slow down the growth of NHL-B.

IL-15

IL-15 is biologically similar to IL-2; it acts in many ways as synergist, particularly in LAK-cell induction process. It is produced in response to viral infection and other signals that trigger innate immunity. It is homologous to IL-2. The function of IL-15 is to promote the proliferation of NK cells. It stimulates expansion of NK cells within the first few days after infections. IL-15 increases the antitumoral activities of T-killer and NK cells and can be a chemoattractant for T lymphocytes. Endogenous IL-15 is a key condition for IFN-gamma synthesis.

IL-16

IL-16 acts as a T-cell chemoattractant. It increases the mobility of CD8+ and CD4+ T cells and with IL-2 promotes their activation. It is found in B lymphocytes. High levels are found in patients with stages III and IV cancers. Histamine and serotonin increase the production of IL-16.

IL-17

IL-17 induces granulopoiesis via granulocyte (G)-CSF. It can reinforce the antibody-dependent tumor cell destruction. It takes part in the regulation of many cytokines such as IL-1, IL-4, IL-6, IL-10, IL-12, and IFN-gamma. Histamine and serotonin increase the production of IL-17. IL-17 mimics many of the proinflammatory actions of tumor necrosis factor (TNF)-alpha and TNF-beta.

IL-18

IL-18 acts as a synergist with IL-12 in some of their effects, especially in the induction of IFN-gamma production and inhibition of angiogenesis. A high IFN-gamma production under an integrated effect of IL-18 and IL-12 suppresses tumor growth. IL-18 is structurally homologous to IL-1 and signals by a similar receptor. It has a very different function from IL-1. It stimulates the production of IFN-gamma by NK cells and T cells, and it is synergistic with IL-12 in this response.

IL-19

Lipopolysaccharides and granulocyte-macrophage (GM)-CSF stimulates synthesis of IL-19. The biologic function is similar to that of IL-10. It regulates the functions of macrophages and suppresses the activities of T_H1 and T_H2. It increases the synthesis of bcl-2 protein, thereby influencing apoptosis of tumoral and immune cells.

IL-20

IL-20 plays an important role in skin inflammations. Its biologic activities are similar to those of IL-10 and can stimulate tumor growth.

IL-21

IL-21 regulates hematopoiesis and immune response and influences the development of lymphocytes. It is similar to IL-2 and IL-15 in antitumor defense system. It promotes high production of T lymphocytes, fast growth and maturation of NK-cells, and fast growth of B lymphocytes.

IL-22

IL-22 is similar to IL-10 but does not prohibit the production of proinflammatory cytokines through monocytes in response to LPS. IL-22 is somewhat similar to IFN-alpha, beta, and gamma.

IL-23

This newly discovered cytokine shares some in vivo functions with IL-12, including the activation of the transcription factor STAT4 (signal transducer and activator of the transcription factor-4). IL-23 is composed of the IL-12p40 "soluble receptor" subunit and a novel cytokine-like subunit related to IL-12p35, termed *p19.* Human and mouse IL-23 exhibit some activities similar to IL-12 but differ in their capacities to stimulate particular populations of memory T cells.

IL-25

This cytokine, also called *SF20,* is a novel secreted bone marrow stroma-derived growth factor. This factor is produced by Th2 T cells and is biologically characterized as a member of the IL-17 cytokine family. In vitro assay has revealed that SF20/IL-25 has no detectable myelopoietic activity but supports proliferation of cells in the lymphoid lineage. IL-25 has been demonstrated to be capable of amplifying allergic type inflammatory responses by its actions on other cell types in mice.

Interferons

The IFNs are a group of cytokines discovered in virally infected cultured cells. This interference with viral replication in the cells by another virus led to the name "interferons."

IFNs are one of the body's natural defensive responses to foreign components (e.g., microbes, tumors, and antigens). They may be among the most broadly active physiologic regulators, enhancing the expression of specific genes, inhibiting cell proliferation, and augmenting immune effector cells. IFNs have been demonstrated to act as antiviral agents, immunomodulators, and antineoplastic agents.

Type I IFNs mediate the early innate immune response to viral infections. They are composed of two distinct groups of proteins (IFN-alpha, IFN-beta) that are structurally quite different, but bind to the same cell surface receptor and induce similar biologic responses.

Just over a decade ago, IFN-alpha-2 produced by recombinant-DNA technology was introduced into clinical trials. IFN-alpha-2 was the first pure human protein found to have antitumor activity in the treatment of cancer. IFNs are now licensed in more than 40 countries for at least a dozen therapeutic indications of both viral and neoplastic origin. IFNs have been found to be clinically useful in diseases of diverse pathogenesis and manifestations. This includes the use of IFN-alpha for hairy cell leukemia, laryngeal and genital papillomas, Kaposi's sarcoma in acquired immunodeficiency syndrome (AIDS), and chronic viral hepatitis caused by either hepatitis B or hepatitis C virus. Inhibition of oncogene expression may account for the sustained effectiveness of IFN-alpha-2a in chronic myelogenous leukemia and other myeloproliferative syndromes. In addition, IFN-alpha-2a has been demonstrated to induce the early regression of life-threatening, corticosteroid-resistant hemangiomas of infancy. IFN-beta may have therapeutic usefulness in some stages of multiple sclerosis and for hyperlipidemias. IFN-gamma has properties distinctive from those of IFN-alpha and IFN-beta and is approved as an immunomodulatory treatment for chronic granulomatous disease (CGD). IFN-gamma decreases the frequency of bacterial infections in CGD and may be efficacious either alone or in combination in inhibiting the replication of intracellular microbial pathogens. Promising clinical results with IFNs have also been reported for basal cell carcinoma, cutaneous squamous cell carcinoma, and early human immunodeficiency virus infection. As these and

other examples illustrate, the increasing number of therapeutic applications of these proteins to diverse diseases can be expected to expand their clinical usefulness during the next decade. Future clinical uses of IFNs may emphasize combination therapy with other cytokines, chemotherapy, radiation, surgery, hyperthermia, or hormones. The diversity of the cellular effects of IFNs suggests that they may be useful in a wider range of benign and malignant neoplasms in the future.

IFN-Alpha

IFN-alpha was originally called leukocyte interferon. Because many of the IFN-alpha effects appear to be inhibitory, this protein may be an important immunosuppressive agent in controlling the immune response in a negative manner.

IFN-Beta

IFN-beta was originally called fibroblast IFN or B-cell stimulatory factor 2. Cloning of the gene for this protein revealed that a single molecule was responsible for a variety of functions. The protein was named IL-6. Some of the functional properties of IFN-beta are discussed under IL-6.

IFN-Gamma

IFN-gamma is the principal macrophage-activating cytokine and serves a critical function in innate immunity and in specific cell-mediated immunity. It stimulates expression of class I and class II MHC molecules and costimulates antigen-presenting cells, promotes the differentiation of naïve CD4+ T cells to the T_H1 subset and inhibits the proliferation of T_H2 cells. In addition, IFN-gamma acts on B cells to promote switching to certain IgG subclasses, activates neutrophils, and stimulates the cytolytic activity of NK cells. It is also antagonistic to IL-4. IFN-gamma is of most immunologic interest because of its diverse effects on the immune response. It is the ability of IFN-gamma to augment the activity of many cytokines that has resulted in clinical trials in a number of different diseases. IFN-gamma is being administered alone or in combination with other cytokines for the treatment of arthritis, cancer, and AIDS.

Tumor Necrosis Factor

TNF is the principal mediator of the acute inflammatory response to gram-negative bacteria and other infectious microbes. It is responsible for many of the systemic complications of severe infections. The TNF receptor family either stimulates gene transcription or induces apoptosis in a wide variety of cells. The gene-encoding TNF-alpha is located in the HLA region between the HLA-DR and HLA-B loci.

TNF is also called TNF-alpha for historical reasons and to distinguish it from the closely related TNF-beta (lymphotoxin). TNF-alpha and TNF-beta share similar activities. TNF also possesses many of the same activities as IL-1. However, TNF differs from IL-1 in that TNF is not able to stimulate T-cell proliferation, and IL-1 has only limited ability to lyse tumor cells.

The principal physiologic functions of TNF are:
- To stimulate the recruitment of neutrophils and monocytes to sites of infection
- To activate these cells to eradicate microbes

In low concentrations, TNF acts on leukocytes and endothelium to induce acute inflammation. At moderate concentrations TNF mediates the systemic effects of inflammation. In severe infections TNF is produced in large amounts and causes clinical and pathologic abnormalities (e.g., septic shock). When they gain access to the circulation during infection, they mediate a series of reactions that induce shock and can result in death. The syndrome, septic shock, is a complication of severe gram-negative bacterial sepsis.

The potential exists for TNF to be used as an antitumor agent. However, these cytokines are extremely potent. Therefore TNFs have the potential beneficial characteristic of destroying tumor cells, but also have the potential for lethal side effects.

Some studies suggest that the concentration of serum TNF may be predictive of the outcome of severe gram-negative infections. In addition, cerebrospinal fluid levels of tumor TNF-alpha are higher in patients with chronic progressive multiple sclerosis than in patients with stable disease, and cerebrospinal fluid levels of TNF-alpha are correlated with disease progression in chronic progressive multiple sclerosis.

TNF-beta (lymphotoxin) is also a mediator of the acute inflammatory response and provides a link between T-cell activation and inflammation. Biologic effects of TNF-beta are the same as those for TNF-alpha. TNF-beta is usually a locally acting cytokine but not a mediator of systemic injury because of the low concentrations secreted.

HEMATOPOIETIC STIMULATORS

Stem Cell Factor (c-Kit Ligand)

Stem cell factor is a cytokine (Table 5-12) that interacts with a tyrosine kinase membrane receptor, the protein product of the cellular oncogene *c-kit*. The cytokine that interacts with this receptor is called c-kit ligand or stem cell factor because it acts on immature stem cells.

Stem cell factor is believed to be needed to make bone marrow stem cells responsive to other CSFs, but it does not cause colony formation by itself. Stem cell factor may also play a role in sustaining the viability and proliferative capacity of immature T cells in the thymus and mast cells in mucosal tissues.

Colony-Stimulating Factors

A variety of CSFs such as G-CSF and GM-CSF are also made by T cells. These pathways provide a link between the lymphoid and the hematopoietic systems. For example, G-CSF and GM-CSF regulate the production of granulocytes and monocytes, thus enabling the T-cell system to promote the inflammatory response.

The biologic activity of CSF is measured by its ability to stimulate hematopoietic progenitor cells to form colonies in semisolid medium. These proteins are necessary for the survival, proliferation, and differentiation of precursor cells of the immune system.

CSFs are potentially important in the treatment of human disease. GM-CSF is being used in a number of clinical trials to increase circulating leukocytes in patients with AIDS, patients with other immunocompromised conditions (e.g., patients recovering from chemotherapy), and bone marrow transplant recipients.

Transforming Growth Factor-Beta

Like the IFNs, transforming growth factors (TGFs) were identified as products of virally transformed cells. These factors were found to induce phenotypic transformation in nonneoplastic cells and subsequently were named transforming growth factors. TGF-beta is a group of five cytokines released by many cell types, including macrophages and

TABLE 5-12	Hematopoietic Cytokines		
Cytokines	**Main Cellular Source(s)**	**Main Cellular Target(s)**	**Type of Cell Induced**
Stem cell factor (c-kit ligand)	Bone marrow stromal cells	Pluripotent stem cells	All
Granulocyte CSF (G-CSF)	Macrophages, fibroblasts, endothelial cells	Committed progenitor	Granulocytes
Monocyte CSF (M-CSF)	Macrophages, endothelial cells, bone marrow cells, fibroblasts	Committed progenitor	Monocytes
Granulocyte-monocyte CSF (GM-CSF)	T cells, macrophages, endothelial cells, fibroblasts	Immature and committed progenitors, mature macrophages	Granulocytes, monocytes, macrophage activation
IL-3 (see Table 5-9)			
IL-7 (see Table 5-9)			
IL-9 (see Table 5-9)			
IL-11 (see Table 5-9)			

Modified from Abbas AK, Lichtman AH, Pober JS: *Cellular and molecular immunology,* ed 4, Philadelphia, 2000, WB Saunders.
CSF, Colony-stimulating factor.

platelets. TGF-beta is known to be a potent inhibitor of IL-1-induced T-cell proliferation.

The principal action of TGF-beta in the immune system is to inhibit the proliferation and activation of lymphocytes and other leukocytes. It inhibits the proliferation and differentiation of T cells and the activation of macrophages. In mice, it stimulates the production of IgA. TGFs are important in inflammation, tumor defense, and cell growth, including wound healing. The ability of TGF-beta to augment certain aspects of the immune response while suppressing others suggests that this cytokine may play an important role in chronic inflammatory disorders.

Chemokines

Chemokines are a large family of structurally homologous cytokines that stimulate transendothelial leukocyte movement from the blood to tissue site of infection and regulate the migration of polymorphonuclear leukocytes and mononuclear leukocytes within tissues (see Chapter 3). The word *chemokine* is a contraction of chemotactic cytokine.

About 50 different chemokines have been identified. The group includes: IL-8, platelet factor-4, membrane cofactor protein, CD46 (MCP-1), MIP-1-alpha, MIP-1-beta, and RANTES. Different chemokines act on different cells (e.g., CXC chemokine IL-8 recruits neutrophils preferentially and CC chemokine eotaxin recruits eosinophils). Chemokines appear to control the phased arrival of different cell populations at sites of inflammation.

Although chemokines were discovered based on their activities as a chemoattractant, they also are responsible for many important functions in the immune and other body systems. Chemokines cause rapid shape changes in leukocytes, which results in pseudopod formation. They stimulate alternating polymerization and depolymerization of actin filaments, leading to the movement of leukocytes and their migration toward the chemical gradient of the cytokines. Some of the other functions of various chemokines include:

- Increasing the affinity of leukocyte integrins for their ligands on endothelium (e.g., ICAM-1, ICAM-2, VCAM-1)
- Regulating the traffic of lymphocytes and other leukocytes through peripheral lymphoid tissues
- Maintaining normal migration of immune cells into lymphoid organs, or other specialized cells, to particular sites

Assessment of Cytokines

Traditional methods for assessment of cytokines include:
- Bioassays
- Enzyme-linked immunosorbent assay (ELISA)
- Intracellular staining
- Ribonuclease protection assay
- Polymerase chain reaction (PCR)

Some new methods of measurement include:
- Multiplexed assay using the FlowMetrix-quantify multiple cytokines simultaneously
- Intracellular staining using flow cytometry
- Cord blood mononuclear cells stimulated by allergens (celELISA)
- Real-time PCR for lymph nodes or spleen
- Eli spot assays
- Enhanced immunoassays for cytokines
- Biotrak assay-high sensitivity ELISA

ACUTE-PHASE PROTEINS

Overview of Acute-Phase Proteins

The acute phase response is an innate body defense. This response is a nonspecific indicator of an inflammatory process. A group of glycoproteins associated with the response are collectively called acute-phase proteins or acute-phase reactants. The various acute phase proteins rise at different rates and in varying levels in response to tissue injury (e.g., inflammation, infection, malignant neoplasia, various diseases or disorders, trauma, surgical procedures, or a drug response). The increased synthesis of these proteins takes place shortly after a trauma and is initiated and sustained by proinflammatory cytokines.

The main biologic sign of inflammation is an increase in the ESR. In addition to the ESR, measurement of the plasma concentration of acute-phase reactants is, in most circumstances, a good indicator of local inflammatory activity and tissue damage. There are more than 20 acute-phase proteins that have a definable role in inflammation (Box 5-2). These reactants constitute the majority of the serum glycoproteins (Table 5-13). Acute-phase reactants include C-reactive protein (CRP), inflammatory mediators (e.g., complement components C3 and C4), fibrinogen, transport proteins such as haptoglobin, inhibitors (e.g., alpha 1-antitrypsin), and alpha 1-acid glycoprotein. Profiles of inflammatory changes yield detailed information but rarely provide major evidence in the quest of a diagnosis or choice of a treatment.

The ESR serves first and foremost to detect an inflammatory syndrome. CRP is an acute-phase reactant produced by the liver under the control of IL-6. The CRP is a parameter of inflammatory activity. Serum concentrations can increase 1000-fold with an acute inflammatory reaction. Persistent increases in CRP can also occur in chronic inflammatory disorders (e.g., autoimmune disease or malignancy).

CRP is prominent among the acute-phase proteins because its changes show a great sensitivity. Changes in CRP are independent of those of ESR and parallel the inflammatory process. CRP is a direct and quantitative measure of the acute-phase reaction and, as a result of its fast kinetics, provides adequate information of the actual clinical situation. In contrast, the ESR is an indirect measure of the acute-phase

---

Box 5-2	Major Applications of Acute-Phase Protein Measurements

Monitoring the progress of diagnosed disease activity

Assessing response to therapy in inflammatory diseases (e.g., rheumatoid arthritis, juvenile chronic arthritis, ankylosing spondylitis, Reiter's syndrome, psoriatic arthropathy, vasculitis, and rheumatic fever)

Detection of complications of a known disease (e.g., immune complex deposition, postsurgical infection)

reaction. It reacts much slower to changes of inflammatory activity and is influenced by a number of other factors. The ESR can be falsely normal in conditions such as polyglobulinemia, cryoglobulinemia, and hemoglobinopathy. It may also be spuriously high in the absence of inflammation in patients with anemia or hypergammaglobulinemia.

Synthesis and Catabolism of Acute-Phase Proteins

All of the acute-phase proteins are synthesized rapidly in response to tissue injury. The elevation is twofold to fivefold in certain disease states. In addition, strenuous exercise triggers an inflammatory response having some similarity to the response occurring in sepsis. Indices of the inflammatory response—especially to exercise—include leukocytosis, release of inflammatory mediators and acute-phase reactants, tissue damage, priming of various white blood cell lines, production of free radicals, activation of complement, coagulation, and fibrinolytic cascades.

Acute-phase proteins have different kinetics of variation and various degrees of increase. Some, the so-called "negative" acute-phase proteins, actually decrease, possibly resulting from a loss of protein from the vascular space. In addition, acute-phase proteins can be modified by causes other than inflammation (e.g., low fibrinogen in intravascular coagulation, very low haptoglobin in hemolysis, raised alpha 1-acid glycoprotein [orosomucoid] in renal insufficiency and elevated transferrin in iron deficiency). In addition, liver insufficiency or leakage through the kidney or gut lesions can lower these reactants.

The rate of change and peak concentration of separate acute-phase reactants vary with the component and the clinical situation. In acute inflammation, CRP and alpha 1-antichymotrypsin levels become elevated within the first 12 hours. The complement components, C3 and C4, and ceruloplasmin do not rise for several days.

Acute-phase proteins do not always change in parallel. This mismatch in acute-phase protein levels is most commonly the result of increased catabolism and elimination from the circulation of certain proteins. Differences may also be caused by discrepancies in rates of synthesis. Most acute-phase proteins have half-lives of 2 to 4 days, but CRP has a half-life of 5 to 7 hours. For this reason, CRP falls much more rapidly than the other acute-phase proteins when the patient recovers.

C-Reactive Protein

Traditionally CRP has been used clinically for monitoring infection, autoimmune disorders, and more recently healing after a myocardial infarction. Levels of CRP parallel the course of the inflammatory response and return to lower, undetectable levels as the inflammation subsides. CRP demonstrates a large incremental change, with as much as a 100-fold increase in concentration in acute inflammation, and is the fastest responding and most sensitive indicator of acute inflammation. CRP increases faster than the ESR in responding to inflammation, whereas the leukocyte count may remain within normal limits despite infection. An elevated CRP can signal infection many hours before it can be confirmed by culture results; therefore treatment can be prompt. Because of these characteristics, CRP is the method of choice for screening for inflammatory and malignant organic diseases and monitoring therapy in inflammatory diseases.

Elevations of CRP occur in nearly 70 disease states, including septicemia and meningitis in neonates, infections in immunosuppressed patients, burns complicated by infection, serious postoperative infections, myocardial infarction, malignant tumors, and rheumatic disease. Measurement of CRP may add to the diagnostic procedure in selected cases (e.g., in the differentiation between a bacterial and a viral infection). An extremely elevated CRP (procedure described later in this chapter) is suggestive of a possible bacterial infection. In general, the CRP is advocated as an indicator of bacterial infection in at-risk patients in whom the clinical assessment of infection is difficult to make, but a lack of specificity rules out CRP as a definitive diagnostic tool.

CRP levels rise after tissue injury or surgery. In uncomplicated cases the level of CRP peaks about 2 days after surgery and gradually returns to normal levels within 7 to 10 days. If the CRP level is persistently elevated or returns to an increased level, it can be suggestive of underlying sepsis preceding clinical signs and symptoms and should alert the clinician to postoperative complications.

TABLE 5-13	Examples of Clinically Useful Acute-Phase Proteins		
Protein	Normal Concentration (g/L)	Concentration in Acute Inflammation (g/L)	Response Time (Hours)
C-reactive protein	0.0008-0.004	0.4	6-10
Alpha$_1$-antichymotrypsin	0.3-0.6	3.0	10
Alpha$_1$-antitrypsin	2.0-4.0	7.0	24
Orosomucoid	0.5-1.4	3.0	24
Haptoglobin	1.0-3.0	6.0	24
Fibrinogen	2.0-4.5	10.0	24
C3	0.55-1.2	3.0	48-72
C4	0.2-0.5	1.0	48-72
Ceruloplasmin	0.15-0.6	2.0	48-72

In clinical practice CRP is particularly useful when serial measurements are performed. The course of the CRP level may be useful for monitoring the effect of treatment and for early detection of postoperative complications or intercurrent infections. In rheumatoid arthritis CRP reflects both short- and long-term disease activity. Monitoring of CRP levels allows for early prediction of response to a particular drug—often several months before clinical and radiologic confirmation is possible. In disorders such as rheumatoid arthritis, CRP can be used to assess the effect of antiinflammatory drugs (e.g., aspirin) and the nature of their action. Aspirin-like drugs do not suppress acute-phase proteins in inflammation. This permits a patient to have optimal therapy in the shortest possible time and minimizes ongoing inflammation and joint damage. Assessment of CRP is also valuable in monitoring therapy and disease activity in other arthritides. Rheumatic fever and Crohn's disease can also be monitored by CRP. In addition, CRP assessment has been found to enhance the value of traditional enzyme measurements in myocardial infarction.

In a number of chronic inflammatory diseases, however, CRP is an unreliable indicator. CRP values may be normal when other acute-phase proteins are altered in disorders such as SLE, dermatomyositis, and ulcerative colitis. SLE shows little or no CRP response despite apparently active inflammation.

Both C-reactive protein and low-density lipoprotein (LDL) cholesterol are known to be elevated in persons at risk for cardiovascular disease. Newly published research (Ridker and colleagues) suggests that the level of CRP is a stronger predictor of cardiovascular events than the LDL cholesterol, an established benchmark of cardiovascular risk.

Case Study

Signs and Symptoms

A 39-year-old woman was admitted for a cholecystectomy. She had a history of chronic cholecystitis; recent x-ray studies revealed stones in the gallbladder and a large stone in the biliary duct (Figure 5-3). During surgery a large stone was removed from the duct, and a cholangiogram was taken in the operating room. It showed no further obstructions of the hepatic or common bile ducts.

The patient became febrile 1 day after surgery. A 48-hour postoperative complete blood count (CBC) and CRP were ordered (Figure 5-4). On the seventh postoperative day, she had abdominal pain and began vomiting. A CBC, ESR, CRP, and blood culture were ordered at that time. The patient was started on a broad-spectrum antibiotic and discharged on the thirteenth hospital day.

Laboratory Data

At 48 hours after surgery, the CBC was within normal limits and the CRP was 11 g/L. A repeat CRP on the sixth day after surgery was 7 g/L.

Results after the episode of abdominal pain showed a normal CBC and ESR and a CRP value of 15 g/L. The blood culture was positive for *Pseudomonas* sp.

Questions

1. Which test was the most rapid and sensitive indicator of infection?
2. Is the CRP diagnostic?
3. Why was the CRP elevated immediately after surgery?

Discussion

1. The CRP was the most sensitive indicator of infection and was consistent with the patient's febrile state. Neither the white blood count nor the ESR was elevated.
2. No, the CRP is suggestive of inflammation and/or infection, but it is not diagnostic. The growth of *Pseudomonas* sp. in the blood culture was diagnostic of sepsis.
3. The CRP was elevated after surgery because any tissue trauma will cause an elevation. The level of acute-phase proteins such as CRP should decline within a few days after surgery.

Diagnosis

Postoperative Infection

The Significance of Other Acute-Phase Reactants

Alpha 1-antitrypsin is an acute-phase protein that increases in acute inflammatory reactions. Generalized vasculitis, such as occurs in immune complex disease, may result in inappropriately low levels of alpha 1-antitrypsin, probably resulting from increased elimination of complexes with leukocyte lysosomal enzymes.

Defects in the complement components C3a and C5a and the opsonin C3b result in serious infections. In addition, immune complex disease and gram-negative bacteremia result in low levels of complement components, particularly C3 and C4, because the components are consumed during complement activation. Acute inflammation leads to normal or slightly elevated levels. If both disorders are present, complement consumption may be masked, making it deceptive to use complement measurement as the only index of immune complex deposition in disease. The detection of complement breakdown products is more useful than the measurement of total complement component concentrations. It is more desirable to measure C3 breakdown products than total C3 in conditions such as peritonitis or pancreatitis.

Lymphomas may result in a marked increase in C1 esterase inhibitor with little other change.

Ceruloplasmin, often measured as serum copper, is used to monitor Hodgkin's disease. Increases are considered to be a specific indication of relapse. Although it has not been definitely established, ceruloplasmin monitoring may provide similar information in non-Hodgkin's lymphoma.

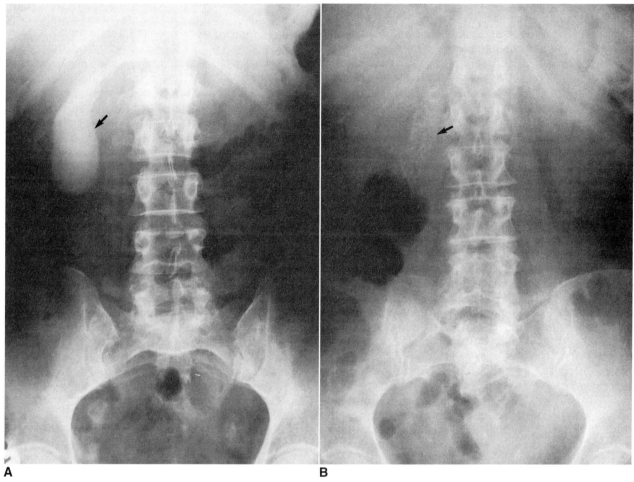

Figure 5-3 **A,** The arrow points to a normal gallbladder (contrast dye x-ray). **B,** The arrow points to a gallbladder filled with stones (contrast dye x-ray).

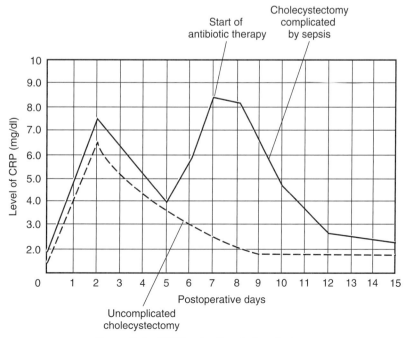

Figure 5-4 CRP levels after cholecystectomy.

Acute-Phase Reactant Assessment Methods

Inflammation almost always follows acute tissue damage. Diagnostic categories of acute inflammation can include bacterial causes and nonbacterial causes such as trauma, chronic inflammation, or viral disease. Many laboratory tests have been advocated for early diagnosis of acute inflammation: total white blood cell count (including the absolute count and the percentage of band and segmented neutrophils as determined by a 100-cell differential count on a peripheral blood smear), acute-phase proteins, and the ESR.

The ESR, or sedrate, is a nonspecific indicator of disease with increased sedimentation of erythrocytes seen in acute and chronic inflammation and malignancies. Although this procedure is nonspecific, it is one of the most frequently performed laboratory tests.

In addition to these hematologic tests, several tests are of direct value in immunologic testing. These procedures include a simple phagocytic cell function test and the determination of CRP.

C-Reactive Protein Rapid Latex Agglutination Test*

Principle

The CRP agglutination test is based on the reaction between patient serum containing CRP as the antigen and the corresponding antihuman (CRP) antibody coated to the treated surface of latex particles. The coated particles enhance the detection of an agglutination reaction when antigen is present in the serum being tested. The clinical applications of CRP evaluation include detecting inflammatory diseases, particularly infections. It is also a useful indicator in screening for organic disease, both inflammatory and malignant disease, and in monitoring therapy in inflammatory diseases. Because CRP is more rapidly synthesized than other acute-phase proteins, assays of CRP are the measurement of choice in suspected inflammatory conditions.

Specimen Collection and Preparation

No special preparation of the patient is required before specimen collection. The patient must be positively identified when the specimen is collected, and the specimen should be labeled at the bedside. Specimen labels shall include the patient's full name, the date, the patient's hospital identification number, and the phlebotomist's initials.

Blood should be drawn by an aseptic technique. A minimum of 2 mL of clotted blood (red-top evacuated tube) is required. The specimen should be centrifuged promptly and an aliquot of serum removed. Lipemia, hemolysis, or contamination with bacteria render a specimen unsuitable for testing. Although icteric and turbid specimens have given valid results, fresh non-heat–inactivated serum is recommended for use in the test.

If the test cannot be performed immediately, the specimen should be refrigerated (2° to 8° C) for no longer than 24 hours. If additional delay occurs, the serum should be frozen at –20° C or below. Frozen serum should be thawed rapidly at 37° C. Repeat freezing and thawing must be avoided. If the specimen is turbid on thawing, it should be centrifuged to clear it before use.

Preliminary Specimen Preparation

Serum must be at room temperature. Prepare a 1:5 dilution of patient serum by pipetting 0.1 mL of serum into a test tube and adding 0.4 mL of the commercially prepared glycine-saline buffer diluent. Mix the contents thoroughly.

Reagents, Supplies, and Equipment

Materials provided in IMMUNEX kit: latex reagent, concentrated diluent 20×, positive control, negative control, glass slide.

Materials required but not provided in kit: stirrers, conventional test tubes, distilled water, serologic pipettes.

Reagents

IMMUNEX CRP Latex Reagent (latex particles sensitized with antihuman CRP [sheep]); contains buffer and preservative; sodium azide 0.1%

NOTE: Store at 2° to 8° C. Shake gently and thoroughly before use.

Do not freeze CRP latex reagent. Properly stored reagent is stable until expiration date indicated on the label. Reagent that does not produce appropriate quality control results should be discarded after verification by repeat testing.

Concentrated diluent (glycine-saline buffer in kit); contains preservative sodium azide 2%. Prepare a 1:20 dilution of the concentrated diluent by mixing the contents of the concentrated diluent vial with 190 mL of distilled water.

NOTE: Store the prepared diluent at 2° to 8° C. Properly stored reagent is stable until expiration date indicated on the label. Reagent that does not produce appropriate quality control results should be discarded after verification by repeat testing. Discard if contaminated (i.e., evidence of cloudiness or particulate material in solution).

Supplies and Equipment

Capillary pipettes
Applicator sticks
Glass slide (in kit) (Clean only with distilled water; DO NOT USE detergent.)
Stopwatch or timer
12 × 75-mm test tubes
Serologic pipettes (1 mL graduated) and safety pipetter
Calibrated pipetter (optional)

---

*Source: CRP Wampole Laboratories, Cranbury, NJ.

Quality Control

Positive Control Serum (Human)

Provided in kit

Contains buffer, stabilizer and preservative, sodium azide 0.1%

Store at 2° to 8° C

NOTE: Failure to observe a positive reaction with this serum is indicative of deterioration of the latex reagent and/or positive control.

Negative Control Serum (Human)

Provided in kit

Contains buffer, stabilizer and preservative, sodium azide 0.1%

Store at 2° to 8° C.

NOTE: A smooth or slightly granular reaction must be observed with the negative control. If agglutination is exhibited with this control, the test should be repeated. If repeat testing produces the same results, the reagents should be replaced.

A positive and a negative control must be tested with each unknown patient specimen.

CAUTION: Because the control sera are derived from human sources, they should be handled at Biosafety Level 2 in the same manner as clinical serum specimens (see Universal Blood and Body Fluid Precautions in Chapter 6).

Procedure

NOTE: All reagents and specimens must be at room temperature before testing.

Reagent Check Test

1. Place one drop of POSITIVE CONTROL on a section of the slide and 1 drop of NEGATIVE CONTROL on another section.
2. Test each control according to "procedure" beginning with step 4.
3. Observe results immediately at 2 minutes.
4. The POSITIVE CONTROL must show agglutination, whereas the NEGATIVE CONTROL should appear uniformly turbid.

Procedure

1. Specimens should be tested undiluted and diluted 1:10 with the prepared DILUENT.
2. Place 1 drop (~50 µL) of undiluted specimen into one of the rings on the slide and 1 drop (~50 µL) of the diluted 1:10 specimen into another ring.
3. Place 1 drop each of the POSITIVE and NEGATIVE CONTROLS into two more rings on the slide.
4. Resuspend the CRP latex reagent by gently mixing until the suspension is homogeneous. Using the dropper provided, add 1 drop of the CRP latex reagent to each serum specimen and to each control.
5. Using separate applicator sticks, mix each specimen and each control thoroughly. The contents of the mixtures should be spread evenly over the entire area of their respective divisions on the slide.

6. Tilt the slide back and forth, slowly and evenly 8 to 10 times per minute, for 2 minutes. Place the slide on a flat surface and observe immediately for macroscopic agglutination using a direct light source.
   WARNING: The latex reagent, controls, and buffer contain sodium azide as a preservative. Sodium azide may react with lead and copper plumbing to form highly explosive metal azides. On disposal, flush with a large volume of water to prevent azide buildup.

Reporting Results

In patients who are free of inflammation and/or tissue necrosis, CRP is absent from the serum or present in concentrations below 0.5 mg/dl. Reference range mean values are 0.01 mg/dL in newborns and <0.05 mg/dL in adult males and nonpregnant females.

Positive Reaction

Agglutination of the latex suspension is a positive result. A positive reaction is reported when either the undiluted or 1:5 diluted specimen demonstrates agglutination or when both exhibit agglutination.

Negative Reaction

The absence of visible agglutination and the presence of opaque fluid constitute a negative reaction. A negative reaction is reported only when both the undiluted and 1:5 diluted specimen exhibit no visible agglutination.

Procedure Notes

Specimen collection and handling are important to the quality of the test. Strict adherence must be paid to technique, with a special emphasis on drop size, complete mixing, reaction time, and temperature of reagents.

The strength of a positive reaction may be graded as follows:

1+ Very small clumping with an opaque fluid background

2+ Small clumping with a slightly opaque fluid background

3+ Moderate clumping with a fairly clear fluid background

4+ Large clumping with a clear fluid background

Sources of Error

False-positive results may be observed if serum specimens are lipemic, hemolyzed, or heavily contaminated with bacteria. If the reaction time is longer than 2 minutes, a false-positive result may also be produced from a drying effect.

False-negative results may be observed in undiluted serum specimens because of high levels of CRP (antigen excess). A 1:5 dilution of serum is also tested for this reason.

Clinical Applications

Usually with the onset of a substantial inflammatory event such as infection, myocardial infarction, or surgery, the CRP level increases very significantly (>10-fold) above the reference range values for healthy individuals.

The test is clinically useful in early detection of inflammatory diseases particularly infections, as an indicator in screening for organic diseases, and in monitoring patient progress.

Limitations

Because the latex slide agglutination test is a qualitative and semiquantitative procedure, other methods such as nephelometry should be used for quantitative determination of the level of CRP when indicated. The strength of the agglutination reaction is not always indicative of the CRP concentration. Weak reactions may be produced in samples with either elevated or low CRP values. Results may vary depending on the condition of a patient.

This 2-minute slide latex agglutination test has a detection level of 1 $\pm$ mg CRP/dl; therefore patients with CRP values of <1 mg/dl CRP may be undetected. The sensitivity of the procedure has been assessed at 93%.

CHAPTER HIGHLIGHTS

The complement system is a heat-labile series of 18 plasma proteins, many of which are enzymes or proteinases. Complement plays a major role in the immune system as a potent mediator of inflammation. Normally, complement components are present in the circulation in an inactive form.

Complement is composed of three interrelated enzyme cascades: the classic, the alternative, and the mannose-lectin binding pathways. The classic pathway is initiated by the complexing of antigen to its specific antibody, either IgG or IgM, and is the primary amplifier of the biologic effects of humoral immunity. The alternative pathway is activated by contact with a foreign surface such as the polysaccharide coating of a microorganism, and it amplifies nonimmune defense against microbial infection and other biologic alterations. Mannose-binding lectin is a member of a family of calcium-dependent lectins and is homologous in structure to C1q.

Complement levels may be abnormal in certain disease states. Increased complement levels are often associated with inflammatory conditions, trauma, or acute illness. Separate complement components (e.g., C3) are acute-phase proteins. These elevations, however, are common and nonspecific. In contrast, deficiencies of complement account for a small percentage of primary immunodeficiencies, but depression of complement levels frequently coexists with SLE and other disorders associated with an immunopathologic process. A deficiency of mannose-binding lectin is due to one of three point mutations in the gene for mannose-binding lectin, each of which reduces levels of the lectin. The biologic functions of the complement system fall into two general categories: cell lysis by the MAC or biologic effects of proteolytic fragments of complement.

During immune complex reactions, certain complement proteins become physically bound to the tissue in which the immunologic reaction is occurring. These proteins can be demonstrated in tissue by appropriate immunopathologic stains. The most frequent evaluation of complement, however, is by serum/plasma assay. Complement components (i.e., C3 and C4) can be assessed by nephelometry. These assays are useful in diagnosis and monitoring of patients.

OTHER SOLUBLE MEDIATORS OF THE IMMUNE RESPONSE

Cytokines are a family of proteins that are synthesized and secreted by the cells associated with innate and adaptive immunity in response to microbial and other antigen exposure. As cytokines are discovered and characterized, they are assigned a number using a standard nomenclature (i.e., IL-1 through IL-22). Many cytokines are released in response to specific antigens; however, they are nonspecific in the sense that their chemical structure is not determined by the stimulating antigen. Most cytokines have multiple activities and act on numerous cell types. The CSFs and ILs have been shown to play important roles in normal proliferation, differentiation, and activation of several hematopoietic and lymphoid lineages. Cytokines also have a variety of roles in host defense. In innate immunity, cytokines mediate early inflammatory reactions to microbial organisms and stimulate adaptive immune responses. In contrast, in adaptive immunity, cytokines stimulate proliferation and differentiation of antigen-stimulated lymphocytes and activate specialized effector cells (e.g., macrophages).

The interferons are a group of cytokines discovered in virally infected cultured cells. IFNs are one of the body's natural defensive responses to foreign components (e.g., microbes, tumors, and antigens). They may be among the most broadly active physiologic regulators, enhancing the expression of specific genes, inhibiting cell proliferation, and augmenting immune effector cells. IFNs have been demonstrated to act as antiviral agents, immunomodulators, and antineoplastic agents.

Tumor necrosis factor is the principal mediator of the acute inflammatory response to gram-negative bacteria and other infectious microbes. It is responsible for many of the systemic complication of severe infections. TNF is also called TNF-alpha for historical reasons and to distinguish it from the closely related TNF-beta (lymphotoxin).

Hematopoietic stimulators include stem cell factor, a cytokine that acts on immature stem cells. Stem cell factor is believed to be needed to make bone marrow stem cells responsive to other CSFs, but it does not cause colony formation by itself. A variety of CSFs such as granulocyte CSF and granulocyte-monocyte CSF are also made by T cells. These pathways provide a link between the lymphoid and the hematopoietic systems.

Like the IFNs, transforming growth factors were identified as products of virally transformed cells. TGF-beta is a group of five cytokines released by many cell types, including macrophages and platelets. TGF-beta is known to be a potent inhibitor of IL-1 induced T-cell proliferation.

Migratory inhibitory factor was the first cytokine activity to be described. MIF is a T-cell derived activity that immobilizes macrophage migration. This effect may cause phagocytes to be retained and accumulate at sites of inflammation.

Chemokines are a large family of structurally homologous cytokines that stimulate transendothelial leukocyte movement from the blood to tissue site of infection and regulate the migration of polymorphonuclear leukocytes and mononuclear leukocytes within tissues. Chemokines appear to control the phased arrival of different cell populations at sites of inflammation.

ACUTE-PHASE PROTEINS

The acute-phase response is an innate body defense. This response is a nonspecific indicator of an inflammatory process. Various acute-phase proteins rise at different rates and in varying levels in response to tissue injury (e.g., inflammation, infection, malignant neoplasia, various diseases or disorders, trauma, surgical procedures, drug response). Increased synthesis of these proteins takes place shortly after a trauma and is initiated and sustained by proinflammatory cytokines. Acute-phase proteins have different kinetics of variation and various degrees of increase. Some, the so-called "negative" acute-phase proteins, actually decrease, possibly resulting from a loss of protein from the vascular space.

C-REACTIVE PROTEIN

Traditionally CRP has been used clinically for monitoring infection, autoimmune disorders, and more recently healing after a myocardial infarction. Levels of CRP parallel the course of the inflammatory response and return to lower, undetectable levels as the inflammation subsides. CRP demonstrates a large incremental change, with as much as a 100-fold increase in concentration in acute inflammation, and is the fastest responding and most sensitive indicator of acute inflammation.

REVIEW QUESTIONS

1. The complement system is
   A. a heat-labile series of plasma proteins
   B. composed of many proteinases
   C. composed of three interrelated pathways
   D. all of the above

2. All of the below are complement-controlling proteins except
   A. C1 (INH)
   B. factor I
   C. factor H
   D. C3

3. Various cell types express surface membrane glycoproteins that react with one or more of the fragments of

   _____ produced during complement activation and degradation.
   A. C1
   B. C3
   C. C5
   D. C8

4. All of the following result from complement activation except
   A. decreased cell susceptibility to phagocytosis
   B. blood vessel dilation and increased vascular permeability
   C. production of inflammatory mediators
   D. cytolysis or hemolysis

Questions 5-8. Complete the following activation sequence of the classic complement pathway: C1-C_(5)-C_ _(6)-_ _ -C3-_C(7) _-C6-C7- C_(8) _ _-C9

   A. 2
   B. 4
   C. 5
   D. 8

9. Which complement component is present in the greatest quantity in plasma?
   A. 2
   B. 3
   C. 4
   D. 8

Questions 10-12. Arrange the three stages of the classic complement pathway in their correct sequence.

10. _____

11. _____

12. _____

   A. enzymatic activation
   B. membrane attack
   C. recognition

13. Fixation of the C1 complement component is related to each of the following factors except
   A. molecular weight of the antibody
   B. the presence of IgM antibody
   C. the presence of most IgG subclasses
   D. spatial constraints

14. At which stage does the complement system reach its full amplitude?
   A. C1q, C1r, C1s complex
   B. C2
   C. C3
   D. C4

15. Which of the following is not a component of the membrane attack complex?
   A. C3b
   B. C6
   C. C7
   D. C8

16. The final steps (C8 and C9) in complement activation lead to
    A. cell lysis
    B. phagocytosis
    C. immune opsonin adherence
    D. virus neutralization

Questions 17-20. Select the appropriate pathway response.

17. activated by antigen-antibody complexes

18. generates a C3 convertase

19. activated by microbial and mammalian cell surfaces

20. terminates in a membrane attack complex
    A. classic pathway
    B. alternate pathway
    C. both A and B

21. The alternate complement pathway is/can be
    A. initiated by the formation of antigen-antibody reactions
    B. predominantly a nonantibody-initiated pathway
    C. activated by factors such as endotoxins
    D. both B and C.

22. Which of the following conditions can be associated with hypercomplementemia?
    A. myocardial infarction
    B. systemic lupus erythematosus
    C. glomerulonephritis
    D. subacute bacterial endocarditis

Questions 23-26. Match the following complement deficiency states in humans with their respective deficient components. (Use an answer only once.)

23. _____ C2

24. _____ C5

25. _____ C6

26. _____ C7

    A. Neisseria infections
    B. Leiner's disease
    C. Raynaud's phenomenon
    D. recurrent pyogenic infections

27. A (the) nonspecific component(s) of the immune system is (are)
    A. complement
    B. T cells
    D. both A and B

Questions 28-31. Match the following.

28. _____ interleukin-1 (IL-1)

29. _____ interleukin-2 (IL-2)

30. _____ interleukin-3 (IL-3)

31. _____ interleukin-5 (IL-5)

    A. T-cell growth factor
    B. lymphocyte-activating factor
    C. B cell growth factor 2
    D. multicolony-stimulating factor

Questions 32-35. Match the following.

32. _____ interleukin-6 (IL-6)

33. _____ interleukin-7 (IL-7)

34. _____ interleukin-8 (IL-8)

35. _____ interleukin-12 (IL-12)

    A. NK cell stimulatory factor
    B. monocyte-derived neutrophil chemotactic factor
    C. interferon beta-2
    D. lymphopoietin-1

Questions 36-39. Match the following.

36. _____ interleukin-1 (IL-1)

37. _____ interleukin-2 (IL-2)

38. _____ interleukin-3 (IL-3)

39. _____ interleukin-4 (IL-4)

    A. enhances cytolytic activity of lymphokine-activated killer cells (LAK)
    B. potent mediator in acute-phase response
    C. stimulates hematopoietic cells
    D. enhances production of IgG and inhibits production of IgE by activated B cells

Questions 40-43. Match the following.

40. _____ interleukin-5 (IL-5)

41. _____ interleukin-6 (IL-6)

42. _____ interleukin-7 (IL-7)

43. _____ interleukin-8 (IL-8)

    A. induction of secretion of Ig
    B. inflammatory cytokine
    C. stimulates early B-cell progenitor cells
    D. shares many activities with IL-4

Questions 44-47. Match the following.

44. _____ interleukin-9 (IL-9)

45. _____ interleukin-10 (IL-10)

46. _____ interleukin-11 (IL-11)

47. _____ interleukin-12 (IL-12)

    A. inhibits cytokine synthesis
    B. increases the number of IgG-secreting B lympho-cytes
    C. stimulates proliferation of T cells and mast cells
    D. enhances the activity of cytotoxic effector T cells

Questions 48-51. Match the following.

48. _____ interleukin-13

49. _____ interleukin-14

50. _____ interleukin-15

51. _____ interleukin-16

    A. inhibits activation of macrophages
    B. promotes proliferation of NK cells
    C. acts as a T-cell chemoattractant
    D. acts as a B-cell growth factor

Questions 52-55. Match the following.

52. _____ interleukin-17

53. _____ interleukin-18

54. _____ interleukin-19

55. _____ interleukin-20

    A. acts as a synergist with IL-12
    B. suppresses activities of TH1 and TH2
    C. associated with skin inflammations
    D. induces granulopoiesis

Questions 56 and 57. Match the following:

56. _____ interleukin 21

57. _____ interleukin 22

58. _____ interleukin 23

59. _____ interleukin 25

    A. promotes increased production of T cells
    B. somewhat similar to IFN-alpha, IFN-beta, and IFN-gamma
    C. also called SF20
    D. shares some in vivo functions with IL-12

Questions 60-63. Indicate true statements with the letter "A," and false statements with the letter "B."

60. _____ Cytokines secreted by lymphocytes are also called lymphokines.

61. _____ Cytokines are polypeptide products of activated cells.

62. _____ Cytokines are released only in response to specific antigens.

63. _____ Most cytokines have multiple activities and act on numerous cell types.

Questions 64-67. Match each term to its appropriate description. (Use each answer only once.)

64. _____ interleukins

65. _____ interferons

66. _____ tumor necrosis factor

67. _____ colony-stimulating factors

    A. unable to stimulate T cell proliferation
    B. act(s) between leukocytes
    C. discovered in virally infected cells
    D. provide(s) a link between the lymphoid hematopoi-etic system

68. Transforming growth factors:
    A. are products of virally transformed cells
    B. in their beta form, can be a potent inhibitor of IL-1 induced T-cell proliferation
    C. are important in inflammation, tumor defense, and cell growth
    D. all of the above

69. An activity associated with interferon is
    A. enhances phagocytosis
    B. enhances expression of specific genes
    C. promotes complement-mediated cytolysis
    D. retards bacterial multiplication

70. Tumor necrosis factor (TNF) differs from IL-1 in that it is not able to
    A. mediate an acute inflammatory reaction
    B. increase the expression of IL-2 receptors
    C. enhance the proliferation and differentiation of B lymphocytes
    D. stimulate T-cell proliferation

Questions 71-73. Match the following.

71. _____ tumor necrosis factor

72. _____ colony-stimulating factors

73. _____ transforming growth factors

    A. stimulates hematopoietic growth factor
    B. encoding gene located in HLA region between HLA-DR and HLA-B loci
    C. induce phenotypic transformation in non-neoplastic cells

BIBLIOGRAPHY

Alper CA, Rosen FS: Clinical applications of complement assays. In Stollerman GH, editor: *Advances in internal medicine,* vol 20, Chicago, 1975, Year Book Medical Publishers.

Anderson KC et al: Interleukin-11 promotes accessory cell-dependent B-cell differentiation in humans, *Blood* 80(11):2797-2804, 1992.

Ashman RF: Rheumatic diseases. In Lawlor GJ, Fischer TJ, editors: *Manual of allergy and immunology,* ed 2, Boston, 1988, Little, Brown.

Baron S et al: The interferons, *JAMA* 266(10):1375-1383, 1991.

Beezhold DH: Immune regulation, *Guthrie J* 59(1):5, 1990.

Bertagnolli MM et al: IL-12 augments antigen-dependent proliferation of activated T lymphocytes, *J Immunol* 149(12):3778-3783, 1992.

Borden EC: Interferons-expanding therapeutic roles, *N Engl J Med* 326(22):1491-1493, 1992.

Claman HN: The biology of the immune response, *JAMA* 268(20):2790-2796, 1992.

D'Andrea AD: Cytokine receptors in congenital hematopoietic disease, *N Engl J Med* 330(12):839-846, 1994.

Desai BB et al: IL-12 receptor, *J Immunol* 148(10):3125-3132, 1992.

Dinarello CA: The role of interleukin-1 in disease, *N Engl J Med* 328(2):106-113, 1993.

Donahue RE, Yang Y-C, Clark SC: Human P40 T-cell growth factor (interleukin-9) supports erythroid colony formation, *Blood* 75(12):2271-2275, 1990.

Ezekowitz RA, Mulliken JB, Folkman J: Interferon alpha-2a therapy for life-threatening hemangiomas of infancy, *N Engl J Med* 326(22):1456-1463, 1992.

Fearon DT, Austen KF: Current concepts in immunology: the alternative pathway of complement-a system for host resistance to microbial infection, *N Engl J Med* 303:259-263, 1980.

Fort MM et al: IL-25 induces IL-4, IL-5, and IL-13 and Th2-associated pathologied in vivo, *Immunology* 5-6:985-995, 2001.

Frank MM: Complement in the pathophysiology of human disease, *N Engl J Med* 316:1525, 1987.

Frigas E: Angioedema with acquired deficiency of the C1 inhibitor: a constellation of syndromes, *Mayo Clinic Proc* 64:1269-1275, 1989.

Frucht DM: IL-23: a cytokine that acts on memory T cells, *Sci STKE 2002* 114:PE1, 2002.

Gabay C, Kushner I: Acute-phase proteins and other systemic responses to inflammation, *N Engl J Med* 340(6):448-454, 1999.

Gruss H-J et al: Interleukin-9 is expressed by primary and cultured Hodgkin and Reed-Sternberg cells, *Cancer Res* 52:1026-1031, 1992.

Holaday RJ et al: Potential role for interleukin-10 in the immunosuppression associated with kala azar, *J Clin Invest* 92(6):2626-2632, 1993.

Hurst SD et al: New IL-17 family members promote Th1 or Th2 responses in the lung: in vivo function of the novel cytokine IL-25, *J Immunol* 169(1):443-453, 2002.

Kelleher K et al: Human interleukin-9, *Blood* 77(7):1436-1441, 1991.

Keller DC et al: Interleukin 11 inhibits adipogenesis and stimulates myelopoiesis in human long-term marrow cultures, *Blood* 82(5):1428-1435, 1993.

Knutsen AP, Fischer TJ: Immunodeficiency diseases. In Lawlor GJ, Fischer TJ, editors: *Manual of allergy and immunology,* ed 2, Boston, 1988, Little, Brown.

Kobayashi S et al: Interleukin-11 acts as an autocrine growth factor for human megakaryoblastic cell lines, *Blood* 81(4):889-893, 1993.

Larchmann PJ, Rosen FS: Genetic defects of complement in man, *Springer Semin Immunopathol* 1:339-353, 1978.

Larson RS, Springer TA: Structure and function of leukocyte integrins, *Immunol Rev* 18:181-217, 1990.

Liblau RS, Fugger L: Tumor necrosis factor-alpha and disease progression in multiple sclerosis, *N Engl J Med* 326(4):272, 1992.

MacKay IR, Rosen RS: Allergy and allergic diseases," *N Engl J Med* 344:109-113, 2001.

Medzhitov R, Janeway C Jr: Innate immunity, *N Engl J Med* 343:338-344, 2000.

Merz H et al: Interleukin-9 expression in human malignant lymphomas: unique association with Hodgkin's disease and large cell anaplastic lymphoma, *Blood* 78(5):1311-1317, 1991.

Muller-Eberhardt HJ: Complement abnormalities in human disease, *Hosp Pract* 13(12):65-76, 1978.

National Institute of Child Health and Human Development: website: http://156.40.88.3

Noti JD: Laboratory of molecular biology, *Guthrie J* 63(2):51-53, 1994.

Parham C et al: A receptor for the heterodimeric cytokine IL-23 is composed of IL-23R beta 1 and a novel cytokine receptor subunit, IL-23R, *J Immunol* 168(11):5699-5708, 2002.

Pedrazzi AH: Acute phase proteins: clinical and laboratory diagnosis. A review, *Ann Pharm Fr* 56(3):108-114, 1998.

Peter JB: *The use and interpretation of tests in medical laboratory immunology,* ed 8, Los Angeles, 1991-92, Specialty Laboratories, Inc.

Ridker et al: Comparison of C-reactive protein and low-density lipoprotein cholesterol levels in the prediction of first cardiovascular events, *N Engl J Med* 347:1557-1565, 2002.

Rlav JY et al: Serum interleukin-10 in non-Hodgkin's lymphoma: a prognostic factor, *Blood* 82(7):2169-2174, 1993.

Roberts WL et al: Evaluation of four automated high-sensitivity C-reactive protein methods: implications for clinical and epidemiological applications, *Clin Chem* 46(4):461-468, 2000.

Ruddy S: Complement. In Rose NR, Friedman H, Fahey JL, editors: *Manual of clinical laboratory immunology,* ed 3, Washington, DC, 1986, American Society of Microbiology.

Ruddy S: Complement. In Stein J, editor: *Internal medicine,* ed 4, Boston, 1994, Little, Brown.

Ruddy S: Complement measurement. In Stein J, editor: *Internal medicine,* ed 4, Boston, 1994, Little, Brown and Co.

Schoenhaut DS et al: Cloning and expression of murine IL-12, *J Immunol* 148(11):3433-3440, 1992.

Soiffer R et al: Interleukin-12 augments cytolytic activity of peripheral blood lymphocytes from patients with hematologic and solid malignancies, *Blood* 82(9):2790-2796, 1993.

Taga K, Mostowski H, Tosato G: Human interleukin-10 can directly inhibit T cell growth, *Blood* 81(11):2964-2971, 1993.

Tizmann SE, Daniels JC, editors: *Serum protein abnormalities,* Boston, 1975, Little, Brown.

Tulin EE et al: SF20/IL-25, a novel bone marrow stroma-derived growth factor that binds to mouse thymic shared antigen-1 and supports lymphoid cell proliferation, *J Immunol* 167(11):6338-6347, 2001.

Turgeon ML: *Fundamentals of immunohematology,* ed 3, Baltimore, 1999, Williams & Wilkins.

van Leeuwen MA, van Rijswijk MH: Acute phase proteins in the monitoring of inflammatory disorders, *Baillieres Clin Rheumatol* 8(3):531-552, 1994.

Waldmann TA: The multichain interleukin 2 receptor, *JAMA* 263(2):272-274, 1990.

Walport MJ: Complement, *N Engl J Med* 344:1058-1065, 2001.

Walport MJ: Complement, *N Engl J Med* 344:1140-1144, 2001.

Zeiss CR et al: A hypocomplementemic vasculitic urticarial syndrome, *Am J Med* 68:867-875, 1980.

Part Two

The Theory of Immunologic and Serologic Procedures

Chapter 6

Safety and Basic Techniques in the Immunology-Serology Laboratory

LEARNING OBJECTIVES

At the conclusion of this chapter, the reader should be able to:
- Discuss the occupational transmission of hepatitis B virus (HBV) and human immunodeficiency virus (HIV).
- Describe the practice of Universal Blood and Body Fluid Standards.
- Explain the proper handling of hazardous material and waste management, including infectious waste, chemicals, and radioactive waste.
- Describe the principles of immunologic-serologic testing, including written procedural protocol, accuracy in testing, and blood specimen preparation.

In the immunology-serology laboratory, precautions must be taken to prevent accidental exposure to infectious disease. In addition, laboratories using radioactive test protocols must adhere to strict safety standards. Clinical laboratory personnel are routinely exposed to hazardous chemicals in their day-to-day activities. Many laboratory accidents result in chemical-related illnesses ranging from skin and eye irritations to pulmonary edema.

SAFETY PRACTICES

All laboratories need programs to minimize risks to the health and safety of employees, volunteers, and patients. Suitable physical arrangements, an acceptable work environment, and appropriate equipment need to be available to maintain safe operations.

Each laboratory must have an up-to-date safety manual. This manual should contain a comprehensive listing of approved policies, acceptable practices, and precautions including Universal Blood and Body Fluid Standards. Specific regulations that conform to current state and federal requirements such as Occupational Safety and Health Administration (OSHA) regulations must be included in the manual. Other sources of mandatory and voluntary standards include the Joint Commission on Accreditation of Healthcare Organizations (JCAHO), the College of American Pathologists (CAP), and the Centers for Disease Control and Prevention (CDC).

The recognition and rapid increase in the number of patients identified with HIV-1 have generated new policies from the CDC and mandated regulations by OSHA. Compliance with the OSHA Blood-borne Pathogens Standard and the Occupational Exposure Standard is required to provide a safe work environment. OSHA mandates that the employer:

- Educate and train all health care workers in Universal Standards and in preventing blood-borne infections
- Provide proper equipment and supplies (e.g., gloves)
- Monitor compliance with the protective biosafety policies

According to the CDC concept of Universal Standards, all human blood and other body fluids are treated as potentially infectious for HIV-1, HBV, or other blood-borne microorganisms that can cause disease in humans.

UNIVERSAL BLOOD AND BODY FLUID STANDARDS

The rapid increase in the number of patients identified with HIV was partially responsible for a change in the initial recommendations issued in 1983 by the CDC in regard to the handling of blood and body fluids from patients suspected of or known to be infected with a blood-borne pathogen. Current safety guidelines for the control of infectious disease are based on the original CDC publication, "Recommendations for Prevention of HIV Transmission in Health-Care Settings" (*MMWR,* Suppl 2S, 1987). Clarifications of safety practices appear in the 1988 CDC clarifications of the original guidelines (*MMWR* 37(24), 1988), as well as in the Department of Labor, Occupational Safety and Health Administration's "Occupational Exposure to Blood-borne Pathogens": Part 1910 to title 29 of the Code of Federal Regulations, 64175-64182, (*Fed Reg* 56(235), 1991); also in the U.S. Department of Health and Human Services "Regulations for Implementing the Clinical Laboratory Improvement Amendments of 1988: A Summary" (*MMWR* 41(RR-2), 1992). Laboratory personnel should also remain alert to further updates of these policies.

Universal Blood and Body Fluid Standards or Universal Standards have been instituted in clinical laboratories to prevent parenteral, mucous membrane, and nonintact skin exposures of health care workers to blood-borne pathogens such as HIV and HBV. Universal Standards state that the blood and most body fluids of all patients should be treated as potentially infectious (Box 6-1).

Although HIV has been isolated from blood, semen, vaginal secretions, saliva, tears, breast milk, cerebrospinal fluid (CSF), amniotic fluid, and urine, only blood, semen, vaginal secretions, and breast milk have been implicated in transmission of HIV to date. HIV has been found in saliva and tears in very low quantities from some AIDS patients.

Box 6-1	**Potentially Infectious Body Fluids***

SPECIFIC HUMAN FLUIDS

Amniotic fluid
Bile
Blood
Bloody fluids
Breast milk
Cerebrospinal fluid
Colostrum
Feces
Nasal secretions (?)
Nasopharyngeal washings
Pericardial fluid
Peritoneal fluid
Pleural fluid
Pus and purulent discharge
Saliva (?)
Semen
Sweat (?)
Synovial fluid
Tears (?)
Urine (?)
Vaginal secretions

OTHER MATERIALS

Any body fluid visibly contaminated with blood
All body fluids in situations in which it is difficult or impossible to differentiate between body fluids
Unfixed tissue or organs (other than intact skin from a human—living or dead)
HIV-containing cell or tissue culture
Organ cultures of HIV-containing culture medium

From US Department of Health and Human Services, Centers for Disease Control and Prevention: Updated US Public Health Services Guidelines for the management of occupational exposures to HBV, HCV and HIV and recommendations for postexposure prophylaxis, June 29, 2001, p 4.
*Most body fluids are not efficient vehicles of transmission because they contain low quantities of infectious viruses (e.g., hepatitis B virus).

But it is important to realize that finding a small amount of HIV in a body fluid does not necessarily mean that HIV can be transmitted by that body fluid. HIV has not been recovered from the sweat of HIV-infected persons. Contact with saliva, tears, or sweat has never been shown to result in transmission of HIV.

OCCUPATIONAL TRANSMISSION OF HBV AND HIV

Medical personnel should be aware that HBV and HIV are totally different diseases caused by completely unrelated viruses. The most feared hazard of all, the transmission of HIV through occupational exposure, is among the least likely to occur if proper safety practices are followed. Occupational exposure is defined as a percutaneous injury, for example, from a needlestick or cut with a sharp object, or from contact with mucous membranes or nonintact skin with blood, tissues, blood-stained body fluid to which

TABLE 6-1	Risk of Occupationally Transmitted HIV Infection to Health Care Workers	
	Route of Exposure	
Occupation	**Documented**	**Possible**
Laboratory Technician, Clinical	48	5

From Centers for Disease Control and Prevention: *HIV/AIDS Surveillance Report* vol 10, no 2, 1998.
*Both percutaneous and mucocutaneous exposure (2), unknown route (2).

Universal Standards apply, or concentrated virus. Among health care personnel with documented occupationally acquired HIV infection, percutaneous exposure was the most prevalent.

Exposure to HIV is uncommon, but cases of occupational transmission to health care personnel with no other known high-risk factors have been documented (Table 6-1). Although HIV is an unlikely work-related hazard, it cannot be underrated because at the present time, it is considered to be a fatal disease.

The cumulative total of persons in the United States reported to be living with HIV infection and AIDS reported to the CDC through June 2001 was 466,023.

Based on the number of reported percutaneous and mucocutaneous blood exposures, phlebotomists represent 4%, and clinical laboratory workers (nonphlebotomists) register 3.7% of the total percentage of blood exposures by occupation in the United States.

Exposure to blood constitutes the major source of infection in the reported cases of occupationally acquired HIV. However, bloody fluid, unspecified fluid, and exposure to the live virus in the laboratory also account for exposure in additional cases.

The transmission of HBV can also be fatal, and it is more probable than transmission of HIV. OSHA estimates that occupational exposures account for 5900 to 7400 cases of HBV infection annually. Although the number of cases has sharply declined since hepatitis B vaccine became available in 1982, approximately 800 health care workers become infected with HBV each year after occupational exposure.

Blood is the single most important source of HIV, HBV, and other blood-borne pathogens in the occupational setting. HBV can be present in extraordinarily high concentrations in blood, but HIV is usually found in lower concentrations. HBV may be stable in dried blood and blood products at 25° C for up to 7 days. HIV retains infectivity for more than 3 days in dried specimens at room temperature and for more than a week in an aqueous environment at room temperature. The likelihood of infection after exposure to blood infected with HBV or HIV depends on a variety of factors, including:
- Concentration of HBV or HIV virus. Viral concentration is higher for HBV than for HIV
- Duration of the contact
- Presence or skin lesions or abrasions on the hands or exposed skin of the health care worker
- Immune status of the health care worker for HBV

HBV and HIV may be directly transmitted by various portals of entry (Table 6-2). In the occupational setting, however, the following list of situations may lead to infection:
- Percutaneous (parenteral) inoculation of blood, plasma, serum, or certain other body fluids from accidental needlesticks and so forth.
- Contamination of the skin with blood or certain body fluids without overt puncture, as a result of scratches, abrasions, burns, weeping, or exudative skin lesions.
- Exposure of mucous membranes (oral, nasal, or conjunctiva) to blood or certain body fluids, as the direct result of pipetting by mouth, splashes, or spattering.
- Centrifuge accidents or the improper removal of rubber stoppers from test tubes, thereby producing droplets. If these aerosol products are infectious and come in direct contact with mucous membranes or nonintact skin, direct transmission of virus can result.

HBV and HIV may be indirectly transmitted. Viral transmission can result from contact with inanimate objects such as work surfaces or equipment contaminated with infected blood or certain body fluids. If the virus is transferred to the skin or mucous membranes by hand contact between a contaminated surface and nonintact skin or mucous membranes, it can produce viral exposure.

PROTECTIVE TECHNIQUES FOR INFECTION CONTROL

Universal Standards are intended to supplement rather than replace recommendations such as hand washing for routine infection control. Infection control efforts for HIV, HBV, and other blood-borne pathogens must focus on prevention of exposure to blood. It is a possible and wise preventive measure to be vaccinated against HBV. The risk of nosocomial transmission of HBV, HIV, and other blood-borne pathogens can be minimized if laboratory personnel are aware of and adhere to essential safety guidelines.

Selection and Use of Gloves

Gloves for medical use are either sterile surgical or nonsterile examination gloves made of vinyl or latex. There are no reported differences in barrier effectiveness between intact latex and intact vinyl gloves. Tactile differences have been observed between the two types of gloves, with latex gloves providing more tactile sensitivity; however, either type is

TABLE 6-2	Risk of HIV in Health Care Settings			
Portal of Entry	**Type of Risk**	**Risk of Getting to Site**	**Risk of Viral Entry**	**Risk of Inoculation**
Blood				
Blood products*	Medically required	High	High	High
Shared needles†	Choice	High	High	Very high
Needle injury†	Accidental	Low	High	Low
Traumatic wound	Accidental	Moderate	High	High
Conjunctiva	Accidental	Moderate	Moderate	Very low
Nasal Mucosa	Accidental	Low	Low	Very low
Oral Mucosa	Accidental/choice	Moderate	Moderate	Low
Perinatal	Accidental	High	High	High
Respiratory (lower)	Accidental	Very low	Very low	Very low
Sexual				
Anus	Choice	Very high	Very high	Very high
Penis	Choice	High	Low	Low
Ulcers	Choice	High	High	Very high
Vagina	Choice	Low	Low	Medium
Skin				
Intact	Accidental	Very Low	Very low	Very low
Broken	Accidental	Low	High	High

Data from Recommendations for prevention of HIV transmission in health care settings, *MMWR* 36:35, August 21, 1987; Update: Universal Precautions for prevention of transmission of HIV, hepatitis B virus, and other blood-borne pathogens in the health care settings, *MMWR* 37:377, June 24, 1988.
HIV, Human immunodeficiency virus.
*Unscreened donors and/or untreated products.
†If the needles are contaminated with virus-infected blood.

usually satisfactory for phlebotomy and as a protective barrier when performing technical procedures. Latex-free gloves should be available for personnel with sensitivity to usual glove material. Rubber household gloves may be used for cleaning procedures.

General guidelines related to the selection and general use of gloves include:

- Use sterile gloves for procedures involving contact with normally sterile areas of the body or during procedures where sterility has been established and must be maintained. Use nonsterile examination gloves for procedures that do not require the use of sterile gloves.
- Wear gloves when processing blood specimens, reagents, or blood products. Gloves should be changed frequently and immediately if they become visibly contaminated with blood or certain body fluids or if physical damage occurs.
- Do not wash or disinfect latex or vinyl gloves for reuse. Washing with detergents may cause increased penetration of liquids through undetected holes in the gloves. Rubber gloves may be decontaminated and reused, but disinfectants may cause deterioration. Rubber gloves should be discarded if they have punctures, tears, or evidence of deterioration or if they peel, crack, or become discolored.

As a result of the CDC modifications published in June 1988, some institutions have relaxed recommendations for using gloves for phlebotomy procedures by skilled phlebotomists in settings where the prevalence of blood-borne pathogens is known to be very low. Institutions or organizations that choose to modify the policy of requiring gloves for all phlebotomies must periodically reevaluate their policy and must provide gloves to all personnel who wish to use them for phlebotomy. However, the guidelines for the use of gloves during phlebotomy procedures include:

- Gloves must be used by phlebotomists who have cuts, scratches, or other breaks in their skin. The presence of skin lesions will increase the likelihood of infection subsequent to skin exposure.
- Gloves should be worn when the phlebotomist judges that hand contamination may occur (e.g., when performing phlebotomy on an uncooperative patient).
- Gloves must be worn when performing fingersticks and/or heelsticks on infants and children.
- Gloves must be worn when receiving phlebotomy training.
- Gloves should be changed between each patient contact.

Gloves as a Barrier Protection During Testing

Vinyl gloves should be worn when:

- Handling human blood, serum, plasma, or certain body fluids.
- Handling human blood or potentially infectious blood products (e.g., antiseras of human origin and reagent red blood cells).

- Testing human serum, plasma, or red blood cells.
- Using items potentially contaminated with human blood or certain body fluids (e.g., specimen containers, laboratory instruments, countertops).

Care must be taken to avoid indirect contamination of work surfaces or objects in the work area. Gloves should be properly removed or covered with an uncontaminated glove or paper towel before answering the telephone, handling laboratory equipment, or touching door knobs.

Facial Barrier Protection and Occlusive Bandages

Facial barrier protection should be used if there is a potential for splashing or spraying of blood or certain body fluids. Masks and/or facial protection should be worn if mucous membrane contact with blood or certain body fluid is anticipated. All disruptions of exposed skin should be covered with a water-impermeable occlusive bandage. This includes defects on the arms, face, and neck.

Laboratory Coats or Gowns as Barrier Protection

A color-coded, two-laboratory coat or equivalent system should be used whenever laboratory personnel are working with potentially infectious specimens. The garment worn in the laboratory must be changed or covered with an uncontaminated coat when leaving the immediate work area. Garments should be changed immediately if grossly contaminated with blood or body fluids to prevent seepage through to street clothes or skin. Contaminated coats or gowns should be placed in an appropriately designated biohazard bag for laundering. Disposable plastic aprons are recommended if there is a significant possibility that blood or certain body fluids may be splashed. Aprons should be discarded into a biohazard container.

The introduction of the use of water-retardant gowns has formed the biggest change in many personal protective equipment practices.

Important Safety Practices

Hand Washing

Frequent hand washing is an important safety precaution. It should be performed after contact with patients and laboratory specimens. Gloves should be used as an adjunct to, not a substitute for, hand washing.

The efficacy of hand washing in reducing transmission of microbial organisms has been demonstrated. At the very minimum, hands should be washed with soap and water (if visibly soiled) or with soap and water or by hand antisepsis with an alcohol-based hand rub (if hands are not visibly soiled):

- After completing laboratory work and before leaving the laboratory.
- After removing gloves. The Association for Professionals in Infection Control and Epidemiology reports extreme variability in the quality of gloves, with leakage in 4% to 63% of vinyl gloves and 3% to 52% of latex gloves.
- Before eating, drinking, applying make up, and changing contact lenses, and before and after using the lavatory.

TABLE 6-3	Preparation of Diluted Household Bleach		
Volume of Bleach	Volume of H_2O	Ratio	% Sodium Hypochlorite
1 mL	9 mL	1:10	0.5

- Before all activities that involve hand contact with mucous membranes or breaks in the skin.
- Immediately after accidental skin contact with blood, body fluids, or tissues. If the contact occurs through breaks in gloves, the gloves should be removed immediately, and the hands thoroughly washed. If accidental contamination occurs to an exposed area of the skin or because of a break in gloves, one must wash first with a liquid soap, rinse well with water, and apply a 1:10 dilution of bleach or 50% isopropyl or ethyl alcohol. The bleach or alcohol is left on skin for at least 1 minute before final washing with liquid soap and water.
- Two important points in the practice of hand hygiene technique are:
  1. When decontaminating hands with a waterless antiseptic agent (e.g., alcohol-based hand rub), apply product to the palm of one hand and rub hands together, covering all surfaces of hands and fingers, until hands are dry. Follow the manufacturer's recommendations on the volume of product to use. If an adequate volume of an alcohol-based hand rub is used, it should take 15 to 25 seconds for hands to dry.
  2. When washing with a nonantimicrobial or antimicrobial soap, wet hands first with warm water, apply 3 to 5 mL of detergent to hands, and rub hands together vigorously for *at least* 15 seconds, covering all surfaces of the hands and fingers. Rinse hands with warm water and dry thoroughly with a disposable towel. Use the towel to turn off the faucet.

The Department of Health and Human Services (CDC) issued a draft guide in 2001 for Hand Hygiene in Health Care Settings (Box 6-2).

Decontamination of Work Surfaces, Equipment, and Spills

All work surfaces should be cleaned and sanitized at the beginning and end of the shift with a 1:10 dilution of household bleach (Table 6-3). Instruments such as scissors or centrifuge carriages should be sanitized daily with a diluted solution of bleach. Diluted household bleach prepared daily inactivates HBV in 10 minutes and HIV in 2 minutes. Disposable materials contaminated with blood must be placed in containers marked "Biohazard" and properly discarded.

All blood spills should be treated as potentially hazardous. In the event of a blood spill, this procedure for cleaning up the spill should be used:

1. Wear gloves and a laboratory coat.
2. Absorb the blood with disposable towels. Bleach solutions are less effective in the presence of high concentrations of protein. Remove as much liquid blood or serum as possible before decontamination.

Box 6-2   Guidelines for Hand Washing and Hand Antisepsis in Health Care Settings

RECOMMENDATIONS

- Wash hands with a nonantimicrobial soap and water or an antimicrobial soap and water when hands are visibly dirty or contaminated with proteinaceous material.
- If hands are not visibly soiled, use an alcohol-based waterless antiseptic agent for routinely decontaminating hands in all other clinical situations.
- Waterless antiseptic agents are highly preferable, but hand antisepsis using an antimicrobial soap may be considered in settings where time constraints are not an issue and easy access to hand hygiene facilities can be ensured, or in rare instances when a caregiver is intolerant of the waterless antiseptic product used in the institution.
- Decontaminate hands after contact with a patient's intact skin,
- Decontaminate hands after contact with body fluids or excretions, mucous membranes, nonintact skin, or wound dressings, as long as hands are not visibly soiled.
- Decontaminate hands if moving from a contaminated body site to a clean body site during patient care.
- Decontaminate hands after contact with inanimate objects in the immediate vicinity of the patient.
- Decontaminate hands before caring for patients with severe neutropenia or other forms of severe immune suppression.
- Decontaminate hands after removing gloves.

U.S. Department of Health and Human Services, Center for Disease Control and Prevention (CDC): Draft guideline for hand hygiene in health care settings, *Fed Reg* 66(218):56680, Nov. 9, 2001; USDHHS: Guidelines for hand hygiene in health-care settings, *MMWR* 51(RR16):1-44, Oct 25, 2002.

3. Using a diluted bleach solution, clean the spill site of all visible blood.
4. Wipe down the spill site with paper towels soaked with diluted bleach.
5. Place all disposable materials used for decontamination into a biohazard container.

Needle Precautions

OSHA estimates that approximately 600,000 to 1 million needlestick injuries, the majority of which are unreported, occur in the United States each year. To prevent needlestick injuries, needles should never be recapped, separated from syringes, or otherwise manipulated by hand. Used needles should be placed intact into specifically designated red, puncture-proof, biohazard containers. The same criteria should be applied to used scalpel blades and any other sharp device that may be contaminated with blood. The container should be located as close as possible to the work area. Phlebotomists should carry red, puncture-resistant containers in their collection trays. Needles should not project from the top of the container. To discard the containers, close and place them into the biohazard waste. An accidental needlestick must be reported to the supervisor or other designated individual.

Other Safety Precautions

A variety of other safety practices should be adhered to reduce the risk of inadvertent contamination with blood or certain body fluids. These practices include:

- All devices in contact with blood that are capable of transmitting infection to the donor or recipient must be sterile and nonreusable.
- Food and drinks should not be consumed in work areas or stored in the same area as specimens. Containers, refrigerators, or freezers used for specimens should be marked as containing a biohazard.
- Specimens needing centrifugation should be capped and placed into a centrifuge with a sealed dome.
- Slowly and carefully open test tubes with rubber stoppers with a 2 × 2 gauze square placed over the stopper to minimize aerosol production (the introduction of substances into the air).
- Use safety bulbs for pipetting. Pipetting by mouth of any clinical material must be strictly forbidden.

Compliance with Universal Standards

A clear policy on institutionally required Universal Standards is needed. For usual laboratory activities, personal protective equipment consists of gloves and a laboratory coat or gown. Other equipment such as masks would normally not be needed.

Compliance with the enforcement of Universal Standards also requires relevant training programs. The OSHA categories of risk classifications are now obsolete, but the Public Health Service (PHS) Biosafety Levels 1, 2, and 3 describe the relative risk that may be encountered in a work area. Biosafety Level 1 is the least threatening. The PHS biosafety levels of risk that may be encountered in a work area are as follows:

Level 1

Work that involves agents of no known or of minimal potential hazard to laboratory personnel and the environment.

Level 2

Work that involves agents of moderate potential hazard to personnel and the environment. NOTE: Most work with blood requires Biosafety Level 2 precautions (Box 6-3). Exceptions may be appropriate if no open specimens will be encountered.

Level 3

Work that involves indigenous or exotic agents that may cause serious or potentially lethal disease as a result of exposure by inhalation.

Prophylaxis, Medical Follow-up, and Records of Accidental Exposure

Vaccination against hepatitis B and compliance with Universal Standards are the best prophylaxis against blood-borne pathogens. If an individual has not been vaccinated, hepatitis B immune globulin (HBIG) is usually given concurrently with hepatitis B vaccine postexposure to penetrating injuries. If administered in accordance with the manufacturer's directions, both products are considered safe and have been proven free of any risk of infection with HBV or HIV.

If a known or suspected parenteral exposure takes place, a technician or technologist may request follow-up monitoring for HBV or HIV antibodies. This monitoring and follow-up counseling must be provided free of charge. If voluntary informed consent is obtained, the source of the potentially infectious material and the technician/technologist should be tested immediately. The technician/technologist should also

Box 6-3	**Summary of Minimum Biosafety Level 2 Precautions**

- Decontaminate bench tops daily.
- Use biosafety cabinet to contain aerosols or wear gloves, gown, goggles, and mask.
- Use gowns and gloves routinely.
- Do not pipette by mouth.
- Transport specimens properly.
- Dispose of infectious waste properly.
- Do not eat, drink, smoke, or apply cosmetics or contact lenses in work areas.
- Conduct high-risk activities in restricted areas.
- Practice needle precautions.
- Immediately report accidental exposure to suspected or actual hazardous material.

be tested at intervals after exposure. An injury report must be filed after parenteral exposure.

HAZARDOUS MATERIAL AND WASTE MANAGEMENT

The control of infectious, chemical, and radioactive waste is regulated by a variety of government agencies, including OSHA and the Food and Drug Administration (FDA). Legislation and regulations that affect laboratories include the Resource Recovery and Conservation Act, the Toxic Substances Control Act, clean air and water laws, "right to know" laws, and HAZCOM (chemical hazard communication). Laboratories should implement applicable federal, state, and local laws that pertain to hazardous material and waste management by establishing safety policies. Laboratories with multiple agencies should follow the guidelines of the most stringent agency. Safety policies should be reviewed and signed annually or whenever a change is instituted. Employers are responsible for ensuring that personnel follow the safety policies.

Infectious Waste

Infectious waste such as contaminated gauze squares and test tubes must be discarded into proper biohazard containers. These containers should:
- Be conspicuously marked "Biohazard" and bear the Universal Biohazard symbol.
- Be of the universal color—orange, orange and black, or red.
- Be rigid, leak proof, and puncture-resistant. Cardboard boxes lined with leak-proof plastic bags are available.
- Be used for blood and certain body fluids,* as well as disposable materials contaminated with them.

---

*Some local health codes currently permit blood and other body fluids to be disposed of by being poured down the sink into the sanitary sewerage system. If disposal by this method is used, care must be taken to prevent splashing. Water should not be running in the sink, and facial protection and a plastic apron should be worn in addition to gloves and a laboratory coat. Sinks used for hazardous waste disposal should not be used for hand washing.

If the primary infectious waste containers are red plastic bags, they should be kept in secondary metal or plastic cans. Extreme care should be taken not to contaminate the exterior of these bags. If they do become contaminated on the outside, the entire bag must be placed into another red plastic bag. Secondary plastic or metal cans should be decontaminated regularly and immediately after any grossly visible contamination with an agent such as a 1:10 solution of household bleach.

Terminal disposal of infectious waste should be by incineration; however, an alternate method of terminal sterilization is autoclaving. If incineration is not done in the health care facility or by an outside contractor, all contaminated disposables should be autoclaved before leaving the facility for disposal with routine waste.

Chemical Hazards

OSHA recommends that all chemically hazardous material be properly labeled with the hazardous contents and severity of the material, as well as bear a hazard symbol. The chemical hygiene plan is the core of the OSHA safety standard. A written plan (to be developed by each employer) must specify the training and information requirements of the standard. It also establishes appropriate work practices, standard operating procedures, methods of control, measures for appropriate maintenance and use of protective equipment, medical examinations, and special precautions for working with particularly hazardous substances. Existing safety and health plans may meet the requirements.

Chemical hazard precautions legislation such as state "right to know" laws and OSHA document 29 CFR 1910 sets the standards for HAZCOM and determines the types of documents that must be on file in a laboratory. For example, a yearly physical inventory of all hazardous chemicals must be performed, and material safety data sheets (MSDs) should be made available in each department of use. Each institution should also have at least one centralized area where all MSDs are stored.

Many toxic chemicals now have limits that must be met within the laboratory, specifically threshold limit values (TLVs) and permissible exposure limit (PEL). TLVs are the maximum safe exposure limits as set down by the federal government. PEL is the personal allowable limit per time.

Recent government regulations require that all employees who handle hazardous material and waste must be trained to use and handle these materials. Chemical hazard education sessions must be presented to new employees and conducted annually for all employees. Each laboratory is required to evaluate the effectiveness of its plan at least annually and to update it as necessary. The written plan must be available to employees.

Radioactive Waste

The Nuclear Regulatory Commission regulates the methods of disposal of radioactive waste. Radioactive waste associated with the radioimmunoassay (RIA) laboratory must be disposed of with special caution. In general, low-level RIA radioactive waste can be discharged in small amounts into the sewer with copious amounts of water. This will probably be illegal in the future; therefore the best method of disposal is to store the used material in a locked, marked room until the background count is down to 10 half-lives for I^{125}. It can then be disposed with other refuse. Meticulous records are required to document the amounts and methods of disposal.

BASIC SEROLOGIC PROCEDURES

Procedures Manual

The procedures manual must be a complete document of current techniques and approved policies, available at all times in the immediate bench area of laboratory personnel. It is extremely important for all personnel to periodically review this manual. The manual should comply with the National Commission for Clinical Laboratory Standards format standards for a procedures manual (Box 6-4). The procedural format found in this text follows these guidelines.

Alternate techniques can be included with each procedure if more than one technique is acceptable. New pages must be dated and initialed when inserted, and removed pages must be retained for 5 years, with the date of removal and the reason for removal indicated. It may be legally necessary to identify the procedure followed for a particular reason.

Accuracy in Testing

For elimination of the most frequent source of pretesting error, a patient must be positively identified when a blood specimen is obtained. This specimen must be properly collected and labeled. In general, hemolyzed specimens should not be used for serologic testing.

Inaccuracies in testing can be systematic or sporadic. Systematic errors can be eliminated by a continuing quality-assurance program that monitors equipment, reagents, and so on. Reagents should be checked for turbidity or an abnormal appearance at each time of use. Contaminated reagents can produce erroneous results. Test protocols must be strictly followed, and techniques must be exact.

Sporadic or isolated errors in technique can produce false-positive and/or false-negative results. Depending on the tech-

nique used for testing, possible causes of technical errors include:

Possible causes of false-positive errors:
- Addition of the wrong reagent to a test tube
- Overcentrifugation of a serum-cell mixture
- Dirty glassware
- Hemolyzed patient serum
- Inadequate dispersal of centrifuged serum-cell mixture
- Extended incubation

Possible causes of false-negative errors:
- Omitting patient serum from the test mixture
- Omitting reagent from the test mixture
- Undercentrifugation of a serum-cell mixture
- Vigorous shaking of a centrifuged serum-cell mixture

Possible causes of false-positive or false-negative errors:
- Incorrect labeling of test tubes
- Addition of the wrong reagent
- Erroneously reading or interpreting results
- Inaccurately recording results
- Expired or improperly stored reagents

Blood Specimen Preparation

After blood has been obtained from a patient, it should be allowed to clot, and the serum should be promptly removed for testing. Clotting and clot retraction should take place at room temperature or in the refrigerator, depending on the protocol for the specific procedure. Complete clot retraction normally takes about an hour. After clot retraction, the clot should be loosened from the sides of the test tube with an applicator stick and centrifuged for 10 minutes at a moderate speed. After centrifugation, serum can be transferred to a labeled tube with a Pasteur pipette and rubber bulb. If the serum is contaminated with erythrocytes, it should be recentrifuged. The serum-containing tube should be sealed. Testing should be promptly conducted, or the serum should be frozen at -20° C. Universal Precautions must be followed when blood specimens are handled.

Inactivation of Complement

Some procedures require the use of inactivated serum. Inactivation is the process that destroys complement activity. Complement is known to interfere with the reactions of certain syphilis tests and complement components such as C1q. It can agglutinate latex particles and cause a false-positive reaction in latex passive agglutination assays. Complement may also cause lysis of the indicator cells in hemagglutination assays.

Complement in body fluids can be inactivated by heating to 56° C for 30 minutes. When more than 4 hours has elapsed since inactivation, a specimen can be reinactivated by heating it to 56° C for 10 minutes.

Pipettes

Pipettes are used in the immunology-serology laboratory for the quantitative transfer of reagents and the preparations of serial dilution of specimens such as serum. Although semi-automated micropipettes have replaced traditional glass pipettes in the laboratory, there may be occasions when traditional methods are needed.

Box 6-4	Written Procedural Protocol*

Procedure name
Name of the test method
Principle and purpose of the test
Specimen collection and storage
Quality control
Reagents, equipment, and supplies
Procedural protocol
Expected or normal (reference) values
Procedural notes:
    Sources of error
    Limitations
    Clinical applications

*Summary of NCCLS Approved Guideline GP2-A2, *Clinical Laboratory Technical Procedure Manual*, ed 2, Villanova, Pa; National Committee for Clinical Laboratory Standards, 1992.

The type of pipette used in manual procedures is the serologic pipette. It is recognized by a frosted ring at the noncalibrated end with calibrations extending to the tip. The letters T.D. (to deliver) appear on the pipette, and for quick recognition, each size of pipette has an imprinted, color-coded band that indicates the volume. The serologic pipette is usually allowed to empty by gravity. Depending on the calibration, the remaining drop needs to be expelled to deliver the full volume.

Each serologic pipette is marked with identifying numerals (e.g., 10 mL in 1/10). The first of these numbers represents the total capacity of the pipette. The second number represents the smallest gradation into which the pipette is divided. In the example cited, therefore, the total pipette volume is 10 mL. Markings then divide it into 1-mL sections, and each mL is further divided into tenths. Sizes of serologic pipettes most frequently used are the following: 10 mL in 1/10, 5 mL in 1/10, 2 mL in 1/10, 2 mL in 1/100, 1 mL in 1/10, and 1 mL in 1/100. For greatest accuracy, the smallest pipette that will hold the desired volume should be used.

Before use, glass pipettes should be inspected for broken or chipped ends or contamination. A safety bulb must be used to aspirate liquid into the pipette, as well as to dispense it. Liquid should be aspirated to about 1 inch above the top (zero) line of the pipette. After a liquid is aspirated, the pipette should be raised vertically to avoid the introduction of air bubbles, and the exterior surface must be wiped off with a clean gauze or tissue square. Working at eye level, slowly lower the liquid so the meniscus is at zero. The contents of the pipette can then be aspirated into the appropriate test tube or vessel. Gloves should be worn during pipetting procedures in compliance with universal precautions.

PRINCIPLES OF IMMUNOLOGIC-SEROLOGIC TESTING

Procedures used in immunology apply many techniques common to other scientific disciplines such as chemistry and immunohematology. In the field of immunology, however, many serologic techniques are used to detect the interaction of antigens with antibodies. These methods are suitable for the detection and quantitation of antibodies to infectious agents (see Part Three), as well as microbial and nonmicrobial antigens.

Antibodies can be detected in various ways. The purpose of Part Two is to present the various methods of antibody or antigen detection. In some cases antibodies to an agent may be detected in more than one way, but different procedures may not detect the same antibody.

Serum for detection of antibodies should be drawn during the acute phase of illness or when first discovered, and again during convalescent period, usually 2 weeks later. A difference in antibody titer may be noted when the acute and convalescent specimens are tested concurrently. Some infections, however, such as legionnaires' disease or hepatitis, may not manifest a rise in titer until months after the acute infection.

A central concept of serologic testing is the manifestation of a rise in titer. The titer or concentration of an antibody is the reciprocal of the highest dilution of the patient's serum in which the antibody is detectable. Therefore a high titer indicates that a considerable amount of antibody is present in the serum.

Determination of the concentration of antibody (titer) for a specific antigen involves two steps:

1. Preparing a serial dilution of the antibody-containing solution (e.g., serum).
2. Adding an equal volume of antigen suspension to each dilution.

A serial dilution represents progressive and regular increments of serum. Most commonly, serial dilutions are twofold (i.e., each dilution is half as concentrated as the preceding one) (Table 6-4). The total volume in each tube is the same. The generation of normal reference ranges is established for each type of test. Titers are usually reported as the reciprocal of the last dilution demonstrating the desired results, such as a color change or agglutination.

For most pathogens an increase in the patient's titer of 2 doubling dilutions (e.g., from a positive result of 1:8 to a positive result of 1:32 over several weeks) is considered to be diagnostic of a current infection. This is called a fourfold rise in titer.

CHAPTER HIGHLIGHTS

In the immunology-serology laboratory, precautions must be taken to prevent accidental exposure to infectious disease. In addition, laboratories using radioactive test protocols must adhere to strict safety standards. The rapid increase in the number of patients identified with HIV was partially responsible for a change in the initial recommendations issued in 1983 by the CDC in regard to the handling of blood and body fluids from patients suspected of or known to be infected with a blood-borne pathogen. Universal Blood and Body Fluid Standards, or Universal Standards, have been instituted in clinical laboratories to prevent parenteral, mucous membrane, and nonintact skin exposures of health care workers to blood-borne pathogens such as HIV and HBV. Universal

TABLE 6-4 An Example of the Preparation of a Serial Dilution

Tube	1	2	3	4	5	6	7	8	9	10
Saline (mL)	1	1	1	1	1	1	1	1	1	1
Patient serum or preceding dilution (mL)	1	1 of 1:2	1 of 1:4	1 of 1:8	1 of 1:16	1 of 1:32	1 of 1:64	1 of 1:128	1 of 1:256	1 of 1:512
Final dilution	1:2	1:4	1:8	1:16	1:32	1:64	1:128	1:256	1:512	1:1024

Standards state that the blood and certain body fluids of all patients should be treated as potentially infectious.

Although HIV has been isolated from blood, semen, vaginal secretions, saliva, tears, breast milk, CSF, amniotic fluid, and urine, only blood, semen, vaginal secretions, and possibly breast milk have been implicated in transmission of HIV to date. Medical personnel should be aware that HBV and HIV are totally different diseases caused by totally unrelated viruses. The most feared hazard of all, the transmission of HIV through occupational exposure, is among the least likely to occur if proper safety practices are followed. Although exposure to HIV is uncommon, a few cases of occupational transmission to health care personnel with no other known high-risk factors have been documented. HBV and HIV may be indirectly transmitted. Viral transmission can result from contact with inanimate objects such as work surfaces or equipment contaminated with infected blood or certain body fluids if the virus is transferred to nonintact skin or mucous membranes by hand contact. Universal Standards are intended to supplement rather than replace recommendations for routine infection control, such as hand washing. Infection control efforts for HIV, HBV, and other blood-borne pathogens must focus on prevention of exposure to blood. It is a possible and wise preventive measure to be vaccinated against HBV. The risk of nosocomial transmission of HBV, HIV, and other blood-borne pathogens can be minimized if laboratory personnel are aware of and adhere to essential safety guidelines.

In addition to establishing a clear policy on the institutionally required Universal Standards previously discussed, compliance with the enforcement of Universal Standards also requires that categories of risk classifications for all routine and reasonably anticipated job-related tasks and personal protective equipment be included with the departmental procedures manual. The control of infectious, chemical, and radioactive waste is regulated by a variety of government agencies, including OSHA and the FDA.

For elimination of the most frequent source of pretesting error, a patient must be positively identified when a blood specimen is obtained. This specimen must be properly collected and labeled. Inaccuracies in testing can be systematic or sporadic. Systematic errors can be eliminated by a continuing quality-assurance program that monitors equipment, reagents, and so forth. Reagents should be checked for turbidity or an abnormal appearance at each time of use. Contaminated reagents can produce erroneous results. Test protocols must be strictly followed, and techniques must be exact. Sporadic or isolated errors in technique can produce false-positive and/or false-negative results, depending on the technique used for testing. Procedures used in immunology apply many techniques common to other scientific disciplines such as chemistry and immunohematology. In the field of immunology, however, many serologic techniques are used to detect the interaction of antigens with antibodies. These methods are suitable for the detection and quantitation of antibodies to infectious agents, as well as microbial and nonmicrobial antigens.

Antibodies can be detected in various ways. In some cases, antibodies to an agent may be detected in more than one way, but different procedures may not detect the same antibody. Serum for detection of antibodies should be drawn during the acute phase of illness or when first discovered, and again during the convalescent period, usually 2 weeks later. A central concept of serologic testing is the manifestation of a rise in titer. The titer, or concentration, of an antibody is the reciprocal of the highest dilution of the patient's serum in which the antibody is detectable. Therefore a high titer indicates a considerable amount of antibody in the serum.

REVIEW QUESTIONS

1. Human immunodeficiency virus (HIV) has been isolated from:
   A. amniotic fluid
   B. urine
   C. blood
   D. all of the above

2. Which of the following body fluids in addition to blood has been positively implicated in the transmission of HIV?
   A. saliva
   B. tears
   C. semen
   D. cerebrospinal fluid

3. HBV may be stable in dried blood specimens at room temperature for up to:
   A. 24 hours
   B. 48 hours
   C. 5 days
   D. 7 days

4. HIV retains infectivity for:
   A. 24 hours
   B. 48 hours
   C. 3 days
   D. 5 days

5. The likelihood of infection after exposure to HBV- or HIV-infected blood or body fluids depends on all of the following factors except:
   A. the source (anatomic site) of the blood or fluid
   B. the concentration of the virus
   C. the duration of the contact
   D. the presence of nonintact skin

6. HBV and HIV may be directly transmitted in the occupational setting by all of the following except:
   A. parenteral inoculation with contaminated blood
   B. exposure of skin to contaminated blood or certain body fluids
   C. exposure of mucous membranes to contaminated blood or certain body fluids
   D. sharing bathroom facilities with an HIV-positive person

7. Universal Standards have been instituted in clinical laboratories to prevent _____ exposures of health care workers to blood-borne pathogens such as HIV and HBV.
   A. parenteral
   B. mucous membrane
   C. nonintact skin
   D. all of the above

8. Exposure to _____ constitutes the major source of HIV and HBV infection in health care personnel.
   A. bloody fluids
   B. blood
   C. urine
   D. semen

9. The transmission of HBV is _____ probable than transmission of HIV.
   A. less
   B. more

10. The likelihood of an infection after exposure to an HIV-infected substance depends on:
    A. the concentration of the virus
    B. the duration of contact
    C. the presence of skin lesions on the hands
    D. all of the above

11. HBV and HIV may be directly transmitted in the occupational setting by:
    A. accidental needlestick with an infected needle
    B. contamination of the skin with abrasions or open lesions
    C. pipetting by mouth
    D. all of the above

12. Gloves for medical use may be:
    A. sterile or nonsterile
    B. latex or vinyl
    C. used only once
    D. all of the above

Questions 13-18. Indicate true statements with the letter "A," and false statements with the letter "B."

13. _____ Wear gloves when processing blood specimens, reagents, or blood products.

14. _____ Wash and disinfect latex or vinyl gloves for reuse.

15. _____ Wear gloves when performing phlebotomy, if a cut or scratch exists in the skin.

16. _____ Change gloves between each patient contact.

17. _____ Carefully recap needles to prevent an accidental needlestick.

18. _____ Hazardous waste should bear the Universal Biohazard symbol.

Questions 19-23. True or False.
A = true
B = false

19. Sterile gloves should be worn when processing specimens.

20. Latex or vinyl gloves can be washed or disinfected for reuse.

21. Gloves should be worn when handling blood, serum, plasma, or certain body fluids.

22. Gloves should be worn when handling antisera of human origin.

23. Your hands should be washed after removing gloves.

24. Diluted household bleach prepared daily inactivates HBV in _____ (24) minutes and HIV in _____ (25) minutes.
    A. 1 minute
    B. 5 minutes
    C. 7 minutes
    D. 10 minutes

25.
    A. 1 minute
    B. 2 minutes
    C. 5 minutes
    D. 7 minutes

26. Diluted bleach for disinfecting work surfaces, equipment, and spills should be prepared daily by preparing a _____ (26) dilution of household bleach. This dilution requires _____ (27) mL of bleach diluted to 100 mL with H_2O.
    A. 1:5
    B. 1:10
    C. 1:20
    D. 1:100

27.
    A. 1
    B. 10
    C. 25
    D. 50

28. Infectious waste must be discarded into containers with all of the following characteristics except:
    A. be marked "Biohazard"
    B. bear the Universal Biohazard symbol
    C. be orange, orange and black, or red in color
    D. be manufactured of sturdy cardboard for landfill disposal

Questions 29-33. Select the appropriate answer for each of the following questions.

29. Omitting patient serum or reagent from the test mixture

30. Dirty glassware

31. Addition of the wrong reagent

32. Inaccurately recording results

33. Hemolyzed patient serum
    A = false-positive
    B = false-negative
    C = false-positive or false-negative

Questions 34-37. Insert the missing elements in the list below, choosing from the following answers.
    A. quality control
    B. sources of error
    C. principle and purpose of the test
    D. procedural protocol

A written procedural protocol should contain this information in the following order:
Procedure name
Name of test method

34. _____ Specimen collection and storage

35. _____ Reagents, supplies and equipment

36. _____ Expected or normal (reference) values

Procedural notes

37. _____ Limitations

Clinical applications

38. Complement can be inactivated in human serum by

    heating to _____ (38)° C for _____ (39) minutes.
    A. 25
    B. 37
    C. 45
    D. 56

39.
    A. 5
    B. 10
    C. 15
    D. 30

40. A specimen should be reinactivated when more than

    _____ hour(s) has/have elapsed since inactivation.
    A. 1
    B. 2
    C. 4
    D. 8

41. If a serial dilution is prepared in 2 dilutions, the final dilution in tube 6 is:
    A. 1:25
    B. 1:32
    C. 1:64
    D. 1:256

42. The most frequent source of pretesting error is:
    A. incorrect patient identification
    B. contaminated reagents
    C. hemolyzed specimens
    D. using the wrong type of anticoagulant

43. Complement is known to:
    A. agglutinate latex particles
    B. cause false-positive reaction in latex passive agglutination assays
    C. cause lysis of the indicator cells in hemagglutination assays
    D. do all of the above

44. Serum for detection of antibodies should be drawn during the:
    A. acute phase of illness only
    B. acute and convalescent phases of illness
    C. convalescent phase of illness only
    D. acute and convalescent phases, as well as 6 months after an illness

45. A central concept of serologic testing is:
    A. antigen-antibody interaction
    B. determination of antibody composition
    C. determination of antigen titer
    D. manifestation of a rise in antibody titer

BIBLIOGRAPHY

Albertson D: Final OSHA regs mandate HIV, HBV protection, *Med Lab Observer* 24(2):17-18, 1992.

Alpert LI: OSHA: new player in the battle against AIDS, *Med Lab Observer* 22(4):49-52, 1990.

Alpert LI: Prevention of device-mediated blood-borne infections, *Med Lab Observer* 24(11):43-46, 1992.

Baer DM: Bleach stability, *Med Lab Observer* 22(4):9, 1990.

Brown JW: Biosafety in the laboratory, *Testrends* 5(1):1-3, 1991.

Centers for Disease Control and Prevention: Surveillance of health care workers with HIV/AIDS, October, 2001, website: www.thebody.com.

DeCraemer D: Postmortem viability of human immunodeficiency virus—implications for the tracking of anatomy, *N Engl J Med* 33(19):1315, 1994.

Duetsch CE, Malley CB: Safety standards and laboratory procedures for exposure to chemicals, *Lab Med* 23(7):482-484, 1992.

Fahey BJ, Henderson DK: Minimizing risks for occupational blood-borne infections, *JAMA* 264(9):1189-1190, 1990.

Ferdinand M: OSHA's blood-borne pathogens standard: enforcement, compliance and comment, *J Health Care Materials Manage* 11(8):12-14, 1993.

Forbes BA, Sahm DF, Weissfeld AS: *Bailey and Scott's Diagnostic microbiology*, ed 11, St Louis, 2002, Mosby.

Girbuding JL: Management of occupational exposures to blood-borne viruses, *N Engl J Med* 332(7):444-451, 1995.

Larson EL: APIC Guideline for hand washing and hand antisepsis in health-care settings, *Am J Infect Control* 23:251-269, 1995.

Mast EE et al: Transmission of blood-borne pathogens during sports: risk and prevention, *Ann Intern Med* 122(4):283-285, 1995.

Miller LE: Recommended concentrations of bleach, *Lab Med* 21(2):116, 1990.

Nace L: Changing health environment no deterrent for proper specimen management, *Adv Med Lab Prof* 7(12):14-16, 1995.

Nace L: OSHA to enforce tighter safety controls, *Adv Med Lab Prof* 7(12):10-11, 1995.

Perry S, Ryan J, Polan HJ: Needlestick injury associated with venipuncture, *JAMA* 276(1):54, 1992.

Pilehach L: Health care goes green, *Lab Med* 26(5):323-328, 1995.

Roberts RL et al: Investigation of patients of health care workers infected with HIV, *Ann Intern Med* 122(9):653-657, 1995.

Schwartlander B et al: Guidelines for designing rapid assessment surveys of HIV seroprevalence among hospitalized patients, *Public Health Rep* 109(1):53-59, 1994.

Turgeon ML: *Fundamentals of immunohematology,* ed 2, Baltimore, 1995, Williams & Wilkins.

Turgeon ML: *Clinical hematology,* ed 3, Boston, 1999, Little, Brown.

US Dept. of Health and Human Services, Centers for Disease Control and Prevention, Update: Universal Precautions for prevention of transmission of human immunodeficiency virus, hepatitis B virus, and other blood-borne pathogens in health-care settings, *MMWR* 37(24):377-388, 1988.

US Department of Health and Human Services, Centers for Disease Control and Prevention: Guidelines for prevention of transmission of human immunodeficiency virus and hepatitis B virus to health-care and public safety workers, *MMWR* 38(S-6):4, 5, 9, 11, 1989.

US Department of Health and Human Services, Centers for Disease Control and Prevention: Regulations for implementing the Clinical Laboratory Improvement Amendments of 1988: a summary, *MMWR* 41(RR-2):1, Feb 28, 1992.

US Department of Health and Human Services, Centers for Disease Control and Prevention: Surveillance for occupationally acquired HIV infection—United States, 1981-1992, *MMWR* 41(43): 823-825, 1992.

US Department of Health and Human Services, Centers for Disease Control and Prevention: Draft guideline for hand hygiene in health care settings, *Fed Reg* 66(218:56680), Nov. 9, 2001.

US Department of Health and Human Services, Centers for Disease Control and Prevention: *Exposure to blood: what health-care workers need to know,* Washington, DC, 2001, CDC.

US Department of Health and Human Services, Centers for Disease Control and Prevention: HIV/AIDS Surveillance report, year end 2001, vol 13, no 2, Sept 25, 2002.

US Department of Labor, Occupational Safety and Health Administration: Occupational Exposure to Blood-borne Pathogens: Part 1910 to title 29 of the Code of Federal Regulations, *Fed Reg* 56(235):64175-64182, 1991.

Voldish K: The "dirty dozen"—12 common violations of OSHA's blood-borne pathogens standard, *Lab Med* 24(5):305-306, 1993.

Wong ES et al: Are universal precautions effective in reducing the number of occupational exposures among health care workers? *JAMA* 265(9):1123-1128, 1991.

Chapter 7

Agglutination Methods

LEARNING OBJECTIVES

At the conclusion of this chapter, the reader should be able to:
- Describe the principles of agglutination.
- Name and compare the characteristics of at least five agglutination methods.
- Explain methods for enhancing agglutination.
- Describe the characteristics of graded agglutination reactions.
- Discuss the principles of pregnancy testing, including sources of error.

PRINCIPLES OF AGGLUTINATION

Precipitation and agglutination are the visible expression of the aggregation of antigens and antibodies through the formation of a framework in which antigen particles or molecules alternate with antibody molecules (Figure 7-1). Precipitation is the term applied to aggregation of soluble test antigens. Agglutination is the term used to describe the aggregation of particulate test antigens.

Agglutination of particles to which soluble antigen has been absorbed produces a serum method of demonstrating precipitins. Examples of artificial carriers include latex particles and colloidal charcoal. Cells unrelated to the antigen, such as erythrocytes coated with antigen in a constant amount, can be used as biologic carriers. Whole bacterial cells can contain an antigen that will bind with antibodies produced in response to that antigen when it was introduced into the host.

The quality of test results depends on a variety of factors, including:
- Time of incubation with the antibody source (i.e., patient serum)
- Amount and avidity of an antigen conjugated to the carrier
- Conditions of the test environment (e.g., pH and protein concentration)

Agglutination tests are easy to perform and in some cases are the most sensitive tests currently available. These tests have a wide range of applications in the clinical diagnosis of noninfectious immune disorders and infectious diseases.

LATEX AGGLUTINATION

In latex agglutination procedures (Box 7-1), antibody molecules can be bound to the surface of latex beads. Many antibody molecules can be bound to each latex particle, increasing the potential number of exposed antigen-binding sites. If an antigen is present in a test specimen such as the C-reactive protein, the antigen will bind to the combining sites of the antibody exposed on the surface of the latex beads, forming visible cross-linked aggregates of latex beads and antigen (Figure 7-2). In some test systems (e.g., pregnancy testing

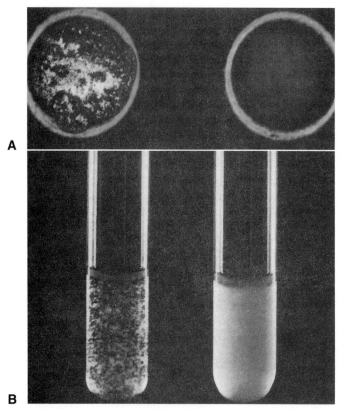

Figure 7-1 Agglutination patterns. **A,** Slide agglutination of bacteria with known antisera or known bacteria. A positive reaction is demonstrated by the specimen on the left, a negative reaction by the specimen on the right. **B,** Tube agglutination. A positive reaction is demonstrated by the specimen on the left, a negative reaction by the specimen on the right. (From Barrett JT: *Textbook of immunology,* ed 5, St Louis, 1988, Mosby.)

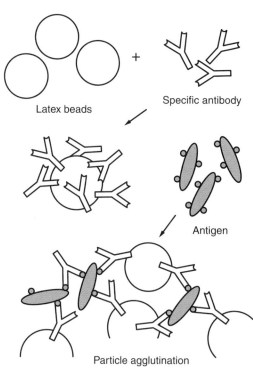

Figure 7-2 Alignment of antibody molecules bound to the surface of a latex particle and latex agglutination reaction. (Redrawn from Forbes BA, Sahm DF, Weissfeld AS: *Bailey and Scott's diagnostic microbiology,* ed 11, St Louis, 2002, Mosby.)

Box 7-1	Examples of Immunologic Assays Performed by Latex Particle Agglutination

C-Reactive protein
Immunoglobulin G rheumatoid factors
Immunoglobulin M rheumatoid factors
Rubella antibody

[see pregnancy test procedure later in this chapter] or rubella antibody testing), latex particles can be coated with antigen. In the presence of serum antibodies, these particles agglutinate into large, visible clumps.

Procedures based on latex agglutination must be performed under standardized conditions. The amount of antigen-antibody binding is influenced by factors such as pH, osmolarity, and ionic concentration of the solution.

Coagglutination and liposome-enhanced latex agglutination are variations of latex agglutination (Figure 7-3). Coagglutination uses antibodies bound to a particle to enhance the visibility of agglutination. It is a highly specific method

but may not be as sensitive as latex agglutination for detecting small quantities of antigen.

FLOCCULATION TESTS

Flocculation tests for antibody detection are based on the interaction of soluble antigen with antibody, which results in the formation of a precipitate of fine particles. These particles are macroscopically or microscopically visible only because the precipitated product is forced to remain in a confined space.

Two variations of flocculation testing can be used in syphilis serologic testing (see Chapter 15). These tests are the Venereal Disease Research Laboratory (VDRL) and the rapid plasma reagin (RPR) tests. In the VDRL test an antibody-like protein, reagin, binds to the test antigen, cardiolipid-lecithin-coated cholesterol particles, and produces the particles that flocculate. In the RPR test, the antigen, cardiolipid-lecithin-coated cholesterol with choline chloride, also contains charcoal particles that allow for macroscopically visible flocculation.

DIRECT BACTERIAL AGGLUTINATION

Direct whole pathogens can be used to detect antibodies directed against pathogens. The most basic tests are those

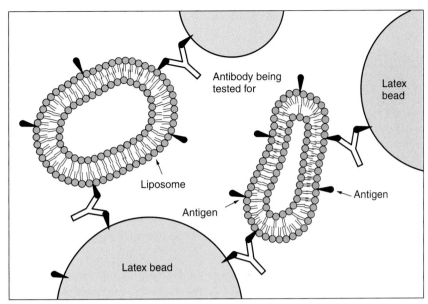

Figure 7-3   Diagram of liposome-latex agglutination reactions. (Redrawn from Neo-Planotest Ducoclox Slide Test, Organon Teknika Corp., Durham, NC.)

that measure the antibody produced by the host to determinants on the surface of a bacterial agent in response to infection with that bacterium. In a thick suspension of the bacteria, the binding of specific antibodies to surface antigens of the bacteria causes the bacteria to clump together in visible aggregates. This type of agglutination is called bacterial agglutination.

The formation of aggregates in solution is influenced by electrostatic and other forces; therefore certain conditions are usually necessary for satisfactory results. The use of sterile physiologic saline with free positive ions in the agglutination procedure enhances the aggregation of bacteria because most bacterial surfaces exhibit a negative charge that causes them to repel each other. Because tube testing allows more time for antigen-antibody reaction, it is considered to be more sensitive than slide testing. The small volume of liquid used in slide testing requires rapid reading before the liquid evaporates.

INDIRECT OR PASSIVE HEMAGGLUTINATION

Hemagglutination, agglutination of red blood cells, tests for antibody detection. In the indirect or passive hemagglutination technique, erythrocytes are coated with substances such as extracts of bacterial cells, rickettsiae, pathogenic fungi, or protozoa, or with purified polysaccharides or proteins. Erythrocytes of animals such as sheep or rabbits, or from group O humans, function as carriers for detecting and titrating the corresponding antibodies by agglutination. This technique is called indirect hemagglutination or passive hemagglutination (PHA) testing because it is not the antigen of the erythrocytes themselves but the passively attached antigens that are bound by antibody. In PHA techniques such as some rubella antibody procedures, erythrocytes are coated with rubella antigen. In the presence of

<table>
<tr><td>**Box 7-2**</td><td>**Examples of Immunologic Assays Performed by Indirect Hemagglutination**</td></tr>
</table>

Antinuclear ribonucleoprotein
Anti-Sm
Antithyroglobulin and antithyroid microsome
Rubella antibodies
Sheep cell agglutination titer

antibody, agglutination occurs. Control specimens are necessary to ensure that positive results are caused by antibodies against the absorbed antigen rather than by natural antierythrocyte antibodies.

HEMAGGLUTINATION

The hemagglutination method of testing detects antibodies to erythrocyte antigens. The antibody-containing specimen can be serially diluted and a suspension of red cells added to the dilutions. If a sufficient concentration of antibody is present, the erythrocytes are cross-linked and agglutinated. If nonreacting antibody or an insufficient quantity of antibody is present, the erythrocytes will fail to agglutinate.

By binding different antigens to the red cell surface in indirect hemagglutination or PHA, the hemagglutination technique can be extended to detect antibodies to antigens other than those present on the cells (Box 7-2). Chemicals such as chromic chloride, tannic acid, and glutaraldehyde can be used to cross-link antigens to the cells.

Some antibodies (e.g., immunoglobulin G [IgG]) do not directly agglutinate erythrocytes. This incomplete or blocking type of antibody may be detected by using an enhancement medium such as antihuman globulin reagent. If antihuman globulin reagent is added, this second antibody binds to the antibody present on the erythrocytes.

Mechanism of Agglutination

Agglutination is the clumping of particles that have antigens on their surface, such as erythrocytes, by antibody molecules that form bridges between the antigenic determinants. This is the end point for most tests involving erythrocyte antigens. Agglutination is influenced by a number of factors and is believed to occur in two stages: sensitization and lattice formation.

Sensitization

The first phase of agglutination, sensitization, represents the physical attachment of antibody molecules to antigens on the erythrocytic membrane. In this initial reversible interaction, antibodies combine rapidly with antigenic particles. The amount of antibody that will react is affected by the equilibrium constant, or affinity constant, of the antibody. In most cases the higher the equilibrium constant, the higher the rate of association and the slower the rate of dissociation of antibody molecules. The degree of association of antigen with antibody is affected by a variety of factors and can be altered in some cases in vitro by altering some of these factors. The factors influencing antigen-antibody association include:

- The antigen-antibody ratio, or the number of antibody molecules in relation to the number of antigen sites per cell
- Physical conditions such as pH, temperature, and length of time of incubation; ionic strength; and steric hindrance

Decreased Antigen-Antibody Ratio. Under conditions of antibody excess, a surplus exists of molecular antigen-combining sites not bound to antigenic determinants. The outcome of excessive antibody concentration is known as the prozone phenomenon, which can result in false-negative reaction. This phenomenon can be overcome by serially diluting the antibody-containing serum until optimum amounts of antigen and antibody are present in the test system.

pH. Although the optimum pH for all reactions has not been determined, a pH of 7.0 is used for routine laboratory testing. It is known that some antibodies react best at a lower pH.

Temperature and Length of Incubation. The optimum temperature needed to reach equilibrium in an antibody-antigen reaction differs for different antibodies. IgM antibodies are cold-reacting (thermal range 4° to 22° C), and IgG antibodies are warm-reacting, with an optimum temperature of reaction at 37° C. The length of time of incubation required to achieve maximum results depends on the rate of association and dissociation of each specific antibody. In laboratory testing, incubation times range from 15 to 60 minutes. The optimum time of incubation varies, depending on the class of immunoglobulin and how tightly an antibody attaches to its specific antigen.

Ionic Strength. The concentration of salt in the reaction medium has an effect on antibody uptake by the membrane-bound erythrocyte antigens. Sodium (Na^+) and chloride (Cl^-) ions in a solution have a shielding effect. These ions cluster around and partially neutralize the opposite charges on antigen and antibody molecules, which hinders the association of antibody with antigen. By reducing or lowering the ionic strength of a reaction medium (e.g., using low-ionic-strength saline), antibody uptake is enhanced.

Steric Hindrance. Steric hindrance is an important physiochemical effect that influences antibody uptake by cell surface antigens. If dissimilar antibodies with approximately the same binding constant are directed against antigenic determinants located close to each other, they will compete for space in reaching their specific receptor sites. The effect of this competition can be mutual blocking, steric hindrance, and neither antibody type will be bound to its respective antigenic determinant. Steric hindrance can occur whenever a conformational change in the relationship of an antigenic receptor site to the outside surface occurs. In addition to antibody competition, competition with bound complement, other protein molecules, or the action of agents that interfere with the structural integrity of the cell surface can produce steric hindrance. The combination of antigen and antibody is a reversible chemical reaction. Altering the physical conditions can result in the release of antibody from the antigen-binding site. When physical conditions are purposely manipulated to break the antigen-antibody complex, with subsequent release of the antibody into the surrounding medium, the procedure is referred to as an elution procedure.

Lattice Formation

Lattice formation, or the establishment of cross-links between sensitized particles (e.g., erythrocytes) and antibodies resulting in aggregation (clumping), is a much slower process than the sensitization phase. The formation of chemical bonds and resultant lattice formation depends on the ability of a cell with attached antibody on its surface to come close enough to another cell to permit the antibody molecules to bridge the gap and combine with the antigen receptor site on the second cell. Cross-linking is influenced by factors such as the zeta potential.

Methods of Enhancing Agglutination

Several techniques can be used to enhance agglutination. These techniques include:

- Centrifugation
- Treatment with proteolytic enzymes
- The use of colloids
- Antihuman globulin (AHG) testing

Treatment with proteolytic enzymes and the use of colloids or AHG techniques are common techniques in blood banking. These methods, however, can also be applied in the immunology laboratory. Centrifugation attempts to overcome the problem of distance by subjecting sensitized cells to a high gravitational force that counteracts the repulsive effect and physically forces the cells together. Enzyme treatment alters the zeta potential or dielectric constant to enhance the chances of demonstrable agglutination. Mild proteolytic enzyme treatment can strip off some of the negative charges on the cell membrane by removing surface sialic acid residues (cleaving sialoglycoproteins from the cell surface), which reduces the surface charge of cells, lowers the zeta potential, and permits cells to come closer together for chemical linking by specific antibody molecules. Some IgG antibodies will agglutinate if the zeta potential is carefully adjusted by the addition of colloids and salts. In some cases antigens may be so deeply embedded in the membrane surface that the previously described techniques will not bring the antigens and antibodies close enough to cross-link. The antihuman globulin test is frequently incorporated into the protocol of many laboratory techniques to facilitate agglutination. The direct antiglobulin test can be used to detect disorders such as hemolytic disease of the newborn, transfusion reactions, and differentiation of Ig from complement coating of erythrocytes.

Graded Agglutination Reactions

Observation of agglutination is initially made by gently shaking the test tube containing the serum and cells and viewing the lower portion, the button, with a magnifying glass as it is dispersed. Because agglutination is a reversible reaction, the test tube must be treated delicately and hard shaking must be avoided; however, all of the cells in the button must be resuspended before an accurate observation can be determined. Attention should also be given to whether discoloration of the fluid above the cells, the supernatant, is present. If the erythrocytes have been ruptured or hemolyzed, this is as important a finding as agglutination.

The strength of agglutination (Table 7-1), called grading, uses a scale of 0 or negative (no agglutination) to 4+ (all of the erythrocytes are clumped).

Pseudoagglutination, or false appearance of clumping, may rarely occur because of the presence of rouleaux formation. Rouleaux formation can be encountered in patients with high or abnormal types of globulins in their blood, such as in multiple myeloma, or after receiving dextran as a plasma expander. If this condition is present, on microscopic examination the erythrocytes will appear as rolls resembling stacks of coins. To disperse the pseudoagglutination, a few drops of physiologic sodium chloride (saline) can be added to the reaction tube, remixed, and reexamined. This procedure, saline replacement, should be performed carefully after pseudoagglutination is suspected. It should never be done before the initial testing protocol is followed, for a false-negative result may occur from the dilutional effect of the saline.

TABLE 7-1 Grading Agglutination Reactions

Grade	Description
Negative	No aggregates
Mixed field	Few isolated aggregates, mostly free-floating cells, supernatant appears red
Weak (+/−)	Tiny aggregates that are barely visible macroscopically, many free erythrocytes, turbid and reddish supernatant
1+	A few small aggregates just visible macroscopically, many free erythrocytes, turbid and reddish supernatant
2+	Medium-sized aggregates, some free erythrocytes, clear supernatant
3+	Several large aggregates, some free erythrocytes, clear supernatant
4+	All erythrocytes are combined into one solid aggregate; clear supernatant

Microplate Agglutination Reactions

Serologic testing has usually been performed by slide or test tube techniques, but the increased emphasis on cost containment has stimulated interest in microtechniques as an alternative to conventional methods. Capillary tubes and microplates have been used in some laboratories for a long time. Microtesting for typing lymphocytes was introduced 20 years ago. This method has been adopted internationally and is basically the only method used today for typing lymphocytes. Micromethods for red cell antigen and antibody testing are either hemagglutination or solid-phase adherence assays. These methods are also considered simpler to perform. Use of microplates allows for the performance of a large number of tests on a single plate, which eliminates time-consuming steps such as labeling test tubes.

A microplate is a compact plate of rigid or flexible plastic with multiple wells. The wells may be U-shaped or have a flat-bottom configuration. The U-shaped well has been the most commonly used in immunohematology. The volume capacity of each well is approximately 0.2 mL, which prevents spilling during mixing. Samples and reagents are dispensed with small-bore Pasteur pipettes. These pipettes are recommended because they deliver 0.025 mL, which prevents splashing. After the specimens and reagents are added to the wells, they are mixed by gentle agitation of the plates. The microplate is then centrifuged for an immediate reading. Countertop or floor model centrifuges are suitable if they are equipped with special rotors that can accommodate microplate centrifuge carriers and are capable of speeds between 400 and 2000 rpm. Smaller plates can be centrifuged in serologic centrifuges with an appropriate adapter.

After centrifugation the cell buttons are resuspended either by gently tapping the microplate or by using a flat-topped mechanical shaker. A shaker provides a more consistent and standard resuspension of the cells than manual tapping. After the cells are resuspended, the wells are examined with an optical aid or over a well-lit surface. A positive reaction will settle in a diffuse, uneven button; negative reactions are manifested by a smooth, compact button. Detection of weakly positive reactions is enhanced by allowing the red cells to settle.

HEMAGGLUTINATION INHIBITION TECHNIQUE

Many human viruses have the ability to bind to surface structures on erythrocytes from different species. The rubella virus, for example, can bind to human group O, goose, or chicken red blood cells and cause agglutination of these cells. For the detection of some viral antibodies, hemagglutination inhibition (HAI) is the standard against which other screening and diagnostic tests are measured.

Serologic tests for the presence of viral antibodies such as rubella exploit the agglutinating properties of the virus particles. Serum suspected of containing disease-causing virus is pretreated with a substance such as kaolin to remove nonspecific inhibitors such as beta lipoproteins (of red cell agglutination and nonspecific antibodies to the red cells). A known quantity of rubella viral antigen is mixed with dilutions of the patient's serum, to which red blood cells are added. If the serum lacks antibody, the virus will spontaneously attach to the red cells, link together, and agglutinate. If antibodies to the virus are present, all of the virus particles will be bound by antibody, which prevents or inhibits hemagglutination. The serum is therefore positive for HAI antibodies. The highest dilution of serum that totally inhibits agglutination of red cells determines the antibody titer of the serum.

The HAI detects a combination of IgG and IgM class antibodies. If IgG antibodies are separated from IgM antibodies by techniques such as sucrose density gradient fractionation or protein absorption, HAI can be used to test for IgM antibodies.

Disadvantages of this technique include the time-consuming nature of the procedure with the requirement of pretreatment of the serum, the fact that the method is highly technique-dependent for accuracy, and the need for visual interpretation of results. Subjective interpretation can influence results, and this type of variability may lead to a finding of seroconversion when none has occurred.

Negative results do not always indicate the absence of antibody. In some cases false-negative results can result from a low titer of antibody or the removal of antibody by the pretreatment process. False-positive results can be caused by nonspecific inhibitors. The lack of a procedural control removes the assurance that all nonspecific inhibitors have been removed.

PREGNANCY TESTING

The principle of antigen and antibody interaction has been applied to pregnancy testing since the first agglutination tests were developed in the 1960s. These assays replaced animal testing.

Biochemical Detected by Testing

Pregnancy tests are designed to detect minute amounts of human chorionic gonadotropin (hCG), a glycoprotein hormone secreted by the trophoblast of the developing embryo that rapidly increases in the urine or serum during early stages of pregnancy.

This glycoprotein hormone consists of two noncovalently linked subunits, alpha and beta. The alpha unit is identical to that found in luteinizing hormone, follicle-stimulating hormone, and thyroid-stimulating hormone. The beta subunit has a unique carboxy-terminal region. Using antibodies made against the beta subunit will cut down on cross-reactivity with the other three hormones. Accordingly, many pregnancy test kits contain monoclonal antibody directed against the beta subunit to increase the specificity of the reaction.

Physiology of Human Chorionic Gonadotropic Hormone

For the first 6 to 8 weeks after conception, hCG helps to maintain the corpus luteum and stimulate the production of progesterone. As a general rule, the level of hCG should double every 2 to 3 days. Pregnant women usually attain serum concentrations of 10 to 50 mIU of hCG in the week following conception. If a test is negative at this stage, the test should be repeated within a week. Peak levels are reached approximately 2 to 3 months after the last menstrual period.

Principle of Agglutination Inhibition

The determination of in vitro agglutination inhibition depends on incubation of the patient's specimen with anti-hCG, followed by the addition of latex particles coated with hCG. If hCG is present, it neutralizes the antibody; thus no agglutination of latex particles is seen. If no hCG is present, agglutination occurs between the anti-hCG and hCG-coated latex particles.

> ### ▪ Pregnancy Testing Protocols

Principle

Rapid latex slide agglutination test for detection of hCG is based on the principle of agglutination inhibition.

Specimen

The first morning urine specimen is required because it contains the highest concentration of hormone. It should have a specific gravity of at least 1.015. Collect the urine specimen in a clean glass or plastic container. It may be refrigerated for up to 2 days or frozen at −20° C for at least 1 year. Thaw frozen samples by placing the frozen specimen in a water bath at 37° C and then mixing thoroughly before use. If turbidity or precipitation is present after thawing, filtering or centrifuge is recommended. Specimens containing blood, large amounts of protein, or excessive bacterial contamination should not be used. Do not refreeze.

Materials

Anti-hCG serum
hCG-coated latex particles
Positive and negative controls
Stirrers, disposable pipettes, black glass slides, filter paper, centrifuge

Sample Procedure

1. Ensure that all reagents are at room temperature.
2. On clean slide, label positive control, negative control, and patient sample.
3. Using the disposable pipette provided, place 1 drop of patient urine in the central circle on the glass slide. Place 1 drop of negative control and 1 drop of positive control into the circles on either side of the patient sample, using a new disposable pipette for each.
4. Add 1 drop of antiserum reagent on each circle.
5. Add 1 drop of well-shaken latex antigen reagent to each circle.
6. Mix well, using a new stirrer for each circle. Spread the mixture over the entire circle.
7. Rock the slide gently back and forth for 3* minutes.

---

*NOTE: The length of time may vary.

8. Observe immediately for agglutination, using a light source held directly above the slide.

Technical Sources of Error

Reagents should never be expired; latex reagent must be well shaken, and agglutination should be read within 3 minutes to avoid erroneous results caused by evaporation.

Results

Agglutination represents a negative reaction.
No agglutination represents a positive reaction.

False-Positive Results

If a patient has been given an hCG injection (e.g., Profasi or Pregnyl) to trigger ovulation or to lengthen the luteal phase of the menstrual cycle, trace amounts can remain in the patient's system for as long as 10 days after the last injection. This will produce a false-positive result. Two consecutive quantitative hCG blood assays can circumvent this problem. If the hCG level increases by the second test, the patient is probably pregnant.

Chorioepithelioma, hydatidiform mole, or excessive ingestion of aspirin may give false-positive results. In men, a test identical to the one used for pregnancy may be performed to detect the presence of a testicular tumor. If monoclonal antibody against the beta subunit is not used, other hormones with the same alpha unit may cross-react and cause a false-positive reaction.

False-Negative Results

Testing before reaching detectable levels of hCG will yield false negative results.

Alternate Procedural Protocols

Latex agglutination slide tests have been replaced in some circumstances (e.g., home testing) by one-step chromatographic color-label immunoassays for the qualitative detection of hCG in urine (e.g., CLEARVIEW HCG II and CLEARVIEW HCG EASY [Wampole Laboratories, Princeton NJ]). The test procedure is simple, and each device has an internal control feature—a line appears in the Reference/Control Region to indicate that the test procedure has been performed correctly. These assays detect >25-mIU of hCG/mL in urine or serum. The procedure is CLIA waived for use with urine.

Another variation is one-step chromatographic color-label immunoassay for use with urine or serum (e.g., Wampole PreVue HCG Stick or Cassette, or STATUS HCG [Wampole Laboratories, Princeton, NJ]). The advantage of STATUS compared to PreVue or other similar products is that STATUS detects >15 mIU of hCG/mL in urine or serum.

CHAPTER HIGHLIGHTS

Agglutination of particles to which soluble antigen has been adsorbed produces a serum method of demonstrating precipitins. Examples of artificial carriers include latex particles and colloidal charcoal. Cells unrelated to the antigen, such as erythrocytes coated with antigen in a constant amount, can be used as biologic carriers.

In latex agglutination procedures, antibody molecules can be bound to the surface of latex beads. If an antigen is present in a test specimen, the antigen will bind to the combining sites of the antibody exposed on the surface of the latex beads, forming visible cross-linked aggregates of latex beads and antigen.

Flocculation tests for antibody detection are based on the interaction of soluble antigen with antibody, which results in the formation of a precipitate of fine particles.

Direct bacterial agglutination can be used to detect antibodies directed against pathogens.

In the indirect or PHA technique, erythrocytes are coated with substances such as extracts of bacterial cells, rickettsiae, pathogenic fungi, or protozoa, or with purified polysaccharides or proteins. This technique is called indirect hemagglutination or PHA testing because it is not the antigen of the erythrocytes themselves but the passively attached antigens that are bound by antibody.

REVIEW QUESTIONS

1. The quality of test results in an agglutination reaction depends on all of the following except:
   A. length of incubation
   B. amount of antigen conjugated to the carrier
   C. avidity of antigen conjugated to the carrier
   D. whether the carrier is artificial or biologic

2. Flocculation procedures differ from latex agglutination procedures because:
   A. antigen is bound to a carrier
   B. antibody is bound to a carrier
   C. soluble antigen reacts with antibody
   D. they are only qualitative procedures

3. Indirect hemagglutination is:
   A. also referred to as passive hemagglutination
   B. a system that uses passively attached antibody
   C. a system that uses passively attached antigen
   D. both A and C

4. In the hemagglutination technique, antihuman globulin is used as an enhancement medium to detect

   _____ type antibodies.

   A. IgM
   B. IgG
   C. IgD
   D. IgE

5. The prozone phenomenon can result in a (an)

   _____ .

   A. false-positive
   B. false-negative
   C. enhanced agglutination
   D. diminished antigen response

6. The effect of competing antibodies seeking to attach to antigen sites is called:
   A. prozone phenomenon
   B. ionic strength
   C. steric hindrance
   D. sensitization

7. All of the following are methods that can be used to enhance agglutination of IgG type antibodies except:
   A. centrifugation
   B. treatment with proteolytic enzymes
   C. acidifying the mixture
   D. using colloids

Questions 8-11. Match the following grades of agglutination with the appropriate description.

8. _____ Mixed field

9. _____ 1+

10. _____ 2+

11. _____ 4+

   A. all of the erythrocytes are combined into one solid aggregate, clear supernatant
   B. few isolated aggregates, supernatant appears red
   C. medium-sized aggregates, clear supernatant
   D. a few small aggregates, turbid and reddish supernatant
   E. several large aggregates, clear supernatant

12. A classic technique for the detection of viral antibodies is:
   A. passive hemagglutination
   B. indirect hemagglutination
   C. hemagglutination inhibition
   D. latex particle agglutination

Questions 13-17. Match each term to its definition.

13. _____ precipitation

14. _____ agglutination

15. _____ coagglutination

16. _____ flocculation

17. _____ hemagglutination

   A. aggregation of particulate test antigens
   B. aggregation of soluble test antigens
   C. uses antibodies bound to a particle to enhance visibility of agglutination
   D. agglutination of erythrocytes in tests for antibody detection
   E. based on the interaction of soluble antigen with antibody, resulting in formation of a precipitate of fine particles

18. Artificial or biologic carriers that can be used in an agglutination reaction include:
   A. latex particles
   B. colloidal charcoal
   C. erythrocytes coated with antigen in a constant amount
   D. all of the above

Questions 19 and 20. Identify the components of a latex agglutination reaction in the figure below.

Latex beads   +   19 _____

20 _____

Particle agglutination

(Redrawn from Forbes BA, Sahm DF, Weissfeld AS: *Bailey and Scott's diagnostic microbiology*, ed 11, St Louis, 2002, Mosby.)

   A. antigen
   B. specific antibody

21. Sensitization:
    A. is the first phase of agglutination
    B. represents the physical attachment of antibody molecules to antigens on the RBC membrane
    C. is an irreversible reaction
    D. both A and B

22. Agglutination can be used to enhance reactions by every means listed below except:
    A. decreasing the ionic strength of the reaction
    B. centrifugation
    C. increasing the pH of the reaction
    D. the use of colloids and antihuman globulin (AHG) testing

Questions 23-25. Match each grade of agglutination with its respective description below:

23. _____ negative

24. _____ weak (+/−)

25. _____ 3+

    A. tiny aggregates that are barely visible macroscopically
    B. several large aggregates
    C. all erythrocytes combined into one solid aggregate
    D. no aggregates

26. All of the following statements are correct regarding human pregnancy testing except:
    A. tests detect human chorionic gonadotropic hormone (hCG)
    B. the hCG is secreted by the trophoblast of the developing embryo
    C. the presence of hCG rapidly increases in urine or serum
    D. the presence of hCG in maternal urine or serum persists throughout pregnancy

27. All of the following statements are correct regarding human chorionic gonadotropic hormone (hCG) except:
    A. it helps to maintain the corpus luteum
    B. it stimulates production of progesterone
    C. it is detectable within 72 hours after the last expected menstrual period
    D. it reaches peak levels at 2 to 3 months after the last menstrual period

28. The most common laboratory method for detecting human hCG is:
    A. latex agglutination
    B. enzyme-linked immunosorbent assay
    C. immunofluorescence
    D. antibody titration

29. In the latex agglutination method for the detection of hCG, no agglutination indicates:
    A. absence of hCG
    B. presence of hCG
    C. absence of hCG, a positive test
    D. presence of hCG, a negative test

30. A urine specimen for pregnancy testing _____ be frozen.
    A. may
    B. may not

31. A false-positive reaction in a latex agglutination test for hCG can be caused by all of the following except:
    A. chorioepithelioma
    B. hydatidiform mole
    C. taking birth control pills
    D. excessive ingestion of aspirin

BIBLIOGRAPHY

Aloisi RM: *Principles of immunology and immuno-diagnostics,* Philadelphia, 1988, Lea & Febiger.

Baines W, Noble P: Sensitivity limits of latex agglutination tests, *Am Clin Lab* 12(3):14-15, 1993.

Forbes BA, Sahm DF, Weissfeld AS: *Bailey and Scott's diagnostic microbiology,* ed 11, St Louis, 2002, Mosby.

Henry JB, editor: *Clinical diagnosis and management,* ed 18, Philadelphia, 1991, WB Saunders.

Peacock JE, Tomar RH: *Manual of laboratory immunology,* Philadelphia, 1980, Lea & Febiger.

Turgeon ML: *Fundamentals of immunohematology,* ed 2, Baltimore, 1995, Williams & Wilkins.

Chapter 8

Electrophoresis Techniques

LEARNING OBJECTIVES

At the conclusion of this chapter, the reader should be able to:
- Describe the electrophoresis technique.
- Name the number of fractions that serum proteins can be divided into by electrophoresis.
- Describe the characteristics of immunoelectrophoresis.

- Explain the characteristics of immunofixation electrophoresis.
- State the clinical applications of immunoelectrophoresis.
- Compare immunoelectrophoresis and immunofixation electrophoresis.

IMMUNOELECTROPHORESIS

Serum electrophoresis results in the separation of proteins into five fractions on cellulose acetate. This separation is based on the rate of migration of these individual components in an electrical field. By comparison, immunoelectrophoresis (IEP) involves the electrophoresis of serum or urine followed by immunodiffusion. The size and position of precipitin bands provide the same type of information regarding equivalence or antibody excess as the double immunodiffusion method. Proteins, however, are differentiated not only by their electrophoretic mobility but by their diffusion coefficient and antibody specificity.

Although double-diffusion produces a separate precipitation band for each antigen-antibody system in a mixture, it is often difficult to determine all of the components in a very complex mixture. IEP separates the antigen mixture by electrophoresis before performing immunodiffusion.

Principle

IEP is a combination of the techniques of electrophoresis and double immunodiffusion. IEP consists of two phases: electrophoresis and diffusion. In the first phase, serum is placed in an appropriate medium (e.g., cellulose acetate or agarose), then electrophoresed to separate its constituents according to electrophoretic mobilities: albumin, $alpha_1$, $alpha_2$, beta, and gammaglobulin fractions. In the second phase after electrophoresis, the fractions are allowed to act as antigens and to interact with their corresponding antibodies. Antiserum, polyvalent or monovalent, is deposited in a trough cut into the gel to one side and parallel to this line of separated proteins. Incubation allows double immunodiffusion of these antigens and antibodies toward each other to take place. Each antiserum diffuses outward, perpendicular to the trough, and each serum protein diffuses outward from its point of electrophoresis. When a favorable antigen-to-antibody ratio exists (equivalence point), the antigen-antibody complex becomes visible as precipitin lines or bands. Diffusion is halted by rinsing the plate in 0.85% saline. Unbound protein is washed from the agarose with saline, and the antigen-antibody precipitin arcs are stained with a protein-sensitive stain.

Each line represents one specific protein. Proteins are thus differentiated not only by their electrophoretic mobility but by their diffusion coefficient and antibody specificity. Antibody diffuses as a uniform band parallel to the antibody trough. If the proteins are homogeneous, the antigen diffuses in a circle, and the antigen-antibody precipitation line resembles a segment or arc of a circle. If the antigen is heterogeneous, the antigen-antibody line assumes an elliptical shape. One arc of precipitation forms for each constituent in the antigen mixture. This technique can be used to resolve the protein of normal serum into 25 to 40 distinct precipitation bands. The exact number depends on the strength and specificity of the antiserum used.

Normal Appearance of Precipitin Bands

Immunoprecipitation bands should be of normal curvature, symmetry, length, position, intensity, and distance from the antigen well and antibody trough (Figure 8-1). In normal serum, immunoglobulin (Ig)G, IgA, and IgM are present in sufficient concentrations of 10 mg/mL, 2 mg/mL, and 1 mg/mL, respectively, to produce precipitin lines. The normal concentrations of IgD and IgE are too low to be detected by IEP.

A normal IgG precipitin band is elongated, elliptical, slightly curved, and clearly visible in undiluted and in 1:10 diluted serum. An IgG band is located cathodic to the antigen well in the alpha area of the electrophoretogram; if monospecific serum is used, it is fused with a thin precipitin line positioned midway between the antigen well and antibody trough and extending into the beta area. The IgM and IgA bands are visible in undiluted serum but disappear at a 1:10 dilution of serum. The IgA band is a flattened, thin arc, slightly cathodic to the well in the alpha-beta position. The IgM line is a barely visible, thin line, slightly cathodic to the antigen well.

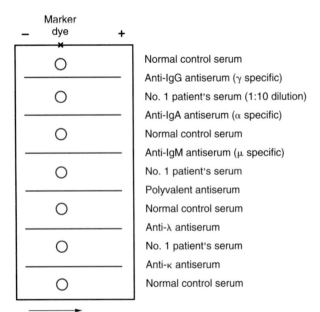

Marker
dye
−   +

○   Normal control serum

Anti-IgG antiserum (γ specific)

○   No. 1 patient's serum (1:10 dilution)

Anti-IgA antiserum (α specific)

○   Normal control serum

Anti-IgM antiserum (μ specific)

○   No. 1 patient's serum

Polyvalent antiserum

○   Normal control serum

Anti-λ antiserum

○   No. 1 patient's serum

Anti-κ antiserum

○   Normal control serum

Electrophoresis direction

Figure 8-1   Suggested sequence of antigen-antiserum combinations used in immunoelectrophoresis (IEP). (Redrawn from Bauer JD: *Clinical laboratory methods,* ed 9, St Louis, 1982, Mosby.)

Clinical Applications of IEP

IEP is a reliable and accurate method for detecting both structural abnormalities and concentration changes in proteins. It is possible to identify the absence of a normal serum protein such as a congenital deficiency of some complement components or alterations in serum proteins. This method can be used for screening for circulating immune complexes, characterization of cryoglobulinemia and pyroglobulinemia, recognition and characterization of antibody syndromes, and recognition and characterization of the various forms of dysgammaglobulinemias.

The most common application of IEP is in the diagnosis of a monoclonal gammopathy, a condition in which a single clone of plasma cells produces elevated levels of a single class and type of Ig. The elevated Ig is referred to as a monoclonal protein, M protein, or paraprotein. Monoclonal gammopathies may indicate a malignancy such as multiple myeloma or macroglobulinemia. Antikappa and antilambda antisera are necessary for complete typing of the Ig in the evaluation of the ratio and for the diagnosis of monoclonal M proteins. The class (heavy [H] chain) and type (light [L] chain) must be established because a patient's prognosis, and treatment may differ depending on the Ig identified. Differentiation must also be made between monoclonal and polyclonal gammopathies. A polyclonal gammopathy is a secondary condition caused by disorders such as liver disease, collagen disorders, rheumatoid arthritis, and chronic infection. It is characterized by elevation of two or more (often all) Igs by several clones of plasma cells. Polyclonal increases of proteins are usually twice the normal levels.

The most important application of IEP of urine is the demonstration of Bence Jones (BJ) protein. IEP detects very low concentrations of BJ protein (about 1 to 2 mg/dL). If BJ protein is present in a urine specimen, precipitin lines will form with either kappa or lambda antilight chain antisera because BJ protein is composed of homogeneous light chains of a single antigen type, either kappa or lambda. Normal light chains are heterogeneous and include equal concentrations of kappa and lambda.

Abnormal Appearance of Precipitin Bands

The size and position of precipitin bands provide the same type of information regarding equivalence or antigen-antibody excess as double immunodiffusion systems. The position and shape of precipitin bands in the IEP assay of serum are relatively stable and reproducible. Virtually any deviation is abnormal. These abnormalities can be detected by evaluating the following features of the precipitin bands:

- Position of the band in relationship to electrophoretically identified protein fractions
- Position of the band between the antigen well and the antibody trough
- Distortion of the curvature or arc formation
- Thickening (density) and elongation of a band
- Shortening (inhibition), thinning, or doubling

Position of the Band

The precipitin band may be displaced compared with its normal position in the control serum because molecular charges in the abnormal protein may affect its speed of migration in the electrophoresis phase of IEP. A precipitin band may form a line of fusion or partial fusion with another protein, indicating the presence of proteins immunologically similar but electrophoretically distinct. A distinct abnormality in the position of the band is seen in cases of monoclonal IgA gammopathy. The monoclonal IgA band is closer to the antibody trough than normal IgA.

Distortion of Curvature or Arc

An abnormal curvature of the precipitin band can be observed with M proteins because of an antigen excess. The monoclonal IgG band shows an arc of a circle rather than the elongated, elliptical shape of a normal band. This distortion of IgG reflects the homogeneous nature and limited electrophoretic mobility of the abnormal protein.

Normal IgM and IgD bands are hardly visible, but the monoclonal IgM or IgD bands are skewed arcs of a circle.

Thickening and Elongation

Thickening and elongation can be seen in the presence of M proteins because excess antigen diffuses a greater distance. Monoclonal IgM, IgG, IgD, and IgA all demonstrate denser-than-normal bands. In addition, monoclonal IgG touches the antisera trough.

Shortening, Thinning, or Doubling

A band may be shortened and incomplete because of inhibition of a segment resulting from the antibody's reacting with only a portion of the abnormal protein. Monoclonal IgE elevation leads to a short, thick arc in the antigen well area extending to the anodal side.

Polyvalent and Monovalent Antisera

Polyvalent antiserum confirms the presence or absence of major protein fractions. Monospecific antisera for specific individual Igs identify only the corresponding proteins. If the nonspecific antisera have combining sites for H and L chains, the combining sites will react with L chains of other Igs or with the free L chains of BJ protein. H chain-specific sera do not cross-react with other proteins.

 Immunoelectrophoresis

Principle

The patient specimen (e.g., serum) is placed on an appropriate medium and electrophoresed to separate its constituents according to electrophoretic mobilities. After electrophoresis, antiserum, polyvalent or monovalent, is deposited in a trough cut into the gel to one side and parallel to the line of separated proteins. Incubation allows double immunodiffusion of these antigens and antibodies toward each other to take place. When an equivalence point is reached, bands become visible as precipitin lines. Diffusion is halted, unbound protein is washed away, and the antigen-antibody precipitin arcs are stained with a protein-sensitive stain. This technique can be used to identify the protein of normal serum into 25 to 40 distinct precipitation bands.

Specimen Collection and Preparation

Fresh human serum or urine is the specimen of choice. No special preparation of the patient is required before specimen collection. The patient must be positively identified when the specimen is collected, and the specimen should be labeled at the bedside. Specimen labels should include the patient's full name, the date, the patient's hospital identification number, and the phlebotomist's initials.

Blood should be drawn by an aseptic technique. A minimum of 2 mL of clotted blood (red top evacuated tube) is required. The specimen should be centrifuged promptly and an aliquot of serum removed. Hemolysis or contamination with bacteria renders a specimen unsuitable for testing.

Urine specimens should be tested in both unconcentrated and concentrated (10× to 50×) forms because of the wide range of light chain concentrations.

Serum and urine samples for assay should be fresh. If the test cannot be performed immediately, the specimen can be refrigerated (2° to 8° C) for up to 5 days after collection.

Reagents, Supplies, and Equipment

Reagents and supplies for gel electrophoresis are commercially available from Helena Laboratories, Beaumont, TX.

1. 0.85% saline solution.
2. Barbital buffer (sodium barbital, pH 8.3 to 8.7). Packaged, dry buffer should be stored at room temperature (15° to 30° C) and is stable until the expiration date on the package. Discard packaged buffer if the material shows signs of dampness or discoloration.

    Prepare the buffer by transferring one prepackaged packette to a 1-L volumetric flask and dilute to the calibration mark with purified water. The buffer is ready for use when it is completely dissolved. Transfer the reconstituted buffer to a clean storage bottle. Label the bottle with the appropriate identification, warning, and date of preparation. Reconstituted buffer solution is stable for 6 months at 15° to 30° C. Discard buffer solution if it becomes turbid.

    CAUTION: Barbital can be toxic if ingested.
3. Destaining solution. Prepare by measuring and adding 675 mL of 95% ethanol (denatured with either methanol or isopropanol) and 675 mL of purified water to a 1-L volumetric flask. Mix. NOTE: Wear safety glasses and perform the next step under a hood. Measure and add 150 mL of glacial acidic acid. Mix thoroughly and transfer to a clean, labeled bottle with a cap.
4. IEP stain (Coomassie brilliant blue). Dry stain should be stored at room temperature (15° to 30° C) and is stable until the expiration date indicated on the package.

    Prepare by adding one packette of stain to a 1-L volumetric flask. Measure and add 450 mL of 95% ethanol (denatured with either methanol or isopropanol). Mix thoroughly to dissolve all of the stain. Add 450 mL of purified water and mix.

NOTE: Wear safety glasses and perform the next step under a hood. Measure and add 100 mL of glacial acidic acid. Mix thoroughly and transfer to a clean, labeled bottle with a cap.

Stain solution is stable for 6 months when stored at room temperature (15° to 30° C) in a tightly closed container. The stain can be returned to the bottle and reused. If the stain shows signs of deterioration (i.e., evidence of precipitate), it should be discarded.

5. Albumin marker. Albumin marker is 0.5% bromphenol blue in aqueous solution. The bromphenol blue binds with the albumin in the control. The tagged albumin allows for verification of protein mobility. The solution should be stored at 15° to 30° C and is stable until the expiration date indicated on the vial. Discard if the solution color changes from yellow to brown.

6. IEP normal human serum control contains pooled normal human serum with 0.1% sodium azide as a preservative. It is in liquid form and ready for use as packaged. Before using, add 2 drops of albumin marker to the control vial. Store at 2° to 6° C. The solution is stable until the expiration date indicated on the vial. Stability is not affected by the addition of albumin marker. Control should be light yellow and slightly hazy before the addition of the marker.

CAUTION: Because the control sera is derived from human sources, it should be handled in the same manner as clinical serum specimens (see Universal Blood and Body Fluid Precautions in Chapter 6).

WARNING: Sodium azide is used as a preservative. To prevent the formation of toxic vapors, do not mix with acidic solutions. Sodium azide may react with lead and copper plumbing to form highly explosive metal azides. On disposal, flush with a large volume of water to prevent azide buildup. In addition to purging pipes with water, occasionally decontaminate plumbing with 10% NaOH.

7. Gel plates. Titan gel IEP plates containing 1% agarose (w/v) in barbital-sodium barbital buffer with 0.1% sodium azide as a preservative. They are ready to use as packaged and should be stored flat at 2° to 6° C in the protective packaging in which they are shipped.

CAUTION: Do not freeze the plates or expose them to excessive heat.

The plates are stable until the expiration date indicated on the label unless signs of deterioration are apparent. If the plates do not have a smooth, clear agarose surface, deterioration has occurred. Discard plates that are cloudy, exhibit bacterial growth, or have been exposed to freezing (a cracked or bubbled surface) or excessive heat (a dried, thin surface).

8. Antiserum for assay (commercially prepared). Depending on the desired assay, one of the following should be used:
   a. An antiserum to human IgG, IgM, IgA, or IgD; IgE trivalent antiserum to human Igs (heavy chain specific for IgG, IgA, IgM); or antiserum to human kappa or lambda light chain.
   b. Antisera, supplied in liquid form, are prepared in horse, sheep, goat, donkey, or rabbit. Each vial contains 0.1% sodium azide as a preservative. The antisera should be stored at 2° to 6° C and are stable until the expiration date indicated on the vial; they should be colorless to light yellow in color.

9. Gel blotter C
10. Gel blotter E
11. Serologic rotator
12. Gel-staining set
13. Humidity chamber
14. Microdispenser tubes (1 to 10 μL) or (1 to 25 μL)
15. Gel chamber
16. Sponge wicks
17. Digital power supply
18. Incubator/dryer
19. Development weight
20. Viewbox (optional)
21. Immunocamera (optional)

Quality Control

The normal human serum control with albumin marker added should be used as a control for each antiserum specificity used. It should be tested with each test run.

Procedure

Preparation of Gel Chamber

1. Measure 200 mL of barbital buffer in a graduated cylinder. (The buffer may be reused one time by reversing the polarity of the chamber. The plates must then be placed with the wells on the left side [formerly the anodic side].) Add 100 L of the buffer to each outer section of the chamber.
2. Place a long IEP sponge wick in each buffer-filled compartment. Allow the sponges to become saturated with buffer. Place the sponges against the chamber walls.
3. Cover the chamber until ready to use.

Sample Application

1. Remove the gel plates from the refrigerator and allow the plates to come to room temperature while still in the protective packaging.
2. Remove the needed number of plates from the protective packaging and save the plastic holder for later use in the incubation chamber.
3. Using a microdispenser, apply 2 μL of the control to the wells labeled "C." The sample should be applied with care to avoid damaging the wells during sample application.
4. Using a microdispenser, apply 2 μL of the patient sample to wells labeled "P." The sample should be applied with care to avoid damaging the wells during sample application.

Electrophoresis

1. Quickly put the plate(s) in the electrophoresis chamber, agarose side down, with the wells toward the

cathode (−). Make sure that the agarose is in good contact with the sponge wicks. Two plates may be electrophoresed in one chamber.
2. Put the cover on the electrophoresis chamber and wait 30 to 60 seconds before applying current. This allows the plate(s) to equilibrate with the buffer.
3. Electrophorese the plate(s) at 100 volts for a migration distance of 35 mm or greater. This requires approximately 40 to 50 minutes. Migration distance can be verified by observing the position of the albumin marker.

Antisera Application

1. Remove the plate(s) from the chamber and put it on a flat surface, agarose side up.
2. Apply 25 μL of the appropriate antiserum to each trough in the plate. Fill the troughs by placing the tip of a microdispenser in the end of the trough farthest from the sample well. While holding the microdispenser in place, slowly depress the plunger and dispense the antiserum into the trough. The antiserum will flow down the trough by capillary action. The troughs easily hold 25 μL of antiserum without overflowing. Severe overfilling may cause antisera to contaminate other troughs, yielding erroneous results.
3. Before moving the plates, allow the antisera to absorb for approximately 3 to 5 minutes.
4. Put each plate in the protective packaging previously removed from the gel plate.
5. Stack the plates (within the holders) in a humidity chamber containing a moist paper wick.
6. Incubate the plate(s) at room temperature (15° to 30° C) for 18 to 24 hours. The minimum incubation time is 18 hours. Optimum precipitation will occur between 2 μL of sample and at least 25 μL of antiserum after 18 to 24 hours. If less than 25 μL of antiserum is used, diffuse precipitin arcs will result, interfering with pattern interpretation.

Washing and Staining the Gel Plate(s)

1. At the end of the incubation period, remove the plate(s) from the plastic packaging and put it in 0.85% saline. The saline stops the diffusion reaction and washes out unbound protein.
2. Wash and press-dry the plate using a quick wash (described below), 6-hour wash, or overnight wash.

Quick Wash

Press-dry the plate for 5 minutes using the following procedure:
1. Lay the plate on a flat surface, agarose side up. Place one blotter C directly on the plate, followed by 2 blotter Es. Then place a development weight on top of the plate and blotters for 5 minutes.
2. Remove the weight and discard the blotters.
3. Wash the plate in 0.85% saline for 5 to 10 minutes.
4. Repeat the press-and-wash steps two more times. After the third wash, press again.

Completion of Procedure

1. After washing and pressing, place the plate on a blotter, agarose side up, in a drying oven at 60° to

75° C for 3 to 5 minutes or until dry. The plate must be completely dry to stain and destain it properly.
2. Fill a staining chamber with staining solution.
3. Fill three destaining chambers with destaining solution.
4. Place the dried plate(s) in a staining rack and lower into the staining chamber. Stain the plate(s) for 4 minutes.
5. Remove the staining rack containing the plate(s) and put it on a paper towel to drain off surplus stain.
6. Raise and lower the rack four times in the first destaining chamber to further remove excess stain.
7. In the second destaining chamber, raise and lower the rack four times to further remove excess stain. The background should be clear after this wash; if not, put the plate(s) in the third destaining chamber until the background is clear, no more than 2 to 3 minutes. Do not destain further if the stain in the IgM arc will be lost. Plates can be restained if necessary.
8. Remove the plate(s) from the rack and put each plate on a blotter, agarose side up.
9. Dry the plate(s) in a laboratory drying oven at 60° to 70° C for 3 to 5 minutes or until dry. A stained and dried gel plate is stable for an indefinite period.

Reporting Results

Formation of a precipitin arc between a well containing a test specimen and a trough containing antiserum indicates the presence of the protein specific to the antisera. Lack of a precipitin arc indicates that a detectable amount of the protein is not present in the test specimen. The size, location, and shape of the precipitin arc, as compared with the control, are indications of the amount of protein in the test specimen.

When protein concentrations are below normal, precipitin arcs are shortened and located farther from the antiserum trough than the corresponding arc in the control. When protein concentrations are above normal, precipitant arcs are thicker and located closer to the antiserum trough than the control. Figure 8-2 is a sample Ig profile. The pattern of precipitin arcs are interpreted by comparing the patient sample to the control. In the illustration the patient serum forms a dense, bowed arc against IgG antiserum. There appears to be a diminished IgA level and virtually no IgM in the patient serum when compared to the IgA and IgM in the control. The abnormal IgG band is also visible against both human and univalent antisera. The patient specimen reveals a bowed, abnormal kappa arc and a decreased lambda arc. This composite is indicative of an IgG monoclonal gammopathy, kappa type.

Reference ranges to be considered include patient age, sex, history, and clinical presentation, which will affect Ig levels.

Procedure Notes

Interpretation of IgM light chain reactions is often difficult because of the umbrella effect of IgG. IgM (19S) can be depolymerized with 2-mercaptoethanol into single molecular (7S) units, which diffuse through the agarose more rapidly. In rare instances, this may be necessary for IgA typing.

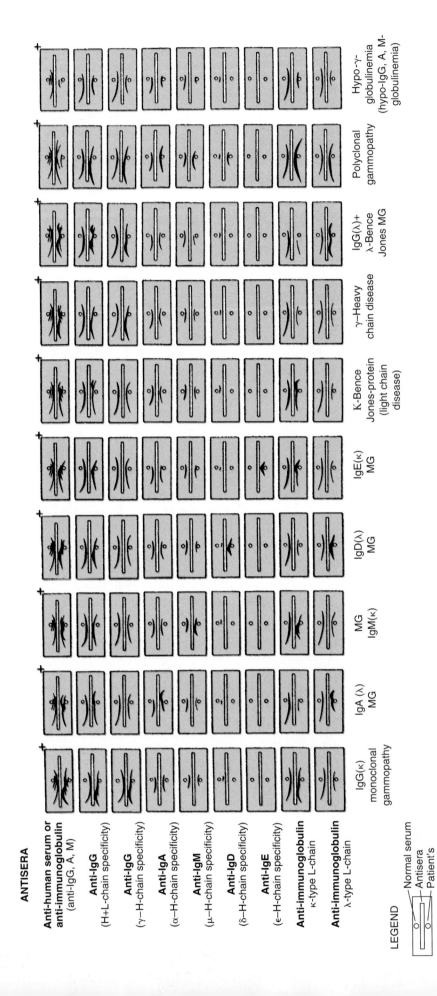

Figure 8-2   Abnormal immunoglobulin pattern (IEP). (Redrawn from Ritzman SE, Daniels JC: *Laboratory notes—serum proteins*, No. 3, Somerville, NJ, 1973, Behring Diagnostics/Hoechst Pharmaceuticals Inc.)

Sources of Error

Prozone is an incomplete precipitin reaction caused by antigen excess (too high an antigen-antibody ratio). Prozoning should be suspected if a precipitin arc appears to "run" into a trough, if a light chain appears fuzzy when a heavy chain is increased, or if an arc appears to be incomplete.

Clinical Applications

IEP is a reliable and accurate method for detecting both structural abnormalities and concentration changes in proteins. The most common application of IEP is in the diagnosis of monoclonal gammopathies.

Limitations

IEP is a semiquantitative technique.

IMMUNOFIXATION ELECTROPHORESIS

Immunofixation electrophoresis (IFE) is a two-stage procedure using agarose gel protein electrophoresis in the first stage and immunoprecipitation in the second. The test specimen may be serum, urine, cerebrospinal fluid, or other body fluids. The primary use of IFE in clinical laboratories is for the characterization of monoclonal Igs.

Applications

Although IFE was first described in 1964, it was introduced as a procedure for the study of Igs in 1976. IEP and IFE are complementary techniques best used in the workup of a patient with a suspected monoclonal gammopathy. The laboratory protocol for ruling out monoclonal gammopathy should include high-resolution electrophoresis, immunoelectrophoresis of both serum and urine, and a quantitative Ig assay. These procedures are usually sufficient to detect and characterize monoclonal proteins with a serum concentration of 1 g or more.

Three variables of protein can be determined using IFE:
1. Antigenic specificity
2. Electrophoretic mobility
3. Quantity or ratio of the test and control proteins

Procedural Protocol

In the first step of the IFE procedure, a single specimen is applied to six different positions on an agarose plate, and the proteins are separated according to their net charge by electrophoresis. In the second phase, monospecific antisera are applied to five of the electrophoresis patterns: IgG, IgA, IgM, and kappa and lambda antisera. A protein fixative solution is applied to the sixth pattern to produce a complete protein reference pattern. The plate is incubated for 10 minutes.

If complementary antigen is present in the proper proportions in the test sample, antigen-antibody complexes form and precipitate. The formation of a stable antigen-antibody precipitate fixes the protein in the gel. After fixation the gel is washed in deproteination solution (e.g., dilute sodium chloride), and nonprecipitated proteins are washed out of the agarose, leaving only the antigen-antibody complex. The protein reference pattern and the antigen-antibody precipitation bands are stained with a protein-sensitive stain.

Comparison of IEP and IFE

IEP is technically simpler and less subject to antigen excess phenomenon than IFE. If IFE-high concentrations of monoclonal protein give no visible reactions, IEP is considered to be a better technique for typing large monoclonal gammopathies. IFE, however, can be optimized to give both greater sensitivity and resolution than IEP. IFE should be reserved for anomalous proteins, which are difficult to characterize by IEP. These include small bands such as those exhibited in the early stages of monoclonal gammopathies or light chain disease, and any multiple, closely spaced bands. IFE is easier to interpret than IEP because interpretation is based on examination of a precipitate pattern directly analogous to routine electrophoresis; it does not depend on detecting slight deviations in the shape of a precipitin arc.

CHAPTER HIGHLIGHTS

Serum electrophoresis results in the separation of proteins into five fractions on cellulose acetate. This separation is based on the rate of migration of these individual components in an electrical field. By comparison, IEP involves the electrophoresis of serum or urine followed by immunodiffusion. The size and position of precipitation bands provide the same type of information regarding equivalence or antibody excess as the double immunodiffusion method. IEP is a combination of the techniques of electrophoresis and double immunodiffusion. IEP consists of two phases: electrophoresis and diffusion. Proteins are thus differentiated not only by their electrophoretic mobility but by their diffusion coefficient and antibody specificity.

The most common application of IEP is in the diagnosis of monoclonal gammopathies. A monoclonal gammopathy is a condition in which a single clone of plasma cells produces elevated levels of a single class and type of Ig.

IFE is a two-stage procedure using agarose gel protein electrophoresis in the first stage and immunoprecipitation in the second. The primary use of IFE in clinical laboratories is for the characterization of monoclonal Igs.

REVIEW QUESTIONS

1. Protein can be separated into _____ fractions by use of serum electrophoresis.
   A. three
   B. four
   C. five
   D. six

2. Which of the following is the most common application of immunoelectrophoresis (IEP)?
   A. identification of the absence of a normal serum protein
   B. structural abnormalities of proteins
   C. screening for circulating immune complexes
   D. diagnosis of monoclonal gammopathies

3. Abnormalities of precipitin bands in an IEP assay can be evaluated by all of the following features except:
   A. position of the band between antigen well and antibody trough
   B. position of the band in relationship to electrophoretically identified protein fractions
   C. general location of the band
   D. distortion of the arc formation

4. Immunofixation electrophoresis is best used in
   A. the workup of a polyclonal gammopathy
   B. the workup of a monoclonal gammopathy
   C. screening for circulating immune complexes
   D. identification of hypercomplementemia

Questions 5-9. True or False

A = True
B = False

5. _____ IEP is technically simpler and less subject to antigen excess phenomenon than IFE.

6. _____ IFE is considered to be a better technique than IEP for typing large monoclonal gammopathies.

7. _____ IFE can be optimized to give both greater sensitivity and resolution than IEP.

8. _____ IFE should be reserved for anomalous proteins that are difficult to characterize by IEP.

9. _____ IEP is easier to interpret than IFE.

10. Immunoelectrophoresis involves:
    A. separation of proteins based on the rate of migration of individual components in an electrical field
    B. electrophoresis of serum or urine
    C. double immunodiffusion following electrophoresis
    D. all of the above

11. In immunoelectrophoresis (IEP), proteins are differentiated by:
    A. electrophoresis
    B. diffusion coefficient
    C. antibody specificity
    D. all of the above

12. Immunoelectrophoresis can divide the proteins of normal serum into _____ distinct precipitation bands.
    A. 5-10
    B. 15-20
    C. 25-40
    D. 45-100

13. IEP is useful for clinically detecting:
    A. structural abnormalities
    B. concentration changes in proteins
    C. congenital deficiency of some complement components
    D. all of the above

14. The most common application of IEP of serum is:
    A. diagnosis of monoclonal gammopathy
    B. diagnosis of polyclonal gammopathy
    C. diagnosis of autoimmune hemolysis
    D. demonstration of Bence Jones (BJ) protein

15. Immunofixation electrophoresis (IFE) can test:
    A. serum and urine
    B. cerebrospinal fluid
    C. whole blood
    D. A and B

16. The primary use of IFE is:
    A. characterization of monoclonal immunoglobulins
    B. characterization of polyclonal immunoglobulins
    C. identification of monoclonal immunoglobulins
    D. identification of polyclonal immunoglobulins

BIBLIOGRAPHY

Killingsworth LM, Warren BM: *Immunofixation for the identification of monoclonal gammopathies,* Beaumont, Tex, 1986, Helena Laboratories.

Ritzmann EE: Immunoglobulin abnormalities. In Ritzman S, editor: *Serum protein abnormalities, diagnostic and clinical aspects,* Boston, 1976, Little, Brown.

Sun T: Immunofixation electrophoresis procedures. In *Protein abnormalities,* vol 1, Physiology of immunoglobulins: diagnostic and clinical aspects, New York, 1982, Alan R Liss.

Chapter 9

Labeling Techniques in Immunoassay

LEARNING OBJECTIVES

At the conclusion of this chapter, the reader should be able to:
- Describe chemiluminescence.
- Name at least three types of labels that can be used in immunoassay.
- Describe and compare chemiluminescence, enzyme immunoassay (EIA), and immunofluorescent techniques.
- Briefly compare direct immunofluorescent, inhibition immunofluorescent assay, and indirect immunofluorescent assays.

- Compare the advantages, disadvantages, and application of quantum dots (Q dots), SQUID technology, luminescent oxygen channeling immunoassay (LOCI), fluorescent in situ hybridization (FISH), signal amplification technology, and magnetic labeling technology.

TYPES OF LABELS

The original technique of using antigen-coated cells or particles in agglutination techniques may be considered the earliest method for labeling components in immunoassays. Ideal characteristics of a label include the quality of being measurable by several methods, including visual inspection. The properties of a label used in an immunoassay determine the ways in which detection is possible. For example, coated latex particles can be detected by various methods: visual inspection, light scattering (nephelometry), and particle counting. The conversion of a colorless substrate into a colored product in enzyme immunoassay (EIA) allows for two methods of detection, colorimetry and visual inspection.

The use of a radioactive label, the radioimmunoassay (RIA) method, that could identify an immunocomponent at very low concentrations was developed by Yalow and Berson in 1959. In the 1960s researchers began to search for a substitute for the successful RIA method because of the inherent drawbacks of using radioactive isotopes as labels (e.g., radioactive waste and short shelf life). Today, chemiluminescent reactions have supplanted most RIAs in the clinical laboratory. This relatively simple, cost-effective technology has sensitivity at least as good as that of RIA. The principles and applications of chemiluminescence, enzymes, and fluorescent substances as labels are presented in this chapter.

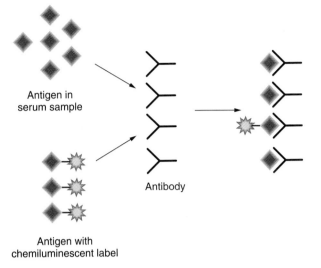

Figure 9-1 Format for competitive immunoassays. (Redrawn from Jandreski MA: Chemiluminescence technology in immunoassays, *Lab Med* 29:557, 1998.)

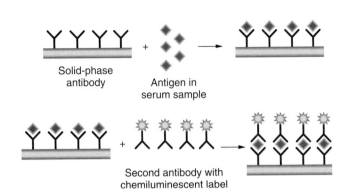

Figure 9-2 Format for sandwich immunoassays. (Redrawn from Jandreski MA: Chemiluminescence technology in immunoassays, *Lab Med* 29:557, 1998.)

CHEMILUMINESCENCE

Chemiluminescence is being pursued as the technology of choice by most immunodiagnostics manufacturers. Chemiluminescence has excellent sensitivity and dynamic range. It does not require sample radiation, and nonselective excitation and source instability are eliminated. Most chemiluminescent reagents and conjugates are stable and relatively nontoxic.

In immunoassays chemiluminescent labels can be attached to an antigen or an antibody. Chemiluminescent labels are being used to detect proteins, viruses, oligonucleotides, and genomic nucleic acid sequences in immunoassay. Two formats are used:

- Competitive
- Sandwich immunoassays

In a competitive immunoassay a fixed amount of labeled antigen competes with unlabeled antigen from a patient specimen for a limited number of antibody-binding sites (Figure 9-1). The amount of light emitted is inversely proportional to the amount of analyte (antigen) measured.

In a sandwich immunoassay, the sample antigen binds to an antibody fixed onto a solid phase; a second antibody, labeled with a chemiluminescent label, binds to the antigen-antibody complex on the solid phase (Figure 9-2). In the sandwich assay the emitted light is directly proportional to the analyte concentration. The detection device for analyses is a simple photomultiplier tube used to detect the emitted light.

Chemiluminescent labels can be divided into five major groups:

- Luminol
- Acridinium esters
- Peroxyoxalates
- Dioxetanes
- Tris (2,2'bipyridyl) ruthenium (II)

The direct labels include luminol, acridinium ester, and electrogenerated luminescence from a $Ru(bpy)_3^{2+}$ complex. These labels are attached directly to antigens, antibodies, or DNA probes, depending on the assay format. The light from direct labels is emitted in the form of a flash lasting 1 to 5 seconds. Peak intensity can be used for the measurement. An alternate method is to use an integrator to measure the entire light output for greater sensitivity.

Enzymes are usually used for indirect labels. Indirect labels are attached to antibodies, antigens, and DNA probes, depending on the assay format. Enzyme labels commonly used in indirect procedures are:

- Alkaline phosphatase
- Horseradish peroxidase
- Beta-galactosidase

ENZYME IMMUNOASSAY

The enzyme immunoassay (EIA) method uses a nonisotopic label that offers the advantage of safety. EIA is usually an objective measurement that provides numeric results. Some EIA procedures provide diagnostic information and measure immune status (e.g., detect either total antibody IgM or IgG).

An enzyme-labeled antibody or enzyme-labeled antigen conjugate is used in immunologic assays for a variety of antigens or antibodies, respectively (Box 9-1). The enzyme with its substrate detects the presence and quantity of antigen or antibody in a patient specimen. In some tissues an enzyme-labeled antibody can identify antigenic locations.

Various enzymes are used in enzyme immunoassay (Table 9-1). The most commonly used enzymes are peroxidase and alkaline phosphatase. To be used in EIA, an enzyme must fulfill a number of criteria, including:

- A high amount of stability
- Extreme specificity

Box 9-1	Examples of Enzyme Immunoassays

Borrelia burgdorferi (IgG and IgM)
Cytomegalovirus (IgG and IgM Ab)
Cytomegalovirus (Ag)
Hepatitis A (Total Ab)
Hepatitis B:
    anti-HBs
    anti-HBc
    anti-HBe
    anti-HBc (IgM)
    HBs Ag
    HBe Ag
Hepatitis delta virus (total Ab)
Hepatitis non-A, non-B
HIV Ab
HIV Ag
HTLV-I Ab
HTLV-II AB
Human B lymphotropic virus Ab
Rubella virus (IgG and IgM Ab)
Toxoplasma gondii (IgG and IgM Ab)

TABLE 9-1 Enzymes Used in Enzyme Immunoassay

Enzyme	Source
Acetylcholinesterase	*Electrophorous electicus*
Alkaline phosphatase	*Escherichia coli*
Beta-Galactosidase	*Escherichia coli*
Glucose oxidase	*Aspergillis niqer*
Glucose-6-phosphate dehydrogenase (G6-PD)	*Leuconostoc mesenteroides*
Lysozyme	Egg white
Malate dehydrogenase	Pig heart
Peroxidase	Horseradish

- Absence from the antigen or antibody
- No alteration by inhibitor with the system

In a representative EIA test, a plastic bead or plastic plate is coated with antigen (e.g., virus) (Figure 9-3). The antigen reacts with antibody in the patient serum. The bead or plate is then incubated with an enzyme-labeled antibody conjugate. If antibody is present, the conjugate reacts with the antigen-antibody complex on the bead or plate. The enzyme activity is measured spectrophotometrically after the addition of the specific chromogenic substrate. For example, peroxidase cleaves its substrate, o-dianisidine, causing a color change. In some cases the test can be read subjectively. The results of a typical test are calculated by comparing the spectrophotometric reading of patient serum to that of a control or reference serum. The advantage of an objective enzyme test is that results are not dependent on a technician's interpretations. In general the EIA procedure is faster and requires less laboratory work than comparable methods.

IMMUNOFLUORESCENT TECHNIQUES

Fluorescent labeling is another method of demonstrating the complexing of antigens and antibodies (Figure 9-4). Fluorescent molecules are used as substitutes for radioisotope or enzyme labels. The fluorescent antibody technique consists of labeling antibody with fluorescein isothiocyanate (FITC), a fluorescent compound with an affinity for proteins, to form a complex (conjugate). This conjugate is able to react with antibody-specific antigen.

Fluorescent techniques are extremely specific and sensitive. Antibodies may be conjugated to other markers in addition to fluorescent dyes; the use of these markers is called colorimetric immunologic probe detection. The use of enzyme-substrate marker systems has been expanded. Horseradish peroxidase, alkaline phosphatase, and avidin-biotin conjugated enzyme labels have all been used as visual tags for the presence of antibody. These reagents have the advantage of requiring only a standard light microscope.

Fluorescent conjugates are used in the following basic methods:
- Direct immunofluorescent assay
- Inhibition immunofluorescent assay
- Indirect immunofluorescent assay

Direct Immunofluorescent Assay

In the direct technique a conjugated antibody is used to detect antigen-antibody reactions at a microscopic level (Figure 9-5). This technique can be applied to tissue sections or in smears for microorganisms. Fluorescein-conjugated antibodies bound to the fluorochrome FITC are used to visualize many bacteria in direct specimens. Peroxidase conjugated to antibody, the immunoperoxidase stain, can be used to detect cytomegalovirus (CMV), other viruses, or nucleic acids in cells. In biotin-avidin, enzyme-conjugated methods, single-stranded nucleic acid probes, antimicrobial antibodies, or antibiotin antibodies can be bound to the small molecule, biotin. These molecules have a strong affinity for the protein avidin, which has four binding sites. Biotin bound to avidin or antibody can be complexed to fluorescent dyes or to color-producing enzymes to form specific detector systems. This system can be applied to the detection of nucleic acids in organisms such as CMV, hepatitis B virus, Epstein-Barr virus, and chlamydia.

The chemical manipulation in labeling antibodies with fluorescent dyes to permit detection by direct microscopic examination does not seriously impair antibody activity (i.e., the ability of the fluorescent antibody conjugate to react specifically with its homologous antigen). Monoclonal antibodies have also been successfully conjugated to fluorescein for the detection of chlamydiae, rabies virus, and other pathogens in directly stained specimens.

A fluorescent substance is one that, when absorbing light of one wavelength, emits light of another (longer) wavelength. In fluorescent antibody microscopy, the incident or exciting light is often blue-green to ultraviolet. The light is provided by a high-pressure mercury arc lamp with a primary

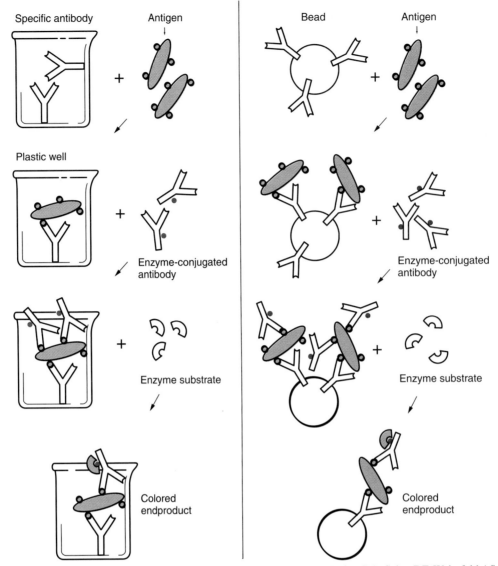

Figure 9-3 Principle of solid-phase enzyme immunosorbent assay. (Forbes BA, Sahm DF, Weissfeld AS: *Bailey and Scott's diagnostic microbiology,* ed 11, St Louis, 2002, Mosby.)

Figure 9-4 Principles of direct and indirect fluorescent techniques. **A,** Direct fluorescence. **B,** Indirect fluorescence. Key: *1* = microscopic slide, *2* = cell (cytoplasm and nucleus), *3* = antiserum, conjugate in A and unconjugate in B, *4* = conjugated antiglobulin serum.

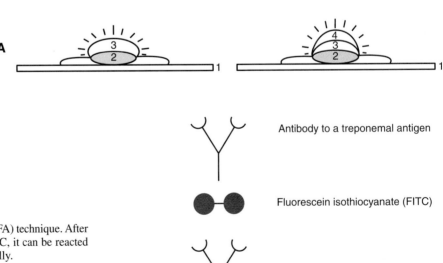

Figure 9-5 Direct fluorescent antibody (DFA) technique. After the labeling of a specific antibody with FITC, it can be reacted with its antigen and identified microscopically.

Antibody to a treponemal antigen

Fluorescein isothiocyanate (FITC)

FITC conjugated antibody

Treponemal antigen to another specificity

Treponema pallidum

(e.g., blue-violet) filter between the lamp and the object that passes only fluorescein-exciting wavelengths. The color of the emitted light depends on the nature of the substance. Fluorescein gives off yellow-green light, and the rhodamines fluoresce in the red portion of the spectrum. The color observed in the fluorescent microscope depends on the secondary or barrier filter used in the eyepiece. A yellow filter absorbs the green fluorescence of fluorescein and transmits only yellow. Fluorescein fluoresces an intense apple-green color when excited.

Inhibition Immunofluorescent Assay

The inhibition immunofluorescent assay is a blocking test in which an antigen is first exposed to unlabeled antibody, then to labeled antibody, and is finally washed and examined. If the unlabeled and labeled antibodies are both homologous to the antigen, there should be no fluorescence. This result confirms the specificity of the fluorescent antibody technique. Antibody in an unknown serum can also be detected and identified by the inhibition test.

Indirect Immunofluorescent Assay

The indirect method is based on the fact that antibodies (immunoglobulins [Igs]) not only react with homologous antigens but can act as antigens and react with antiimmunoglobulins (Box 9-2).

Box 9-2	**Examples of Immunologic Assays Performed by Indirect Fluorescence Antibody Technique**

Antiadrenal antibodies
Antibody (HRANA)
Anticentriole antibodies
Anticentromere antibodies
Antiglomerular basement membrane antibodies
Antiislet cell antibodies
Anti-LKM
Antimitochondrial
Antimyelin
Antimyocardial
Antinuclear antibody
Antiparietal cell
Antiplatelet
Antireticulin
Antiribosome
Antiskin (dermal-epidermal)
Antiskin (interepithelial)
Antismooth muscle
Antistriational
Cytomegalovirus (IgM antibody)
Histone-reactive antinuclear
Human immunodeficiency virus (HIV) total and IgM antibody
IgM antibodies (antigen-specific)
Lymphocyte typing
Rubella virus antibody
Toxoplasma gondii antibody

The serologic method most widely used for the detection of diverse antibodies is the indirect immunofluorescent assay (IFA). Immunofluorescence is used extensively in the detection of autoantibodies and antibodies to tissue and cellular antigens. For example, antinuclear antibodies—a heterogeneous group of circulating Igs that react with the whole nucleus or nuclear components such as nuclear proteins, deoxyribonucleic acid (DNA), or histones in host tissues—are frequently assayed by indirect fluorescence. By using tissue sections that contain a large number of antigens, it is possible to identify antibodies to several different antigens in a single test. The antigens are differentiated according to their different staining patterns.

Immunofluorescence can also be used to identify specific antigens on live cells in suspension (i.e., flow-cell cytometry). When a live stained-cell suspension is put through a fluorescent active-cell sorter (FACS), which measures its fluorescent intensity, the cells are separated according to their particular fluorescent brightness. This technique permits the isolation of different cell populations with different surface antigens (e.g., CD4+ and CD8+ lymphocytes) (see Chapter 4).

In the indirect immunofluorescent assay, the antigen source (such as a whole toxoplasma microorganism or virus in infected tissue culture cells) to the specific antibody being tested is affixed to the surface of a microscope slide. The patient's serum is diluted and placed on the slide to cover the antigen source. If antibody is present in the serum, it will bind to its specific antigen. Unbound antibody is then removed by washing the slide. In the second phase of the procedure, antihuman globulin (directed specifically against IgM or IgG) conjugated to a fluorescent substance that will fluoresce when exposed to ultraviolet light is placed on the slide. This conjugated marker for human antibody will bind to the antibody already bound to the antigen on the slide and will serve as a marker for the antibody when viewed under a fluorescent microscope. One of the biggest problems in interpreting IFA results is background staining. For most IFAs, laboratories must choose a screening dilution because undiluted specimens will show background staining resulting from nonspecific binding or clinically insignificant levels of circulating autoantibodies. The screening dilution plays a critical role—the more dilute the specimen becomes, the less sensitive but more specific the procedure becomes.

EMERGING LABELING TECHNOLOGIES

Quantum Dots (Q dots)

One example of an advanced labeling technique is quantum dots (Q dots). Q dots are semiconductor nanocrystals that are used as fluorescent labeling reagents for biologic imaging. A valuable property of Q dots is that different sizes of crystals produce different signals with a single laser excitation. This seemingly simple physical property implies that different size Q dots could be directed against different analyte targets and the Q dots would fluoresce different colors in a size-dependent manner. This allows for the detection of multiple analytes with a single assay. Q dots are just the next step in the evolution of luminescence-based assays.

SQUID Technology

A novel method of target labeling is to tag antibodies with superparamagnetic particles, allow the tagged antibodies to

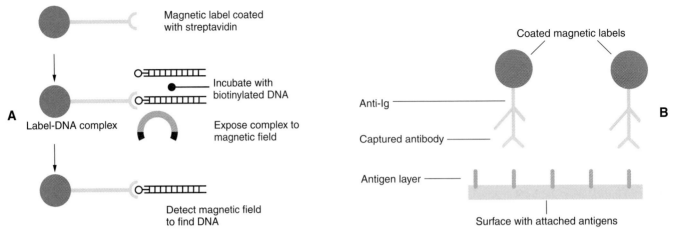

Figure 9-6   A, Detection of deoxyribonucleic acid. **B,** Detection of antibodies. (Redrawn from Adelman L: Laboratory technology: magnetic labeling technology, *Adv Med Lab Admin* 11(6):131, 1999.)

bind with the target antigen, and use a superconducting quantum interference device (SQUID) to detect the tagged antigen-antibody complex. The amplitude of the signal is proportional to the number of bound particles and correspondingly to the amount of target. A current application of this technology is its use in the detection of *Listeria monocytogenes (L. monocytogenes)*.

Luminescent Oxygen Channeling Immunoassay

This novel detection technology is based on two different 200-nm latex particles: a sensitizer particle that absorbs energy at 680 nm with generation of singlet oxygen (the donor bead) and a chemiluminescer molecule that shifts the emission wavelength to 570 nm (the receptor bead). When these particles are in close proximity of one another during excitation, singlet oxygen moves from the donor bead to the receptor bead, where it triggers the generation of a luminescent signal. Luminescent Oxygen Channeling Immunoassay (LOCI) technology is broadly applicable to any molecule that can be determined in a binding assay. The production of endpoint qualitative and quantitative RNA determination by LOCI is currently under investigation.

Signal Amplification Technology

Tyramide signal amplification (TSA) may be used in a wide variety of both fluorescent and colorimetric detection applications. The technique's protocols are simple and require very few changes to standard operating procedures. TSA provides an m-RNA in situ hybridization protocol that is effective in detecting B-cell clonality in plastic-embedded tissue specimens. Immunoglobulin light chain mRNA molecules can be detected directly in paraffin-embedded tissue using fluorescein-labeled oligonucleotide probes. The strength of TSA amplification enables B cells to be detected in tissue sections without additional processing steps and specially prepared sections. Similar in situ hybridization technology can also be used for the de-

tection of cytokines (e.g., interferon gamma and interleukin-4 [IL-4]).

Magnetic Labeling Technology

Magnetic labeling technology (Figure 9-6) is an application of the high resolution magnetic recording technology already developed for the computer disk drive industry. Increased density of microscopic magnetically labeled biologic samples (e.g., nucleic acid on a biochip) translates directly into reduced sample processing times. Magnetic labeling can be applied to automated DNA sequences, DNA probe technology, and gel scanners/electrophoresis. Compared with other nonradioactive labeling systems, magnetic labels are inherently safe, instrumentation is less expensive than competing methods, and signals from magnetic labels are virtually permanent and increased spatial resolution can be applied based on existing disk drive technology. In a magnetic label-based gel electrophoresis application sphere, DNA is analyzed. DNA is separated into bands using electrophoresis and magnetic labels are bound to the DNA in each band. By applying a magnetic field and then removing it, the magnetization of magnetic domains in each label will all be oriented in the same direction, resulting in a net magnetic field in the vicinity of the bands in the direction of the applied field (Figure 9-7).

Fluorescent in situ Hybridization

The rapid expansion in the availability of polyclonal and monoclonal antibodies has fostered a dramatic increase in light microscopic immunohistochemistry and in situ hybridization. Fluorescent in situ hybridization (FISH) is a molecular cytogenetic technique that uses recombinant DNA technology. In metaphase FISH, a specific nucleic acid sequence (probe) is bound to the homologous segment on a metaphase chromosome affixed to a glass slide. The existence of a region-specific DNA sequence in a nondividing cell can be detected using interphase FISH. Clinical applications of FISH in the detection of constitutional and

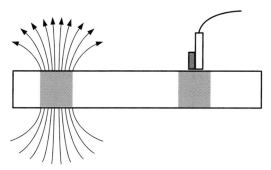

Figure 9-7 A cross section schematic of a small region of the sequencing gel or nylon membrane with magnetic labels bound to DNA that is separated into two bands. The arrows on the left band represent the magnetic field due to the magnetized labels, whereas the band on the right has a sensor very near the surface. (Redrawn from Adelman L. Laboratory technology: magnetic labeling technology, *Adv Med Lab Admin* 11(6):131, 1999.)

acquired chromosomal abnormalities include hematopathology and oncology.

CHAPTER HIGHLIGHTS

The original technique of using antigen-coated cells or particles in agglutination techniques may be considered the earliest method for labeling components in immunoassays. Ideal characteristics of a label include the quality of being measurable by several methods, including visual inspection. The properties of a label determine the ways in which detection is possible. The conversion of a colorless substrate into a colored product in EIA allows for two methods of detection, colorimetry and visual inspection.

Chemiluminescence is being pursued as the technology of choice by most immunodiagnostics manufacturers. Chemiluminescence has excellent sensitivity and dynamic range. In immunoassays chemiluminescent labels can be attached to an antigen or an antibody. Two formats are used: competitive and sandwich immunoassays. Chemiluminescent labels can be divided into five major groups.

The EIA method uses a nonisotopic label, which offers the advantage of safety and shares the specificity, sensitivity, and rapidity of RIA. If the method is intended to detect antibodies, the antigen in question is firmly fixed to a solid matrix such as the inside of the microplate well or the outside of a bead. Such a system is called solid-phase immunosorbent assay.

Fluorescent labeling (direct and indirect) is another method of demonstrating the complexing of antigens and antibodies. Fluorescent molecules are used as substitutes for radioisotope or enzyme labels.

Fluorescent conjugates are used in the basic methods of direct immunofluorescent assay, inhibition immunofluorescent assay, and indirect immunofluorescent assay. In the direct technique, a conjugated antibody is used to detect antigen-antibody reactions at a microscopic level. The indirect method is based on the fact that antibodies (Igs) not only react with homologous antigens but can act as antigens and react with antiimmunoglobulins. Emerging labeling technologies include quantum dots (Q dots), SQUID technology,

LOCI, signal amplification technology, and magnetic labeling technology. FISH technology is becoming popular in hematopathology and oncology.

REVIEW QUESTIONS

1. Chemiluminescence:
   A. has excellent sensitivity and dynamic range
   B. does not require sample radiation
   C. uses unstable chemiluminescent reagents and conjugates
   D. both A and B

Match questions 2 and 3.

2. Competitive immunoassay

3. Sandwich immunoassay

   A. fixed amount of labeled antigen competes with unlabeled antigen from a a patient specimen for a limited number of antibody-binding sites
   B. the sample antigen binds to an antibody fixed onto a solid phase; a second antibody, labeled with a chemiluminescent label, binds to the antigen-antibody complex on the solid phase

4. Enzyme labels commonly used in indirect procedures are:
   A. alkaline phosphatase
   B. horseradish peroxidase
   C. beta-galactosidase
   D. all of the above

Match questions 5 and 6.

5. _____ Enzyme immunoassay (EIA)

6. _____ Immunofluorescent technique

   A. uses a nonisotopic label
   B. uses antibody labeled with fluorescein isothiocyanate (FITC)
   C. uses a colloidal particle consisting of a metal or an insoluble metal compound

Questions 7-9. Match the following.

7. _____ Direct immunofluorescent assay

8. _____ Inhibition immunofluorescent assay

9. _____ Indirect immunofluorescent assay

   A. based on the fact that antibodies can act as antigens and react with antiimmunoglobulins
   B. uses conjugated antibody to detect antigen/antibody reactions
   C. antigen first exposed to unlabeled antibody, then labeled antibody

10. For an enzyme to be used in an EIA immunoassay, it must meet all of the list criteria except:
    A. a high amount of stability
    B. extreme specificity
    C. presence in antigen or antibody
    D. no alteration by inhibitor with the system

Questions 11 and 12. Fill in the blanks below, choosing from the following answers.

Possible answers for question 11.
    A. emitting
    B. absorbing
    C. generating bright
    D. generating dull

Possible answers for question 12.
    A. emits
    B. absorbs
    C. reduces
    D. increases

A fluorescent substance is one that, while (11) _____

light of one wavelength, (12) _____
light of another (longer) wavelength.

Match questions 13-16.

13. _____ Quantum dots (Q dots)

14. _____ SQUID technology

15. _____ luminescent oxygen channeling immunoassay (LOCI)

16. _____ fluorescent in situ hybridization (FISH)

    A. semiconductor nanocrystals
    B. a method of tagging antibodies with superparamagnetic particles
    C. technology based on two different 200-nm latex particles
    D. a molecular cytogenetic technique

BIBLIOGRAPHY

Adelman L: Laboratory technology—magnetic labeling technology, *Adv Med Lab Admin* 11(6):131, 1999.

Forbes BA, Sahm DF, Weissfeld AS: *Bailey and Scott's diagnostic microbiology,* ed 11, St Louis, 2002, Mosby.

Jandreski MA: Chemiluminescence technology in immunoassays, *Lab Med* 29(9):555-560, 1998.

Mark HFL: Fluorescent in situ hybridization as an adjunct to conventional cytogenetics, *Ann Clin Lab Sci* 24(2):153-163, 1994.

Sainato D: The coming revolution in assay technologies, *Clinical Laboratory News* 20:26-27, 2000.

Van Den Berg F. Applications of a signal amplification technique for light microscopy, *Clinical Laboratory News* 15:8-9, 1996.

Chapter 10

Automated Procedures

LEARNING OBJECTIVES

At the conclusion of this chapter, the reader should be able to:
- Describe the principle, advantages, and disadvantages of nephelometry.
- Explain the principle of flow-cell cytometry and its clinical application.

- Discuss current trends in immunoassay.
- List at least three potential benefits of automated immunoassay.

NEPHELOMETRY

Nephelometry has become increasingly more popular in diagnostic laboratories and depends on the light-scattering properties of antigen-antibody complexes (Figure 10-1). The quantity of cloudiness or turbidity in a solution can be measured photometrically. When specific antigen-coated latex particles acting as reaction intensifiers are agglutinated by their corresponding antibody, the increased light scatter of a solution can be measured by nephelometry as the macromolecular complexes form. The use of polyethylene glycol enhances and stabilizes the precipitates, thus increasing the speed and sensitivity of the technique by controlling the particle size for optimal light angle deflection. The kinetics of this change can be determined when the photometric results are analyzed by computer. In immunology, nephelometry is used to measure complement components, immune complexes, and the presence of a variety of antibodies (Box 10-1).

Principle

Formation of a macromolecular complex is a fundamental prerequisite for nephelometric protein quantitation. The pro-

cedure is based on the reaction between the protein being assayed and a specific antisera. Protein in a patient specimen reacts with specific nephelometric antisera to human proteins and forms insoluble complexes. When light is passed through such a suspension, the resulting complexes of insoluble precipitants scatter incident light in solutions. The scattered light can be detected with a photodiode. The amount of scattered light is proportional to the number of insoluble complexes and can be quantitated by comparing the unknown patient values with standards of known protein concentration.

The relationship between the quantity of antigen and the measuring signal at a constant antibody concentration is expressed by the Heidelberger curve. If antibodies are present to excess, a proportional relationship exits between the antigen and the resulting signal. If the antigen overwhelms the quantity of antibody, the measured signal drops.

By optimizing the reaction conditions, the typical antigen-antibody reactions as characterized by the Heidelberger curve are effectively shifted in the direction of high concentration. This ensures that these high concentrations will

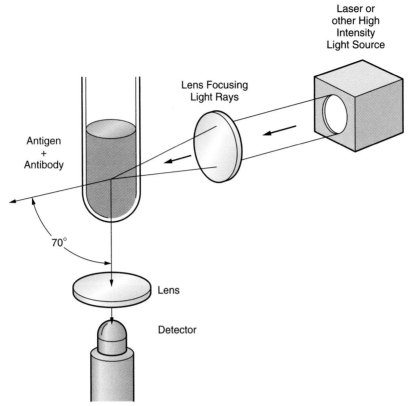

Figure 10-1   Principle of nephelometry for the measurement of antigen-antibody reactions. Light rays are collected in a focusing lens and can ultimately be related to the antigen or antibody concentration in a sample.

Box 10-1	Examples of Immunologic Assays Performed by Nephelometry

Acid alpha 1-glycoprotein
Albumin
Alpha 1-antitrypsin
Alpha 2-macroblobulin
C1 esterase inhibitor (C1 inhibitor)
C3
C3b Inhibitor (C3b inactivator)
C3PA (C3 Proactivator, Properdin factor B)
C4
C6
C7
C8
Ceruloplasmin
Complement components (C1r, C1s, C2, C3, C4, C5, C6, C7, C8)
C-reactive protein (CRP)
Cryofibrinogen
Cryoglobulins
Haptoglobin
Hemopexin
Immunoglobulins
Properdin factor B
Transferrin

---

be measured on the ascending portion of the curve. At concentrations higher than the reference curve, the instrument will transmit an out-of-range warning.

Physical Basis

Nephelometry is based on the principle of light scattered by an homogeneous particulate solution at a variety of angles. Three types of scatter can occur: scatter around the particles, forward scatter because of out-of-phase backscatter, and forward scatter exceeding backward scatter.

Optical System

In the nephelometric method, an infrared high-performance light-emitting diode (LED) is used as the light source. Because an entire solid angle is measured after convergence of this light via a lens system, an intense measuring signal is available when the primary beam is blocked off. In connection with the lens system, this produces a light beam of high collinearity. The wavelength is 840 nm. Light scattered in the forward direction in a solid angle to the primary beam ranges between 13 and 24 feet and is measured by a silicon photodiode with an integrated amplifier. The electrical signals generated are digitalized, compared with reference curves, and converted into protein concentrations.

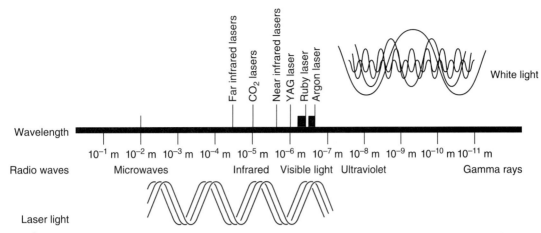

Figure 10-2 The electromagnetic spectrum. YAG = yttrium, aluminum, and garnet. (Redrawn from Turgeon ML: *Clinical hematology: theory and procedures,* ed 3, Philadelphia, 1999, Lippincott Williams & Wilkins.)

Measuring Methods

A fixed-time method is used routinely for precipitation reactions. Ten seconds after all reaction components have been mixed, a cuvette (an initial blank measurement) is taken. Six minutes later a second measurement is taken, and after subtraction of the original 1-second blanking value, a final answer is calculated against the multiple-point or single-point calibration in the computerized program memory for the assay.

Advantages and Disadvantages of Nephelometry

Nephelometry represents an automated system that is rapid, reproducible, relatively simple to operate, and very common in higher volume laboratories. It has many applications in the immunology laboratory. Currently, instruments using a rate method and fixed-time approach are commercially available with tests for the following determinations: immunoglobulin (Ig)G, IgA, IgM, C3, C4, properdin, C-reactive protein, rheumatoid factor, ceruloplasmin, alpha 1-antitrypsin, apolipoproteins, and haptoglobins.

The disadvantages include high initial equipment cost and the fact that interfering substances such as microbial contamination may cause protein denaturation and erroneous test results. Intrinsic specimen turbidity or lipemia may exceed the preset limits. In these cases a clearing agent may be needed before an accurate assay can be performed. In addition, low-molecular-weight Igs, monoclonal Igs, and antibovidae antibodies also may produce spurious results in nephelometry.

FLOW-CELL CYTOMETRY

Fundamentals of Laser Technology

1917 Einstein speculated that under certain conditions atoms or molecules could absorb light or other radiation and then be stimulated to shed this gained energy. Today, lasers have been developed with numerous medical and industrial applications.

The electromagnetic spectrum ranges from long radio waves to short, powerful gamma rays (Figure 10-2). Within this spectrum is a narrow band of visible or white light, composed of red, orange, yellow, green, blue, and violet light. Laser (light amplified stimulated emitted radiation) light ranges from the ultraviolet and infrared spectrum through all of the colors of the rainbow. In contrast to other diffuse forms of radiation, laser light is concentrated. It is almost exclusively of one wavelength or color, and its parallel waves travel in one direction. Through the use of fluorescent dyes, laser light can occur in numerous wavelengths. The types of lasers include glass-filled tubes of helium and neon lasers, the most common; YAG-type (yttrium-aluminum-garnet), an imitation diamond; argon; and krypton.

Lasers sort the energy in atoms and molecules, concentrate it, and release it in powerful waves. In most lasers a medium of gas, liquid, or crystal is energized by high-intensity light, an electrical discharge, or even nuclear radiation. When an atom extends beyond the orbits of its electrons or when a molecule vibrates or changes its shape, they instantly snap back, shedding energy in the form of a photon. The photon is the basic unit of all radiation. When a photon reaches an atom of the medium, the energy exchange stimulates the emission of another photon in the same wavelength and direction. This process continues until a cascade of growing energy sweeps through the medium.

Photons travel the length of the laser and bounce off mirrors. First a few and eventually countless photons synchronize themselves until an avalanche of light streaks between the mirrors. In some gas lasers, transparent disks referred to as Brewster windows are slanted at a precise angle, which polarizes the laser's light. The photons, which are reflected back and forth, finally gain so much energy that they exit as a powerful beam. The power of lasers to pass on energy and information is rated in watts.

Principles of Cell Cytometry

Flow-cell cytometry is a marriage of technologies combining fluid dynamics, optics, laser science, high-speed computers

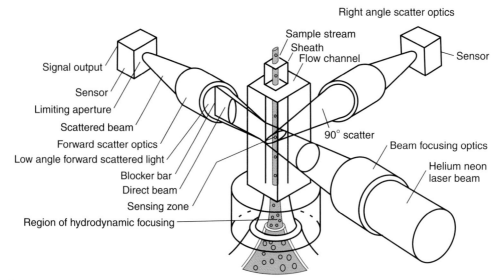

Figure 10-3   Laser-flow cytometry. (Redrawn from Turgeon ML: *Clinical hematology: theory and procedures,* ed 3, Philadelphia, 1999, Lippincott Williams & Wilkins.)

and fluorochrome-conjugated monoclonal antibodies that rapidly classify groups of cells within heterogeneous mixtures. The principle of flow cytometry is based on the fact that cells are stained in suspension with an appropriate fluorochrome, which may be either an immunologic reagent, a dye that stains a specific component, or some other marker with specific reactivity. Fluorescent dyes used in flow cytometry must bind or react specifically with the cellular component of interest (e.g., reticulocytes, peroxidase enzyme, or DNA content). Fluorescent dyes include acridine orange and thioflavin T. Pygon is preferred for fluorescein isothiocyanate (FITC) labeling. Krypton is often used as a second laser in dual analysis systems and serves as a better light source for compounds labeled by tetramethylrhodamine isothiocyanate and tetra-m cyclopropylrhodamine isothiocyanate.

A suspension of stained cells is pressurized using gas and transported through plastic tubing to a flow chamber within the instrument (Figure 10-3). In the flow chamber, the specimen is injected through a needle into a stream of physiologic saline called the sheath. The sheath and specimen both exit the flow chamber through a 75-µm orifice. This laminar flow design confines the cells to the very center of the saline sheath, with the cells moving in single file.

The stained cells next pass through the laser beam. The laser activates the dye, and the cell fluoresces. Although the fluorescence is emitted throughout a 360-degree circle, it is usually collected via optical sensors located at 90 degrees relative to the laser beam. The fluorescence information is then transmitted to a computer. Flow cytometry performs fluorescence analysis on single cells at rates up to 50,000 cells per minute.

The computer is the heart of the instrument; it controls all decisions regarding data collection, analysis, and cell sorting. The major applications of this technology are:
- Identification of cells
- Cell sorting before further analysis

Cell Sorting

In flow cytometry, cells can be sorted from the main cellular population into subpopulations for further analysis (Figure 10-4). Any fresh specimen that can be placed into a single cell suspension is a valid candidate for immunophenotyping (e.g., T cells, B cells, CD34+ stem cells, detection of minimal residual disease in leukemias). Sorting is accomplished using stored computer information.

When the laser strikes a stained cell, the dye creates distinctive colored light that the cytometer recognizes. This fluorescent intensity is recorded and analyzed by the computer, and cells are sorted according to a preprogrammed selection. If the particular cell in the laser beam is of interest, the computer waits an appropriate length of time for the cell to reach the droplet break-off point within the charging collar. At that point the computer signals the charging collar to administer either an electrostatically positive or negative charge to the stream containing the target cell. A droplet containing this cell is then removed from the main stream before the charge has time to redistribute.

This action produces the cell of interest within a liquid drop that has on its surface an electrostatic charge (only the droplet is charged). The droplet falls between a set of deflection plates, which creates an electrical field. The charged droplets are deflected either to the left or right, depending on their polarity, and collected for further analysis.

Four-Color Immunofluorescence

Current methods use four monoclonal antibodies, each directly conjugated to a distinct fluorochrome, per tube of patient cell suspension. The four most commonly used fluorochromes are FITC, phycoerythrin (PE), peridinin chlorophyll protein (PerCP) and allophycocyanin (APC). The first three fluorochromes are excited by the 488-nm line of an argon laser; the fourth fluorochrome is excited by the 633-nm line of a helium-neon laser or diode-laser. Four-color immunofluorescence offers the advantages of greater sensitivity and specificity.

The future of flow cytometry includes clinical use of six and greater antibody analysis as lasers further progress into solid-state form and flow cytometer electronics move

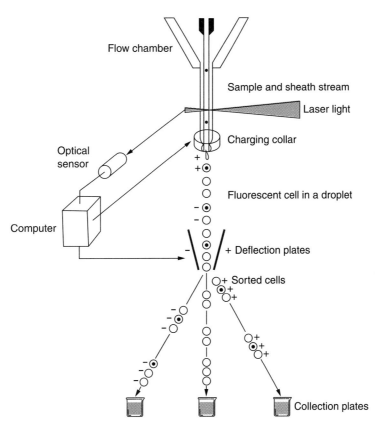

Figure 10-4 Laser and cell-sorting schematic.

from an analog to a digital form. Increased ability to identify and subclassify individual cells is also expected. Improvements in methods and probes may lead to fluorescence in situ hybridization (FISH) in suspension as a routine protocol and enable flow cytometry to operate on a molecular level to simultaneously identify chromosomal abnormalities.

A system that uses a flow cytometer, specific data analysis software and fluorescent latex particles, the Luminex 100 Total System, has been developed by Luminex Technology (Austin, TX). This system combines advances in computing and optics with a new concept in color coding to create a simple, cost-efficient analysis system. Latex beads are coupled to various amounts of two different fluorescent dyes, which are analyzed by the flow cytometer and software to allow the distinct separation of up to 64 slightly different colored bead sets. The color-coded microspheres identify each unique reaction. Hundreds of microspheres sets can be identified at once in a single sample. Advanced computer and optical technology recognizes each microsphere and provides a precise, quantitative measure simply and in real time.

Currently, up to 64 microsphere sets are recognized. The current FlowMetrix System is compatible with the BD (Franklin Lakes, NJ) FACS Vantage SE System and the BD FACSCalibur, the most widely used flow cytometers for cellular analysis. Because the Luminex technology requires fewer steps to assess multiple parameters with a high level of sensitivity and accuracy, it is significantly more cost-effective than current methods of analysis. Some immunologic applications already demonstrated with FlowMetrix are human immunodeficiency virus (HIV) and hepatitis B

seroconversion; multiple cytokine measurement; multiplexed allergy testing; DNA-based tissue typing; herpes simplex viral load; IgG, IgA, and IgM assay; IgG subclassification; autoimmunity pane; epitope mapping; hCG and alpha-fetoprotein, HIV viral load; and the TORCHS (toxoplasmosis, other [viruses], rubella, cytomegalovirus, herpes [viruses], syphilis) panel.

CURRENT TRENDS IN IMMUNOASSAY AUTOMATION

Automated immunoassay instrumentation has progressed more slowly than in other disciplines of medical technology. But technical advances in methodologies, robotics, and computerization has led to expanded immunoassay automation (see Tables 10-1 and 10-2). Newer systems are using chemiluminescent labels and substrates rather than older fluorescent labels and detection systems. Immunoassay systems have the potential to improve turn-around time with enhanced cost-effectiveness (Box 10-2).

Fluorescent Polarization Immunoassay

The fluorescent polarization immunoassay, the IMx System manufactured by Abbott Laboratories, is an automated analyzer designed to perform microparticle enzyme immunoassay, fluorescence polarization immunoassay, and ion capture technologies. This unique combination allows both high- and low-molecular-weight analytes to be measured. This expands the range of available assays to include tests for endocrine function, fertility, cancer, hepatitis, transplant, rubella, and congenital disease.

TABLE 10-1 Examples of Automated Random Access Immunoassay Systems

Company	Instrument	Principle
Abbott Diagnostics	AXSYM	FPIA/MEI
Bayer	Immuno-1	Latex, EIA, ELISA
Beckman Coulter	Access	Chemilum
Boehringer Mannheim	Elecsys	Electro chemilum
Chiron	ACS: 1 80 SE	Chemilum
Chiron	Centaur	Chemilum
Dade	Opus Plus	Fluorescent EUSA
Diagnostic Products	Immulite	Enzyme amplif. chemilum
Diagnostic Products	Immulite 2000	Enzyme amplif. chemilum
Nichols	Advantage	Chemilum
Ortho Diagnostics	Vitros	Chemilum
Tosoh	AIA-1200	Kinetic fluorescence
Tosoh	NexiA	Kinetic fluorescence

Source: Blick K: Current trends in automation of immunoassays, *J Clin Ligand Assoc* 22(1):6-12, Spring 1999.
Chemilum, Chemiluminescence; *EIA,* enzyme immunoassay; *ELISA,* enzyme-linked immunosorbent assay; *FPIA,* fluorescent polarization immunoassay; *MEIA,* microparticle enzyme immunoassay.

TABLE 10-2 Manufacturers of Automated Immunoassay Analyzers

Manufacturer	Instrument	Launch Date/Country
Abbott Diagnostics	Architect I	2000/1999/US
	AxSym	1993 worldwide, 1994/US
ACT Diagnostics	Alpha Prime	2000/France
Bayer Diagnostics	Advia Centaur	1998/US
	ACS: 180SE	1997/US
	Bayer Immuno I	
	Immunoassay System	1993/US
Beckman Coulter, Inc.	Access Immunoassay System	1993/US-France
	Access 2 Immunoassay System	2001/US
The Binding Site, Inc.	DSX Automated System	2000/Guernsey, U.K.
BioChem ImmunoSystems (US), Inc.	Labotech	1996/Italy
	PersonalLab	1998/Italy
BioMérieux Inc.	Vidas & MiniVidas	1989/US
	Coda	1996
Dade Behring, Inc.	Opus Plus	1992/US
	Stratus CS Stat	1998
	Fluorometric Analyzer	1997
	Dimension RxL Chemistry System with Heterogeneous Module (HM)	
Diagnostic Products Corp.	IMMUNLITE	1993
	IMMUNLITE Turbo	1999
	Immunlite	2000/1998/US
Diamedix Corp.	Mago Plus Automated EIA Analyzer	1997/Italy
Diasorin Inc.	ETI-Lab	1996/Italy
	Inbu.	1996/US
Grifols-Quest, Inc.	Triturus	1999/Spain
Hycor Biomedical, Inc.	Hy.Tec 288	1998/US
		1999/Netherlands
	Hy.Tec 480	1994/Switzerland

Source: modified from CAP TODAY, April, 2001.

TABLE 10-2	Manufacturers of Automated Immunoassay Analyzers—cont'd	
Manufacturer	**Instrument**	**Launch Date/Country**
Nichols Institute Diagnostics	CL System ID	1993/Sweden
	Nichols Advantage	
	Specialty System	1997/Germany
Olympus America, Inc.	AU400	1999/Japan
Ortho-Clinical Diagnostics	Vitros Eci	
	Immunodiagnostic System	1997/US
Roche Diagnostics	Elecsys 2010	1996
	Elecsys 1010	1997
Sigma Diagnostics	Aptus Automated EIA System	1998/US
Tosoh Medics, Inc.	AIA Nex.IA	1997/Japan
	AIA-600 II	2000/Japan

Box 10-2	**Potential Benefits of Immunoassay Automation**

Ability to provide better service with less staff

Savings on controls, duplicates, dilutions, and repeats

Elimination of radioactive labels and associated regulations

Better shelf life of reagents with less disposal due to out-dating

Better sample identification with bar-code labels and primary tube sampling

Automation of sample delivery possible

Source: Modified from Blick K: Current trends in automation of immunoassays, *J Clin Ligand Assay* 22(1):6-12, Spring 1999.

CHAPTER HIGHLIGHTS

The quantity of turbidity in a solution can be measured photometrically. When specific antigen-coated latex particles acting as reaction intensifiers are agglutinated by their corresponding antibody, the increased light scatter of a solution can be measured by nephelometry as the macromolecular complexes form. In immunology, nephelometry is used to measure complement components, immune complexes, and the presence of a variety of antibodies. The procedure is based on the reaction between the protein being assayed and a specific antisera. Protein in a patient specimen reacts with specific nephelometric antisera to human proteins and forms insoluble complexes. When light is passed through such a suspension, the resulting complexes of insoluble precipitants scatter incident light in solutions that can be measured. Nephelometry is a rapid and highly reproducible automated method.

Within the electromagnetic spectrum is a narrow band of visible or white light, composed of red, orange, yellow, green, blue, and violet light. Laser (light amplified stimulated emitted radiation) light ranges from the ultraviolet and infrared spectrum through all of the colors of the rainbow. Laser light is almost exclusively of one wavelength or color, and its parallel waves travel in one direction. Through the use of fluorescent dyes, laser light can occur in numerous wavelengths. The principle of flow cytometry is based on the fact that cells are stained in suspension with an appropriate fluorochrome, which may be either an immunologic reagent, a dye that stains a specific component, or some other marker with specified reactivity. Laser light is the most common light source used in flow cytometers because of the properties of intensity, stability, and monochromaticity. The stained cells pass through the laser beam, the laser activates the dye, and the cell fluoresces. The major applications of this technology are identification of cells and cell sorting before further analysis.

Four-color immunofluorescence uses four monoclonal antibodies, each directly conjugated to a distinct fluorochrome, per tube of patient cell suspension. Four-color immunofluorescence offers the advantages of greater sensitivity and specificity.

The future of flow cytometry includes clinical use of six and greater antibody analysis as lasers further progress into solid-state form and flow cytometer electronics move from an analog to a digital form. Increased ability to identify and subclassify individual cells is also expected. Improvements in methods and probes may lead to FISH in suspension as a routine protocol and enable flow cytometry to operate on a molecular level to simultaneously identify chromosomal abnormalities. A system that uses a flow cytometer, specific data analysis software, and fluorescent latex particles has been developed by Luminex Technology. Some immunologic applications are HIV and hepatitis B seroconversion; multiple cytokine measurement; multiplexed allergy testing; DNA-based tissue typing; herpes simplex viral load; IgG, IgA, and IgM assay; IgG subclassification; autoimmunity pane; epitope mapping; hCG and AFP; HIV viral load; and the TORCHS panel.

Newer systems in immunoassay automation use chemiluminescent labels and substrates rather than older fluorescent labels and detection systems. Immunoassay systems have the potential to improve turn-around time with enhanced cost-effectiveness.

REVIEW QUESTIONS

1. Nephelometry measures the light scatter of:
   A. ions
   B. macromolecules
   C. antibodies
   D. soluble antigens

2. LASER is an acronym for:
   A. light amplified stimulated emitted radiation
   B. light augmented stimulated emitted radiation
   C. light amplified stimulated energy radiation
   D. large angle stimulated emitted radiation

3. All of the following are descriptive characteristics of laser light except:
   A. intensity
   B. stability
   C. polychromaticity
   D. monochromaticity

4. In the figure below, identify the most likely contents of the test tube, if nephelometry is being used.

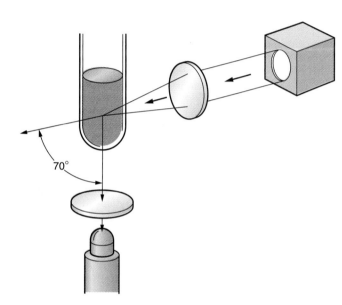

   A. antigen
   B. antigen-coated
   C. latex-coated antibody
   D. antigen-coated latex particles and antibody

5. Nephelometry can be used to assay all of the following except:
   A. IgM
   B. IgG
   C. IgD
   D. IgA

6. A photon is a:
   A. basic unit of light
   B. basic unit of all radiation
   C. component of an atom
   D. component of laser light

7. The major applications of flow cell technology is:
   A. Identification of cells
   B. Cell sorting before further analysis
   C. Diagnosis of autoimmune disease
   D. Both A and B

8. Four-color immunofluorescence commonly uses:
   A. fluorescein isothiocyanate (FITC)
   B. phycoerythrin (PE)
   C. peridinin chlorophyll protein (PerCP)
   D. all of the above

BIBLIOGRAPHY

Bakke AC: The principles of flow cytometry, *Lab Med* 32:207-211, 2001.

Behring nephelometer system folder, Branchburg, NJ, 1987, Behring Diagnostics, Inc.

Blick KE: Current trends in automation of immunoassays, *J Clin Ligand Assay* 22:6-12, 1999.

Hoffman EG: Laboratory evaluation of monoclonal gammopathies, *Can J Med Technol* 49(2):99-115, 1987.

Kaplan LA, Pesce AJ: *Clinical chemistry,* ed 3, St Louis, 1996, Mosby.

Kelliher AS et al: Multiparameter flow cytometry in the clinical lab: present capacities and future projections, *Adv Med Lab Prof* 9-13, 2001.

Lovett EJ et al: Application of flow cytometry to diagnostic pathology, *Lab Invest* 50(2):115-140, 1984.

Smalley D, Aller RD: Picturing tomorrow's system, CAP TODAY, 15:53-84, April, 2001.

Turgeon ML: *Clinical hematology,* ed 3, Philadelphia, 1999, Lippincott Williams & Wilkins.

Chapter 11

Molecular Techniques

LEARNING OBJECTIVES

At the conclusion of this chapter, the reader should be able to:
- Describe the polymerase chain reaction (PCR) amplification technique.
- Compare various PCR modifications.
- Name and briefly describe other amplification techniques.

- Describe the "gold standard" of genetic analysis.
- Compare DNA sequencing and branched DNA protocols.
- Name and compare at least three hybridization techniques.
- Explain how microarrays are applied to immunologic testing.

AMPLIFICATION TECHNIQUES IN MOLECULAR BIOLOGY

Polymerase Chain Reaction

PCR is an in vitro method (Figure 11-1, *A*) that amplifies low levels of specific DNA sequences in a sample to higher quantities suitable for further analysis. To use this technology, the target sequence to be amplified must be known. Typically, a target sequence ranges from 100 to 1000 base pairs in length. Two short DNA "primers" that are typically 16 to 20 base pairs in length are used. Namely, the oligonucleotides (small portions of a single DNA strand) act as a template for the new DNA. These primer sequences are complementary to the 3' ends of the sequence to be amplified.

This enzymatic process is carried out in cycles. Each repeated cycle consists of:
- DNA denaturation—the separation of the double DNA strands into two single strands through the use of heat.
- Primer annealing—the recombination of the oligonucleotide primers with the single-stranded original DNA.
- Extension of the primed DNA sequence—the enzyme DNA polymerase synthesizes new complementary strands by the extension of primers.

Each cycle theoretically doubles the amount of specific DNA sequence present and results in an exponential accumulation of the DNA fragment being amplified (amplicons). In general, this process is repeated approximately 30 times. At the end of 30 cycles the reaction mixture should contain about 2^{30} molecules of the desired product. After cycling is completed, the amplification products can be examined in various ways. Typically the contents of the reaction vessel are subjected to gel electrophoresis. This allows visualization of the amplified gene segments (e.g., PCR products, bands) and a determination of their specificity. Additional product analysis by probe hybridization or direct DNA sequencing is often performed to further verify the authenticity of the amplicon.

The three important applications of PCR are:
1. Amplification of DNA
2. Identification of a target sequence
3. Synthesis of a labeled antisense probe

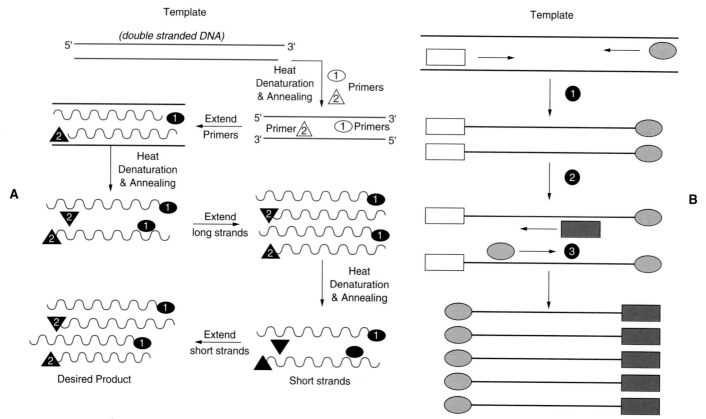

Figure 11-1   **A,** Polymerase chain reaction. **B,** Nested primer polymerase chain reaction. Step 1: Primers anneal to and amplify a broad region of DNA around the gene of interest. Step 2: Nested primers anneal to the specific gene to be amplified. Step 3: Amplification of the desired gene by nested primers occurs. (Redrawn and modified from Warden BA, Thompson E: Apolipoprotein E and the development of atherosclerosis, *Lab Med* 25(7):453, 1994.)

PCR analysis can lead to the detection of gene mutations that signify the early development of cancer, identification of viral DNA associated with specific cancers (e.g., human papilloma virus [HPV], a causative agent in cervical cancer), or the detection of genetic mutations associated with a wide variety of disease (e.g. coronary artery disease associated with mutations of the gene that encodes for the low-density lipoprotein receptor [LDLR]).

Adaptations of the PCR technique (Figure 11-1, *B*) have been developed. One adaptation uses nested primers. This adaptation uses a two-step amplification process. In the first step, a broad region of the DNA surrounding the sequence of interest is amplified. This is followed by a second round of amplification to amplify the specific gene sequence to be studied. Another recent modification of the PCR technique has been used successfully to differentiate alleles of the same gene.

Polymerase Chain Reaction Modifications

Reverse Transcriptase-Polymerase Chain Reaction

If the nucleic acid of interest is RNA rather than DNA, the PCR procedures can be modified to include the conversion of RNA to DNA using reverse transcriptase (RT-PCR) in the initial steps. This technique is useful in the identification of RNA viral agents (e.g. human immunodeficiency virus [HIV] or hepatitis C virus [HCV]).

Multiplex Polymerase Chain Reaction

Multiplex PCR uses numerous primers within a single reaction tube so as to amplify nucleic acid fragments from different targets. Specific nucleic acid amplification should occur if the appropriate target DNA is present in the sample tests. Detection may be accomplished by traditional Southern transfer and subsequent nucleic aid probe, by enzyme immunoassay methods, or by gene-chip analysis. This technology is limited by the number of primers that can be included in a single reaction, primer-primer interference, and nonspecific nucleic acid amplification.

Real-Time Polymerase Chain Reaction

Another method based on PCR is real-time PCR. This PCR variation uses fluorescence resonance energy transfer. The application of this technique is in the quantitation of specific DNA sequences of interest and for identification of point mutations. This PCR variation is particularly appealing because the procedure is less susceptible to amplicon contamination and is more accurate in quantifying the initial copy number.

Other Amplification Techniques

Strand Displacement Amplification

Strand displacement amplification (SDA) is a fully automated method that amplifies target nucleic acid without the use of a thermocycler. A double-strand DNA fragment is created and becomes the target for exponential amplification.

Transcription Mediate Amplification

Transcription mediate amplification (TMA) is another isothermal assay that targets either DNA or RNA, but generates RNA as its amplified product. This method is currently being used to detect microorganisms (e.g., *Mycobacterium tuberculosis*).

Nucleic Acid Sequence-Based Amplification

Nucleic acid sequence-based amplification (NASBA) is similar to TMA, but only RNA is targeted for amplification. Applications of this technique are detection and quantitation of HIV and detection of cytomegalovirus (CMV).

Ligase Chain Reaction Nucleic Acid Amplification

Oligonucleotide pairs hybridize to target sequences within the gene or the cryptic plasmid. The bound oligonucleotides are separated by a small gap at the target site. The enzyme DNA polymerase uses nucleotides in the Ligase chain reaction nucleic acid amplification (LCR) reaction mixture to fill in this gap, creating a ligatable junction. Once the gap is filled, DNA ligase joins the oligonucleotide pairs to form a short single-stranded product that is complementary to the original target sequence. This product can itself serve as a target for hybridization and ligation of a second pair of oligonucleotides present in the LCR reaction mixture. Subsequent rounds of denaturation and ligation lead to the geometric accumulation of amplification product. The amplified products are detected in an LCx analyzer (Abbott Laboratories, Abbott Park, IL) by microparticle enzyme immunoassay.

ANALYSIS OF AMPLIFICATION PRODUCTS

Many of the revolutionary changes that have occurred in research in the biologic sciences, particularly the Human Genome Project, can be directly attributed to the ability to manipulate DNA in defined ways. Molecular genetic testing focuses on examination of nucleic acids (DNA or RNA) by special techniques to determine if a specific nucleotide base sequence is present. Although nucleic acid testing is in its infancy, its applications have expanded, despite higher costs associated with testing, in various areas of the clinical laboratory. Clinical applications include genetic testing, hematopathology diagnosis and monitoring, and identification of infectious agents. The distinct advantages of molecular testing include:

- Faster turnaround time
- Smaller required sample volumes
- Increased specificity and sensitivity

Conventional analysis uses agarose gel electrophoresis after ethidium bromide staining. Other techniques are used to enhance both the sensitivity and specificity of amplification techniques. Probe-based DNA detection systems have the advantage of providing sequence specificity and decreased detection limits. Other techniques include hybridization protection assay, DNA enzyme immunoassay, automated DNA sequencing technology, single-strand conformational polymorphisms, and restriction fragment length polymorphism (RFLP) analysis. The selection of one technique over another is often based on a variety of factors (e.g., sensitivity and specificity profiles, cost, turnaround time, and local experience).

DNA Sequencing

DNA sequencing is considered to be the "gold standard" method by which other molecular methods are compared. DNA sequencing displays the exact nucleotide or base sequence of a fragment of DNA that is targeted. The Sanger method, which uses a series of enzymatic reactions to produce segments of DNA complementary to the DNA being sequenced, is the most frequently used method for DNA sequencing. Automated sequencing techniques use primers with four different fluorescent labels.

1. The first step to sequence a target is usually to amplify it in some way either by cloning or in vitro amplification—usually PCR. Once the amplified DNA is purified from the clinical specimen (the target DNA), it is heat-denatured to separate the double-stranded DNA (dsDNA) into single strands (ssDNA).
2. The second step involves adding primers, short synthetic segments of single-stranded DNA that contain a nucleotide sequence complementary to a short of the target DNA, to the ssDNA. The patient's DNA serves as a template to copy. DNA polymerase catalyzes the addition of the appropriate nucleotides to the preexisting primer. DNA synthesis is terminated when the deoxynucleotide is embodied into a growing DNA chain.

Branched DNA

Branched DNA (b-DNA) represents an alternative quantitative test that uses signal amplification instead of target amplification. Target DNA or RNA is hybridized at different sites by two types of probes. Branched DNA assays are being used to measure the viral load of hepatitis B virus (HBV), hepatitis C virus (HCV), human immunodeficiency virus (HIV-1), cytomegalovirus (CMV), and microbial organisms (e.g., *Trypanosoma brucei*).

VERSANT HIV-1 RNA 3.0 assay (b-DNA), manufactured by Bayer Diagnostics (Bayer Group, Germany), which uses branched DNA technology, is the only viral load assay specifically designed to target multiple sequences of the HIV-1 genome with more than 80 nucleic acid probes.

Hybridization Techniques

Probe-hybridization assays involving the complementary pairing of a probe with a DNA or RNA strand derived from the patient specimen exist in many forms. The common feature of probe hybridization assays is the use of a labeled nucleic acid probe to examine a specimen for a specific, homologous DNA or RNA sequence. The clinical probes are most often labeled with nonradioisotopic molecules such as digoxigenin, alkaline phosphatase, biotin, or a fluorescent compound. The detection systems are conjugate-dependent and include chemiluminescent, fluorescent, and calorimetric methodologies.

Liquid-Phase Hybridization

In the liquid-phase hybridization (LPH) assay both the target nucleic acid and the labeled probe interact in solution. Specific homologous hybrids are subsequently separated from the remaining nucleic acid component, and the hybrids are identified by an appropriate detection system.

Dot Blot and Reverse Dot Blot

These hybridization methods are used in the clinical laboratory for the detection of disorders in which the DNA sequence of the mutated region has been identified (e.g., sickle cell anemia or cystic fibrosis). These techniques are capable of distinguishing homozygous or heterozygous states for a mutation.

Dot Blot. The dot blot hybridization is a method used to detect single-base mutations using allele-specific oligonucleotides (ASOs). Unlike other assays, the dot blot does not require enzyme digestion or electrophoretic separation of DNA fragments. The procedure uses labeled oligonucleotide probes of about 15 to 19 base pairs. DNA is amplified in the region of a known mutation, denatured, and applied to separate areas of a membrane or filter. A probe designed to detect a normal DNA sequence is added to one area; a second probe for the detection of a sequence with the single-base mutation is applied to a second area. Ideally, only the labeled probe whose base sequences perfectly match those of the patient will hybridize.

Reverse Dot Blot. In this variation of the dot blot procedure, the ASO probes are bound to a filter and denatured DNA from the patient is added to the immobilized ASO. Hybridization occurs only if the patient's DNA contains base sequences that are 100% complementary to those of the probe. A common variation of the reverse dot blot procedure is to bind oligonucleotide probes of a slightly longer length than in the reverse dot blot procedure to a 96-well microtiter plate. Biotin is used to label copies of the target sequence. The labeled copies are hybridized in the wells to the bound probes and detected using avidin conjugated to horseradish peroxidase. Subsequent addition of substrate produces a colored reaction that can be read photometrically.

Blotting Protocols

The Southern blot and Northern blot are used to detect DNA and RNA, respectively. These procedures share some common procedural steps: electrophoretic separation of patient's nucleic acid, transfer of nucleic acid fragments to a solid support (e.g., nitrocellulose, hybridization with a labeled probe of known nucleic acid sequence, and autoradiographic or colorimetric detection of the bands created by the probe-nucleic acid hybrid).

Southern Blot. Specimen DNA is denatured, treated with restriction enzymes to result in DNA fragments, and then the single-stranded DNA (ssDNA) fragments are separated by electrophoresis. The electrophoretically separated fragments are then blotted to a nitrocellulose membrane, retaining their electrophoretic position and hybridized with radiolabeled single-stranded DNA fragments with sequences complementary to those being sought. The resulting double-stranded DNA bearing the radiolabel is then, if present, detected by radiography.

The Southern blot procedure has clinical diagnostic applications for diseases/disorders associated with significant changes in DNA, a deletion or insertion of at least 50 to 100 base pairs (e.g., fragile X syndrome or determination of clonality in lymphomas of T- or B-cell origin). If a single-base mutation changes an enzyme restriction site on the DNA resulting in an altered band or fragment size, the Southern blot procedure can be used to detect these changes in DNA sequences (referred to as restriction fragment length polymorphisms). Single-base mutations that can be determined by Southern blot include sickle cell anemia and hemophilia A.

Northern Blot. Messenger RNA (mRNA) from the specimen is separated by electrophoresis and blotted to a specially modified paper support to result in covalent fixing of the mRNA in the electrophoretic positions. Radiolabeled, single-stranded DNA fragments complementary to the specific mRNA being sought are then hybridized to the bound mRNA. If the specific mRNA is present, the radioactivity is detected by autoradiography. The derivation of this technique from the Southern blot used for DNA detection has led to the common usage of the term *Northern blot* for the detection of specific mRNA. The Northern blot is not routinely used in clinical molecular diagnostics.

Western Blot. In comparison to the Southern blot, which separates and identifies RNA fragments and proteins, and the Northern blot, which concentrates on isolating m-RNA, Western blot is a technique in which proteins are separated electrophoretically, transferred to membranes, and identified through the use of labeled antibodies specific for the protein of interest. The Western blot technique (Figure 11-2) is used to detect antibodies to specific epitopes of electrophoretically separated subspecies of antigens. It is a technique in which electrophoresis of antigenic material yields separation of the antigenic components by molecular weight. Blotting the separated antigen to nitrocellulose, retaining the electrophoretic position, and causing it to react with patient specimen will result in the binding of specific antibodies, if present, to each antigenic "band." Electrophoresis of known molecular weight standards allows for the determination of the molecular weight of each antigenic band to which antibodies may be produced. These antibodies are then detected using EIA reactions that characterize antibody specificity. This technique is often used to confirm the specificity of antibodies detected by enzyme-linked immunosorbent assay (ELISA) screening procedures.

Microarrays

Microarray (DNA chip) technology (Figure 11-3) has catapulted into the limelight, promising to accelerate genetic analysis in much the same way that microprocessors have sped up computation. Microarrays are basically the product of bonding or direct synthesis of numerous specific DNA probes on a stationary, often silicon based support. The chip may be tailored to particular disease processes. It is easily performed and readily automated. Microarrays are miniature gene fragments attached to glass chips. These chips are used to examine gene activity of thousands or tens of thousands of gene fragments and to identify genetic mutations, using a hybridization reaction between the sequences on the microarray and a fluorescent sample. After hybridization, the chips are scanned with high-speed fluorescent detectors and the intensity of each spot is quantitated (Figure 11-4). The identity and amount of each sequence are revealed by the location and intensity of fluorescence displayed by each spot. Computers are used to analyze the data (Figure 11-5).

The applications of microarrays in clinical medicine include analysis of gene expression in malignancies (e.g., mutations in BRCA-1, mutations of the tumor-suppressor gene p53, genetic disease testing, and viral resistance mutation detection).

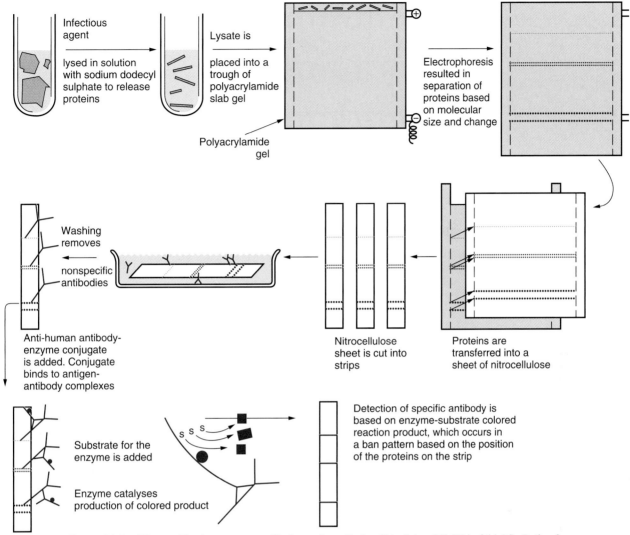

Figure 11-2 Western blot immunoassay. (Redrawn from Forbes BA, Sahm DF, Weissfeld AS: *Bailey & Scott's diagnostic microbiology,* ed 11, St Louis, 2002, Mosby.)

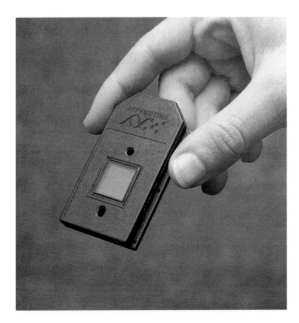

Figure 11-3 Affymetrix GeneChip probe array. (Image courtesy Affymetrix, Inc., Santa Clara, Calif.)

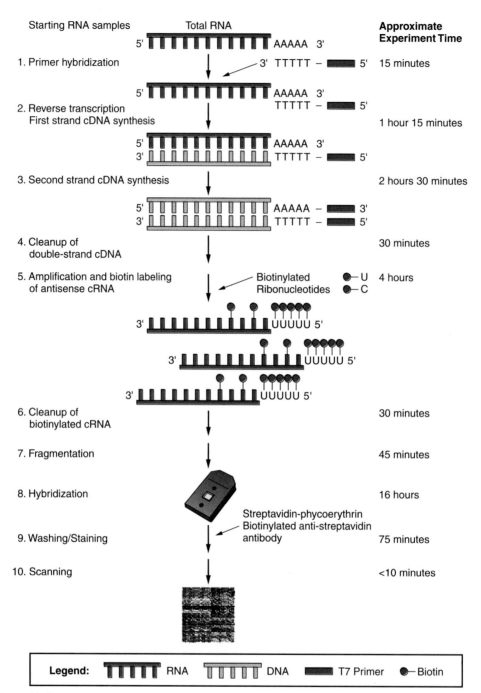

Figure 11-4   An overview of eukaryotic target labeling for GeneChip expression arrays. (Image courtesy Affymetrix, Inc., Santa Clara, CA.)

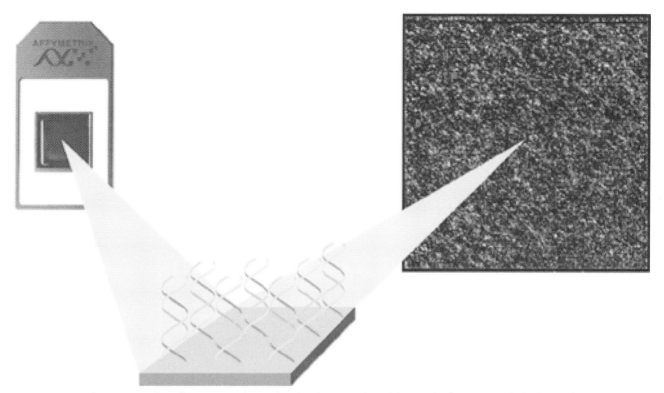

Figure 11-5   Data from an experiment showing the expression of thousands of genes on a single GeneChip probe array. (Image courtesy Affymetrix, Inc., Santa Clara, Calif.)

The Human Genome GeneChip set (HG-U133 Set), (Affymetrix, Inc, Santa Clara, CA) consisting of two GeneChip arrays, contains almost 45,000 probe sets representing more than 39,000 transcripts derived from approximately 33,000 well-substantiated human genes. The sequence clusters were created from the UniGene database and then were refined by analysis and comparison with a number of other publicly available databases, including the Washington University EST trace repository and the University of California, Santa Cruz Golden Path human genome database (April 2001 release). The HG-U133A array includes representation of the RefSeq database sequences and probe sets related to sequences previously represented on the Human Genome U95Av2 array. The HG-U133B array contains primarily probe sets representing EST clusters. The applications of this array include definition of tissue and cell type-specific gene expression, investigation of cellular and tissue responses to their environment (e.g., heat shock; interactions with other cells; exposure to chemical compounds, growth factors, or other signaling molecules). In addition, this array helps to better understand human cell differentiation by determining which transcripts are increased or decreased during distinct stages in cellular differentiation and by detecting what genes are uniquely expressed during different stages of tumorigenesis.

Another genomic microarray (GenoSensor, Vysis, Inc., Downer's Grove, Ill.) enables researchers to screen for abnormal gene amplifications and deletions with the sensitivity to detect single gene-copy change in a variety of specimens. The GenoSensor System simultaneously screens for gene copy number changes in 287 targets spotted in triplicate. This permits the screening of proto-oncogenes, tumor suppressor genes, microdeletion syndrome gene, regions and subtelomeric regions.

CHAPTER HIGHLIGHTS

PCR is an in vitro method that amplifies low levels of specific DNA sequences in a sample to higher quantities suitable for further analysis. To use this technology, the target sequence to be amplified must be known. This enzymatic process is carried out in cycles. Each repeated cycle consists of DNA denaturation, primer annealing, and extension of the primed DNA sequence. Each cycle theoretically doubles the amount of specific DNA sequence present and results in an exponential accumulation of the DNA fragment being amplified (amplicons). The three important applications of PCR are amplification of DNA, identification of a target sequence, and synthesis of a labeled antisense probe.

PCR analysis can lead to the detection of gene mutations that signify the early development of cancer, identification of viral DNA associated with specific cancers (e.g., HPV, a causative agent in cervical cancer), or the detection of genetic mutations associated with a wide variety of disease (e.g., coronary artery disease associated with mutations of the gene that encodes for the LDLR).

Adaptations of the PCR technique have been developed. One adaptation uses nested primers. This adaptation involves a two-step amplification process. In the first step, a broad region of the DNA surrounding the sequence of interest is amplified. This is followed by a second round of amplification to amplify the specific gene sequence to be studied.

PCR modifications include RT-PCR, multiplex PCR, and real-time PCR.

Other amplification techniques include SDA, TMA, NASBA, and LCR nucleic acid amplification:

Clinical applications include genetic testing, hematopathology diagnosis and monitoring, and identification of infectious agents. Conventional analysis is the use of agarose gel electrophoresis after ethidium bromide staining. Probe-based DNA detection systems have the advantage of providing sequence specificity and decreased detection limits. The selection of one technique over another is often based on a variety of factors (e.g., sensitivity and specificity profiles, cost, turnaround time, and local experience).

Probe-hybridization assays, involving the complementary pairing of a probe with a DNA or RNA strand derived from the patient specimen, exist in many forms. LPH, dot blot and reverse dot blot, and blotting protocol are popular methods. The Southern blot and Northern blot are used to detect DNA and RNA, respectively. Single-base mutations that can be determined by Southern blot include sickle cell anemia and hemophilia A. The derivation of this technique from the Southern blot used for DNA detection has led to the common usage of the term *Northern blot* for the detection of specific mRNA. The Northern blot is not routinely used in clinical molecular diagnostics.

Western blot is a technique in which proteins are separated electrophoretically, transferred to membranes, and identified through the use of labeled antibodies specific for the protein of interest. Western blot is used to detect antibodies to specific epitopes of electrophoretically separated subspecies of antigens. This technique is often used to confirm the specificity of antibodies detected by ELISA screening procedures.

Microarray (DNA chip) are basically the product of bonding or direct synthesis of numerous specific DNA probes on a stationary, often silicon-based support. Microarrays are miniature gene fragments attached to glass chips. These chips are used to examine gene activity of thousands or tens of thousands of gene fragments and to identify genetic mutations, using a hybridization reaction between the sequences on the microarray and a fluorescent sample. Applications of microarrays in clinical medicine include analysis of gene expression in malignancies (e.g., mutations in BRCA-1, mutations of the tumor-suppressor gene p53, genetic disease testing, and viral resistance mutation detection).

REVIEW QUESTIONS

1. In comparison to serologic assays, nucleic acid testing offers all of the following benefits, *except:*
   A. reduced cost
   B. enhanced specificity
   C. increased sensitivity
   D. all of the above

2. PCR testing is useful in:
   A. forensic testing
   B. genetic testing
   C. disease diagnosis
   D. all of the above

3. The traditional PCR technique:
   A. extends the length of the genomic DNA
   B. alters the original DNA nucleotide sequence
   C. copies the target region of DNA
   D. amplifies the target region of RNA

4. For the PCR reaction to take place, one must provide which of the following?
   A. oligonucleotide primers
   B. individual deoxynucleotides
   C. thermostable DNA polymerase
   D. all of the above

5. The enzyme reverse transcriptase converts:
   A. mRNA to cDNA
   B. tRNA to DNTP
   C. dsDNA to ssDNA
   D. mitochondrial to nuclear DNA

6. DNA polymerase catalyzes:
   A. primer annealing
   B. primer extension
   C. hybridization of DNA
   D. hybridization of RNA

7. The figure below depicts:

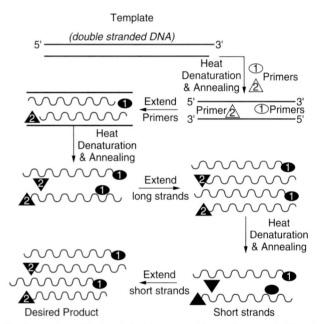

(Redrawn from Warden BA, Thompson E: Apolipoprotein E and the development of atherosclerosis, *Lab Med* 25(7):453, 1994.)

   A. polymerase chain reaction (PCR)
   B. nested primer PCR
   C. Western blot analysis
   D. Southern blot analysis

Questions 8-10. Match the method with the appropriate description.

8. _____ Southern blot immunoassay

9. _____ Northern blot immunoassay

10. _____ Western blot immunoassay

    A. Messenger RNA is studied.
    B. Called immunoblot, it is used to detect antibodies to subspecies of antigens.
    C. Single-stranded DNA is studied.

11. Which of the following techniques uses signal amplification?
    A. b-DNA
    B. TMA
    C. NASBA
    D. RT-PCR

12. Which of the following nucleic acid amplification techniques does not require the use of a thermocycler?
    A. PCR
    B. SDA
    C. NASBA
    D. TMA

BIBLIOGRAPHY

Branca M: One genome—two chips, *Bio-IT World* 1(1):12, 2002.
Capetandes A: Polymerase chain reaction: the making of something big, *Med Lab Observer* 31:26, 1999.
Doty A: Monitoring the quality of nucleic acid testing for infectious disease, *Adv Med Lab Prof* 13(10):12-16, 2001.
Forbes BA, Sahm DF, Weissfeld AS: *Bailey and Scott's diagnostic microbiology,* ed 11, St Louis, 2002, Mosby.
Kazmi S, Krull IS: Proteonomics and the current state of protein separations, *PharmaGenomics* 1(1):14-29, 2001.
Miyake K: Olympus develops DNA computer, *Bio-IT World* 1(1):2, 2002.
Nadder TS: The new millennium laboratory: molecular diagnostics goes clinical, *Clin Lab Sci* 14:252, 2001.
Rohlfs EM, Silverman LM: Molecular diagnosis of inherited disease, *Med Lab Observer* 28:44-52, 1996.
Schena M: *Microarray biochip technology,* Natick, Mass, 2000, A: Eaton Publishing.
Turgeon ML: *Clinical hematology,* ed 3, Philadelphia, 1999, Lippincott Williams & Wilkins.
Tang Y, Procop GW, Persing DH: Molecular diagnostics of infectious diseases, *Clin Chem* 43:2021-2038, 1997.
Uphoff TS: Basic concepts and innovations in molecular diagnosis, *ADV Med Lab Prof* 14(18):13, 2002.
Warden BA, Thompson E: Apolipoprotein E and the development of atherosclerosis, *Lab Med* 25(7): 449-455, 1994.
Weiss RL: *Interpretive data guide,* Salt Lake City, 1999, ARUP Laboratories.
Weiss RL, editor: *ARUP's guide to molecular diagnostics clinical laboratory testing,* ed 2, Salt Lake City, 2001, ARUP Laboratories.
Wisecarver J: Amplification of DNA sequences, *Lab Med* 28:191-196, 1997.

Miscellaneous Techniques

LEARNING OBJECTIVES

At the conclusion of this chapter, the reader should be able to:
- Describe the principle and application of radial immunodiffusion.
- Cite the principle and disadvantages of the radioimmunoassay procedure.

- Define and compare the radioallergosorbent test (RAST) with radioimmunosorbent test (RIST).
- Describe the principles and use of the CH$_{50}$ and complement fixation procedures.
- Explain the neutralization procedure.
- Interpret the results of the cryoglobulin procedure.

Some procedures are used infrequently but are appropriate in some clinical or research circumstances. Various procedures, some of which were very popular in the past, are described in this chapter.

RADIAL IMMUNODIFFUSION

Gel techniques identify antigens and antibodies only qualitatively; however, by further modification and the use of single radial immunodiffusion (RID), they can become quantitative. The RID is a simple and specific method for identification and quantitation of a number of proteins found in human serum and other body fluids (Box 12-1). This technique may be used when the nature of a protein is not readily differentiated by standard electrophoretic procedures.

Principle

The quantitation of proteins by gel diffusion using antibody incorporated in agar was reported in 1957. In the last several decades a wide selection of specific antisera has become available, which allows for the quantitation of their corresponding antigen.

Radial immunodiffusion is based on a technique using a precipitin reaction in which the internal reactants (i.e., specific antibody) are added to a buffered agarose medium. Serum containing standard volumes of the protein (i.e., test antigen) is placed in a well centered in the agarose. When this immunodiffusion system has an unlimited amount of antibody available and no undue restrictions placed on free diffusion of the antigen, the diameter of the resulting pre-

---

Box 12-1   Examples of Immunologic Assays Performed by Radial Immunodiffusion

Alpha 1–acid glycoprotein
Alpha 1–antitrypsin
Haptoglobin
Transferrin
C3
C4
C5
C-reactive protein
Immunoglobulins (IgM, IgG, IgA, and IgD)

---

cipitin zone is related to the concentration of antigen placed in the well. While the precipitin ring is enlarging, the log of the antigen concentration is approximately proportional to the diameter of the end point, and the area (square of the diameter) varies directly with the concentration.

Methods

Two principal RID methods have been developed: the Fahey method and the Mancini method. The difference between the two techniques is that the Fahey method is a kinetic approach in which the ring diameter is read at a specified time, whereas the Mancini method is an end point method in which the ring diameter is read after diffusion is completed. In the Mancini method the quantitative determination of proteins is after 24 hours of diffusion.

After antibody is added to the well cut in the agar gel and fixed volumes of test antigen of different concentrations are put into the wells, the gel plate is allowed to incubate for 18 to 24 hours (Mancini method) in order for the antigen to diffuse out from the wells. Antigen continues to diffuse and bind more antibody until an equivalence point is reached and the soluble complexes precipitate in a ring. If the antibody concentration and gel thickness are uniform and constant, the area within the precipitin ring (measured as the ring diameter squared) is proportional to the antigen concentration. When the diameter of the ring (D^2) is plotted against the antigen concentration, a straight line results based on this equation:

$$D^2 = K(Cag) + So$$

where K = constant; Cag = concentration of antigen; and So = intercept (function of antigen well diameter and of antigen volume)

The concentration of protein in an unknown specimen is derived by interpolation from a standard curve. The whole process may be reversed to determine the concentrations of unknown antibody.

Advantages and Disadvantages

RID requires no special equipment and can be performed in many clinical laboratories. The procedure is considered to be sensitive, rapid, and accurate. In addition, for many smaller laboratories it is an economical and practical method of performing quantitative studies.

One limitation of the procedure is that it is limited by the assay ranges of the plate. The precision of the assay as expressed by the coefficient of variation is about 10%. In addition, idiotypically related differences in the immunologic reactivity to immunoglobulin (Ig)G, IgA, or IgM may result in differences in the quantitative values obtained with the RID method. Multiple myeloma or other disorders involving monoclonal gammopathies may yield values either higher or lower than those reported with other methods.

RID Protocol

Principle

A qualitative relationship exists between the concentration of a protein deposited in a well, cut into a thin agarose layer containing the corresponding monospecific antiserum. The wells are filled with unknown serum or a suitable standard and incubated in a moist environment at room temperature. After the optimal point of diffusion has been reached, the diameters of the precipitin rings are measured. The diameter of the ring is related to the concentration of the constituent (e.g., Ig) (Figure 12-1). RID is intended for the quantification of specific proteins such as IgM, IgG, IgA, alpha 1 antitrypsin, transferrin, and complement components (e.g., C3).

Specimen Collection and Preparation

No special preparation of the patient is required before specimen collection. The patient must be positively identified when the specimen is collected, and the specimen should be labeled at the bedside. Specimen labels should include the patient's full name, the date, the patient's hospital identification number, and the phlebotomist's initials.

Blood should be drawn by an aseptic technique. A minimum of 2 mL of clotted blood (red top evacuated tube) is required. The specimen should be centrifuged promptly and an aliquot of serum removed. Lipemia, hemolysis, or contamination with bacteria renders a specimen unsuitable for testing. Although icteric and turbid specimens have given valid results, fresh non-heat-inactivated serum is recommended for use in the test.

If the test cannot be performed immediately, the specimen should be refrigerated (2° to 8° C) for no longer than 72 hours. If additional delay occurs, the serum should be frozen at –18° C or below. Frozen serum should be thawed rapidly at 37° C.

Reagents, Supplies, and Equipment

- RID plates (available commercially)
- Three standard serum dilutions
- Microliter dispenser
- Semilog and linear graph paper
- Ruler

Quality Control

Reference sera with known values should be tested simultaneously.

CAUTION: Because the control sera is derived from human sources, it should be handled in the same manner as clinical serum specimens (see Universal Blood and Body Fluid Precautions in Chapter 6).

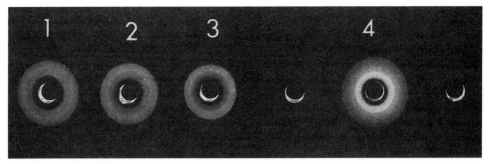

Figure 12-1   Quantitation of IgG by radial immunodiffusion. Increasing diameters of precipitin rings reflect increasingly larger protein concentrations. Wells 1 through 3 are known IgG standards; well 4 is an unknown serum. (From Bauer JD: *Clinical laboratory methods,* ed 9, St Louis, 1982, Mosby.)

■ *Radial Immunodiffusion*

1. Remove plate from envelope and allow to stand open for about 5 minutes to allow any moisture to evaporate.
2. Label the wells on the outer margin of the plate and on a card to identify sera and controls to be deposited into the wells.
3. Fill three wells with 2 to 20 μL (in accordance with manufacturer's instructions) with the standards supplied.
4. Fill the remaining groups of two or three wells with diluted or undiluted patient's sera (follow manufacturer's instructions).
5. Tightly close plate and place into envelope sealed with tape to prevent loss of moisture.
6. Store the plate in a horizontal position at room temperature for a minimum of 6 to 12 hours (Fahey-McKelvey technique) or for about 50 hours (Mancini technique), depending on the type of Ig assayed.
7. After the appropriate time (see below), measure the diameter (D) of the precipitin ring (in millimeters) of the unknown and standards to an accuracy of 0.1 mm using a calibrated magnifier and a light source beneath the plate.

Calculations

Square the diameter reading (D^2) and construct a standard curve. Two methods are available for the construction of the standard curve and the calculation of patient values.

Fahey-McKelvey Method

The early readout method of Fahey measures the precipitin rings (unknown and standards) before they reach maximal size, after about 6 to 12 hours. In this method the logarithm of the antigen concentration is proportional to the area of the precipitin ring (D^2). Plot the squared diameter (D^2) of the precipitin rings obtained from three standards on the ordinate of semilog graph paper, and enter the corresponding concentrations of the standards (in milligrams/deciliter) on the abscissa. Because the concentrations are plotted on semilog paper, a straight line is obtained.

Mancini Method

This method is based on the fact that after a certain time, depending on the concentration and the molecular weight of the protein, a precipitin ring reaches a maximal value and further incubation fails to increase its size. The area of the precipitin ring (square of its diameter) is linearly proportional to the antigen concentration in the well. Plotting these values on linear graph paper produces a straight line. The maximal ring diameter is obtained in about 24 hours by IgG in normal concentration and in about 50 hours by IgM in normal concentration. The linear relationship between the area (in square millimeters) and concentration is not established until the rings (standard and unknown) reach their maximal size. The end point method has a high degree of accuracy, reproducibility, and sensitivity but requires time.

1. Plot the squared diameter (D^2) of the precipitin rings obtained from the three standards on ordinate of linear graph paper, and enter the corresponding concentrations of the standards (in milligrams/deciliter) on the abscissa. Connecting the three reference points should result in a straight line. The patient's value is obtained by reference to this calibration curve.
2. If diluted patient's serum is used, multiply the concentration by the dilution factor to obtain the value for whole serum.

Reporting Results

Method is sensitive (10 to 20 mg protein/dL, depending on the protein).

Procedure Notes

Sources of Error

Sources of technical error include:
1. Specimen contamination
2. Spilling of the antigen
3. Inadequate filling of the wells
4. Damaged or out-of-date gel

Clinical Applications

If the procedure is used for Ig assay, hypogammaglobulinemia, or hypergammaglobulinemia may be detected.

Limitations

The precision of the Ig assay (cv) is about 10%.

RADIOIMMUNOASSAY

The radioimmunoassay (RIA) method continues to be used for some immunologic assays, primarily by reference laboratories. Radioisotopes can be used to measure the concentration of antigen or antibody in serum samples. The basis of the RIA procedure relies on the principle of competitive binding.

If antibody concentration is being measured, the principle of the procedure is that radioactive-labeled antibody competes with patient unlabeled antibody for binding sites on a known amount of antigen. When all three components are present in the system, an equilibrium exists.

A typical RIA procedure begins with antigen in saline being incubated on a microplate or in a test tube. Small quantities of the antigen become absorbed onto the plastic surface. After incubation, free antigen is washed away. The plate may then be blocked with an excess amount of an irrelevant protein, which prevents any subsequent binding of proteins.

Test antibody, which binds to the antigen, is then added. Unbound proteins are washed away, and the antibody is detected by a radiolabeled ligand. The ligand may be a molecule such as staphylococcal protein A (which binds to the Fc region of IgG) or, more often, another antibody specific to the test antibody. Unbound ligand is washed away, and the radioactivity of the plate or tube is counted on a gamma counter.

As the amount of test antibody increases, the counts per minute rise from a background level through a linear range to a plateau. Antibody titers can be detected correctly only within the linear range. Typically the plateau binding rate is 20 to 100 times the background count. A reduction in radioactivity of the antigen-antibody complex compared to the radioactive counts measured in the control test with no antibody is used to quantitate the amount of patient antibody bound to the antigen.

The main advantage of the RIA method is the extreme sensitivity and ability to detect trace amounts of antigen or antibody. In addition, a large number of tests can be performed in a relatively short time period. The disadvantages, as previously cited, are the hazards and instability of isotopes.

RADIOALLERGOSORBENT TEST

The radioallergosorbent (RAST) test measures antigen-specific IgE in a radioimmunoassay when the ligand is a labeled anti-IgE antibody. The steps are identical to the standard radioimmunoassay except that the antigen (allergen) is covalently bonded to a cellulose polymer sponge rather than noncovalently to a radioimmunoassay plate. Having much more antigen available on the disc permits the high sensitivity necessary to bind the small quantities of IgE present in serum.

Allerprint's results are generated from a reference curve calibrated with the World Health Organization standard for Total IgE. Allerprint uniquely provides a single report with quantitative units (kU/L) and modified RAST counts and classes allowing physicians to use the scoring method they prefer.

Esoterix Allergy and Asthma (www.esoterix.com) offers an advanced in vitro allergy assay called Allerprint SM. Allerprint is an ultrasensitive, quantitative assay that identifies levels of specific IgE associated with hypersensitivity to allergens.

In vitro allergy testing (sometimes referred to as RAST testing) has become a common procedure in the diagnosis of allergies. The demand for quantitative reporting capabilities has been driven by Pharmacia Diagnostics, a manufacturer of in vitro assay systems that has been successful in the branding of the ImmunoCAP assays, the first to be cleared by the Food and Drug Administration for the quantitative measurement of specific IgE.

RADIOIMMUNOSORBENT TEST

The radioimmunosorbent test (RIST) is a competition radioimmunoassay for total serum IgE. The plate is sensitized with anti-IgE, and increasing amounts of labeled IgE are added to the plate to determine the maximum amount of IgE that the plate can bind. A quantity of labeled IgE equivalent to approximately 80% of the plateau binding is chosen. In the test experiment, this amount of labeled IgE is mixed with the serum containing the IgE to be tested. The test IgE competes with the labeled IgE. Therefore the more IgE that is present in the test serum, the less the amount of labeled IgE that binds.

COMPLEMENT

CH$_{50}$ Assay

This test assesses the hemolytic activity of the complement system, a natural protein found in the blood. Monitoring CH$_{50}$ is useful in following the course of immune complex disease, in screening for genetic deficiencies of the complement system, and in diagnosing hereditary angioneurotic edema. Low levels confirm complement activation or in vitro degradation.

Complement Decay Rate

A decrease of CH$_{50}$ activity in plasma at 37° C causes 10% to 20% decay. A decay rate greater than 50% is abnormal and is consistent with, but not diagnostic of C1 esterase inhibitor deficiency.

A traditional method for determination of functional complement activity is the total hemolytic (CH$_{50}$) assay. This assay measures the ability of a test sample to lyse 50% of a standardized suspension of sheep erythrocytes coated with antierythrocyte antibody. Both the classic activation pathway and the terminal complement components are measured during this reaction. Total complement activity is usually abnormal if any component is defective. Individual component abnormalities or abnormalities in the alternative pathway, however, can exist despite a normal CH$_{50}$ value.

Acquired complement deficiencies are frequently encountered in active systemic lupus erythematosus and other autoimmune diseases, a variety of kidney and liver diseases, subacute bacterial endocarditis, cryoglobulinemia, and allograft rejection. Assaying and monitoring specific components, especially C3, C4, and C3 activator for the classic and alternate pathways, provide a valuable guide to the management of such patients. The C4 level often provides the most sensitive indicator of disease activity. C4 is destroyed only when the classic pathway is activated. Although C3 lies at the junction of the two pathways, it is much more severely depressed when activation occurs via the alternative pathway. Reduction of C3 and C4 components implies that activation of the classic pathway has been initiated.

■ CH₅₀ Total Hemolytic Complement

Principle

The CH_{50} total hemolytic complement assay measures the ability of a test sample to lyse 50% of a standardized suspension of sheep erythrocytes coated with anti-erythrocyte antibody. Antibody-coated erythrocytes are incubated with the test specimen. Activation of complement results in cell lysis and release of hemoglobin. The degree of hemolysis is proportional to the total hemolytic complement activity.

Both the classic activation pathway and the terminal complement components are measured during this reaction. Low levels of complement confirm complement activation (or degradation in vitro). Assessment of CH_{50} is useful in screening for genetic deficiencies of the complement system, in diagnosing hereditary angioneurotic edema, and in monitoring the progress of patients with immune complex disease.

Specimen Collection and Preparation

No special preparation of the patient is required before specimen collection. The patient must be positively identified when the specimen is collected and labeled at the bedside. Specimen labels must include the patient's full name, the date the specimen is collected, the patient's hospital identification number, and the phlebotomist's initials.

Blood should be drawn using an aseptic technique. A minimum of 2 mL of clotted blood (red top evacuated tube) is required. The specimen should be allowed to clot at room temperature, and the serum should be separated by centrifugation at 4° C. The serum should be removed from the clot and kept at 4° C. Testing should be conducted immediately after collection and separation, or the serum should be frozen at –70° C until the time of testing. Hemolysis renders a specimen unsuitable for testing.

Reagents, Supplies, and Equipment

The following components are supplied in the CH_{50} assay kit commercially available from Sigma Diagnostics, St. Louis, MO:

1. Sensitized sheep red blood cells: a standardized concentration of sheep erythrocytes coated with antisheep erythrocytes suspended in buffer, pH 7.3 with stabilizer. Sodium azide 0.02% is added as a preservative. It is stored under refrigeration (2° to 6° C). The cells are stable until the expiration date shown.

2. Reference standard CH_{50}: a lyophilized human serum containing a known CH_{50} value. The total hemolytic complement activity (unit/mL) is indicated on the label. Dry vials are stored in the freezer (–20° C). Vial label bears expiration date.

Immediately before use, the contents of the vial are reconstituted by adding 0.3 mL deionized water, then mixed gently until dissolution is complete. Within 30 minutes of reconstitution, aliquot and store any remaining solution at –70° C or in liquid nitrogen. If such storage means are not available, discard contents of the vial.

WARNING: Sodium azide may react with lead and copper plumbing to form highly explosive metal azides. On disposal, flush with a large volume of water to prevent azide buildup. Sodium azide is also toxic, so care should be taken to avoid ingestion.

Additional Required Equipment and Supplies

1. Refrigerated centrifuge
2. Spectrophotometer and cuvettes
3. Pipetting device
4. Timer

Quality Control

CH_{50} low activity control and CH_{50} high-activity control (Sigma Diagnostics, St. Louis, Mo.) should be tested with the patient specimen.

Immediately before use, reconstitute the contents of each vial by adding 0.3 mL of deionized water. Mix gently until dissolution is complete. Within 30 minutes of reconstitution, aliquot and store any remaining solutions at –70° C or in liquid nitrogen. If such storage means are not available, discard contents of the vials.

The reconstituted controls should be treated in the exact manner as a test specimen. The total hemolytic complement activity should be within ±10% of the value indicated on the vials.

CAUTION: Because the reference standard and control sera are derived from human sources, they should be handled in the same manner as clinical serum specimens (see Universal Blood and Body Fluid Precautions, Chapter 6).

Procedure

Preliminary preparation: Allow the sensitized sheep red blood cells to warm to room temperature before use. Immediately before use, resuspend the cells by repeated inversions. Reconstitute or defrost the reference standard and controls.

1. For each test sample and control, label one tube of sheep cells. Label one tube for the reference standard and one tube "Lysis Control" (spontaneous lysis).
2. Remove the tube caps and pipette 0.005 μl (5 μl) of test sample, controls, or reference standard to the appropriately labeled tube. No sample is added to the lysis control.
3. Replace caps and mix immediately by inverting each tube two or three times.

4. Incubate the tubes at room temperature (18° to 26° C) for 60 ± 5 minutes.
5. Mix the contents of all tubes again by inverting two or three times.
6. Centrifuge all tubes at approximately 600 × g for 10 minutes.
7. Transfer the supernatant fluid to a cuvette.
8. Read absorbance of the supernatants at 415 nm within 15 minutes after centrifugation. Zero the instrument using a water blank. Read and record the absorbance of the Lysis Control ($A_{control}$). Zero the instrument using the Lysis Control as a blank. Read and record the absorbance value of the Reference Standard ($A_{standard}$) and of each test specimen and the controls ($A_{specimen}$).

Calculations

The CH_{50} value of each specimen or control is calculated as follows:

CH_{50} value of a specimen = $A_{specimen}/A_{standard} \times CH_{50}$ value of standard.

Example:
Stated CH_{50} value of the standard = 192 U/mL
Absorbance value of $A_{specimen}$ = 1.104
Absorbance value of $A_{standard}$ = 0.901
CH_{50} value of a specimen = 1.104/0.901 = × 192 = 235 U/mL

Reporting Results

The reference CH_{50} titer is about 200 CH_{50} U/mL.

Procedure Notes

The concentration of sensitized cells has been adjusted to yield 50% hemolysis in the presence of 5 mL of normal human serum (i.e., 1 CH_{50} U).

Because the assay is nearly linear over a broad range, a single point can be used for calibration of this method.

The absorbance value of the lysis control when read against water at 415 nm should be less than 0.15 using a spectrophotometer with a 1-cm lightpath. If the $A_{control}$ exceeds 0.15, the assay results will not be valid and the assay must be repeated with new sensitized sheep cells.

Sources of Error

Only serum, not plasma, should be used in the assay. Proper collection, handling, and storage of the serum are essential to accuracy.

Clinical Applications

Increases in complement levels occur because of increased synthesis. An increased rate of complement is part of the acute-phase reactant response. Elevations in total hemolytic activity can be associated with:
- Acute inflammatory conditions
- Leukemia
- Hodgkin's disease
- Sarcoma
- Behçet's disease

Decreases in complement levels, hyposynthesis, can be caused by a variety of conditions. These conditions include:
- Congenital defects
- Liver disease
- Nutritional imbalance
- Hypocatabolism

In addition, complement fixation can result from the presence of tissue or cell-bound immune complexes, or when circulating immune complexes are displayed. Bound immune complexes can be associated with chronic glomerulonephritis, rheumatoid arthritis, hemolytic anemia, and graft rejection. Circulating immune complexes are characteristically associated with systemic lupus erythematosus, acute glomerulonephritis, subacute bacterial endocarditis, and cryoglobulinemia.

Limitations

The limitations of this procedure should be noted:
1. Results of the CH_{50} assay, which are a quantitative value, represent the functional total hemolytic complement activity. Values achieved with this method can be used to determine the presence of abnormal whole complement levels but cannot identify the abnormal component. In cases of abnormal values, the serum must be assayed for the value of each of the individual (C1-C9) components.
2. The measurement of total CH_{50} hemolytic activity cannot exclude all acquired or congenital abnormalities of individual components.
3. The procedure has been developed to aid in diagnosis but is not diagnostic in itself.

Complement Fixation

Complement fixation (CF) is a classic method for demonstrating the presence of antibody (e.g., antistreptolysin O) in serum; however, more sensitive and less demanding systems for the detection of antibodies have replaced the complement fixation procedure.

The CF method consists of two components. The first component is an indicator system consisting of a combination of sheep red blood cells, complement-fixing antibody (IgG) produced against the sheep red cells in another animal, and an exogenous source of complement, usually guinea pig serum. When these three components are combined in an optimum concentration, the antisheep cell antibody, hemolysin, can bind to the surface of the red cells. Complement can subsequently bind to this antigen-antibody complex and cause cell lysis. The second component consists of a known antigen and patient serum, which are added to a suspension of sheep erythrocytes, hemolysin, and a complement.

The two components of the complement fixation procedure are tested in sequence (Figure 12-2). Patient serum is first added to the known antigen, and complement is added to the solution. If the serum contains antibody to the antigen, the resulting

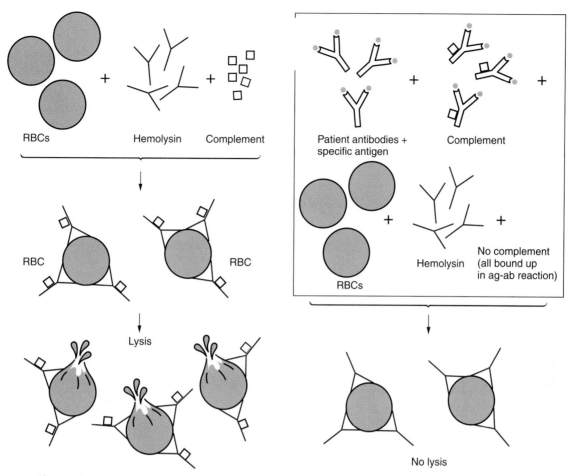

Figure 12-2   Complement fixation test. (Redrawn from Forbes BA, Sahm DF, Weissfeld AS: *Bailey and Scott's diagnostic microbiology,* ed 11, St Louis, 2002, Mosby.)

antigen-antibody complexes will bind all of the complement. Sheep red cells and hemolysin are then added. If complement has not been bound by an antigen-antibody complex formed from the patient serum and known antigen, it is available to bind to the indicator system of sheep cells and hemolysin.

Lysis of the indicator sheep cells indicates both a lack of antibody and a negative complement fixation test. If the patient's serum does contain a complement-fixing antibody, a positive result will be demonstrated by the lack of hemolysis, intact red cells.

NEUTRALIZATION PROCEDURES

The evaluation of neutralizing antibodies, which destroy the infectivity of viruses, can be measured by the neutralization method. In this procedure patient serum is mixed with a suspension of infectious virus particles of the same type as those suspected of causing disease in the patient. A control suspension of virus is mixed with normal serum and then inoculated into an appropriate cell culture. If the patient serum contains antibody to the virus, the antibody will bind to the virus particles and prevent them from invading the cells in culture and neutralizing the infectivity of the virus. Disadvantages of this procedure are that it is technically demanding and time consuming. It is restricted to laboratories that routinely perform viral cultures.

CRYOGLOBULINS

Cryoglobulin analysis is frequently requested when patient symptoms such as pain, cyanosis, Raynaud's phenomenon, or skin ulceration on exposure to cold temperatures are present. Cryoglobulins are proteins that precipitate or gel when cooled to 0° C and dissolve when heated. In most cases, monoclonal cryoglobulins are IgM or IgG. Occasionally the macroglobulin is both cryoprecipitable and capable of cold-induced anti-i–mediated agglutination of red cells.

Cryoglobulins can have a monoclonal protein component, and, when detected, normally prompt a clinical investigation to determine whether an underlying disease exists. Cryoglobulins are classified as follows:

- Type I—the cryoprecipitate is a monoclonal IgG, IgA, or IgM.
- Type II—the cryoprecipitate is mixed, containing two classes of immunoglobulins, at least one of which is monoclonal.
- Type III—the cryoprecipitate is mixed, and no monoclonal protein is found.

To test for the presence of cryoglobulins, blood is collected, placed in warm water, and centrifuged at room temperature. The serum is then put into a graduated centrifuge tube and placed in a 4° C environment for 7 days. If a gel or precipitate is observed, the tube is centrifuged, then the precipitate is washed at 4° C, redissolved at 37° C, and evaluated by double diffusion and immunoelectrophoresis for the content of the cryoglobulin.

CHAPTER HIGHLIGHTS

RID is a simple and specific method for identification and quantitation of a number of proteins found in human serum and other body fluids. This technique may be used when the nature of a protein is not readily differentiated by standard electrophoretic procedures. Radial immunodiffusion is based on a technique using a precipitin reaction in which the internal reactants (i.e., specific antibody) are added to a buffered agarose medium and the area (square of the diameter) varies directly with the concentration.

RIA can be used to measure the concentration of antigen or antibody in serum samples. The basis of the RIA procedure relies on the principle of competitive binding. The main advantage of the RIA method is the extreme sensitivity and ability to detect trace amounts of antigen or antibody. The major disadvantages are the hazards and instability of isotopes.

RAST or its equivalent expression measures antigen-specific IgE in a radioimmunoassay when the ligand is a labeled anti-IgE antibody. The steps are identical to the standard radioimmunoassay except that the antigen (allergen) is covalently bound to a cellulose disc rather than noncovalently to a radioimmunoassay plate. In vitro allergy testing (sometimes referred to as RAST testing) has become a common procedure in the diagnosis of allergies.

RIST is a competition radioimmunoassay for total serum IgE. The plate is sensitized with anti-IgE, and increasing amounts of labeled IgE are added to the plate to determine the maximum amount of IgE that the plate can bind.

CH_{50} assesses the hemolytic activity of the complement system, a natural protein found in the blood. Monitoring CH_{50} is useful in following the course of immune complex disease, in screening for genetic deficiencies of the complement system, and in diagnosing hereditary angioneurotic edema. Low levels confirm complement activation or in vitro degradation.

CF is a classic method for demonstrating the presence of antibody (e.g., antistreptolysin O) in serum; however, more sensitive and less demanding systems for the detection of an-

tibodies have replaced the complement fixation procedure. Lysis of the indicator sheep cells indicates both a lack of antibody and a negative complement fixation test. If the patient's serum does contain a complement-fixing antibody, a positive result will be demonstrated by the lack of hemolysis, intact red cells.

The evaluation of neutralizing antibodies, which destroy the infectivity of viruses, can be measured by the neutralization method. In this procedure patient serum is mixed with a suspension of infectious virus particles of the same type as those suspected of causing disease in the patient.

Cryoglobulin analysis is frequently requested when patient symptoms such as pain, cyanosis, Raynaud's phenomenon, or skin ulceration on exposure to cold temperatures are present. Cryoglobulins are proteins that precipitate or gel when cooled to 0° C and dissolve when heated. In most cases, monoclonal cryoglobulins are IgM or IgG. Occasionally the macroglobulin is both cryoprecipitable and capable of cold-induced anti-i–mediated agglutination of red cells. Cryoglobulins can have a monoclonal protein component, and, when detected, normally prompt a clinical investigation to determine whether an underlying disease exists.

REVIEW QUESTIONS

1. Radial immunodiffusion (RID) is:
   A. used only to identify antigens and antibodies qualitatively
   B. used to functionally assay proteins in human serum
   C. used to identify and quantitate proteins only in human serum
   D. used to identify and quantitate proteins in human serum and other body fluids

2. Radioisotopes are used in:
   A. radioimmunoassay (RIA)
   B. radioallergosorbent test (RAST)
   C. radioimmunosorbent test (RIST)
   D. all of the above

3. The figure below depicts the _____ assay.

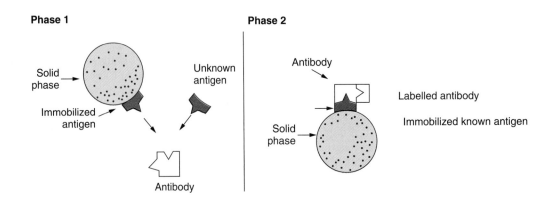

A. RIA
B. RAST
C. RIST
D. EIA

4. The RIST assay measures serum:
   A. IgM
   B. IgG
   C. IgD
   D. IgE.

5. In the RIA procedure, a reduction in radioactivity in the test specimen compared to the radioactive counts measured in the control test is used to quantitate the amount of patient antibody bound to the antigen with:
   A. a labeled amount of antibody
   B. a labeled amount of antigen
   C. no antibody
   D. no antigen

6. The main advantage of the RIA method is:
   A. isotope stability
   B. extreme sensitivity
   C. ability to detect trace amounts of antigen or antibody
   D. both B and C

7. If the test result in the CH_{50} assay is low or below normal, which may be the cause?
   A. in vitro degradation
   B. complement activation
   C. inflammation
   D. both A and B

8. In the complement fixation procedure, a negative result is manifested by:
   A. antigen binding
   B. lysis of guinea pig cells
   C. lysis of sheep red blood cells
   D. agglutination of sheep red blood cells

9. The neutralization assay is used for:
   A. evaluation of antibodies that destroy infectivity of viruses
   B. evaluation of antibodies that destroy infectivity of bacteria
   C. quantitation of complement
   D. quantitation of immune complexes

10. Cryoglobulins are proteins that precipitate or gel when cooled to _____ ° C.
    A. –18° C
    B. 0° C
    C. 4° C
    D. 18° C

Questions 11-13. Match the following types of cryoglobulin with their respective descriptions.

11. _____ type I

12. _____ type II

13. _____ type III

   A. contains two classes of immunoglobulins, at least one of which is monoclonal
   B. mixed, no monoclonal protein found
   C. Monoclonal IgG, IgA, or IgM

14. Complement fixation demonstrates:
    A. the presence of antigen in serum
    B. the presence of antibody in serum
    C. agglutination of antigen and antibody
    D. a negative result if hemolysis occurs

15. Neutralization procedures are used for evaluation of neutralizing antibodies, which destroy the infectivity of:
    A. bacteria
    B. parasites
    C. viruses
    D. fungi

16. Cryoglobulin analysis can be useful in the diagnosis of:
    A. hypothermia
    B. Raynaud's phenomenon
    C. infectious hepatitis
    D. rheumatoid arthritis

BIBLIOGRAPHY

Aloisi RM: *Principles of immunology and immunodiagnostics,* Philadelphia, 1988, Lea & Febiger.

Baron EJ, Peterson LR, Finegold SM: *Bailey and Scott's diagnostic microbiology,* ed 9, St Louis, 1994, Mosby.

Fahey JL, McKelvey EM: Quantitative determination of serum immunoglobulin in antibody-agar plate, *J Immunol* 94:84-94, 1965.

Feinbert JG: Identification, discrimination and quantification in Ouchterlony gel plates, *Int Arch Allergy* 11:129-152, 1957.

Henry JB, editor: *Clinical diagnosis and management,* ed 18, Philadelphia, 1991, WB Saunders.

Mancini G, Carbonara AO, Heremans JF: Immuno-chemical quantitation of antigens by single radial immunodiffusion, *Immunochemistry* 2:235-254, 1965.

Turgeon ML: *Clinical hematology,* ed 3, Philadelphia, 1999, Lippincott Williams & Wilkins.

Warden BA, Thompson E: Apolipoprotein E and the development of atherosclerosis, *Lab Med* 25(7):449-455, 1994.

Part Three

Immunologic Manifestations of Infectious Diseases

Chapter 13

The Immune Response in Infectious Diseases

Characteristics of Infectious Diseases
Development of Infectious Diseases
Immunity to Infectious Diseases
    Bacterial Diseases
    Parasitic Diseases
    Fungal Diseases
    Viral, Rickettsial, and Mycoplasmal Diseases

Laboratory Detection of Immunologic Responses
Chapter Highlights
Review Questions
Bibliography

LEARNING OBJECTIVES

At the conclusion of this chapter, the reader should be able to:
- Describe important characteristics in the acquisition and development of infectious diseases.
- Explain how the body develops immunity to bacterial, parasitic, fungal, viral, rickettsial, and mycoplasmal diseases.

- Briefly describe the laboratory detection of immunologic responses.

CHARACTERISTICS OF INFECTIOUS DISEASES

The acquisition of an infectious disease (e.g., viral, bacterial, parasitic, fungal) is influenced by factors related to both the microorganism and the host. Factors that can influence the exposure to and actual development of an infectious disease include:
- The immune status of an individual (immunocompromised individuals have a much higher rate of microbial disease)
- Overall incidence of an organism in the population
- Pathogenicity or virulence of the agent
- Actual presence of a large enough dose of the agent or organism to produce an infection
- Appropriate portal of entry

In many cases the successful dissemination of a microorganism results from the fact that the microorganism can be spread over long distances by insect vectors or rapidly from country to country by travelers in the jet age. Other considerations in microbial disease development include the abili-

ties of some microorganisms to multiply in an intracellular habitat, such as in macrophages, and the abilities of others to display antigen variation, which makes it difficult for a normal immune mechanism to control.

Host factors such as the general health and age of an individual influence the likelihood of developing an infectious disease and are important determinants of its severity. The very young and the older population develop infectious diseases more frequently than individuals in other age groups. In addition, a history of previous exposure to a disease or the harboring of an organism such as a virus in a dormant condition is also a determining factor in the development of a variety of diseases.

DEVELOPMENT OF INFECTIOUS DISEASES

For an infectious disease to develop in a host, the organism must penetrate the skin or mucous membrane barrier, the first line of defense, and survive other natural and adaptive body defense mechanisms (see Chapter 1). These mechanisms include phagocytosis, antibody and cell-mediated immunity or complement activation, and associated interacting effector mechanisms. Phagocytosis and complement activation may be initiated within minutes of the invasion of a microorganism; however, unless primed by previous contact with the same or similar antigen, antibody and cell-mediated responses do not become activated for several days. It also should be noted that complement and antibodies are the most active constituents against microorganisms free in the blood or tissues, but cell-mediated responses are most active against those microorganisms that are cell associated. The most effective mechanism of body defense in a healthy host depends on factors such as an appropriate portal of entry and the characteristics of each individual microorganism. The routes of infection or portals of entry can include transmission through oral routes such as food- or water-borne contamination; maternal-fetal transmission; insect vectors; sexual transmission; parenteral routes such as the injection or transfusion of infected blood; and respiratory transmission. Development of infectious disease, therefore, occurs only if a microorganism can evade, overcome, or inhibit the body defense mechanisms that normally are operational.

IMMUNITY TO INFECTIOUS DISEASES

Bacterial Diseases

The presence of substances such as the natural antibiotic lysozyme and phagocytosis represents major immunologic defense mechanisms against bacteria. A microorganism, however, is able to survive phagocytosis if it possesses a capsule that impedes attachment, a cell wall that interferes with digestion, and/or the release of exotoxins, which damage phagocytic and other cells. Most capsules and toxins are strongly antigenic, but antibodies can overcome many of their effects; this is the basis of the majority of antibacterial vaccines. Examples of representative bacterial diseases of importance in the study of immunology and serology are presented in Chapters 14 through 16.

Parasitic Diseases

Parasites are relatively large, may have resistant body walls, and may avoid being phagocytized because of their ability to migrate away from an inflamed area. These differences set parasitic infections apart from bacterial and viral infections, to which some forms of natural and adaptive immunity afford protection. (Toxoplasmosis, a representative disease, is discussed in Chapter 17.)

Effectors, however, are present against parasitic disease. These immune responses to parasitic infections include immunoglobulins (Igs); complement; antibody-dependent, cell-mediated cytotoxicity; and cellular defenses such as eosinophils and T cells. Some cestodes, especially in their larval stages, may be eradicated by complement-fixing IgG antibodies. In addition, some antibodies may cross-react with other parasitic antigens. Demonstrating the protective effect of IgA has been difficult. Increased levels of IgE may be noted in many helminth infections. Activation of both the classic and alternate complement pathways may take place

in some cases of schistosomiasis, and the alternate pathway of activation may kill larvae in the absence of antibody.

Phagocytosis may have some direct activity against parasitic organisms, but the most effective protection in some parasitic infections is provided by antibody-dependent, cell-mediated cytotoxicity. Macrophages, neutrophils, and eosinophils may demonstrate direct toxicity or phagocytosis toward parasites. The actual attachment of the cytotoxic cells is most frequently mediated by IgG, although IgE may be effective. The role of eosinophils is complex. They may phagocytize immune complexes and act as effector cells in mediating local (type I) reactions, primarily in tissue-stage parasites. T cells are frequently involved in body defenses against parasites. Sequestration of microorganisms is a classic T-cell-dependent hypersensitivity response. In addition, helper T cells may sensitize B cells to specific parasitic antigens.

Other protective nonspecific factors such as nonstimulated monocytes are a major protective mechanism against parasites such as *Giardia* species. Natural killer cells also have a direct activity against cancer cells and some parasites. Delayed hypersensitivity may be helpful in preventing some parasitic infections but may cause disease in other cases. Deposition of antigen-antibody complexes, demonstrated by Raji cell assays, is responsible for severe pathologic lesions in some parasitic infections. In addition, high levels of circulating IgE may cause hypersensitivity reactions in helminth and cestode infections. Anaphylaxis is a clear risk in echinococcal infections, especially with spontaneous or surgical rupture of a hydatid cyst.

Fungal Diseases

Fungal infections are normally superficial, but a few fungi can cause serious systemic disease, usually entering through the respiratory tract in the form of spores. Disease manifestation depends on the degree and type of immune response elicited by the host. Fungi (e.g., *Candida albicans)* are common and harmless inhabitants of skin and mucous membranes under normal conditions. In immunocompromised hosts, however, *Candida* species and other fungi become opportunistic agents that take advantage of the host's weakened resistance. Manifestations of fungal disease may range from unnoticed respiratory episodes to rapid fatal dissemination of a violent hypersensitivity reaction. Survival mechanisms of fungi that successfully invade the body are similar to bacterial characteristics; these include the presence of an antiphagocytic capsule, resistance to digestion within macrophages, and destruction of phagocytes such as neutrophils. Some types of yeast activate complement via the alternative pathway, but it is unknown if this activation has any effect on the microorganism's survival.

Fungal infections are increasing worldwide for a variety of reasons. These include the use of immunosuppressive drugs and the development of diseases such as AIDS that produce a condition of immunocompromise. Serologic tests (Table 13-1) often play an important role in the diagnosis of these fungal or mycotic infections.

Several species of fungi are associated with respiratory diseases in humans. These diseases are acquired by inhaling spores from exogenous reservoirs, including dust, bird droppings, and the soil. This section focuses on a variety of these diseases.

TABLE 13-1	Methods of Testing
Fungus	**Procedural Methods**
Aspergillosis	Immunocap system (solid phase, two site fluorescent enzyme immunoassay with covalently immobilized antigens)
	IgG to *A. fumigatus* ≤110 mg/L—85% of farmers + some persons with no evidence of disease
Histoplasmosis	Complement fixation, immunodiffusion, PCR (sputum, blood, tissue)
	Fungus media nucleic acid probe
Coccidiosis	Complement fixation using coccidioidin (blood and spinal fluid)
Blastomycosis	Complement fixation (<50% positive in proven cases), immunodiffusion
Sporotrichosis	Latex particle agglutination, EIA, IgG, IgM, IgA on cerebrospinal fluid
Cryptococcus	Latex agglutination (serum or cerebrospinal fluid)

EIA, Enzyme immunoassay; *Ig,* Immunoglobulin; *PCR,* polymerase chain reaction.

Histoplasmosis

Histoplasma capsulatum can be found in soil contaminated with chicken, bird, or bat excreta. Inhalation of spore-laden dust is the source of the disease.

Signs and Symptoms. Histoplasmosis can be difficult to diagnose and can range from asymptomatic to chronic pulmonary disease. In addition, a disseminated form manifesting hepatosplenomegaly with diffuse lymphadenopathy is usually present in varying degrees of severity because of the propensity of the fungus to invade the cells of the mononuclear phagocyte system. Disseminated disease is characterized by fever, anemia, leukopenia, weight loss, and lassitude.

Diagnosing Histoplasmosis. Definite diagnosis requires isolation in culture and microscopic identification of the fungus, as well as serologic evidence. If an immunodiffusion technique is used, H and M bands appearing together indicate active infection. If only an M band is present, it indicates early infection, chronic infection, or a recent reactive skin test. An H band appears later than the M band and disappears earlier. Disappearance of an H band suggests regression of the infection.

Delayed hypersensitivity skin testing is confirmed by a rise in complement-fixing antibodies to *Histoplasma* antigens. Titers of 8 and 16 (dilution 1:8, 1:16) are highly suggestive of infection. A titer of 32 or greater usually indicates active infection. A rising titer indicates progressive infection; a decreasing titer suggests regression. Some disseminated infections are nonreactive in complement fixation tests. In addition, recent skin tests in individuals who have prior exposure to *H. capsulatum* will produce a rise in the complement-fixation titer in 17% to 20% of patients. Cross-reactions in the complement fixation test occur in patients having aspergillosis, blastomycosis, and coccidioidomycosis, but the titers are

usually lower. Several follow-up serum samples should be tested at 2- to 3-week intervals.

Aspergillosis

Another opportunistic mycotic infection that can occur in humans is aspergillosis.

Signs and Symptoms. Aspergillosis can be allergic, invasive, or disseminating, depending on pathologic findings in the host. It is usually secondary to another disease. Allergic bronchopulmonary aspergillosis is characterized by allergic reactions to the toxins and endotoxins of the *Aspergillus* species.

Laboratory Methods for Diagnosing Aspergillosis. Species identification of aspergillosis can be made microscopically. Serologically, skin reactions and immunodiffusion are useful tools for identification, especially if the culture is negative.

Immunodiffusion antibody test with reference antisera and known antigen is a frequently used test for the identification of *Aspergillus* species in nearly all clinical types of aspergillosis. Precipitin formation by immunodiffusion is useful in identifying patients with pulmonary eosinophilia, severe allergic aspergillosis, and aspergillomas. The presence of one or more precipitin bands is suggestive of active infection. The precipitin bands correlate with complement-fixation titers. In this test the greater the number of bands, the higher the titer. In addition, the enzyme immunoassay can be used to detect IgE and IgG antibodies.

Hypersensitivity testing is characterized by both immediate and delayed-type hypersensitivity reactions, as a result of the presence of *Aspergillus*-specific Ig. IgE titers are greatly increased in allergic bronchopulmonary aspergillosis.

Coccidioidomycosis

Coccidioidomycosis is also known as desert fever, San Joaquin fever, or valley fever. The disease may assume several forms, including primary pulmonary, primary cutaneous, or a disseminated form.

Contracting Coccidioidomycosis. The disease is contracted from inhalation of soil or dust containing the arthrospores of *Coccidioides immitis.*

Skin Testing in the Diagnosis of Coccidioidomycosis. Hypersensitivity testing using intradermal injections of coccidioidin or spherulin are useful in screening for *C. immitis.* It is usually the first immunologic test to be positive in both asymptomatic and symptomatic cases. Skin testing does not differentiate between recent or past exposures to *C. immitis.* A positive skin test should be followed by other serodiagnostic tests. A negative test in a previously positive person can indicate a disseminated infection and a state of anergy.

Laboratory Methods of Diagnosis. The fluorescent antibody test can be applied directly to clinical specimens. This procedure is invaluable for making a rapid and specific identification of fungal structures. In addition to culturing the organism, a variety of serologic tests can be used to confirm the diagnosis of coccidioidomycosis. These procedures include the tube precipitin test, immunodiffusion, complement fixation, and latex agglutination. The complement fixation test is the most widely used quantitative serodiagnostic test to identify infection with *C. immitis.* It is very effective in detecting disseminated disease. The tube precipitin test is positive in more than 90% of primary symptomatic cases.

Immunodiffusion is equivalent to complement fixation; it can be used as a screening test, but the results should be confirmed by complement fixation. Latex agglutination is not usually a recommended method because it lacks specificity. This creates many false-positive results.

Antibody Development in Coccidioidomycosis. Two antigens have been developed for the serologic identification of circulating antibodies to *C. immitis*. IgM appears in 1 to 3 weeks after infection in 90% of symptomatic patients. IgG develops in 3 to 6 months after the onset of symptoms. Titers of 1:2 to 1:4 are presumptive evidence of an early infection and should be repeated in 3 to 4 weeks. Titers of 1:8 to 1:16 are evidence of active infection, particularly when accompanied by a positive immunodiffusion test. Titers greater than 1:16 occur in 90% to 95% of patients with disseminated coccidioidomycosis.

Other Mycotic Diseases

North American Blastomycosis. This is a chronic fungal disease usually secondary to pulmonary involvement. Blastomyces dermatitidis causes tumors in the skin or lesions in the lungs, bones, subcutaneous tissues, liver, spleen, and kidneys.

Laboratory Methods for Diagnosing Blastomycosis. Serologic diagnosis is problematic because of high cross-reactivity with antigenic components of the organism. Although both immunodiffusion and complement fixation methods are used, immunodiffusion is considered the better of the two. Complement fixation titers of 8 and 16 are highly suggestive of active infection, and titers of 32 and greater are diagnostic. A decreasing titer is indicative of regression; however, most patients with blastomycosis have negative complement fixation tests.

Sporotrichosis. This is a chronic, progressive, subcutaneous lymphatic mycosis. It is caused by *Sporothrix schenckii*. The disease takes three forms: lymphatic (which is the most common), disseminated, and respiratory. It is characterized by a sporotrichotic chancre at the site of inoculation, followed by the development and formation of subcutaneous nodules along the lymphatics, draining the primary lesions. Infection is associated with injuries caused by thorns or splinters. Handlers of peat moss are particularly susceptible to the disease, especially when working in rose gardens.

Laboratory Methods for Diagnosing Sporotrichosis. Laboratory methods of identification include cultures, serologic techniques, and fluorescent antibody-staining technique. Two of the most sensitive tests are yeast cell and latex particle agglutination test. Titers of 80 or more usually indicate active infection.

Skin testing is also available. Patients with cutaneous infection usually demonstrate negative tests; patients with extracutaneous infections present positive tests.

Cryptococcosis. *Cryptococcus neoformans* is the etiologic agent of this disease. Infected pigeons are the chief vector. The disease is acquired by inhaling yeast. It may initially be asymptomatic or may develop as a symptomatic pulmonary infection. Any organ or tissue of the body may be infected, but localization outside the lungs or brain is relatively uncommon. The disease can be serious in immunocompromised or debilitated patients.

Laboratory Methods for Diagnosing Cryptococcosis. Antigen tests take less time to perform and are more specific than antibody detection. Latex agglutination antigen tests can be performed on serum or spinal fluid. Titers of 1:2 suggest infection, although such findings have been found in individuals with no evidence of cryptococcosis. Titers of 1:4 or greater are evidence of an active infection. Higher titers also indicate more severe infections. Positive titers are found in cerebrospinal fluid in 95% of cases with involvement of the central nervous system.

The indirect fluorescent antibody test detects antibodies to *C. neoformans*. It is most valuable when antigen tests are negative and can even be combined with an antigen test to determine a patient's prognosis. A positive test suggests a present or recent infection.

Complement fixation is the most specific antibody detection test, but it is very insensitive. Tube agglutination test, using serum or spinal fluid that demonstrates a titer of 1:2 or greater, is suggestive of a current or recent infection with *C. neoformans*.

As the disease progresses, antigens begin to appear, along with a decrease in antibody production. After treatment, a decrease in antigen titer and the reappearance of antibodies indicates a good prognosis.

Viral, Rickettsial, and Mycoplasmal Diseases

The characteristic process associated with viral infections is cellular replication, which may or may not lead to cell death. Interferon plays a major role in body defenses against viral infections. Antibodies are valuable in preventing entry and blood-borne spread of some viruses, but the ability of other viruses to spread from cell to cell places the burden of adaptive immunity on the T-cell system, which specializes in recognizing altered "self" histocompatibility (histocompatibility leukocyte antigen) antigens. Macrophages may also play a role in immunity. Some of the most virulent viruses to humans are zoonoses (e.g., rabies). Other viruses, however, can persist for years without symptoms and then be reactivated to cause serious disease, possibly including tumors.

In this decade we are recognizing that new viruses can cause old diseases and, conversely, old viruses can cause new diseases (see Chapters 18 to 22 for representative examples of immunologically important viral diseases). The mutation rates of viruses, especially the RNA viruses such as HIV, are extraordinarily high. Consequently, RNA viruses evolve far more rapidly under selective conditions than their hosts, and it is speculated that contemporary RNA viruses may have descended from a common ancestor only relatively recently. The survival of influenza A and B viruses as new viruses seems to depend on a continual evolution of mutants able to escape patient immunity as a result of preceding viruses. The most frequent cause of "new" viral infections is old viruses that are not natural infections of humans but are accidentally transmitted from other species as zoonoses.

Organisms intermediate between viruses and bacteria are those obligatory intracellular organisms with cell walls (Rickettsiae) and those without cell walls but capable of extracellular replication (*Mycoplasma*). Immunologically, the former are closer to viruses, the latter to bacteria.

Herpesviruses

Two of the members of the human herpesviruses, cytomegalovirus (CMV) and Epstein-Barr virus, are described in detail in Chapters 18 and 19. The other members of the human herpesvirus family—herpes simplex type 1, herpes simplex type 2, varicella zoster, and human herpesvirus-6—are briefly presented here.

The Herpesviruses. All of the human herpesviruses are large, enveloped DNA viruses that replicate within the cell's nucleus. The virus gains an envelope when the virus buds through the nuclear membrane, which has been altered to contain specific viral proteins.

The viruses of the herpes family produce a number of clinical diseases, although they share the basic characteristic of being cell-associated, which may, in part, account for their ability to produce subclinical infections that can be reactivated under appropriate stimuli.

The Epidemiology of Herpes Simplex Virus (HSV). HSV can be cultured from the oropharynx in about 1% of healthy adults and from the genital tract of slightly less than 1% of asymptomatic adult women who are not pregnant.

HSV is widespread. Humans are the only natural hosts or known reservoir of infection for the human herpesviruses. The incubation period is 2 to 12 days. Incidence of seropositivity rises to almost 100% in some populations by age 45 years. Antibody prevalence in adults varies greatly with socioeconomic class (30% to 50% of upper socioeconomic class adults have detectable antibody to HSV, as compared with 80% to 100% of adults in lower socioeconomic groups).

Manifestations of HSV Infection. The most usual manifestation of HSV infection is the common cold sore or fever blister. HSV has been shown to be related to a wide variety of clinical syndromes, as well as to subclinical infection, occurring with either primary or recurrent disease. Recurrent HSV disease usually occurs as a result of reactivation of latent virus resting in paraspinal or cranial nerve ganglia that innervate the site of primary infection. Distant sites may be involved. Activated virus presumably travels down the axon to the skin (or other site) and induces disease. In some cases, exogenous reinfection can occur. Recurrence with cell-to-cell spread of virus occurs in the presence of serum-neutralizing antibodies.

Two cross-reacting antigen types of HSV have been identified, known as herpes simplex type 1 (HSV-1) and herpes simplex type 2 (HSV-2). HSV-1 is generally found in and around the oral cavity and in skin lesions that occur above the waist. HSV-2 is isolated primarily to the genital tract and skin lesions below the waist.

Characteristics of Neonatal and Congenital Infection. Malnutrition, severe illness, many kinds of acute childhood illnesses, and prematurity predispose infants and young children to disseminated primary infection. Neonatal HSV infections may be acquired in the antenatal or perinatal period. Active lesions in the mother's genital tract at the time of birth present the greatest risk of infection to the newborn. The spectrum of disease occurring in an infected newborn varies from subclinical to severe. In cases of overwhelming generalized infection, the infant may develop encephalitis and respiratory failure, or hepatic failure with increasing jaundice and adrenal insufficiency may occur. Infants who survive severe infection are frequently left with some neurologic damage and may have recurrent vesicular skin lesions for many years.

Laboratory Detection of HSV Infection. Several methods for the laboratory diagnosis of HSV are available, including isolation of the virus and the direct detection of antigen in tissues or cytologic preparation through the use of immunofluorescence or immunoenzyme methods. In addition, detection of the virus in body fluids (using monoclonal antibodies) can be performed using immunoassays or immunoblot techniques. Serologic diagnosis of primary infections can be demonstrated when a fourfold or greater rise in titer occurs. Titers may rise significantly in early recurrent infection but usually become stable at moderately high levels after multiple recurrences.

Varicella-Zoster Virus

Varicella-zoster (V-Z) virus is the cause of two different types of clinical diseases resulting from the same virus infection. Primary infection with the virus results in the clinical manifestations of chickenpox. After a primary infection, the virus enters a latent phase, presumably within nuclei in the dorsal root ganglia. Reactivation of the virus results in the clinical manifestation characteristic of (zoster) shingles.

Epidemiology of V-Z. Humans are the only natural hosts of the V-Z virus. Varicella primarily affects children between 2 and 5 years old. The virus is endemic and highly contagious. Periodic epidemics do occur. It is presumed that the mode of transmission is by the respiratory tract.

Zoster is less communicable than varicella. This sporadic disease occurs most frequently in middle-age persons. Antibodies to varicella do not protect against reactivation and/or clinical zoster. The reactivation of V-Z virus is associated with a depressed host immune response. Patients with AIDS, older adults, and immunocompromised persons are at high risk of developing disease. In addition, manipulation of the spinal cord, local radiation therapy, or therapy that suppresses cellular immunity have all been associated with triggering the onset of zoster.

Disease Development of V-Z. Varicella has an incubation period of 14 to 17 days. There may be a 1- to 3-day prodromal period of fever, headache, and malaise. This precedes the eruption of the characteristic red macular rash, which progresses to papules, vesicles, and pustules that crust over and shed without scarring. Successive crops of lesions continue to appear for 2 to 6 days; therefore multiple lesions in various stages of development are present at any one time.

Diseases Caused by V-Z Virus. The name of the virus reflects two associated diseases: varicella (chickenpox) and zoster (shingles). Primary infection with the virus results in the clinical manifestation of chickenpox. After this, the virus enters a latent phase, presumably within nuclei of neutrons in dorsal root ganglia or cranial nerve sensory ganglia. The reactivity of the virus results in the clinical manifestations characteristic of zoster.

Complications of V-Z virus can include pneumonitis, encephalitic complications, nephritis, hepatitis, myocarditis, arthritis, and Reye syndrome. Susceptible individuals who are immunosuppressed have a greater risk of complications after V-Z virus exposure. Another complication can include febrile purpura, which can occur a few days after the onset of the rash and is seen in both children and adults. This complication is characterized by thrombocytopenia and hemorrhage into the vesicles. Postinfection purpura, which begins 1 to 2 weeks after the appearance of the rash, is characterized by thrombocytopenia with gastrointestinal, genitourinary, cutaneous, and mucous membrane hemorrhage. More severe hemorrhagic complications include malignant varicella with purpura and purpura fulminants.

Signs and Symptoms of Zoster Infection. Zoster infection is characterized by neuralgia lasting from a few days to weeks, followed by the characteristic eruption typically confined to one or two adjacent dermatomes. The distribution of zoster occasionally involves multiple dermatomes. Persistent neuralgia in older patients can be severe and last several months to a year.

Neonatal Varicella Infection. Neonatal varicella may be acquired in utero or in the perinatal period. This can result in congenital abnormalities in the infant. The infant is at greatest risk if the mother's illness occurs 4 days or less before delivery.

Laboratory Diagnosis of V-Z Infection. Laboratory diagnosis is similar to HSV methods. Serologic methods that can be used include indirect immunofluorescence, which detects antibodies to specific membrane antigens, or enzyme immunoassay. Complement fixation may be useful in confirming recent infection, but it is relatively insensitive.

Rapid preliminary diagnosis can also be made by direct immunofluorescence to detect viral antigens in vesicular lesions. A Tzanck smear of cells taken from lesions enables direct examination. A presumptive diagnosis can be made by examining scrapings from the base of a vesicular lesion and histologically observing multinucleated giant cells containing intranuclear inclusion, or observing virus particles by electron microscopy. The best way to confirm infection is to recover the virus in human diploid fibroblast cell cultures.

Antibodies to varicella are detectable within several days of the onset of rash and peak at 2 to 3 weeks. Antibodies to zoster increase more rapidly and are detectable at the onset of clinical symptoms. Because of the rapid turnaround time and correlation with clinical symptoms, serologic methods are preferable to viral isolation methods. In addition, enzyme-linked immunosorbent assay (ELISA) methods are valuable for assessing the immune status of adults.

Human Herpesvirus-6

A "new" virus classified as a herpesvirus because of its shape, size, and in vitro behavior has been recently identified. Genomic analysis shows the virus to be molecularly unrelated to other human herpesviruses. Initially the virus was called B-lymphotropic virus, but subsequent studies indicated that T cells are the primary target of infection. This viral agent is currently classified as human herpesvirus-6 (HHV-6).

Signs and Symptoms of HHV-6 Infection. Patients with serologic evidence of acute HHV-6 infection are reported to experience mild, nonspecific symptoms and cervical lymphadenopathy. The same agent has been implicated as the cause of roseola infantum. Up to 75% of infants develop antibody to HHV-6 by 10 to 11 months old, which suggests a high rate of seropositivity in the general population.

Laboratory Diagnosis of HHV-6 Infection. Laboratory methods include direct examination by immunofluorescence or immunoperoxidase staining of cells taken from lesions. In addition, polymerase chain reaction, DNA probes, and serologic methods (e.g., ELISA, radioimmunoassay, indirect immunofluorescence, and latex agglutination) can be used.

Culture methods include the cocultivation of the patient's peripheral blood cells with cord blood mononuclear cells and examination of these cultures after 5 to 10 days by electron

TABLE 13-2	TORCH Antibodies IgM
Infectious Agent	**Interpretation of Assay**
Cytomegalovirus antibody, IgM	Positive—IgM antibody to CMV detected, which may indicate a current or recent infection.
Herpes simplex virus type 1 and/or 2 antibodies, IgM by ELISA	>1.09 IV: Positive—IgM antibody to HSV detected, which may indicate a current or recent infection.
Rubella antibody, IgM	Positive—IgM antibody to rubella detected, which may indicate a current or recent infection or immunization.
Toxoplasma gondii antibody, IgM	Positive—Significant level of antibody detected and may indicate a current or recent infection.

Modified from Associated Regional and University Pathologists, Inc ARUP Test Reference Guide, 2002, website: www.arup-lab.com.

TORCH, Toxoplasma, other [virus], rubella, CMV, and herpes; *Ig,* immunoglobulin; *ELISA,* enzyme-linked immunosorbent assay.

microscopy and anticomplement immunofluorescence. Anticomplement immunofluorescence of infected cell culture has also been used for antibody detection and titration.

LABORATORY DETECTION OF IMMUNOLOGIC RESPONSES

Because IgM is usually produced in significant quantities during the first exposure of a patient to an infectious agent, the detection of specific IgM can be of diagnostic significance. This immunologic characteristic is particularly important in diseases that do not manifest decisive clinical signs and symptoms (e.g., toxoplasmosis) or under those conditions in which a rapid therapeutic decision may be required (e.g., rubella). Procedures that specifically evaluate the presence of IgM or IgG are frequently used to detect CMV, herpesviruses (type 1 and/or 2), *Toxoplasma gondii,* and rubella. The names of the tests have been grouped under the acronym TORCH (toxoplasma, other [virus], rubella, CMV, and herpes) (Tables 13-2 and 13-3).

In many diseases there exists a spectrum of responses from infected individuals. Some patients may develop and manifest antibodies from a subclinical infection or after colonization of an agent without actually developing disease. In these cases the presence of antibody in a single serum specimen or a comparative titer of antibody in paired specimens may merely indicate past contact with the agent; the presence of antibodies cannot be used to accurately diagnose a recent disease. In comparison, some patients may respond to an antigenic stimulus by producing antibodies that can cross-react with other antigens. These antibodies are nonspecific and may lead to misinterpretation of serologic tests.

In most cases a serologic procedure for the diagnosis of recent infection using acute and convalescent specimens is

TABLE 13-3   TORCH Antibodies IgG

Infectious Agent	Interpretation of Assay
Cytomegalovirus antibody, IgG	Positive: IgG antibody to CMV detected which may indicate a current or previous CMV infection.
Herpes simplex virus type 1 and/or 2 antibodies, IgG by ELISA	Positive: IgG antibody to HSV detected which may indicate a current or previous HSV infection.
Rubella antibody, IgG	Positive: IgG antibody to rubella detected which may indicate a current or previous exposure/immunization to rubella.
Toxoplasma gondii antibody, IgG	6-200 IU/mL: Significant level of antibody present. Results indicate long-standing immunity or early phase of seroconversion. >200 IU/mL: High level of antibody present. Results indicate recent seroconversion or demonstrate a persistent high level of immunity.

Modified from Associated Regional and University Pathologists, Inc ARUP Test Reference Guide, © 2002, website: www.arup-lab.com.
CMV, Cytomegalovirus, *ELISA,* enzyme-linked immunosorbent assay; *HSV,* herpes simplex virus; *Ig,* immunoglobulin; *TORCH, Toxoplasma,* other [virus], rubella, CMV, and herpes.

the method of choice. Except for the detection of IgM or in diseases in which no chance of developing an immune response exists, such as rabies virus or the toxin of botulism, the testing of a single specimen is not usually recommended. In a number of circumstances, however, when only one specimen is tested to determine immune status, antibody to past infection or to immunization can be determined.

Throughout this section, various testing protocols are described for the immunologic detection of representative infectious diseases. These protocols are examples of the types of procedures commonly encountered in the serology/immunology laboratory.

CHAPTER HIGHLIGHTS

The acquisition of an infectious disease is influenced by factors related to both the microorganism and the host. These factors can influence the exposure to and actual development of an infectious disease.

For an infectious disease to develop in a host, the organism must penetrate the skin or mucous membrane barrier and survive other natural and adaptive body defense mechanisms. Phagocytosis and complement activation may be initiated

within minutes of the invasion of a microorganism; however, unless primed by previous contact with the same or a similar antigen, antibody and cell-mediated responses do not become activated for several days. Development of infectious disease, therefore, occurs only if a microorganism can evade, overcome, or inhibit the body defense mechanisms that are normally operational.

The mechanism of body defense most effective in a healthy host depends on the type of microorganism. Defenses such as phagocytosis are highly effective in bacterial immunity but are relatively ineffective in the prevention of parasitic disease. T cells, however, are frequently involved in body defenses against parasites. Sequestration of microorganisms is a classic T-cell-dependent hypersensitivity response.

Because IgM is usually produced in significant quantities during the first exposure of a patient to an infectious agent, the detection of specific IgM can be of diagnostic significance and is a frequently used serologic method in the detection of infectious disease. Procedures that specifically evaluate the presence of IgM are frequently used to detect CMV, herpesviruses, *Toxoplasma gondii,* or rubella. The names of the tests for these agents have been grouped under the acronym TORCH (toxoplasma, other [viruses], rubella, CMV, and herpes). In most cases a serologic procedure for the diagnosis of recent infection using acute and convalescent specimens is the method of choice. The testing of a single specimen is not usually recommended.

REVIEW QUESTIONS

1. Factors that influence the development of an infectious disease include all of the following except the:
   A. immune status of the individual
   B. incidence of an organism in the population
   C. pathogenicity of the agent
   D. sole presence of the agent or microorganism

Questions 2-5. Match the appropriate immunologic defense mechanism with the class of microorganism.

2. _____ bacteria

3. _____ yeast

4. _____ viruses

5. _____ parasites

   A. interferon
   B. lysozymes and phagocytosis
   C. immunoglobulins, complement, antibody-dependent, cell-mediated cytotoxicity, and cellular defenses
   D. possibly the activation of complement

6. The detection of _____ can be of diagnostic significance during the first exposure of a patient to an infectious agent.
   A. IgM
   B. IgG
   C. IgA
   D. IgD

7. Serologic procedures for the diagnosis of recent infection should include:
   A. only an acute specimen
   B. only a convalescent specimen
   C. an acute and convalescent specimen
   D. an acute, convalescent, and 6-month postinfection specimen

8. Important among the factors affecting microbial disease development is/are:
   A. the ability of some microorganisms to multiply in an intracellular habitat
   B. the display of antigen variation
   C. the presence of a related microorganism
   D. both A and B

9. For an infectious disease to develop in a host, the organism must initially:
   A. survive phagocytosis
   B. be in the log phase of multiplication
   C. penetrate the skin or mucous membrane barrier
   D. be present in the host for 7 to 10 days

Questions 10-12. Match each type of infectious disease to the appropriate description below.

10. _____ bacterial disease
11. _____ viral disease
12. _____ parasitic disease

A. affected by such immune responses as immunoglobulin; complement; and antibody-dependent, cell-mediated cytotoxicity
B. inhibited by antibiotics, lysozymes, and phagocytosis
C. stimulates production of, and is in turn inhibited by, interferon

13. The first type of antibody that may be apparent in the immune response to an infectious disease is:
   A. IgM
   B. IgG
   C. IgD
   D. IgA

14. A distinguishing characteristic of the herpesviruses is that they are:
   A. cell-associated
   B. enveloped RNA
   C. humans are the only known reservoir of infection
   D. both A and C

15. Up to _____ % of infants develop antibody to HHV-6 by 10 to 11 months of age.
   A. 25
   B. 50
   C. 75
   D. 95

16. Varicella-zoster virus causes:
   A. chickenpox
   B. shingles
   C. measles
   D. both A and B

17. Varicella-zoster virus can be reactivated in patients with:
   A. AIDS
   B. elderly persons
   C. immunocompromised persons
   D. all of the above

18. Rapid preliminary diagnosis of varicella-zoster can be made in the laboratory by:
   A. direct immunofluorescence
   B. viral isolation
   C. ELISA method
   D. complement fixation

19. Histoplasmosis is caused by:
   A. a bacteria
   B. a parasite
   C. a fungus
   D. a virus

20. Aspergillosis is:
   A. an opportunistic organism
   B. caused by a parasite
   C. a cause of skin infections
   D. a relatively mild disease

21. The first test to be positive in coccidiomycosis is:
   A. fluorescent antibody
   B. hypersensitivity testing
   C. complement fixation
   D. culture of the organism

Questions 22-24. Match the following, using each answer only once.

22. _____ blastomycosis
23. _____ sporotrichosis
24. _____ cryptococcosis

A. subcutaneous lymphatic mycosis
B. vector in infected pigeons
C. chronic fungal disease

BIBLIOGRAPHY

Davidson RA: Immunology of parasitic infections, *Med Clin North Am* 69(4):751-757, 1985.

Forbes BA, Sahm DF, Weissfeld AS: *Bailey and Scott's diagnostic microbiology,* ed 11, St Louis, 2002, Mosby.

Kilbourne ED: New viral diseases, *JAMA* 264(1):68-70, 1990.

Pastuszak AL et al: Outcome after maternal varicella infection in the first 20 weeks of pregnancy, *N Engl J Med* 330(13):901-906, 1994.

Playfair JHL: *Immunology at a glance,* Oxford, 1979, Blackwell Scientific Publications.

Turgeon ML: Bloodborne infectious diseases. In Turgeon ML, editor: *Fundamentals of immunohematology,* ed 2, Baltimore, 1996, Williams & Wilkins.

Chapter 14

Streptococcal Infections

LEARNING OBJECTIVES

At the conclusion of this chapter, the reader should be able to:
- Describe the etiology, epidemiology, signs and symptoms, and complications of streptococcal infection.
- Discuss the immunologic manifestations and diagnostic evaluation of streptococcal infection.

- Explain the principle of the rapid latex agglutination antistreptolysin-O procedures.
- Analyze and apply laboratory data to a case study.

ETIOLOGY

Most streptococci that contain cell wall antigens of Lancefield group A are known as (*Streptococcus pyogenes*). Members of this species are almost always beta-hemolytic. *S. pyogenes* is the most common causative agent of pharyngitis and its resultant disorder, scarlet fever, and the skin infection, impetigo. In terms of human morbidity and mortality worldwide, however, the role of *S. pyogenes* in the subsequent development of complications such as acute rheumatic fever and poststreptococcal glomerulonephritis is more important. Other *S. pyogenes*–associated infections include otitis media in children, sinusitis in adults, and osteomyelitis, septic arthritis, neonatal septicemia, and rare cases of pneumonia. Particularly virulent serotypes of given bacterial strains produce proteolytic enzymes that cause

necrotizing fasciitis in a wound or lesion on an extremity. A more pathogenic response to these infections is rapid progression to toxic shock or sepsis.

Morphologic Characteristics

S. pyogenes is a gram-positive cocci and the serotype most frequently associated with human infection. Lancefield divided these beta-hemolytic streptococci into serogroups A through O on the basis of the immunologic action of the cell wall carbohydrate (Figure 14-1). Structures called fimbriae arise near the plasma membrane and project through the cell wall and capsule. These processes contain important surface components of the streptococcus. Lipoteichoic acid found on the fimbriae is important in the adherence

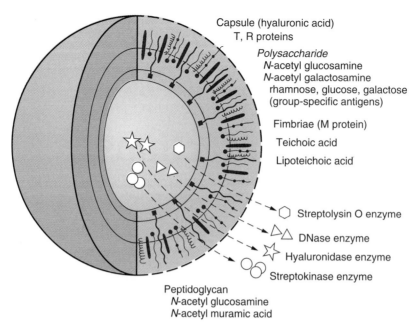

Capsule (hyaluronic acid)
T, R proteins

Polysaccharide
N-acetyl glucosamine
N-acetyl galactosamine
rhamnose, glucose, galactose
(group-specific antigens)

Fimbriae (M protein)

Teichoic acid

Lipoteichoic acid

Streptolysin O enzyme

DNase enzyme

Hyaluronidase enzyme

Streptokinase enzyme

Peptidoglycan
N-acetyl glucosamine
N-acetyl muramic acid

Cytoplasmic membrane

Figure 14-1 *Streptococcus pyogenes* contains many antigenic structural components and produces several antigenic enzymes, each of which may elicit a specific antibody response from the infected host. (Redrawn from Forbes BA, Sahm DF, Weissfeld AS: *Bailey and Scott's diagnostic microbiology,* ed 11, St Louis, 2002, Mosby.)

of the organism to human epithelium and the initiation of infection. The M and R antigens, which are structurally similar but immunologically distinct, are also found on the fimbriae. R antigen has no known biologic role. M protein, a cell protein found in association with the hyaluronic capsule, is a major virulence factor of *S. pyogenes*. Strains of *S. pyogenes* that lack M protein cannot cause infection. M protein inhibits phagocytosis, and antibody synthesized against M protein provides type-specific immunity to group A streptococci. In addition, M protein is the basis for a subclassification of group A streptococci into more than 60 M serotypes.

Extracellular Products

Extracellular products are important in the pathogenesis of disease and in the serologic diagnosis of streptococcal disease. Antibodies produced in response to these substances provide evidence of recent streptococcal infection. Two hemolysins (which have the ability to damage human and animal erythrocytes), polymorphonuclear leukocytes and platelets, are produced by most group A strains. Streptolysin O, an oxygen-labile enzyme, binds to sterols in the red cell membrane, causing stearic rearrangement. This rearrangement produces submicroscopic holes in the red cell membrane, and hemoglobin diffuses from the cells. Streptolysin O is antigenic; the antibody response to it is the most commonly used serologic indicator of recent streptococcal infection. The other hemolysin, streptolysin S, an oxygen-stable enzyme, is responsible for the beta (clear-appearing)-hemolysis on the surface of a blood agar culture plate. Streptolysin S disrupts the selective permeability of the red cell membrane, causing osmotic lysis. It is not antigenic.

Other substances produced by group A streptococci presumably facilitate rapid spread through subcutaneous or deeper soft tissues. These include:

- Hyaluronidase, also called spreading factor, which breaks down hyaluronic acid found in the host's connective tissue
- Four immunologically distinct DNases (A, B, C, D), which degrade deoxyribonucleic acid
- Streptokinase, an enzyme that dissolves clots by converting plasminogen to plasmin
- Other extracellular products that can elicit an antibody response, such as NADase, proteinase, esterase, and amylase
- Erythrogenic toxi, elaborated by scarlet fever-associated strains; it is responsible for the characteristic rash

EPIDEMIOLOGY

S. pyogenes is one of the most common and ubiquitous of human pathogens. It is found in the respiratory tract of humans and is always considered a potential pathogen. Upper respiratory infections caused by *S. pyogenes* occur most frequently in school-age children and are uncommon in children less than 3 years old. No sexual or racial predilection has been described.

Infection is spread by contact with large droplets produced in the upper respiratory tract. Although not as common, food-borne and milk-borne epidemics do occur. Crowding enhances the spread of microorganisms.

A number of individuals, particularly school-age children, carry *S. pyogenes* without signs of illness. Carriers have positive cultures without serologic evidence of infection. If a person carries the organisms in the pharynx for prolonged periods after untreated infection, the number of organisms carried and their ability to produce M protein decline during carriage. This results in a progressive decline in the likelihood of spreading infection to others.

The incidence of the complication of *S. pyogenes,* rheumatic fever, has decreased in the United States. It occurs primarily in the rural South and in areas of crowding and lower socioeconomic status. The incidence of rheumatic fever is 2% to 3% in epidemics and 0.1% to 1% after sporadic cases of streptococcal infection. The probability of developing rheumatic fever is age related, with younger patients more likely to develop carditis than older ones. Rheumatic fever and resultant valvular heart disease, however, are syndromes of major importance among children in developing nations. Patients with a history of rheumatic heart disease resulting from rheumatic fever are at a significantly increased risk of developing cardiac malfunction and endocarditis at a later time. The risk of recurrent rheumatic fever depends on factors such as the age of the patient at the time of previous recurrences, the length of time since the last recurrence, and the presence of carditis. In addition, patients who develop streptococcal glomerulonephritis are at risk of later developing renal failure.

SIGNS AND SYMPTOMS

S. pyogenes causes a wide variety of infections, the most frequent of which are acute pharyngitis (strep throat) and upper respiratory infection, and impetigo (pyoderma). Other manifestations of infection with *S. pyogenes* include sinusitis, otitis, peritonsillar and retropharyngeal abscess, pneumonia, scarlet fever, erysipelas, cellulitis, puerperal sepsis, and gangrene. There is concern that group A streptococcus may be acquiring greater virulence.

Upper Respiratory Infection

The clinical manifestations of *S. pyogenes*–associated upper respiratory infection are age-dependent. If the patient is an infant or young child, the infection is characterized by an insidious onset of rhinorrhea, coughing, fever, vomiting, and anorexia. Cervical adenopathy may also be present. Rhinorrhea is sometimes purulent. This syndrome is called streptococcosis.

The classic syndrome of streptococcal pharyngitis is seen in children over 3 years old. It begins with a sudden onset of sore throat and fever, which rapidly progress in severity. Pharyngeal erythema with purulent tonsillar exudate and petechiae may be observed on the palate, posterior pharynx, and tonsils. Younger children may have abdominal pain, nausea, and vomiting. Most cases, however, do not manifest the classic syndrome. It is more common for a child with *S. pyogenes* pharyngitis to have a fever, mild sore throat, and pharyngeal erythema without exudate. Viral pharyngitis can produce many of the same symptoms and cannot be reliably differentiated from streptococcal pharyngitis on the basis of clinical examination.

Impetigo and Cellulitis

Impetigo is a skin infection that begins as a papule (Figures 14-2 and 14-3). The lesion may itch and will eventually crust over and heal. Cellulitis caused by subcutaneous infection with group A streptococci is associated with a warm, red, tender area

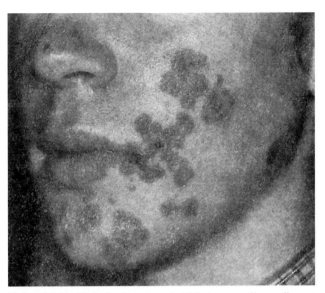

Figure 14-2   Vesicular impetigo. A thick, honey-yellow, adherent crust covers the entire eroded surface. (From Habif TP: *Clinical dermatology: a color guide to diagnosis and therapy,* St Louis, 1985, Mosby.)

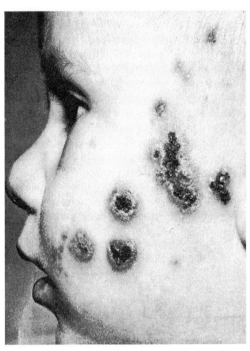

Figure 14-3   Impetigo. Older lesions are dark and encrusted. (From Wehrle PF, Top FH: *Communicable and infectious diseases,* ed 9, St Louis, 1981, Mosby.)

that may be mildly swollen. Erysipelas, a distinct cellulitis syndrome, usually involves the face and may be associated with pharyngitis. This syndrome is characterized by toxicity and a high fever. If left untreated, erysipelas can be fatal.

Scarlet Fever

Scarlet fever is the result of pharyngeal infection with a strain of group A streptococcus that produces erythrogenic toxin and is responsible for the characteristic rash. The signs and symptoms of scarlet fever are those of streptococcal pharyngitis with the addition of a rash. The rash usually develops on the second day of illness and results in hyperkeratosis with subsequent peeling similar to the rash of toxic shock syndrome. About 1 week after the onset of illness, the skin of the face begins to peel; peeling progresses over the next 2 weeks. Exposure to erythrogenic toxin confers specific immunity, which limits to three the number of episodes of scarlet fever in a person.

Complications of *S. pyogenes* Infection

Not all infections with *S. pyogenes* lead to complications. Acute rheumatic fever, for example, occurs only after upper respiratory tract infection. In contrast, glomerulonephritis occurs after pharyngitis or skin infections (pyoderma). Acute rheumatic fever and poststreptococcal glomerulonephritis are considered nonsuppurative because the organs themselves are not directly infected and a purulent inflammatory response is not present in affected organs such as the heart, joints, blood, and kidneys. The pathogenesis of the disease process has not been fully described, but an autoimmune phenomenon may be operational. It is believed that cross-reactive antibodies, originally directed against streptococcal cell membranes, bind to myosin in human heart muscle cells. It is further believed that other cross-reactive antibodies bind to components of the glomerular basement membrane and form immune complexes at the affected site. These antigen-antibody complexes attract reactive host cells and enzymes that ultimately cause the cellular damage.

All M serotypes that infect the throat appear to be capable of causing rheumatic fever. Researchers have identified a few serotypes, however, that cause a much lower proportion of cases of rheumatic fever than would be expected from their frequency as a cause of pharyngitis. The incidence of rheumatic fever is directly proportional to the strength of the antibody response to streptolysin O (SLO). Prognosis of rheumatic fever is good when carditis is absent during the initial infection.

Glomerulonephritis may follow an infection of the skin or respiratory tract with one of a limited number of nephritogenic M serotypes. These serotypes are defined by antisera against a protein component of the cell wall, the M protein, which is also associated with virulence. Why these serotypes cause glomerulonephritis is unknown.

IMMUNOLOGIC MANIFESTATIONS

S. pyogenes is an example of a pathogen that induces production of several different antibodies. This coccus contains antigenic structural components and produces antigenic enzymes, each of which may elicit a specific antibody response from the infected host. In the course of an infection, the extracellular products act as antigens to which the body responds by producing specific antibodies (indications of infection). The majority of infected patients will demonstrate an increase in the concentration of antibody against SLO. The concentration of antibody (titer) begins to rise about 7 days after the onset of infection and reaches a maximum after 4 to 6 weeks. A rise in titer of 50 Todd units in a 1- to 2-week period is of greater diagnostic significance than a single titer. An elevated titer is indicative of a relatively recent infection. Peak titers are seen at the time of acute polyarthritis of acute rheumatic fever, but these titers are no longer at their peak during the carditis of acute rheumatic fever. A patient

may demonstrate an elevated antibody titer for up to a year after infection; therefore the time of infection is not precisely determined by this technique. Low titers of antistreptolysin O (ASO) can be exhibited by apparently healthy persons because of the frequency of subclinical streptococcal infections, but persistently low titers rule out *S. pyogenes* infection.

Half the patients with *S. pyogenes*–related acute glomerulonephritis display a normal ASO titer but demonstrate an elevated titer to one of the other streptococcal substances (e.g., DNAse and NADase). Anti-DNase B antibody appears to be the most reliable measure of recent *S. pyogenes* skin infection. Titers of anti-DNase B are elevated in more than two thirds of patients with recent streptococcal impetigo. Anti-NADase antibodies are a particularly good marker in patients who develop nephritis after pharyngitis.

DIAGNOSTIC EVALUATION

In addition to cultures such as throat cultures in cases of pharyngitis, antibodies to bacterial toxins and other extracellular products that display measurable activity can be tested. ASO and anti-DNase B (ADN-B) are the standard serologic tests. The ability of a patient's serum to neutralize the erythrocyte-lysing capability of SLO (ASO procedure) has been used for many years as a detection method for previous streptococcal infection. After an infection such as pharyngitis with SLO-producing strains, most patients show a high titer of the antibody ASO. The use of particle agglutination (e.g., latex particle agglutination or assay by nephelometry) for the presence of antibodies has replaced the use of the classic ASO procedure in many laboratories.

Streptococci produce the enzyme, deoxyribonuclease B (DNase B). A neutralization test that prevents the activity of this enzyme, the anti-DNase B test, is also a standard serologic method for demonstrating recent or previous *S. pyogenes* infection. Antistreptokinase and antihyaluronidase titers (AHTs) have also been used to diagnose streptococcal infection retrospectively.

Serologic testing should compare acute and convalescent sera collected 3 weeks apart. ASO becomes elevated in acute/convalescent paired specimens in 80% to 85% of patients with acute rheumatic fever. ADN-B and AHT levels are elevated in the remaining 15% to 20% of patients. In many cases no acute serum specimen is available; therefore the antibody titer of the convalescent serum specimen is compared to a reference range value. Reference ranges vary with age, season, and geographic area. False-positive ASO results may be demonstrated because of beta-lipoprotein, contamination of the serum specimen by bacterial growth products, or oxidation of ASO. These errors are not encountered with the ADN-B procedure, which is the serologic test of choice for acute rheumatic fever and acute glomerulonephritis after *S. pyogenes* infection.

Other methods of testing include a PRC-based assay, the Rapid-Cycle Real Timer Polymerase Chain Reaction (Roche Diagnostics, Pleasanton, CA), which uses a unique LightCycler technology to repeat copying and amplification of the two strands of DNA of the *Streptococcous pharyngitis* gene sequence and provides results in 1.5 hours. Another nucleic-acid based test is the Group A Strep Direct probe test manufactured by Gen-Probe Inc. (San Diego, CA). The test is a DNA chemiluminescence probe assay targeted at Group A strep rRNA in a specimen. These emerging technologies underscore the demand to speed up the detection of Group A strep by replacing traditional testing methods, particularly the 48-hour throat culture, which has always been the gold standard.

STREPTOCOCCAL TOXIC SHOCK SYNDROME

There has been a marked increase in the recognition and reporting of highly invasive group A streptococcal infections with or without necrotizing fasciitis associated with shock and organ failure. This streptococcal infection is known as the *toxic streptococcal syndrome* or *streptococcal toxic shocklike syndrome (STSS)*. Although STSS was officially recognized in 1987, outbreaks of similar serious *Streptococcus* infections may have occurred since the seventeenth century. Today, STSS is still considered a new or "emerging" illness, related to the same strains of *Streptococcus* that have been nicknamed "flesh-eating bacteria."

Etiology

Strains of group A streptococci isolated from patients with STSS have been predominantly M types 1 and 3 that produce pyrogenic exotoxin A or B or both.

The portal of entry of streptococci cannot be proven in at least half the cases and can only be presumed in many others. Patients with symptomatic pharyngitis rarely develop STSS. Virus infections (e.g., varicella and influenza) have provided a portal in some cases. In other cases the use of nonsteroidal antiinflammatory agents may have either masked the early symptoms or predisposed the patient to more severe streptococcal infection and shock.

Immunologic Mechanisms

Pyrogenic exotoxins cause fever in humans and animals and also help induce shock by lowering the threshold to exogenous endotoxin. Streptococcal pyrogenic exotoxins A and B induce human mononuclear cells to synthesize not only tumor necrosis factor-alpha (TNF-α) but also interleukin-1-beta (IL-1-beta) and interleukin-6 (IL-6), suggesting that TNF could mediate the fever, shock, and tissue injury observed in patients with STSS.

M protein contributes to invasiveness through its ability to impede phagocytosis of streptococci by human polymorphonuclear leukocytes. Conversely, type-specific antibody against the M protein enhances phagocytosis. Research studies suggest that this exotoxin and a number of staphylococcal toxins (toxic shock syndrome toxin-1 [TSST-1] and staphylococcal enterotoxins A, B, and C) can stimulate T-cell responses through their ability to bind to both the Class II major histocompatibility ability complex of antigen-presenting cells and the Vb region of the T-cell receptor. The net effect would be to induce T-cell stimulation with production of cytokines capable of mediating shock and tissue injury. Quantitation of such T-cell subsets in patients with acute STSS has demonstrated deletion rather than expansion, suggesting that perhaps the life span of the expanded subset was shortened by apoptosis. In addition, an as yet undefined superantigen may play a role.

Cytokine production by less exotic mechanisms likely contributes as well to the genesis of shock and organ failure. Exotoxins such as SLO are also potent inducers of TNFa and IL-1-beta. Pyrogenic exotoxin B, a proteinase precursor, has the ability to cleave pre-IL-1-beta to release preformed IL-1.

Finally, SLO and exotoxin A together have additive effects in the induction of IL-1-beta by human mononuclear cells. Whatever the mechanisms, induction of cytokines in vivo is likely the cause of shock, and these two exotoxins, cell wall components, and the like, are potent inducers of TNF and IL-1.

Epidemiology

The rates of STSS are highest in young children and older adults. More than half of patients have an underlying chronic illness. STSS is also associated with a substantial risk of transmission in households and health care institutions. The mortality rate of an outbreak of *S. pyogenes* that progresses to toxic shock can be as high as 70%. The illness is classified as a rare infection because it affects only about 300 people per year. Most often, STSS appears after *Streptococcus* bacteria have invaded areas of injured skin (e.g., cuts and scrapes or surgical wounds). It almost never follows a simple *Streptococcus* throat infection.

Signs and Symptoms

The symptoms of STSS include shock, fever, a blotchy rash, and an area of infected skin that is red, swollen, and painful. The average incubation period for STSS is 2 to 3 days usually after minor nonpenetrating trauma.

Pain, the most common initial symptom of STSS, is abrupt in onset, severe, and usually precedes tenderness or physical findings. The pain usually involves an extremity but may also mimic peritonitis, pelvic inflammatory disease, pneumonia, acute myocardial infarction, or pericarditis. In all 20% of patients have an influenza-like syndrome characterized by fever, chills, myalgia, nausea, vomiting, and diarrhea. Fever is the most common early sign, although hypothermia may be present in patients with shock.

A total of 80% of patients have clinical signs of soft tissue infection, such as localized swelling and erythema, which in 70% of patients progressed to necrotizing fasciitis or myositis and required surgical debridement, fasciotomy, or amputation. An ominous sign is the progression of soft tissue swelling to the formation of vesicles, then bullae, which appear violaceous or bluish.

Laboratory Data

The case definition of STSS and necrotizing fasciitis includes serologic confirmation of group A streptococcal infection by a fourfold rise against SLO and DNAse B. Although initial laboratory studies usually demonstrate only mild leukocytosis, the mean percentage of immature neutrophils can reach 40% to 50%. Blood cultures are positive in 60% of cases.

Renal involvement is indicated by the presence of hemoglobinuria and by serum creatinine values that are, on average, more than 2.5 times normal. Renal impairment precedes hypotension in approximately 40% to 50% of patients. Hypoalbuminemia is associated with hypocalcemia on admission and throughout the hospital course. The serum creatinine kinase level is useful in detecting deeper soft-tissue infections; when the level is elevated or rising, there is a good correlation with necrotizing fasciitis or myositis.

Treatment

STSS can be deadly and needs immediate treatment. Intravenous fluids and medications to maintain a normal blood pressure are required in acutely ill patients. Penicillin and other beta-lactam antibiotics are the most efficacious against rapidly growing bacteria. After recovery, the skin may peel as the rash heals. Surgery may be necessary to remove areas of dead skin and muscle around an infected wound.

GROUP B STREPTOCOCCAL DISEASE

Group B streptococcus (GBS), *Streptococcus agalactiae* infections cause serious disease in adults and neonates. This bacterium causes substantial morbidity and mortality in adults. The case-fatality rate ranges from 26% to 70% among men and nonpregnant women with GBS disease. GBS is most frequently isolated from blood. The most common clinical finding is skin and soft tissue infection.

Because of the gravity of GBS disease, especially in those who are older and those who have chronic diseases, the development of a vaccine is being pursued. Determining the incidence of adult disease and groups at greatest risk will help in focusing prevention efforts. Intrapartum antibiotics can prevent early-onset neonatal GBS disease, but they have not been widely used.

 Rapid Latex Agglutination Antistreptolysin O Procedure

Principle

Group A streptococci produce two hemolytic exotoxins. One of these toxins SLO, is highly antigenic. Antibodies produced in response to this antigenic stimulation are called streptolysin O antibodies or antistreptolysin O. If polystyrene latex particles are coated with streptolysin O antigen, visible agglutination will be exhibited in the presence of the corresponding antistreptolysin (ASO) antibody. Group A streptococci can be responsible for postinfection complications such as rheumatic fever and the accompanying cardiac abnormalities, as well as acute glomerulonephritis.

Specimen Collection and Preparation

The patient does not need to be specially prepared before specimen collection. The patient must be positively identified when the specimen is collected; the specimen should be labeled at the bedside. Specimen labels should include the patient's full name, the date, the patient's hospital identification number, and the phlebotomist's initials.

Blood should be drawn by an aseptic technique. A minimum of 2 mL of clotted blood (red top evacuated tube) is required. The specimen should be centrifuged promptly, and an aliquot of serum removed. Serum specimens are reportedly stable up to 8 days at 2° to 8° C or for up to 3 months if frozen (at or below –25° C) within 24 hours of venipuncture and if the specimen is not repeatedly thawed and refrozen. Lipemia or contamination with bacteria renders a specimen unsuitable for testing.

Reagents, Supplies, and Equipment

RaPET (Stanbio Laboratory, Inc, San Antonio, TX) contains the following components and positive and negative controls:

1. ASO latex reagent coated with streptolysin O. This is a suspension of polystyrene latex particles coated with streptolysin O in a saline buffer. Reagent is stable until the expiration date printed on the package when stored at 2° to 8° C. Do not freeze. Mix well before use.
2. Glycine-Saline Buffer (20×) Concentrate. A solution of glycine and sodium chloride, pH 8.2 ± −0.1
3. Glass slide with six cells. Use only the glass slide provided in the kit. It should be rinsed in distilled water and thoroughly dried with a soft cloth or tissue after each use.
4. Disposable pipette/mixers

Other materials required but not provided in the kit:
1. Timer
2. 12 × 75-mm test tubes and racks (semiquantitative test only)
3. Serologic pipettes and safety bulb (semiquantitative test only)
4. High-intensity direct light

WARNING: The latex reagent and controls contain sodium azide as a preservative. Sodium azide may react with lead and copper plumbing to form highly explosive metal azides. On disposal, flush with a large volume of water to prevent azide buildup.

Quality Control

Positive control serum: a prediluted serum containing at least 200 U/mL of ASO. This control should exhibit visible agglutination (clumping) at the end of the 2-minute test period.

Negative control serum: a prediluted serum containing less than 100 U/mL of ASO. This control should exhibit a smooth or slightly granular appearance at the end of the 3-minute test period.

A positive and negative control should be tested and read concurrently with each group of patient sera.

CAUTION: Because the control sera are derived from human sources, they should be handled in the same manner as clinical serum specimens (see Universal Blood and Body Fluid Precautions in Chapter 6).

Procedure

Screening Test

NOTE: All reagents and specimens must be at room temperature before testing.

Gently shake the reagent vial to disperse and suspend the latex particles. DO NOT SHAKE VIGOROUSLY.

1. Using a dispensing pipette provided, add one drop of the nondiluted patient serum on to a separate cell on the glass slide. Also place one drop of the positive control and one drop of the negative control on separate cells of the test slide.
2. Gently mix the contents of the latex reagent including the contents of the glass dropper. Fill the dropper with the well-mixed latex suspension and place one drop next to the drop of serum sample on each of the separate cells in use.
3. Mix both drops with the mixer provided, covering the whole surface of each of the cells.

4. Tilt the slide back and forth for 2 minutes manually so that the mixture rotates slowly inside the cells or place the slide on an automatic rotator set at 80 to 100 rpm.
5. Rotate the slide for exactly 2 minutes. Examine immediately with a bright source of direct light.

Reporting Results

Positive: agglutination
Negative: no agglutination

Procedure Notes

Agglutination demonstrates 200 U/mL or more of ASO. Positive results should be retested quantitatively. In semiquantitative testing, the U/mL of the highest dilution of serum to produce visible agglutination is the reported value.

Preparation of patient serum should be as follows:

Dilution	U/mL
1:2	≥ 400
1:4	≥ 800
1:8	≥ 1600
1:16	≥ 3200

Sources of Error

False-positive reactions can result from bacterial contamination of the specimen or if the reaction is observed after 2 minutes. Markedly lipemic serum or plasma may produce nonspecific reactions.

Clinical Applications

Signs and symptoms of streptococcal infection often resemble those of other diseases. For example, rheumatic fever can be confused with rheumatoid arthritis at certain stages of the illness. However, in rheumatoid arthritis the ASO is normal. An elevated titer suggests the presence of group A (beta-hemolytic) streptococcal infection. Eighty percent of streptococcal infections are associated with a rise in ASO titer.

When the ASO is repeated at appropriate intervals, the following can be determined:

1. A rising titer suggests an increase in the severity of the infection.
2. A declining titer suggests a trend toward recovery.
3. A constant (low) titer suggests that a streptococcal infection is not current but that the patient has had a past infection.

Limitations

Streptococcal skin infections and glomerulonephritis can produce very low titers of ASO. If a streptococcal infection is suspected but the ASO titer does not exceed the reference range, an anti-DNase B (ADN-B) should be performed. Because of the subjective reading of results, discrepancies in interpretation may result.

Reference

Stanbio raPET ASO Procedure No. 1125 product insert, 2002.

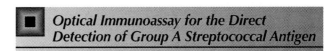

■ Optical Immunoassay for the Direct Detection of Group A Streptococcal Antigen

Principle

The new rapid surface immunoassay (Optical Immuno-Assay) allows for the direct visual detection of the physical change in thickness of thin films resulting from binding reactions between antigens and antibodies (Figure 14-4). Polyclonal anti-group A streptococcal antigen (GAS) antibody is attached to a thin silicon wafer. Light reflected from the surface after passing through this thin film results in a gold color. When a liquid sample containing antigen is placed on the surface, binding occurs between the antigen and the immobilized antibody. When a substrate that binds only to the antigen-antibody complex is added, there is an increase in the thickness of the film, changing the optical path. This causes the reacted surface to appear purple. No color change occurs in the absence of antigen binding.

Specimen Collection and Preparation

A sterile swab must be used to properly collect a specimen from the throat or nasopharynx. The swab must be Dacron or rayon (synthetic) tipped on a plastic shaft.

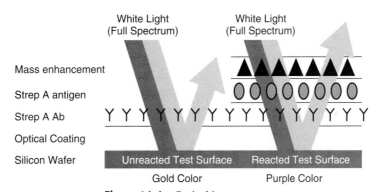

Figure 14-4 Optical immunoassay.

Acceptable transport media for the swab can be either modified Stuart's liquid or semisolid medium, or Amies liquid or semisolid medium. Transport of a wet or dry swab may be in a paper wrapper and transported unrefrigerated in a dry sterile tube or in a sleeve containing acceptable transport medium. Swabs may be stored unrefrigerated and should be processed within 72 hours of collection.

If a culture is to be conducted in addition to the STREP A OIA assay, an additional swab should be collected and handled by conventional methods for culture. If only a single swab is available, perform the culture first, then process the swab in the STREP A OIA test procedure.

Handling precautions: All throat swabs should be handled as though they were capable of transmitting disease. Observe established precautions against microbiologic hazards throughout all procedures and dispose of swabs and reagent tubes in biohazard containers. Washing hands after performing the test is recommended.

Reagents, Supplies, and Equipment

1. OIA test kit containing: Reagents 1-5, test device, and positive control
2. Transfer pipettes
3. Test kit procedure insert
4. Stopwatch

The test kit should be stored at 2° to 8° C. The reagent tray may be stored at room temperature for up to 12 hours and then returned to refrigeration after use. Reagents should not be used beyond the expiration date printed on the label.

Safety Precautions

The test kit is intended for in vitro diagnostic use only. Reagents are not interchangeable between lots and kits. Do not interchange caps between reagents. Reagent 1 is an irritant.

Quality Control

A positive GAS antigen control is incorporated into each test device. This internal control appears as a small purple dot near the center of each test surface after the completion of a properly performed test.

Procedure

Follow the test procedure as described in the package insert. On completion of each test, the test surface should be examined under a bright light source. The light must be reflected off the test surface to observe test results.

Reporting Results

Positive control: a small blue/purple dot in the center of the test surface on completion of each test

Negative test: only the internal positive control will be reactive

Positive test: shows the internal positive control within the reaction circle

Strong positive test: the procedure control may be less apparent within the reaction circle

Positive Result

A solid blue/purple colored reaction circle of any intensity appears in the center of the test surface.

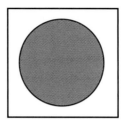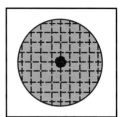

Negative Result

No blue/purple colored reaction circle of any intensity appears on the test surface. The positive control dot is in the center of the test surface.

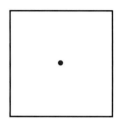

Invalid Result

No blue/purple positive control dot or a solid blue/purple color over entire test surface. The procedure should be repeated if an invalid test result occurs.

Procedure Notes

The reacted test surface and the color change associated with a positive reaction will not deteriorate over time. The test device may be considered a permanent record and should be closed for storage.

In general, direct GAS detection products are relatively inexpensive, rapid, and easy to perform but have poor sensitivity compared with conventional reference culture techniques. The STREP A OIA procedure manufactured by BioStar in Boulder, Colorado has been reported to have overcome problems related to sensitivity and specificity. This method is reported to have 98% specificity and 95% sensitivity. This exceeds the reported sensitivity of the latex method (43%) and appears to be as sensitive as culture technique.

Sources of Error

Whole blood, serum, white blood cells, saliva, and sheep blood agar do not interfere with the test methodology.

Clinical Applications

Traditional rapid gas antigen-detection methods and culture techniques have had little influence on patient management in most clinical settings because of inherent test limitations. The OIA method appears to be a reliable and easily interpretable method for the detection of group A streptococcal antigen from clinical specimens (e.g., pharyngeal swabs).

Limitations

As with other diagnostic procedures, the results obtained with this kit should be used as an adjunct to other clinical observations and information available to the physician. If a negative result is obtained with this assay and the symptoms persist, follow-up testing is recommended to determine other nongroup a streptococcal causes of pharyngitis. This test is not intended to differentiate carriers of group A streptococcus from those with streptococcal infections.

References

STREP A Optical ImmunoAssay Kit, BioStar, Boulder, Colorado, 1995.

Case Study

This 19-year-old woman went to the Emergency Department (ED) with swelling and redness of her right leg. She had fallen down while rollerblading and had a number of abrasions on the skin of her leg. She also had a body temperature of 37.8° C. The ED physician ordered a culture of her leg wound, gave her a prescription for an antibiotic, and discharged her from treatment.

The following evening she collapsed onto the floor of her bedroom. Her roommate found her and called 911. On arrival, the paramedics found an unconscious female with a blood pressure of 80/40 and pronounced redness and swelling of her right leg. She was rushed to the ED and admitted to the intensive care unit where she was immediately placed on IV fluids and medications to raise her blood pressure.

Questions and Discussions

1. Is there any relationship between this patient's problem with her leg and her collapse on the floor?
    Yes. Her infected wound and sudden hypotension could suggest streptococcal toxic shock syndrome (STSS).
2. What are the symptoms of STSS?
    Along with the symptoms of shock, patients can manifest fever, blotchy rash, and an area of infected skin that is red, swollen, and painful.
3. What is the source of this patient's STSS?
    Most often, STSS appears after *Streptococcus* bacteria have invaded areas of injured skin (e.g., cuts

and scrapes or surgical wounds). It almost never follows a simple *Streptococcus* throat infection.
4. Are there any immunologic/serologic manifestations of STSS?
    Yes. Serologic confirmation of group A streptococcal infection can be demonstrated by a fourfold rise against streptolysin O and DNase B.

Diagnosis

Streptococcal Toxic Shock Syndrome

CHAPTER HIGHLIGHTS

Most streptococci that contain cell wall antigens of Lancefield group A are known as *S. pyogenes*. Members of this species are almost always beta-hemolytic. In terms of human morbidity and mortality worldwide, however, the role of *S. pyogenes* in the subsequent development of complications such as acute rheumatic fever and poststreptococcal glomerulonephritis is more important. Lancefield divided these beta-hemolytic streptococci into serogroups A through O on the basis of the immunologic action of the cell wall carbohydrate. Strains of *S. pyogenes* that lack M protein cannot cause infection.

Extracellular products are important in the pathogenesis of disease and in the serologic diagnosis of streptococcal disease. Antibodies produced in response to these substances provide evidence of recent streptococcal infection. Two hemolysins that have the ability to damage human and animal erythrocytes, polymorphonuclear leukocytes and platelets, are produced by most group A strains. SLO, an oxygen-labile enzyme, binds to sterols in the red cell membrane, causing stearic rearrangement. This rearrangement produces submicroscopic holes in the red cell membrane, and hemoglobin diffuses from the cells. SLO is antigenic; the antibody response to it is the most commonly used serologic indicator of recent streptococcal infection. Other substances produced by group A streptococci presumably facilitate rapid spread through subcutaneous or deeper soft tissues. These substances include hyaluronidase, four immunologically distinct DNases, streptokinase, other extracellular products that can elicit an antibody response, and erythrogenic toxin.

REVIEW QUESTIONS

1. *Streptococcus pyogenes* is the most common causative agent of all of the following disorders and complications except:
    A. pharyngitis
    B. gastroenteritis
    C. scarlet fever
    D. impetigo

2. All of the following characteristics are descriptive of M protein except:
    A. no known biologic role
    B. found in association with the hyaluronic capsule
    C. inhibits phagocytosis
    D. antibody against M protein provides type-specific immunity

3. Substances produced by *S. pyogenes* include all of the following except:
   A. hyaluronidase
   B. DNAses (A, B, C, D)
   C. erythrogenic toxin
   D. interferon

4. Laboratory diagnosis of *S. pyogenes* can be made by all of the following except:
   A. culturing of throat or nasal specimens
   B. febrile agglutinins
   C. ASO procedure
   D. anti-DNase (B)

5. False ASO results may be due to all of the following except:
   A. room temperature reagents and specimens at the time of testing
   B. the presence of beta lipoprotein
   C. bacterial contamination of the serum specimen
   D. oxidation of ASO reagent caused by shaking or aeration of the reagent vial

6. Members of the *S. pyogenes* species are almost always

   _____ hemolytic.
   A. alpha
   B. beta
   C. gamma
   D. alpha or beta

7. Long-term complications of *S. pyogenes* infection can include:
   A. acute rheumatic fever
   B. poststreptococcal glomerulonephritis
   C. rheumatoid arthritis
   D. both A and B

8. Particularly virulent serotypes of *S. pyogenes* produce

   proteolytic enzymes that cause _____ in a wound or lesion on an extremity.
   A. necrotizing fasciitis
   B. bone degeneration
   C. burning and itching
   D. severe inflammation

Questions 9-11. Match the substances produced by Group A streptococci with the appropriate description below.

9. _____ hyaluronidase   A. degrades DNA
                                 B. also called "spreading
10. _____ streptokinase   factor"
                                 C. responsible for charac-
11. _____ erythrogenic toxin   teristic scarlet fever rash
                                 D. dissolves clots by con-
                                    verting plasminogen to
                                    plasmin

12. All of the following characteristics of *S. pyogenes* are correct except that it:
   A. is an uncommon pathogen
   B. occurs most frequently in school-age children
   C. is spread by contact with large droplets produced in the upper respiratory tract
   D. has been known to cause food-borne and milk-borne epidemics

13. The clinical manifestations of *S. pyogenes*-associated upper respiratory infection are:
   A. mild and usually unnoticeable
   B. age dependent
   C. associated with cold sores
   D. difficult to detect

14. The most reliable immunologic test for recent *S. pyogenes* skin infection is:
   A. ASO
   B. anti-DNAse B
   C. anti-NADase
   D. antibody to erythrogenic toxin

15. In the rapid agglutination antistreptolysin O procedure, latex particles are coated with:
   A. streptolysin O antigen
   B. antistreptolysin (ASO) antibody
   C. dye for easier-to-read agglutination
   D. A or B

Questions 16-18. Match each ASO titer situation to the appropriate description. (An answer may be used twice.)

16. _____ a rising titer   A. increase in severity of in-
                                   fection
17. _____ a declining titer   B. not a current infection but
                                   indicates a past infection
18. _____ a constant (low)   C. a trend toward recovery
         titer   D. no clinical significance

19. If a streptococcal infection is suspected, but the ASO titer does not exceed the reference range, a (an)

   _____ should be performed.
   A. repeat titer
   B. anti-DNAse B
   C. anti-NADase
   D. throat culture

20. The best standard tests to demonstrate the presence of streptococcal infection are:
   A. ASO and anti-NADase
   B. ASO and anti-DNAse B
   C. anti-NADase and anti-DNAse
   D. both A and B

21. The highest reported levels of sensitivity testing for group A streptococcus are in:
    A. ASO titers
    B. direct latex agglutination tests
    C. surface (optical) immunoassay
    D. A and B, which are equivalent

BIBLIOGRAPHY

Anthony BF et al: Immunospecificity and quantitation of an enzyme-linked immunosorbent assay for group B streptococcal antibody, *J Clin Microbiol* 16:350-354, 1982.

Bisno AL: Group A streptococcal infections and acute rheumatic fever, *N Engl J Med* 325(11):783-793, 1991.

Davies HD et al: Invasive group A streptococcal infections in Ontario, Canada, *N Engl J Med* 335:547-554, 1996.

Farley MM et al: A population-based assessment of invasive disease due to group B streptococcus in nonpregnant adults, *N Engl J Med* 328(25):1807-1812, 1993.

Forbes BA, Sahm DF, Weissfeld AS: *Bailey & Scott's diagnostic microbiology,* ed 11, St Louis, 2002, Mosby.

Hexter DA: Group A streptococcus septicemia in children, *JAMA* 267(1):53-54, 1992.

Hoge CW et al: The changing epidemiology of invasive group A streptococcal infections and the emergence of streptococcal toxic-shock-like syndrome, *JAMA* 269(3):384-391, 1993.

James E: Testing for strep throat, *Adv Medical Lab Prof* (online edition), retrieved 12-02-02, website: www.advanceformLp.com.

Jefferson R: Rapid micro workup key to containing flesh-eating bacteria, *Adv Med Lab Prof* 7(11):6-9, 1995.

Mohle-Boetani JC et al: Comparison of prevention strategies for neonatal group B streptococcal infection, *JAMA* 270(12):1442-1448, 1993.

Schwartz B et al: Invasive group B streptococcal disease in adults, *JAMA* 266(8):1112-1114, 1991.

Smith JM, Bauman MC, Fuchs PC: An optical immunoassay for the direct detection of Group A strep antigen, *Lab Med* 26(6):408-410, 1995.

Stanbio Product Brochure, San Antonio, Tex, 1986, Stanbio Laboratory, Inc.

Turner RB, Hendley JO: *Streptococcus pyogenes* infections. In Stein J, editor: *Internal medicine,* Boston, 1994, Little, Brown.

Syphilis

LEARNING OBJECTIVES

At the conclusion of this chapter, the reader should be able to:

- Describe the etiology, epidemiology, and signs and symptoms of primary, secondary, latent, and late (tertiary) syphilis.
- Describe the origin and manifestations of the condition, congenital syphilis.
- Explain the immunologic manifestations and diagnostic evaluation of syphilis.

- Discuss the principles and clinical applications of the qualitative and quantitative Venereal Disease Research Laboratory (VDRL) procedure and the rapid plasma reagin (RPR) card test
- Discuss the principles and clinical applications of the fluorescent *Treponema pallidum* antibody absorption test (FTA-ABS).

The disease syphilis was reported in the medical literature as early as 1495. In 1905 it was discovered that syphilis was caused by a spirochete type of bacteria, *Treponema pallidum* (originally called *Spirochaeta pallida*). The first diagnostic blood test, the Wassermann test, was developed in 1906. This classic procedure has subsequently been replaced by a variety of methods. In the treatment of syphilis, heavy metals, such as arsenic, were replaced by penicillin in the 1940s. Penicillin continues to remain the drug of choice in the treatment of this disease.

ETIOLOGY

T. pallidum is a member of the order Spirochaetales and the family Treponemataceae (Figure 15-1). The genus *Treponema* includes a number of species that reside in the gastrointestinal and genital tracts of humans. *T. pallidum, T. pertenue,* and *T. carateum* (Table 15-1) are human pathogens responsible for significant worldwide morbidity. Direct examination of the treponemes is most commonly performed with darkfield microscopy. Microscopically these pathogenic

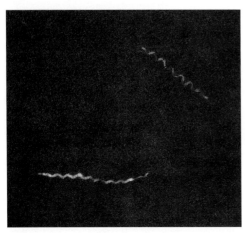

Figure 15-1 *Treponema pallidum.* (From Bauer JD: *Clinical laboratory methods,* ed 9, St Louis, 1982, Mosby.)

TABLE 15-1	**Treponema-Associated Diseases in Humans**
Bacteria	**Associated Disease**
Treponema pallidum	Syphilis
T. pallidum (variant)	Bejel
T. pertenue	Yaws
T. carateum	Pinta

treponemes appear as fine, spiral (8 to 24 coils) organisms approximately 6 to 15 μm long. They have a trilaminar outer membrane similar to that of gram-negative bacteria.

Pathogenic treponemes are not cultivatable with any consistency in artificial laboratory media. Outside of the host, the pathogenic treponemes are extremely susceptible to a variety of physical and chemical agents. Treponemes, however, may remain viable for up to 5 days in tissue specimens removed from diseased animals and from frozen, cryoprotected specimens.

EPIDEMIOLOGY

Pathogenic treponemes are transmitted almost uniformly by direct contact. Syphilis is a venereal disease. The three treponematoses—yaws, pinta, and bejel—are rarely seen in the United States but are prevalent in other countries. These diseases are associated with poverty, overcrowding, and poor hygiene.

Yaws, pinta, and bejel are diseases caused by bacteria closely related to *T. pallidum.* Yaws is common in the Caribbean, Latin America, Central Africa, and the Far East. Pinta is found only in Latin America, and infection is limited to the skin. Bejel is found in the eastern Mediterranean, the Balkans, and the cooler areas of North Africa.

In these infections the skin or oral lesions contain many spirochetes that may be transmitted by personal, but not necessarily venereal, contact. These infections are generally acquired during childhood. In each of these diseases, infection elicits antibodies reactive in nontreponemal and treponemal methods.

Syphilis develops in 30% to 50% of the sexual partners of persons with syphilitic lesions. The risk of acquiring syphilis from a single sexual exposure to an infected partner is unknown. A high percentage of partners, however, do seek medical treatment within 90 days of contact.

In the United States more than 35,600 cases of syphilis were reported by health officials in 1999, including 6650 cases of primary and secondary syphilis (a decline of 5.4% from 1998) and 556 cases of congenital syphilis in newborns. However, more cases of syphilis occur each year than come to the attention of health officials. A total of 265 counties had syphilis rates above the U.S. Public Health Service's Healthy People 2000 objective of 4 cases per 100,000.

In 1999 syphilis occurred primarily in persons ages 20 to 39 years, and the reported rate in men was 1.5 times greater than the rate in women. The incidence of syphilis was highest in women ages 20 to 29 years and in men 30 to 39 years. Some fundamental social problems (e.g., poverty, inadequate access to health care, and lack of education) are associated with disproportionately high levels of syphilis in certain populations. Cases of primary and secondary syphilis in 1999 had the following race or ethnicity distribution: African-Americans, 75%; Caucasians, 16%; Hispanics, 8%; and others, 1%.

Syphilis can be acquired by kissing a person with active oral lesions. Very few cases of transfusion-acquired syphilis have been reported in recent years in the United States. During the first half of this century, however, syphilis was a major blood-borne infectious disease that was easily transmitted through the prevailing method of direct donor-to-patient blood transfusion. The hazard of transmission of syphilis has not disappeared in some tropical countries, where the organization of blood banks is deficient and where direct blood transfusion prevails in emergency situations. Refrigerated blood storage decreases accidental transmission of the microorganism because *T. pallidum* has a short survival period in stored blood. Spirochetes do not appear to survive in units of citrated blood at 4° C for more than 72 hours.

Cases have been reported of children who have acquired syphilis by sharing a bed with an infected parent. In addition, syphilis may be transmitted transplacentally to the fetus. Spirochetes can be transmitted to the fetus during the last trimester of pregnancy, before the mother manifests postpartum evidence of infection.

SIGNS AND SYMPTOMS

Untreated syphilis is a chronic disease with subacute symptomatic periods separated by asymptomatic intervals, during which the diagnosis can be made serologically.

The progression of untreated syphilis is generally divided into stages. Initially, *T. pallidum* penetrates intact mucous membranes or enters the body through tiny defects in the epithelium. On entrance, the microorganism is carried by the circulatory system to every organ of the body. Spirochetemia occurs very early in infection, even before the first lesions have appeared or blood tests become reactive. Before clinical or serologic manifestations develop, patients are said to be "incubating syphilis." The incubation period usually lasts about 3 weeks but can range from 10 to 90 days.

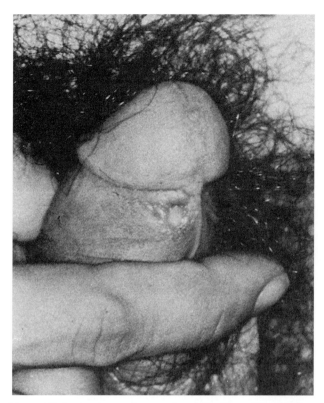

Figure 15-2   A primary chancre of syphilis. (From Kaye D, Rose LF: *Fundamentals of internal medicine,* St Louis, 1983, Mosby.)

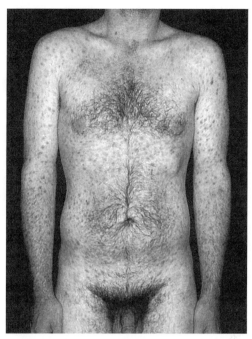

Figure 15-3   Secondary syphilis. (From Habif TP: *Clinical dermatology,* ed 2, St Louis, 1990, Mosby.)

Primary Syphilis

At the end of the incubation period, a patient develops a characteristic primary inflammatory lesion called a chancre at the point of initial inoculation and multiplication of the spirochetes. The chancre begins as a papule and erodes to form a gradually enlarging ulcer with a clean base and indurated edge (Figure 15-2). Generally it is relatively painless. In most cases only a single lesion is present, but multiple chancres are not rare.

Chancres are commonly located around the genitalia, but in about 10% of cases lesions may appear almost anywhere else on the body (e.g., throat, lip, hands). In males, spirochetes are present in the lesion on the penis or discharged from deeper sites with semen. In females, infected lesions are commonly located in the perineal region or on the labia, vaginal wall, or cervix. If the lesion is located inside the urethra, the only symptom may be a scanty serous urethral discharge.

Of patients with primary syphilis of the external genitals, 50% to 70% will subsequently develop inguinal adenopathy. Inguinal adenopathy, however, is less common with chancres involving the cervix or proximal part of the vagina because these sites are drained by the iliac nodes. Regional adenopathy may accompany primary inoculation at other sites (e.g., cervical adenopathy may accompany a syphilitic lesion of the oral cavity). Even without treatment, the primary chancre will persist for 1 to 5 weeks and will heal completely within about 4 to 6 weeks. Regional adenopathy will also resolve itself.

Secondary Syphilis

Within 2 to 8 weeks (but occasionally as long as 6 months) after the appearance of the primary chancre, a patient may develop the signs and symptoms of secondary syphilis. In some cases primary and secondary syphilis overlap, and the chancre is still obvious. In other situations some patients never notice the primary chancre and initially have manifestations of secondary syphilis (Figure 15-3).

The secondary stage is characterized by a generalized illness that usually begins with symptoms suggesting a viral infection: headache, sore throat, low-grade fever, and occasionally a nasal discharge. Blood tests reveal a moderate increase in leukocytes with a relative increase in lymphocytes.

The disease progresses with the development of lymphadenopathy and lesions of the skin and mucous membranes. Approximately 75% of syphilitic patients suffer from generalized adenopathy. Skin lesions are demonstrated by 80% of infected patients. These lesions contain a large number of spirochetes, and when located on exposed surfaces, are highly contagious. Macular lesions are common, and a rash invariably involves the genitalia and often is prominent on the palms and soles. Patients may also develop condylomata lata, flat lesions resembling warts in moist areas of the body (e.g., around the anus or vagina). These lesions do not reflect areas of inoculation but appear to be caused by hematogenous dissemination of spirochetes. The central nervous system (CNS) is asymptomatically involved in about one third of patients. About 2% of cases manifest themselves as acute syphilitic meningitis. Early involvement of CNS

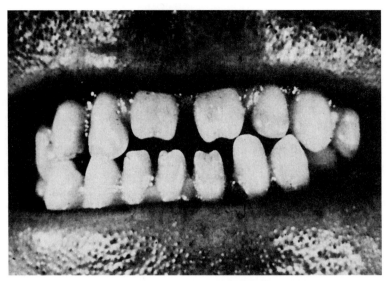

Figure 15-4   Congenital syphilis (hutchinsonian triad). (From Kaye D, Rose LF: *Fundamentals of internal medicine,* St Louis, 1983, Mosby.)

may progress to neurosyphilis if untreated. Hepatitis and immune complex glomerulonephritis occasionally accompany secondary syphilis. Secondary syphilis usually resolves itself within 2 to 6 weeks, even in the absence of therapy.

Latent Syphilis

After resolution of untreated secondary syphilis, the patient enters a latent noninfectious state in which diagnosis can be made only by serologic methods. During the first 2 to 4 years of infection, one fourth of patients will have one or more mucocutaneous relapses in which the manifestation of secondary syphilis reappears. During these relapses, patients are infectious, and the underlying spirochetemia may be passed transplacentally to the fetus. Relapses are extremely rare after 4 years of latency. About one third of patients entering latency are eventually spontaneously cured of the disease, one third will never develop further clinical manifestation of the disease, and the remaining one third will eventually develop late syphilis.

Late (Tertiary) Syphilis

The first manifestations of late syphilis are usually seen from 3 to 10 years after primary infection. About 15% of untreated syphilitic individuals eventually develop late benign syphilis, characterized by the presence of destructive granulomas.

These granulomas, or gummas, may produce lesions resembling segments of circles that often heal with superficial scarring. The skeletal system is frequently affected, but treponemes are rarely seen.

Of untreated patients 10% develop cardiovascular manifestations. *T. pallidum* may directly affect the aortic endothelium. Weakening of the blood vessels can occur as a syphilitic aneurysm, usually of the aortic arch.

In about 8% of untreated patients, late syphilis involves the CNS. Initially CNS disease is asymptomatic and can be detected only by examination of cerebrospinal fluid (CSF). CSF should be examined in all patients being treated for syphilis of unknown duration or who have had syphilis for more than 1 year. Meningovascular syphilis usually mani-

fests itself as a seizure or cerebrovascular accident (stroke). Spirochetes may also involve the brain tissues and cause general paresis, personality changes, dementia, and delusional states. Tabes dorsalis results from involvement of the posterior columns and dorsal roots of the spinal cord and is characterized by a broad-based gait. Impotence and bladder dysfunction are common in this disorder.

Congenital Syphilis

Congenital syphilis is caused by maternal spirochetemia and transplacental transmission of the microorganism. Congenital syphilis is diagnosed in three fourths of the cases in patients over 10 years old. Late congenital syphilis may manifest the hutchinsonian triad: Hutchinson's teeth (Figure 15-4), interstitial keratitis, and nerve deafness. Other characteristics include fissuring around the mouth and anus, skeletal lesions, perforation of the palate, and the collapse of nasal bones to produce a saddle-nose deformity.

In 2000, 529 cases of congenital syphilis were reported for a rate of 13.4 per 100,000 live-born infants compared with rates of 14.5 in 1999 and 27.8 in 1997, a 7.6% and 51.8% decrease from 1999 and 1997, respectively. In 2000 racial/ethnic minority populations had the highest rates: 49.3 among African-Americans, 22.6 among Hispanics, 13.2 among American Indians/Alaska Natives, and 5.9 among Asians/Pacific Islanders, compared with 1.5 among non-Hispanic Caucasians. Compared with 1997, these rates represent a decline of 59.7% among African-Americans, 32.5% among Hispanics, 29.8% among Asians/Pacific Islanders, and 58.3% among non-Hispanic Caucasians. Among American Indians/Alaska Natives, the rate increased by 20%; this represented a change from four cases reported in 1997 to five cases in 2000.

In 2000, 83.2% of mothers of infants with congenital syphilis were less than 35 years old, compared with 84.3% in 1997. In 2000 the maternal age group with the highest rate (16.0 per 100,000 live-born infants) of infants with congenital syphilis was adolescent mothers who delivered at an age less than 19 years. This was a decrease of 45.5% from 1997 when the rate was 29.4.

IMMUNOLOGIC MANIFESTATIONS

In the treponemes, two classes of antigen have been recognized: those restricted to one or a few species and those shared by many different spirochetes. Specific and nonspecific antibodies are produced in the immunocompetent host. Specific antibodies against *T. pallidum* and nonspecific antibodies against the protein antigen group common to pathogenic spirochetes are formed. Specific antitreponemal antibodies in early or untreated early latent syphilis are predominantly immunoglobulin (Ig)M antibodies. The early immune response to infection is rapidly followed by the appearance of IgG antibodies, which soon become predominant. The greatest elevation in IgG concentration is seen in secondary syphilis.

Nontreponemal antibodies, often called reagin antibodies, are produced by infected patients against components of their own or other mammalian cells. Although these antibodies are almost always produced by patients with syphilis, they are also produced by patients with other infectious diseases. Infectious diseases in which reagin can be demonstrated include measles, chickenpox, hepatitis, infectious mononucleosis, leprosy, tuberculosis, leptospirosis, malaria, rickettsial disease, trypanosomiasis, and lymphogranuloma venereum. Reagin can also be exhibited by patients with noninfectious conditions such as autoimmune disorders, drug addiction, old age, pregnancy, and recent immunization.

Delayed hypersensitivity immune mechanisms also contribute to the pathophysiology of syphilis. It is suggested that the granulomatous reactions, or gummas, result from delayed hypersensitivity in the immune host. In addition, the manifestations of congenital syphilis apparently result in part from an immune-inflammatory reaction. Antigen-antibody complexes have been detected in the blood of patients with secondary syphilis and are responsible for the syphilis-associated glomerulonephritis. Suppression of the various aspects of cell-mediated immunity have been noted in syphilis and may contribute to prolonged survival of *T. pallidum*.

DIAGNOSTIC EVALUATION

The diagnosis of syphilis depends on clinical skills, demonstration of microorganism in a lesion, and serologic testing. A wide variety of diagnostic procedures for syphilis is available. Classic serologic methods for syphilis measure the presence of two types of antibodies: treponemal and nontreponemal.

Serologic procedures for syphilis include:
- Nontreponemal methods (e.g., VDRL, RPR)
- Treponemal methods (e.g., FTA-ABS and microhemagglutination *T. pallidum* [MHA-TP]).

Darkfield Microscopy

For symptomatic patients with primary syphilis, darkfield microscopy is the test of choice. A darkfield examination is also suggested for immediate results in cases of secondary syphilis with a VDRL titer follow-up test.

Nontreponemal Methods

The RPR is the most widely used nontreponemal serologic procedure, although the classic serologic procedure, the VDRL, continues to be available in some clinical and refer-

ence laboratories. Each is a flocculation (or agglutination) test in which soluble antigen particles coalesce to form larger particles visible as clumps when they are aggregated by antibody.

The VDRL procedure is recommended when a patient suspected of having syphilis has a negative darkfield microscopy result or when atypical lesions are present. It is further recommended that a quantitative VDRL assessment be made quarterly for 1 year after treatment for syphilis, or that the adequacy of treatment in both early and latent syphilis be monitored. The VDRL procedure can be performed on CSF for the detection of neurosyphilis. The RPR test can be performed on unheated serum or plasma using a modified VDRL antigen suspension of choline chloride with ethylenediaminetetraacetic acid (EDTA). The RPR card test antigen also contains charcoal for macroscopic reading. There are three versions of the RPR test. The original RPR method used unmeasured amounts of plasma and was used as a field procedure for screening large numbers of people. It was about 10% more reactive than the VDRL slide test. The modified RPR uses the unheated serum reagin test and is performed on measured volumes of unheated serum. This version has a somewhat lower level of reactivity than the VDRL slide test. The RPR (circle) card test uses unheated serum, and less frequently plasma, for testing. It is about as specific as, and possibly more sensitive than, the VDRL slide test.

Treponemal Methods

The FTA-ABS and MHA represent treponemal methods. The *T. pallidum* immobilization (TPI) test is obsolete. Reactive (positive) reagin tests can be confirmed with these two specific treponemal antigen tests. These procedures, however, should not be used as primary screening methods. Procedures such as the FTA-ABS and MHA can be used to confirm that a positive nontreponemal test result has been caused by syphilis rather than one of the other biologic conditions that can produce a positive VDRL; or they can determine quantitative titers of antibody, which is useful for following response to therapy. An enzyme-linked immunosorbent assay (ELISA) procedure for syphilis antibody is available, but it is not widely used at present. The ELISA method, however, does offer a sensitive and specific alternative to existing methods.

The FTA-ABS uses a killed suspension *of T. pallidum* spirochetes as the antigen. This procedure is performed by overlaying whole treponemes fixed to a slide with serum from patients suspected of having syphilis because of a previously positive VDRL or RPR test. The patient's serum is first absorbed with non–*T. pallidum* treponemal antigens to reduce nonspecific cross-reactivity. Fluorescein-conjugated antihuman antibody reagent is then applied as a marker for specific antitreponemal antibodies in the patient's serum.

The microhemagglutination assay for *T. pallidum* is based on agglutination by specific antibodies in the patient's serum with sheep erythrocytes sensitized to *T. pallidum* antigen. The MHA method uses treated red cells coated with treponemal antigens from a turkey or other animal. The presence of specific antibody produces red cell agglutination exhibited by the formation of a flat mat across the bottom of a microdilution well in which the test is performed. If their VDRL is positive, selected asymptomatic persons (including all pregnant women, persons with proven contacts, and persons in demonstrated high-risk groups) should be tested with the MHA-TP.

TABLE 15-2	Sensitivity of Commonly Used Serologic Tests for Syphilis		
		Stage	
Test*	**Primary**	**Secondary**	**Late**
Nontreponemal (Reagin Tests)			
Venereal Disease Research Laboratories (VDRL)	70%	99%	1%†
Rapid Plasma Reagin (RPR)	80%	99%	
Automated reagin test (ART)			0%
Specific Treponemal Tests			
Fluorescent treponemal antibody absorption test (FTA-ABS)	85%	100%	95%
T. pallidum hemagglutination assay (TPHA-TP)	65%	100%	95%
Treponemal immobilization (TPI)	50%	97%	

From Tramont E: *Treponema pallidum.* In Mandell GL, Douglas RG Jr, Bennett JE, editors: *Principles and practice of infectious diseases,* ed 2, New York, 1985, John Wiley & Sons.
*Percentage of patients with positive serologic tests in treated or untreated primary or secondary syphilis.
†Treated late syphilis.

Sensitivity of Commonly Used Serologic Tests for Syphilis

Detection of syphilis by serologic methods is related both to the stage of the disease and to the test method (Table 15-2). In the primary stage, about 30% of cases become serologically active after 1 week, and 90% of patients demonstrate reactivity after 3 weeks. Reagin titers increase rapidly during the first 4 weeks of infection and then remain stationary for approximately 6 months. Patients in the secondary stage of syphilis are serologically positive. During latent syphilis there is a gradual return of nonreactive serologic manifestations with nontreponemal method. About one third of patients in the latent stage will remain seroreactive and presumably infectious. In late syphilis, treponemal tests are generally reactive; nontreponemal methods are nonreactive.

SYPHILIS SEROLOGY

■ *Venereal Disease Research Laboratory (VDRL) Qualitative Slide Test*

Principle

During the period of infection with syphilis, reagin, a substance with the properties of an antibody, appears in the serum of affected patients. Reagin has the ability to combine with a colloidal suspension extracted from animal tissue and clump together to form visible masses, a process known as flocculation.

In the VDRL procedure the patient's heat-inactivated serum is mixed with a buffered saline suspension of cardiolipin-lecithin-cholesterol antigen. This serum-antigen mixture is microscopically examined for flocculation. Positive or reactive sera can be serially diluted and titrated. Syphilis and disorders such as pinta, yaws, bejel, and other treponemal diseases can produce positive reactions.

Specimen Collection and Preparation

No special preparation of the patient is required before specimen collection. The patient must be positively identified when the specimen is collected. The specimen is to be labeled at the bedside and must include the patient's full name, date the specimen is collected, and patient's hospital identification number. The phlebotomist's initials should also appear on the label.

Blood should be drawn by an aseptic technique. The required specimen is a minimum of 2 mL of clotted blood (red top evacuated tube). The specimen should be promptly centrifuged and an aliquot of the serum removed. Severely lipemic or hemolyzed serum is unsuitable for testing. Before testing, the serum must be heat inactivated at 56° C for 30 minutes. Inactivated serum should be reheated at 56° C for 10 minutes if tested more than 4 hours after the original inactivation.

Cerebrospinal fluid is also an appropriate fluid for testing.

Reagents, Supplies, and Equipment

1. VDRL antigen—a colorless, alcoholic solution containing 0.03% cardiolipin, 0.9% cholesterol, and sufficient purified lecithin to produce standard reactivity. Each lot must be serologically standardized by comparison with an antigen of known reactivity. Ampules should be stored in the dark at either 6° to 10° C or at room temperature. Antigen that contains precipitate should be discarded.
2. VDRL-buffered saline contains 1% sodium chloride, pH 6.0 ± 0.1, available commercially. pH must be checked—discard if out of range, then store in screw-capped or glass-stoppered bottles.

Working Antigen Suspension

NOTE: The temperature of the buffered saline and antigen should be in the range of 23° to 29° C. The antigen suspension must be used on the day of preparation.

1. Add 0.4 mL of buffered saline to the bottom of the 30-mL, round, glass-stoppered bottle.
2. Rapidly add 0.5 mL of antigen drop by drop (from the lower half of 1-mL pipette graduated to the tip) directly to the saline while continuously and gently rotating the bottle in a circular motion on a flat surface. The pipette tip should remain in upper third of the bottle. Take care to avoid splashing saline on the pipette. Blow the last drop of antigen from the pipette without touching the pipette to the saline.
3. Continue to rotate the bottle for 10 seconds.
4. Add 4.1 mL of buffered saline from a 5-mL pipette.
5. Place the top on the bottle and shake up and down approximately 30 times in 10 seconds. The antigen suspension is ready for use, but it must be gently mixed at the time of use. Do not force back and forth through the needle and syringe. NOTE: A double volume of antigen may be prepared.
   a. Water bath, 56° C.
   b. Mechanical rotator (180-rpm) that circumscribes a circle three-fourths inch in a diameter on a horizontal plane.
   c. 18-gauge hypodermic needle without bevel (this will deliver 60 drops/mL reagent).
   d. Syringe, Lure type, 1 or 2 mL.
   e. Slides with ceramic rings (14 mm in diameter).
   f. Flat-bottom glass bottle (30 mL) with narrow mouth (35 mm in diameter).

Quality Control

1. Include positive control sera of graded reactivity each time serologic testing is performed. The antigen suspension to be used each day is first examined with these control sera. Store control sera frozen at −20° C or liquid form for 7 to 10 days. Thaw, mix thoroughly, and heat inactivate at 56° C before use.
2. Check antigen-dispensing needle at the time of use to be sure that it accurately delivers 60 drops/mL reagent. Clean needles and syringes by rinsing with water, alcohol, and acetone. Remove needle from syringe after cleaning.

Procedure

NOTE: The test should be performed at a temperature range of 23° to 29° C.
1. Pipette 0.5 mL of inactivated patient serum into one of the rings of the ceramic-ringed slide. Pipette additional specimens and controls into additional rings.
2. Add 1 drop of antigen suspension to each serum with a calibrated 18-gauge needle and syringe held in a vertical position.
3. Rotate the slide on a mechanical rotator for 4 minutes. In extremely dry climates cover the slides with a lid containing moistened filter paper to prevent evaporation during rotation.
4. Examine each specimen microscopically with the low (10 ×) objective.

Reporting Results

Nonreactive: no clumping or very slight roughness
Weakly reactive: small clumps
Reactive: medium and large clumps

Procedure Notes
Sources of Error

False-negative reactions can occur in a variety of situations. These conditions include:
1. Technical error (e.g., unsatisfactory antigen or technique).
2. Low antibody titers. Patients may have syphilis, but the reagin concentration is too low to produce a reactive test result. A low concentration of reagin may be caused by several factors: an infection that is too recent to have produced antibodies; the effects of treatment; latent or inactive disease; or patients who have not produced protective antibodies because of immunologic tolerance. These seronegative patients may demonstrate a positive reaction with more sensitive treponemal tests such as the FTA-ABS.
3. The presence of inhibitors in the patient's serum.
4. Reduced ambient temperature (below 23° to 29° C).
5. Prozone reaction.

A prozone reaction is encountered occasionally. This type of reaction is demonstrated when complete or partial inhibition of reactivity occurs with undiluted serum, and minimal reactivity is obtained only with diluted serum. The prozone phenomenon may be so pronounced that only a weakly reactive or rough nonreactive result is produced in the qualitative test by a serum that will be strongly reactive when diluted. It is recommended that all sera producing weak reaction or rough nonreactive results in qualitative testing be retested with a quantitative procedure before a final report of the VDRL slide test is issued.

Weakly reactive results can be caused by:
1. Very early infection
2. Lessening of the activity of the disease after treatment
3. Improper technique or questionable reagents

False-positive reactions can also be observed. Of all positive serologic tests for syphilis, 10% to 30% may be false biologic positive reactions. Nonsyphilitic positive VDRL reactions have been reported with cardiolipin type of antigen in:
1. Lupus erythematosus
2. Rheumatic fever
3. Vaccinia and viral pneumonia
4. Pneumococcal pneumonia
5. Infectious mononucleosis
6. Infectious hepatitis
7. Leprosy
8. Malaria
9. Rheumatoid arthritis
10. Pregnancy
11. Aging individuals

Contaminated or hemolyzed specimens can also produce false-positive results.

Clinical Applications

The purpose of the VDRL procedure is to demonstrate reagin in cases of syphilis. The procedure may also be positive in treponemal diseases such as yaws and pinta. Reagin, however, is found in some patients who are not infected with treponemes, which can be partially explained by the necrotizing effect of spirochetes on tissues and in other conditions and disorders. It is important that results of the VDRL procedure be correlated with patient history, as well as with signs and symptoms.

Limitations

The VDRL procedure is not specific for syphilis but may demonstrate positive reactions in other reagin-producing disorders, autoimmune disorders, infectious diseases, and alterations such as pregnancy or aging in normal physiology.

References

Nicholas L: In Friedman J, Linna TJ, Prier JE, editors: *Immunoserology in the diagnosis of infectious diseases,* Baltimore, 1979, University Park Press.

Olansky S: In Samter M, Alexander HL, editors: *Immunological diseases,* Boston, 1965, Little Brown.

 VDRL Quantitative Slide Test

Principle

Retest quantitatively to an end-point titer all sera that produce reactive, weakly reactive, or questionably nonreactive results in the qualitative VDRL slide test.

Specimen Collection and Preparation

See VDRL qualitative procedure for collecting and processing original undiluted sera.

Preparation of Serial Dilutions

Serial dilutions of serum are prepared as follows:

1. Pipette 0.05 mL of 0.9% saline into ring numbers 2, 3, and 4 on ceramic slide (Figure 15-5). Do not spread the saline.
2. Pipette 0.05 mL of serum to ring numbers 1 and 2. Draw the serum and saline mixture up and down in the pipette tip in ring number 2 to mix. Aspirate 0.05 mL of diluted serum and spread the remaining dilution over the entire area of the circle with the pipette tip.
3. Transfer 0.05 mL of the diluted (1:2) serum in ring number 2 to ring number 3. Draw the serum and saline mixture up and down in the pipette tip in ring number 3 to mix. Aspirate 0.05 mL of diluted serum and spread the remaining dilution over the entire area of the circle with the pipette tip.
4. Transfer 0.05 mL of the diluted (1:4) serum in ring number 3 to ring number 4. Draw the serum and saline mixture up and down in the pipette tip in ring number 3 to mix. Aspirate 0.05 mL of diluted serum and spread the remaining dilution over the entire area of the circle with the pipette tip.

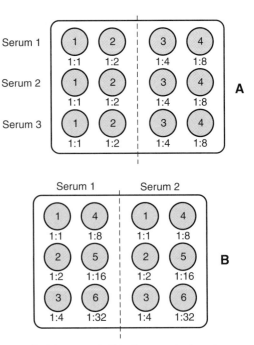

Figure 15-5 **A,** Diagram of slide for quantitative, three-serum, VDRL slide test. **B,** Diagram of slide for quantitative, two-serum VDRL slide test. (Redrawn from Bauer JD: *Clinical laboratory methods,* ed 9, St Louis, 1982, Mosby.)

5. Discard 0.05 mL of the diluted (1:8) serum from ring number 4 unless greater dilutions are needed for strongly reactive serum, and spread the remaining dilution over the entire area of the circle with the pipette tip.

Reagents, Supplies, and Equipment

In addition to reagents, supplies, and equipment required for the qualitative VDRL, the following reagent and piece of equipment are needed:

1. 0.9% saline. Prepare by weighing 0.9 g of sodium chloride (chemical grade) to a 1-L volumetric flask. Dilute to the calibration mark with distilled water.
2. Safety pipette (50 mL or 0.05 mL).

Quality Control (See VDRL Qualitative Procedure)

NOTE: The test should be performed at a temperature range of 23° to 29° C.

1. Add 1 drop of antigen suspension to each diluted serum with a calibrated 18-gauge needle and syringe held in a vertical position.
2. Rotate the slide on a mechanical rotator for 4 minutes. In extremely dry climates, the slides may be covered with a lid containing moistened filter paper to prevent evaporation during rotation.
3. Examine each specimen microscopically (low [10 ×] objective).

Reporting Results

Report the titer in terms of the highest dilution that produces a reactive (not weakly reactive) result. Example:

Serum Dilutions				Result
1:1	1:2	1:4	1:8	
Reactive	Reactive	Weakly reactive	Nonreactive	Reactive, 1:4 dilution or 4 dilutions

Clinical Applications

See VDRL qualitative procedure.

References

See VDRL qualitative procedure.

 VDRL Qualitative Slide Test (Cerebrospinal Fluid)

Principle

See VDRL qualitative procedure.

Specimen Collection and Preparation

Centrifuge and decant the specimen. Spinal fluids that are visibly contaminated or that contain gross blood are unsatisfactory for testing. Specimens of spinal fluid do not need to be heat inactivated before testing.

Reagents, Supplies, and Equipment

See VDRL qualitative procedure for required materials.

Preparation of Working Antigen Suspension

1. Prepare antigen suspension as described for VDRL qualitative slide test.
2. Mix 1 part 10% saline to 1 part VDRL slide test suspension.
3. Mix by gently rotating bottle or inverting tube, and allow to stand for at least 5 minutes but no more than 2 hours before use.

Additional Supplies

1. 22- or 23-gauge hypodermic needle, without bevel. The needle and syringe should dispense 100 ± 2 drops of sensitized antigen suspension per milliliter when the needle and syringe are held vertically.
2. 10% saline. Prepare 10 g sodium chloride/100 mL distilled water.
3. Test slides (2 × 3 inches with concavity measuring 16 mm in diameter and 1.75 mm in depth).

Quality Control

See VDRL qualitative procedure.

Procedure

NOTE: The test should be performed at a temperature range of 23° to 29° C.
1. Pipette 0.05 mL of spinal fluid into a concavity of the slide.
2. Add 1 drop (0.01 mL) of the working antigen suspension to the specimen from a 21- or 22-gauge needle and syringe held in a vertical position.
3. Rotate the slide for 8 minutes on a mechanical rotator at 180 rpm. In extremely dry climates the slides may be covered with a slide containing moistened filter paper to prevent evaporation during rotation.
4. Microscopically examine the slide on low (10×) power.

Reporting Results

Nonreactive: no clumping or very slight roughness
Reactive: definite clumps
A quantitative test should be performed on any reactive specimen.

Clinical Applications

See VDRL qualitative procedure.

References

See VDRL qualitative procedure.

 VDRL Quantitative Slide Test (Cerebrospinal Fluid)

Principle

See VDRL qualitative slide test.

Specimen Collection and Preparation

Diluted Spinal Fluid

Prepare the dilutions as follows:
1. Pipette 0.2 mL of 0.9% saline into each of five or more tubes.
2. Add 0.2 mL of unheated spinal fluid to tube 1, mix, transfer to tube 2.
3. Continue mixing and transferring 0.2 mL from one tube to the next until the last tube is reached. Dilutions: 1:2, 1:4, 1:8, 1:16, 1:32.

Reagents, Supplies, and Equipment

See VDRL qualitative slide test (spinal fluid.)

Quality Control

See VDRL qualitative slide test (spinal fluid).

Examples of Serum Dilutions					Result
1:1	1:2	1:4	1:8	1:16	Reactive,
Reactive	Reactive	Reactive	Reactive	Nonreactive	1:8 dilution
					or 8 dilutions

Procedure

Treat each dilution as if it were undiluted spinal fluid and see VDRL qualitative slide test (spinal fluid) for the procedural protocol.

Reporting Results

Report the titer in terms of the highest dilution that produces a reactive (not weakly reactive) result. See example above.

Clinical Applications

See VDRL qualitative slide test (spinal fluid).

References

See VDRL qualitative procedure.

 Rapid Plasma Reagin (RPR) Card Test

Principle

The RPR test is designed to detect reagin, an antibody-like substance present in serum. In this procedure, serum is mixed with an antigen suspension of a carbon particle cardiolipin antigen. If the specimen contains antibody, flocculation occurs with a coagglutination of the carbon particles of antigen. This flocculation appears as black clumps against the white background of a plastic-coated card. The cards are viewed macroscopically.

This is a nontreponemal testing procedure for the serologic detection of syphilis; however, pinta, yaws, bejel, and other treponemal diseases may produce positive results. Positive reactions are occasionally observed with other acute or chronic conditions.

Specimen Collection and Preparation

No special preparation of the patient is required before specimen collection. The patient must be positively identified when the specimen is collected. The specimen is to be labeled at the bedside and must include the patient's full name, the date the specimen is collected, and the patient's hospital identification number. The phlebotomist's initials should also appear on the label.

Blood should be drawn by an aseptic technique. The required specimen is a minimum of 2 mL of clotted blood (red top evacuated tube). After allowing the blood to clot, centrifuge the specimen and allow the serum to remain in the original tube. Severely lipemic or hemolyzed serum is unsuitable for testing.

NOTE: In special situations when nontreponemal test results are needed rapidly and the specimen is collected in EDTA anticoagulant, plasma can be used for both qualitative and quantitative procedures if the test is performed within 24 hours. Store the specimen at 2° to 8° C and centrifuge before testing.

Reagents, Supplies, and Equipment

NOTE: Except for the antigen, all other components should be stored at room temperature in a dry place in the original kit packaging.

1. The following components are provided in Macro-Vue RPR Card Test Kit.*
   a. RPR card test antigen. This antigen suspension is similar to VDRL antigen: cardiolipin, lecithin, cholesterol, EDTA, Na_2HPO_4, KH_2PO_4, thimerosal (preservative), charcoal, choline chloride, and distilled water.

      If the ampule of antigen is frozen during shipment, it can be reconstituted once by warming to room temperature. Avoid repeated freezing and thawing.

      Store the antigen suspension in ampules or in the plastic dispensing bottle at 2° to 8° C. Unopened ampules have a shelf life of 12 months from the date of manufacture. Before opening, shake the ampule vigorously for 10 to 15 seconds to resuspend the antigen and dispense any carbon particles that may have become lodged in the neck of the ampule. If any carbon should remain in the neck of the ampule after this shaking, no additional effort should be made to dislodge it, as this will only tend to produce a coarse antigen.

      To prepare the antigen, attach the needle to the tapered fitting on the plastic dispensing bottle. Be sure the antigen is below the break line; snap the ampule neck and withdraw all of the antigen into the dispensing bottle by collapsing the bottle and using it as a suction device. Shake the card antigen dispensing bottle gently before each series of antigen droppings. The needle and dispensing bottle should be discarded when the kit reagents are depleted.

      Once the antigen ampule is opened and placed in the dispensing bottle, it is stable for 3 months or the expiration date on the label (if it occurs sooner) if refrigerated at 2° to 8° C. Label dispensing bottle with antigen lot num-

---

*Macro-Vue RPR Card Tests, 18 mm Circle, Brewer Diagnostic Kits Product Insert, BBL Microbiology Systems, Cockeysville, MD.

ber, expiration date, and date antigen is placed in bottle.

Immediate use of refrigerated antigen may result in decreased sensitivity in testing. Allow the antigen to warm to room temperature (23° to 29° C) before use. Do not use beyond expiration date. Avoid bright sunlight.

b. Needle, 18-gauge, without bevel. The needles should deliver 60 ± 2 drops of antigen suspension per milliliter when held in a vertical position. Take care to obtain drops of uniform size. On completion of tests, remove needle from dispensing bottle and rinse needle with distilled or deionized water. Do not wipe needle because this will remove the silicone coating and may affect the accuracy of the drop of antigen being dispensed.

c. Specially prepared, plastic-coated cards, each with ten 18-mm circle spots designed for use with RPR card antigen. Take care not to finger-mark the test areas on the card, as this may result in an oily deposit and improper test results. Avoid scratching the card when spreading the specimen. If the specimen does not spread to the outer perimeter of the test area, use another test area of the card.

d. Dispenstirs, 0.05 mL/drop.

e. Capillary pipettes, 0.05-mL capacity or the following pipettes: 0.2 mL (graduated in 0.01-mL subdivisions), 0.5 mL (graduated in 0.01-mL subdivisions), or 1.0 mL (graduated in 0.01-mL subdivisions). Dispenstirs are provided with the kit for use with the 18-mm circle qualitative test; however, these stirrers may be used only to transfer a specimen to the card surface. New Dispenstirs or capillary tubes must be used for each specimen. Take care to avoid drawing specimen up into the rubber ball attached to the capillary tube.

f. Rubber bulbs.

g. Stirrers.

2. Rotator (100-rpm) circumscribing a circle 2 cm in diameter on a horizontal plane.

3. Humidifier cover containing a moistened sponge.

4. 0.9% saline (for quantitative test). Prepare by adding 0.9 g of sodium chloride (ACS) to 100 mL of distilled water.

Quality Control

1. Controls with established patterns of graded reactivity should be included in each day's testing to confirm optimal reactivity of the antigen suspension. Control sera must be at 23° to 29° C at the time of testing.

CAUTION: Because the control sera are derived from human sources, they should be handled in the same manner as clinical serum.

Serum that is nonreactive to syphilis in 0.9% saline is required for diluting test specimens, producing a reactive result at the 1:16 dilution.

2. A new lot of antigen should be compared with an antigen suspension of known reactivity before being used.

3. The calibration of the delivery needle is an important aspect of quality control. An 18-gauge needle delivers 60 ± 2 drops/mL of reagent. Place the needle on a 2-mL syringe or a 1-mL pipette. Fill the syringe or pipette with the antigen suspension and, holding it in a vertical position, count the number of drops delivered in 0.5 mL. The needle is considered to be satisfactory if 30 ± 1 drops are obtained from 0.5 mL of suspension.

Procedure

Preliminary testing of antigen suspension (see antigen description under Reagents, Supplies, and Equipment).

1. Attach needle hub to tapered fitting on plastic dispensing bottle. Shake antigen ampule to resuspend antigen particles, snap ampule neck at the break line, and withdraw all the RPR card antigen suspension into the dispensing bottle by suction, collapsing the bottle and using it as a bulb. Shake dispenser gently before each series of antigen drops is delivered.

2. Test control sera of graded reactivity each day.

Procedure

1. Place 0.05 mL of unheated serum on an 18-mm circle of the test card with a capillary or serologic pipette. Hold the dispensers in a vertical position directly over the card test area to which the specimen is to be delivered. Do not touch card surface.

2. Spread serum in the circle with an inverted Dispenstir (closed end), stirrer (broad end), or serologic pipette to fill the entire circle. Care must be taken not to scratch the card surface.

3. Gently shake antigen-dispensing bottle before use. Holding it in a vertical position, dispense several drops into the dispensing bottle cap to make sure the needle passage is clear. Add exactly 1 free-falling drop (1/60 mL) or RPR antigen suspension from the 20-gauge (yellow hub) needle to each test area containing serum. Do not stir; mixing is accomplished during rotation.

4. Place card on rotator and cover with humidifier cover. NOTE: The Macro-Vue RPR Card Test (Teardrop Qualitative) Brewer Diagnostic Kit (Hynson, Westcott & Dunning, Div. of Becton Dickinson, Baltimore) can be hand rocked and used where laboratory equipment is not available.

5. Rotate 8 minutes at 100 rpm (95 to 110 rpm acceptable) on mechanical rotator. If below or above range, there is a tendency for the clumping antigen to be less intense in test with undiluted specimen, so that some minimal reactions may be missed.

6. Observe each specimen immediately in the "wet" state under a high-intensity incandescent lamp or strong daylight. Observation should be without magnification. It is permissible to gently rotate or tilt the card by hand (three or four times) to differentiate minimally reactive from nonreactive specimens.

7. Specimens producing questionable reactions should be retested by this method and other serologic methods.

8. When testing is completed, the work area should be cleaned. The dispensing needle should be rinsed in distilled water and air-dried. Avoid wiping the needle because this will remove the silicone coating. Recap the antigen solution and store in the refrigerator.

Reporting Results

Reactive: slight to large agglutination (black clumps)
Nonreactive: no agglutination, or very slight roughness (even light-gray color)

Procedure Notes

All reactive tests should be retested using the quantitative procedure to establish a baseline from which changes in titer can be determined, particularly for evaluating treatment. It is desirable to quantitate specimens that are nonreactive-rough so that an infrequent zonal specimen may be revealed.

18-mm Circle Quantitative Card Test

1. For each specimen to be tested, place 0.05 mL of 0.9% saline onto circle numbers 2 to 5 with a capillary or serologic pipette.

2. Pipette 0.05 mL of serum onto circle number 1 and 0.05 mL of serum onto circle number 2.

3. Prepare a serial twofold dilution by drawing the mixture up and down (avoid formation of bubbles). Transfer 0.05 mL of the dilution to the next circle and repeat procedure to circle number 5. Discard 0.05 mL of the dilution from circle number 5.

4. Beginning with the most dilute specimen (circle number 5), spread the dilution to fill the entire surface of the circle. Use a new stirrer for each circle.

5. Proceed with steps 3 through 8 in the qualitative procedure described above.

Reporting Results

Report the highest dilution producing a minimal to moderate reaction (i.e., circle 1 = 1:1 undiluted, circle 2 = 1:2, circle 3 = 1:4, circle 4 = 1:8, and circle 5 = 1:16). If the 1:16 is reactive, prepare a 1:50 dilution with nonreactive serum in 0.9% saline. This preparation is to be used to prepare subsequent serial dilutions. Pipette 0.05 mL of 1:50 nonreactive serum into each of the circles 2 to 5, pipette 0.05 mL of the 1:16 dilution of test specimen in circle 1, and prepare and test the specimen as described in step 3 above.

Sources of Error

Error can be introduced into test results because of factors such as contamination of rubber bulbs or an improperly prepared antigen suspension.

False-positive biologic reactions have been reported with cardiolipin type of antigens in the following conditions:

1. Lupus erythematosus
2. Rheumatic fever
3. Vaccinia and viral pneumonia
4. Pneumococcal pneumonia
5. Infectious mononucleosis
6. Infectious hepatitis
7. Leprosy
8. Malaria
9. Rheumatoid arthritis
10. Pregnancy
11. Aging individuals

False-negative reactions can result from

1. Poor technique
2. Ineffective reagents
3. Improper rotation

If mechanical rotation is below or above the 95- to 110-rpm acceptable range, there is a tendency for the clumping of the antigen to be less intense in procedures with undiluted specimen, so that some minimal reactions may be missed. In quantitative tests, rotation above 110 rpm tends to produce a decrease in titer—approximately 1 dilution lower.

Clinical Applications

See VDRL qualitative procedure.

Limitations

A diagnosis of syphilis cannot be made based on a single reactive result without clinical signs and symptoms or history. Plasma specimens should not be used to establish a quantitative baseline from which changes in titer can be determined, particularly for evaluating treatment.

RPR cards should not be used for testing CSF. Little reliance should be placed on cord blood serologic testing for syphilis. The RPR procedure has adequate sensitivity and specificity in relation to clinical diagnosis and a reactivity level similar to that of the VDRL slide test.

Reference

Manual of tests for syphilis, Public Health Service Publication, No. 411, 1969.

 FTA-ABS (Fluorescent Treponema pallidum Antibody Absorption Test)

Principle

The FTA-ABS test is a direct method of observation. Although not recommended for screening, it is the most sensitive serologic procedure in the detection of primary syphilis.

Specimen Collection and Preparation

No special preparation of the patient is required before specimen collection. The patient must be positively identified when the specimen is collected. The specimen is to be labeled at the bedside and must include the patient's full name, date the specimen is collected, and patient's hospital identification number. The phlebotomist's initials should also appear on the label.

Blood should be drawn by an aseptic technique. The required specimen is a minimum of 2 mL of clotted blood (red top evacuated tube). The specimen should be centrifuged and the serum removed from the clot. Before testing, the serum should be heated at 56° C for 30 minutes if never inactivated, or for 10 minutes at 56° C if inactivated more than 4 hours before testing. Evidence of hemolysis or bacterial contamination makes the specimen unsuitable for testing.

Reagents, Supplies, and Equipment

1. *T. pallidum* antigen. The antigen for this test is a suspension of *T. pallidum* (Nicols strain) extracted from rabbit testicular tissue, containing a minimum of 30 organisms per high dry field. The antigen may be stored at 6° to 10° C or may be processed by lyophilization. Lyophilized antigen is also stored at 6° to 10° C and is reconstituted for use according to direction when needed. Any antigen that becomes bacterially contaminated or does not give the appropriate reactions with control sera must be discarded. Preparation of *T. pallidum* antigen slides is as follows:
   a. Mix the antigen suspension with a disposable pipette and rubber bulb, drawing the suspension into and expelling it from the pipette at least 10 times to break the treponemal clumps and to ensure an even distribution of treponemes. Check by darkfield examination for even distribution. Additional mixing may be required.
   b. Place one loopful of *T. pallidum* antigen suspension on a glass slide with a wire loop. Spread the suspension into a circle about 1 cm in diameter.
   c. Allow to air-dry for at least 15 minutes.
   d. Fix the smears in acetone for 10 minutes and allow them to air-dry. No more than 60 slides should be fixed with each 200 mL of acetone.
   e. After the slides are thoroughly dry, the smears should be stored in a freezer at −20° C or lower. Fixed, frozen smears can be used indefinitely if satisfactory results are achieved with controls. Antigen smears cannot be thawed and refrozen.
2. FTA-ABS tests sorbent. This is a standardized product prepared from culture of Reiter treponemes. It may be purchased lyophilized or in liquid state and should be stored according to the manufacturer's directions.
3. Fluorescein-labeled antihuman globulin (conjugate). This should be proven quality for FTA-ABS test. Each new lot of conjugate should be tested to ensure its dependability with respect to working titer and to verify that it meets the criteria concerning nonspecific staining and standard reactivity. The lyophilized conjugate should be stored at 6° to 10° C. Rehydrated conjugate should be dispensed in not less than 0.3 mL-quantities and should be stored at −38° C or lower. For practical purposes, a conjugate with a working titer of 1:400 or higher may be diluted 1:10 with sterile phosphate-buffered saline (containing Merthiolate in a concentration of 1:5,000 before storage). When conjugate is thawed for use, it should not be refrozen but should be stored at 6° to 10° C. It may then be used as long as acceptable reactivity is obtained with test controls. If a change in FTA-ABS test reactivity is noted in routine testing, the conjugate should be retitered to determine whether this is the contributing factor.

   CONJUGATE: Prepare serial doubling dilutions of the new conjugate in phosphate-buffered saline (PBS) containing 2% Tween-80 to include the titer indicated by the manufacturer. Examples are the following: (1) 1:2.5, 1:5, 1:10, 1:20, 1:40, 1:80, 1:160; or (2) 1:12.5, 1:25, 1:50, 1:100, 1:200, 1:400, 1:800. Prepare higher dilutions if necessary.

   Test each conjugate dilution with the reactive (4+) control serum diluted 1:5 with PBS (follow the procedure below). Include a nonspecific staining control with each conjugate dilution. A standard conjugate, at its titer, is set up at the same time with a reactive (4+) control serum, a minimally reactive (1+) control serum, and a nonspecific staining control with PBS for the purpose of controlling reagents and test conditions. Table 15-3 illustrates the titration of a new conjugate.

   Read slides in the following order:
   a. Examine the three control slides to ensure that the reagents and testing conditions are satisfactory.
   b. Examine the slides with new conjugate, starting with the lowest dilution of conjugate.
   c. Record readings as graded reactions from negative to 4+.

   The end point of the titration is the highest dilution giving maximal (4+) fluorescence. The working titer of the new conjugate is one doubling dilution below the end point. In Table 15-3, the dilution selected for the working titer is 1:200. The new conjugate should not stain nonspecifically at three doubling dilutions below the working titer of the conjugate. In Table 15-2 the conjugate would meet this criterion, since there is no nonspecific staining with the 1:25 dilution.

   Dispense conjugate in not less than 0.3-mL quantities and store at −20° C or lower. For

TABLE 15-3 New Conjugate Titration

Conjugate	Nonspecific Staining Control (PRS)	Reactive (4+) Control Serum (dil. 1:5)	Reactive (4+) Control Serum
Standard Titer			
1:400	Negative	4+	1+
New Conjugate Titer			
1:12.5	1+	4+	
1:25	Negative	4+	
1:50	Negative	4+	
1:100	Negative	4+	
1:200	Negative	4+	
1:400	Negative	4+	
1:800	Negative	3+	

practical purposes, a conjugate with a working titer of 1:400 or higher may be diluted 1:10 with sterile PBS containing thimerosal (Merthiolate in a concentration of 1:5000) before storage in the freezer. Verify the titer of the conjugate after at least 3 days of storage in the freezer.

CHECK TESTING: If the criterion of acceptability for the nonspecific staining has been met and a working titer has been determined, the new conjugate should be check-tested in parallel with a standard conjugate before being placed in routine use. Testing should be performed on more than one testing day with control sera, individual sera of graded reactivity, and nonreactive sera. Individual sera tested parallel with a standard and a new conjugate are read against the minimally reactive (1+) controls set up with the respective conjugates. A new conjugate is considered to be satisfactory when comparable test results are obtained with both conjugates.

4. PBS, pH 7.2 ± 0.1. Prepare, per liter of distilled water, 7.65 g NaCl, 0.724 g Na_2HPO_4, 0.21 g KH_2PO_4.
5. 2% Tween-80, pH 7.0 to 7.2. Prepare heat PBS and Tween-80 in 56° C water bath. To 98 mL of PBS, add 2 mL of Tween-80. Refrigerate to store. Discard if precipitate forms or if pH is outside the acceptable range (check pH periodically).
6. Mounting medium consisting of one PBS, pH 7.2, plus 9 parts glycerin (reagent quality).
7. Acetone (ACS).
8. Pipettes
9. 12 × 75 test tubes
10. 35° to 37° C incubator
11. Darkfield fluorescent microscope assembly
12. Bibulous paper
13. Slide holder
14. Moist chamber
15. Loop—bacteriologic, standard 2-mm, 26-gauge platinum wire loop

TABLE 15-4 Control Pattern Examples

Control	Reaction
Reactive	
1:5 PBS dilution	Reactive (4+)
1:5 Sorbent dilution	Reactive (3+ to 4+)
Minimally Reactive (1+)	
Nonspecific serum	Reactive (1+)
1:5 PBS dilution	Reactive (2+ to 4+)
1:5 Sorbent dilution	Nonreactive
Nonspecific Staining	
Antigen, PBS and conjugate	Nonreactive
Antigen, sorbent and conjugate	Nonreactive

16. Oil-immersion, low-fluorescence, nondrying
17. Microscope slides—1 × 3 inch
18. Cover slips
19. Dish-stains, glass or plastic with removable slide carriers
20. Glass stirring rods

Quality Control

Control sera must be run concurrently with each set of patient specimens (Table 15-4). Controls should be prepared as follows: reactive (4+) control. This control should demonstrate 4+ fluorescence when diluted 1:5 in PBS and only slightly reduced fluorescence when diluted 1:5 in sorbent. These controls are prepared as follows:

1. PBS dilution. Pipette 0.2 mL of PBS into a small test tube. Add 0.2 mL of reactive (4+) control serum. Mix.
2. Sorbent dilution. Pipette 0.2 mL of sorbent into a small test tube. Add 0.2 mL of reactive (4+) control serum. Mix.

Minimal (1+) Control

Dilutions of reactive serum demonstrating the minimal degree of fluorescence report as reactive for use as a reading standard. The 4+ reactive control may be used for this control when diluted in PBS.

Nonspecific Serum Control

A nonsyphilis serum known to demonstrate at least 2+ nonspecific reactivity in the FTA-ABS test at a dilution of PBS of 1:5 or higher should be used. Prepare as follows:

1. PBS dilution. Pipette 0.2 mL of PBS into a small test tube. Add 0.05 mL of nonspecific control serum. Mix.
2. Sorbent dilution. Pipette 0.2 mL of sorbent into a small test tube. Add 0.05 mL of nonspecific control serum. Mix. Nonspecific staining controls:
   a. Antigen smear treated with 0.03 mL of PBS
   b. Antigen smear treated with 0.03 mL of sorbent

Controls 1, 3, and 4 are included for the purpose of controlling reagents and test conditions. Control 2 (minimally reactive control serum) is included as the reading standard.

Each new lot of reagents should be tested in parallel with reagents that give satisfactory results before being used.

T. Pallidum Antigen

A new lot of antigen should be compared with a standard antigen before being placed in routine use. Testing should be performed on more than one testing day with control sera, individual sera of graded reactivity, and nonreactive sera.

A sufficient number of organisms should remain on the slide after staining so that tests may be read without difficulty. The antigen should not contain background material that stains so as to interfere with the reading of the tests. The antigen should not stain nonspecifically with a standard conjugate as its working titer. Reportable test results on controls and individual sera should be comparable with those obtained with the standard antigen.

FTA-ABS Test Sorbent

A new lot of sorbent should be compared with a standard sorbent before being placed in routine use. Testing should be performed on more than one testing day with control sera, including sera of graded reactivity and nonsyphilitic sera demonstrating nonspecific reactivity. The new sorbent should remove nonspecific reactivity of the nonspecific serum control. The new sorbent should not reduce the intensity of fluorescence of the reactive (4+) control serum to less than 3+. The nonspecific staining control with the new sorbent should be nonreactive. Reportable test results on controls and individual sera should be with those obtained with standard sorbent. The sorbent should be usable when rehydrated to the indicated volume on the label or according to accompanying direction.

Fluorescein-Labeled Antihuman Globulin (Conjugate)

A satisfactory conjugate should not stain a standard antigen nonspecifically at three doubling dilutions below the working titer of the conjugate.

Reportable test results on controls and individual sera should be comparable with those obtained with the standard conjugate. Most manufacturers designate on the label the working titer of the conjugate that was determined under the testing conditions and with the equipment in their laboratories. Because conditions and equipment vary from one laboratory to another, it is necessary to titer and check-test a new lot of conjugate with a fluorescence microscope.

Procedure

1. Label test tubes for patient and control sera.
2. Pipette 0.2 mL into each tube.
3. Using a 0.2-mL pipette, add 0.05 mL of inactivated sera to the appropriately labeled test tubes. Mix eight times.
4. Label a previously prepared antigen suspension slide for each of the patient sera and controls being tested.
5. Cover each antigen preparation with 0.03 mL of a serum dilution (i.e., patient or control).
6. Cover an antigen suspension slide with either 0.03 mL of PBS or sorbent. These are the nonspecific staining controls.
7. Place a moist chamber over the slides to prevent evaporation, and incubate at 35° to 37° C for 30 minutes.
8. Fill two staining dishes with PBS.
9. Place slides in a slide carrier and rinse slides with running PBS for approximately 5 seconds.
10. Place the slides in the staining dish containing PBS solution. Process for 5 minutes. After 5 minutes, dip the slides in and out of the solution at least 10 times.
11. Transfer the slide carrier to the fresh PBS solution in the second staining dish. Process for 5 minutes. After 5 minutes, dip the slides in and out of the solution at least 10 times.
12. Rinse the slides in running distilled water for 5 seconds.
13. Gently blot each smear with bibulous paper to remove all water droplets.
14. Dilute conjugate to its working titer in PBS containing 2% Tween-80.
15. Pipette 0.03 mL of diluted conjugate onto each smear. Spread the conjugate uniformly over the slide with a glass rod.
16. Repeat steps 7 through 13.
17. Mount slides immediately by placing a small drop of mounting medium on each smear, then apply a coverslip to each.
18. Microscopically examine slides as soon as possible. The microscope should be equipped with an ultraviolet light source and a high-power dry objective. A combination of BG 12 exciting filter, not more than 3 mm thick, and OG 1 barrier filter or equivalent has been found to be satisfactory. If a

delay in reading is encountered, place the slides in a darkened room and read within 4 hours.

19. Using the minimally reactive (1+) control slide as the reading standard, record the intensity of fluorescence of the treponemes.

Recording of Fluorescence

Reading	Fluorescence intensity	Report
0	None or vaguely visible	Nonreactive
<1+	Weak reacting	Borderline
1+	Equivalent to 1+ control	Reactive
2+ to 4+	Moderate to strong	Reactive

20. Check nonreactive smears by using illumination from a tungsten light source to verify the presence of treponemes.

Reporting Results
Reporting Protocol

Reading	Repeat Test	Report
0		Nonreactive
<1+	Negative, <1+, or 1+	Borderline
1+	Negative, <1+	Borderline
1+	1+ or greater	Reactive
2+ to 4+		Reactive

Clinical Applications

If a patient has two borderline test results, it is impossible to definitively conclude that the patient has or does not have serologic evidence of syphilitic infection. The attending physician should review the patient's history and physical findings. Diagnosis will rely on the clinical evidence in conjunction with the borderline serologic findings.

The false-positive rate of this test is very low, but it can be associated with autoimmune disorders such as systemic lupus erythematosus. False-positive FTA-ABS results occur in patients suffering from other treponematoses such as pinta, yaws, or bejel, or in those who have high titer of antinuclear antibodies or rheumatoid factor. There is evidence that pregnant women occasionally have false-positive FTA-ABS test results.

Limitations

This test is recommended as a confirmatory procedure for syphilis. Its use is discouraged as a screening test. A reagin test such as the VDRL or RPR is recommended for screening.

References

Hunter EF, Deacon WE, Meyer PC: An improved test for syphilis—the absorption procedure (FTA-ABS), *Public Health Rep* 79:5, 1964.

Jaffe HW et al: Tests for treponemal antibody in CSF, *Arch Intern Med* 138:252, 1978.

Leclerc G et al: Study of fluorescent treponemal antibody test on cerebrospinal fluid using monospecific antiimmunoglobulin conjugates IgG, IgM, and IgA, *Br J Vener Dis* 54:303, 1978.

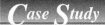

Case Study

History and Physical Examination

A 25-year-old woman comes to an ambulatory center with pain in the right side of her pelvis and a slight temperature. She has a history of two episodes of chlamydia cervicitis and herpes simplex vulvitis.

On physical examination she is found to have abundant mucopurulent cervical discharge and a painless genital lesion. She also has some swelling of her inguinal lymph glands.

Laboratory Data

A stat pregnancy test is ordered. It is positive.

Questions and Discussion

1. What other laboratory tests would you expect to be ordered?

   Cervical cultures for gonorrhea and chlamydia would be appropriate. A direct Gram stain of gonorrhea might also be appropriate. HIV testing and testing for syphilis would also be reasonable.

2. Could this patient have syphilis?

   Yes, this patient could have syphilis. This case is typical of primary syphilis with a painless, indurated ulcer on the genitals and mild inguinal adenopathy. It occurs from 9 to 90 days after exposure, usually at 3 weeks.

3. If syphilis is suspected, what tests should be ordered?

   The etiologic agent of syphilis, *Treponema pallidum*, cannot be easily cultured by routine methods. Diagnosis is made by a combination of clinical and laboratory means. Microorganisms can be visualized by darkfield examination of fluid from the ulcer. Serologic testing is usually positive. This testing involves a screening nontreponemal test (e.g., RPR or VDRL) followed by a confirmatory treponemal test such as the MHA-TP (microhemagglutination test for *T. pallidum*) or FTA-ABS (fluorescent treponemal antibody absorption test). In primary syphilis, the RPR or VDRL is negative, but the treponemal test is positive. Therefore patients who are clinically suspected of having primary syphilis, but who have a negative screening test, should have the treponemal test performed anyway. Serologic follow-up testing is important. Titers of nontreponemal tests are thought to correlate with disease activity. A repeat serology at 3 and 6 months should demonstrate a fourfold drop in titer (2 dilutions). Patients who fail to demonstrate a decline of this amount should undergo a spinal fluid examination to exclude neurosyphilis.

4. Is there risk of a congenital infection in this woman's unborn child?

   Yes, the infant could contract congenital syphilis.

Diagnosis

Syphilis

CHAPTER HIGHLIGHTS

Syphilis is caused by a spirochete *T. pallidum.* In 1906 the first diagnostic blood procedure, the Wassermann test, was developed to detect this disease. The genus *Treponema* contains four principal species: *T. pallidum* (syphilis in humans), *T. pertenue* (yaws), *T. carateum* (pinta), and *T. cuniculi* (syphilis in rabbits). Outside of the host, *T. pallidum* is extremely susceptible to various physical and chemical agents.

Syphilis in humans is ordinarily transmitted by sexual contact. In males the microorganism is transmitted from lesions on the penis or discharged from deeper sites with semen. Lesions in females are commonly located in the perineal region or on the labia, vaginal wall, or cervix. In a small percentage of cases, the primary infection is extragenital and is usually in or around the mouth.

Untreated syphilis is a chronic disease with subacute symptomatic periods separated by asymptomatic intervals, during which the diagnosis can be made serologically. The progression of untreated syphilis is generally divided into stages from the time of contact and initial infection. Primary syphilis is characterized by the presence of chancre, which persists for 1 to 5 weeks and heals spontaneously. During this stage the serum in about one third of cases becomes serologically reactive after 1 week and becomes serologically demonstrable in the majority of cases after 3 weeks. The reagin titer increases rapidly during the first 4 weeks and then remains stationary for approximately 6 months.

Within 2 to 8 weeks after the appearance of the primary chancre, a patient enters the stage of secondary syphilis. This stage is usually characterized by a generalized illness suggestive of a viral infection. Most patients manifest skin lesions that contain a large number of spirochetes and are highly contagious if located on exposed surfaces. These lesions subside spontaneously after 2 to 6 weeks even if untreated. In this noninfectious latent stage, serologic tests for syphilis are positive. Relapses, however, with manifestations of secondary syphilis, occur in about one fourth of patients during the first 2 to 4 years of infection.

The late (tertiary) stage is usually seen from 3 to 10 years after primary infection. Destructive lesions called gummas can appear in about 15% of untreated syphilitic persons who eventually develop late benign syphilis. Complications of this stage of the disease can include lesions of the nervous system, causing tabes dorsalis or cardiovascular complications. Meningovascular syphilis can manifest itself as seizures or as a cerebrovascular accident. In about one fourth of untreated cases, the tertiary stage is asymptomatic and recognized only by serologic testing. Occasionally the lesions heal so completely that even serologic tests become nonreactive.

Classic serologic tests for syphilis measure the presence of two types of antibodies: treponemal and nontreponemal. Treponemal antibodies are produced against the antigens of the organisms themselves. Nontreponemal antibodies, often called reagin antibodies, are produced by infected patients against components of their own or other mammalian bodies. Darkfield microscopy is the test of choice for symptomatic patients with primary syphilis. The widely used nontreponemal serologic test is the RPR method. Both the RPR and VDRL procedures are flocculation methods in which soluble antigen particles are coalesced to form larger particles, visible as clumps when they are agglutinated by antibody. Specific treponemal serologic tests include the FTA-ABS (fluorescent treponemal antibody absorption) test and the MHA (microhemagglutination) test. The TPI (*Treponema pallidum* immobilization) test, yet another procedure, is obsolete.

REVIEW QUESTIONS

Questions 1-4. Match the following *Treponema*-associated diseases in humans with their respective causative organism.

1. _____ *pallidum*

2. _____ *T. pallidum* (variant)

3. _____ *T. pertenue*

4. _____ *T. carateum*

    A. yaws
    B. syphilis
    C. pinta
    D. bejel

Questions 5-8. Match the following stages of syphilis with the appropriate signs and symptoms.

5. _____ Primary syphilis

6. _____ Secondary syphilis

7. _____ Latent syphilis

8. _____ Late (tertiary) syphilis
    A. diagnosis only by serologic methods
    B. presence of gummas
    C. development of a chancre
    D. hutchinsonian triad
    E. generalized illness followed by macular lesions in most patients

9. A term for nontreponemal antibodies produced by an infected patient against components of their own or other mammalian cells is:
    A. autoagglutinins
    B. reagin antibodies
    C. alloantibodies
    D. nonsyphilitic antibodies

Questions 10-13. Match the following:

10. _____ VDRL

11. _____ FTA-ABS

12. _____ MHA-TP

13. _____ RPR

    A. treponemal method
    B. nontreponemal method

14. All of the following are possible causes of a false-negative VDRL reaction except:
    A. inhibitors in patient sera
    B. hemolyzed serum specimen
    C. prozone reaction
    D. low antibody titer

15. In the RPR procedure, a false-positive reaction can result from all of the following except:
    A. infectious mononucleosis
    B. leprosy
    C. rheumatoid arthritis
    D. streptococcal pharyngitis

16. The first diagnostic blood test for syphilis was the

    _____ test.
    A. VDRL
    B. Wassermann
    C. RPR
    D. colloidal gold

17. Syphilis was initially treated with:
    A. Fuller's earth
    B. heavy metals (e.g., arsenic)
    C. sulfonamides (e.g., triple sulfa)
    D. antibiotics (e.g., penicillin)

18. Direct examination of the treponemes is most commonly performed with:
    A. light microscope
    B. darkfield microscopy
    C. VDRL
    D. RPR test

19. Pathogenic treponemes _____ cultivatable with any consistency in artificial laboratory media.
    A. are
    B. are not

20. In infected blood, *Treponema pallidum* does not appear to survive at 4° C for more than:
    A. 1 day
    B. 2 days
    C. 3 days
    D. 5 days

21. The primary incubation period for syphilis *(T. pallidum)* usually lasts about:
    A. 1 week
    B. 2 weeks
    C. 3 weeks
    D. 4 weeks

22. The stage of syphilis that can only be diagnosed by serologic (laboratory) methods is the:
    A. incubation phase
    B. primary phase
    C. secondary phase
    D. latent phase

23. Immunocompetent patients infected with *T. pallidum* produce:
    A. specific antibodies against *T. pallidum*
    B. nonspecific antibodies against the protein antigen group common to pathogenic spirochetes
    C. reagin antibodies
    D. all of the above

24. Which screening procedure can use spinal fluid as a specimen?
    A. VDRL
    B. RPR
    C. FTA-ABS
    D. both A and B

BIBLIOGRAPHY

Angell M, Kassirer JP: Sexually transmitted diseases in the 1990s, *N Engl J Med* 325(19):1368-1373, 1991.

Boyd RF, Hoerl BG: *Basic medical microbiology,* ed 3, Boston, 1986, Little, Brown.

Brown ST et al: Serologic response to syphilis treatment: a new analysis of old data, *JAMA* 253:1296-1299, 1985.

Cerny EH: Adenovirus ELISA for the evaluation of cerebrospinal fluid in patients with suspected neurosyphilis, *Am J Clin Pathol* 85:505-508, 1985.

Division of STD Prevention: *Sexually transmitted disease surveillance,* Atlanta, September 2000, U.S. Dept. of Health and Human Services, Centers for Disease Control and Prevention (CDC).

Farshy CE: Four-step enzyme-linked immunosorbent assay for the detection of *Treponema pallidum* antibody, *J Clin Microbiol* 21:387-389, 1985.

Forbes BA, Sahm DF, Weissfeld AS: *Bailey and Scott's diagnostic microbiology,* ed 11, St Louis, Mosby, 2002.

Gardner MF, Clark ME: The *Treponema pallidum* hemagglutination (TPHA) test, *WHO/VDT/ReS* 75:332, 1975.

Habif TP: *Clinical dermatology,* ed 2, St Louis, 1990, Mosby.

Handsfield HH: Old enemies: combating syphilis and gonorrhea in the 1990s, *JAMA* 264(11):1451-1452, 1990.

Hart G: Syphilis testing in diagnostic and therapeutic decision making, *Ann Intern Med* 104:368-376, 1986.

Hook EW, Marra CM: Acquired syphilis in adults, *N Engl J Med* 326(16):1060-1069, 1992.

Izzat NN et al: Validity of the VDRL test on cerebrospinal fluid contaminated by blood, *Br J Vener Dis* 47:162-164, 1971.

Larson SA et al: Cerebrospinal fluid serologies in syphilis: treponemal and nontreponemal test, International Conjoint STD Meeting, Abstract 166:218, Montreal, 1984.

Mandell GL, Douglas RG, Bennett JE, editors: *Principles and practice of infectious diseases,* ed 2, New York, 1985, John Wiley & Sons.

Muller F: Specific immunoglobulins M and G antibodies in the rapid diagnosis of human treponemal infections, *Diagn Immunol* 4:1-9, 1986.

Muller F, Moskophidis J: Estimation of the local production of antibodies to *Treponema pallidum* in the central nervous system of patients with neurosyphilis, *Br J Vener Dis* 59:80-84, 1983.

1993 sexually transmitted diseases treatment guidelines, *MMWR* 420(No. RR-14):505-535, Sept 24, 1993.

Primary and secondary syphilis—United States, 1981-1990, *MMWR* 40(19):314-322, 1991.

Radolf JD et al: Serodiagnosis of syphilis by enzyme-linked immunosorbent assay with purified recombinant *Treponema pallidum* antigen 4D, *J Infect Dis* 153:1023-1027, 1986.

Rein MF: Infection caused by *Treponema (*syphilis, yaws, pinta, bejel). In Stein J, editor: *Internal medicine,* ed 2, Boston, 1987, Little, Brown.

Rolfs RT, Nakashima AK: Epidemiology of primary and secondary syphilis in the United States, 1981-1989, *JAMA* 264(11):1432-1437, 1990.

Rutherford I, Li T: An evaluation of two hemagglutination tests as alternatives to FTA-ABS in otologic syphilis, *Lab Med* 25(1):22-24, 1989.

Chapter 16

Tick-borne Diseases

Lyme Disease
Etiology
Epidemiology
Signs and Symptoms
Diagnostic Evaluation
Treatment and Prevention

Human Ehrlichiosis
Etiology
Epidemiology
Signs and Symptoms
Diagnostic Evaluation
Treatment and Prevention

Babesiosis
Etiology
Epidemiology
Signs and Symptoms
Diagnostic Evaluation
Treatment and Prevention

Case Studies

Chapter Highlights

Review Questions

Bibliography

LEARNING OBJECTIVES

At the conclusion of this chapter, the reader should be able to:
- Describe the etiology, epidemiology, and signs and symptoms of Lyme disease.
- Discuss the immunologic manifestations and diagnostic evaluation of Lyme disease.
- Explain the treatment and prevention of Lyme disease.
- Describe the etiology, epidemiology, and signs and symptoms of ehrlichiosis.

- Discuss the immunologic manifestations and diagnostic evaluation of ehrlichiosis.
- Explain the treatment and prevention of ehrlichiosis.
- Describe the etiology, epidemiology, and signs and symptoms of babesiosis.
- Discuss the immunologic manifestations and diagnostic evaluation of babesiosis.
- Explain the treatment and prevention of babesiosis.
- Analyze case studies of Lyme disease, ehrlichiosis, and babesiosis.

Since its original description almost 25 years ago, Lyme disease has become recognized as an important infectious disease in the United States. The infection, which is caused by the tick-borne spirochete *Borrelia burgdorferi*, has emerged as a major health hazard for humans and domestic animals. Today, Lyme disease is a global illness. Cases have been recognized on six continents, the exception being Antarctica. It is endemic in more than 15 states in the United States and in Europe and Asia.

In some cases the disease may be transitory and of little consequence, but in others it may become chronic and severely disabling. Accurate diagnosis therefore is of great importance, but laboratory testing techniques still need improvement.

LYME DISEASE

Etiology

Lyme disease (Lyme borreliosis) is caused by a spirochete bacterium. It is a cutaneous-systemic infection that is generally transmitted by a hard-bodied tick (Figure 16-1) and caused by *B. burgdorferi* (Figure 16-2). The causative agent of Lyme borreliosis currently consists of three pathogenic species: *B. burgdorferi, B. afzelii,* and *B. garinii.* Only *B. burgdorferi* strains have been found in the United States. In contrast, most of the illness in Europe is caused by *B. afzelii,* which is associated with the chronica skin condition acrodermatitis chronica atrophicans (ACA), and *B. garinii,* which is associated with

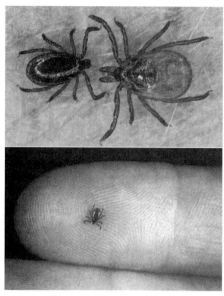

Figure 16-1 The deer tick. (From Habif TP: *Clinical dermatology,* ed 2, St Louis, 1990, Mosby.)

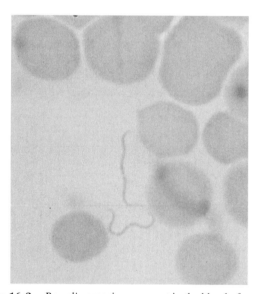

Figure 16-2 *Borrelia* organisms present in the blood of a patient with endemic relapsing fever (Giemsa stain). From Murray PR et al: *Medical microbiology,* ed 4, St Louis, 2002, Mosby.)

neurologic symptoms. Only these two species have been found in Asia. The complete genome of *B. burgdorferi* (strain B31) has now been sequenced.

The spirochete is transmitted by certain ixodid ticks that are part of the *Ixodes ricinus* complex. These include *I. scapularis* (formerly classified as *I. dammini*) in the northeastern and midwestern United States, *I. pacificus* in the western United States, *I. ricinus* in Europe, and *I. persulcatus* in Asia. The vector has not been identified in Australia. Ixodid ticks are also indigenous to Africa and South America.

In the United States the preferred host for both the larval and nymphal states of *I. scapularis* is the white-footed mouse, *Peromyscus leucopus*. White-tailed deer, which are not involved in the life cycle of the spirochete, are the pre-

ferred host for *I. scapuliaris* adult stage, and they seem to be critical to tick survival. Ixodid ticks have also been found on at least 30 types of wild animals and 49 species of birds. Illness is not known to develop in wild animals, but clinical Lyme disease does occur in domestic animals, including dogs, horses, and cattle.

Spirochetes are transmitted from the gut of the tick to human skin at the site of a bite and then migrate outwardly into the skin. This migration causes the unique expanding skin lesion, erythema migrans (EM). Subsequent dissemination of spirochetes to secondary sites may cause major organ system involvement in humans. In dogs the most common symptom is arthritis.

Epidemiology

Retrospectively it appears that the first symptom of Lyme disease was recognized as early as 1908 in Sweden. In the decades that followed, the rash produced by the disease (erythema chronicum migrans [ECM]) was noted elsewhere in Europe, as were other symptoms that seemed to follow ECM's eruption. Secondary symptoms such as impairment of the nervous system were described in France, Germany, and again in Sweden.

In the United States the European rash was virtually unknown until 1969, when a case of a physician bitten by a tick while hunting in Wisconsin was reported. Although a few ECM cases were seen in Americans who had traveled to Europe, there were no further native American cases until 1975, when physicians at the U.S. Navy base in Groton, Connecticut, reported seeing four patients with a rash similar to ECM. At the same time an epidemiologist at the Connecticut State Department of Health and a rheumatologist at Yale were notified of an unusual cluster of cases of arthritis occurring in children in Lyme, Connecticut.

It was not until 1982 that Burgdorfer and Barbour isolated a previously unrecognized spirochete, now called *Borrelia burgdorferi,* from *I. scapularis* ticks and Lyme disease became a recognized vector-borne, infectious disease. Two factors influence the chance that a bitten patient will get the disease: the likelihood that local ixodid ticks carry the Lyme spirochete, and the likelihood of infection after a bite by an infected tick. The probability of infection after an ixodid tick bite in an area of endemic disease is about 3%, but it varies in different regions from less than 1% to as high as 5%. It has been suggested that HLA-DR4 and, secondarily, HLA-DR2 may increase the risk that Lyme arthritis will become chronic and fail to respond to antibiotics.

More than 170,000 cases of Lyme disease have been reported to health authorities in the United States since 1982, when a systematic national surveillance was initiated. Fewer than 18,000 cases of Lyme disease were reported before 1990. Between 1990 and 1999 a total of 122,651 cases were reported to the Centers for Disease Control and Prevention by state health departments (Figure 16-3). A total of 13,452 cases were reported in 2001, which represents a 24% decrease compared to the 17,730 cases reported in 2000.

Lyme disease now accounts for more than 95% of all reported vector-borne illness in the United States. It is a reportable disease and there is a distinctive pattern in which cases remain concentrated in the northeastern, north-central, and Pacific coastal regions (Figure 16-4). Lyme disease cases reported in 2001 were from 50 states,

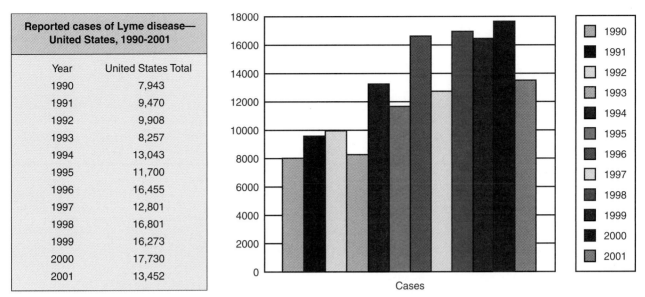

Reported cases of Lyme disease—United States, 1990-2001	
Year	United States Total
1990	7,943
1991	9,470
1992	9,908
1993	8,257
1994	13,043
1995	11,700
1996	16,455
1997	12,801
1998	16,801
1999	16,273
2000	17,730
2001	13,452

Figure 16-3   Reported cases of Lyme disease—United States, 1990-2001. (Redrawn from Centers for Disease Control and Prevention, CDC, 2002.)

REPORTED CASES OF LYME DISEASE, UNITED STATES, 1999*

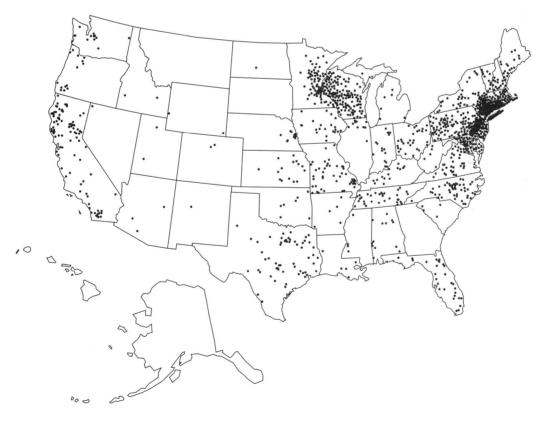

*1 dot = 1 case, placed randomly within county of residence; 16,273 cases

Figure 16-4   Reported cases of Lyme Disease, United States, 1999.

although 11 states (Connecticut, Rhode Island, New Jersey, New York, Delaware, Pennsylvania, Massachusetts, Maryland, Wisconsin, Minnesota, and New Hampshire) accounted for 94% of the nationally reported cases. The greatest number of reported cases, 3688, was reported in upstate New York.

The overall incidence rate of reported cases in the United States is about 5 per 100,000 population, but there is considerable underreporting. The incidence in a few of the most highly endemic communities may reach 1% to 3% per year. Persons of all ages and both genders are equally susceptible. The decrease in the number of Lyme disease cases

TABLE 16-1	Clinical Features of Lyme Disease	
Stage	**Length of Time**	**Common Signs and Symptoms**
I	4 weeks (median) after injection	Cutaneous manifestations (erythema migrans) or other skin eruptions, flulike syndrome, neurologic symptoms
II	Follows a variable latent period	Target organs and systems include the nervous system, heart, eyes, and skin, all of which can manifest abnormalities
III	Weeks to years after infection	Arthritis, late neurologic complications, acrodermatitis chronica atrophicans

in 2001 may reflect heightened awareness of Lyme disease by patients and physicians and an increase in prevention practices by the general public.

Lyme disease is considered an emerging infectious disease because of the impact of changing environmental and socioeconomic factors, such as the transformation of farmland into suburban woodlots favorable for deer and deer ticks. Although pets may represent a spirochete reservoir, it is unlikely that human beings can be infected directly by them. However, in areas of endemic Lyme disease, both adult and nymphal ticks, carried into the household by dogs and cats, may infest humans.

Signs and Symptoms

The basic features of the disease are similar worldwide, but there are regional variations, primarily between the illness found in America and that found in Europe and Asia.

In at least 60% to 80% of patients in the United States, Lyme disease begins with a slowly expanding skin lesion, EM, which occurs at the site of the tick bite. The skin lesion is frequently accompanied by flulike symptoms.

The Centers for Disease Control and Prevention's clinical case definition for Lyme disease includes the presence of EM or at least one objective late-manifestation sign of musculoskeletal, neurologic, or cardiovascular disease and a positive serologic test for antibody to *B. burgdorferi.* Many misdiagnosed patients actually suffer from chronic fatigue syndrome or fibromyalgia, both of which can cause similar symptoms such as joint stiffness or pain, fatigue, and sleep disturbance.

Lyme borreliosis is a multisystem illness that primarily involves the skin, nervous system, heart, and joints (Table 16-1). Lyme disease usually begins during the summer months with EM and flulike symptoms and may be accompanied by right upper quadrant tenderness and a mild hepatitis (stage 1). This stage is followed weeks to months later by acute cardiac or neurologic disease in a minority of untreated individuals (stage 2), and then followed by arthritis and chronic neurologic disease (stage 3) in many untreated patients weeks to years after disease onset. There is considerable overlap between these stages, but Lyme disease is best characterized as an illness that evolves from early to late disease without reference to an arbitrary staging system. However, a patient may have one or all of the stages, and the infection may not become symptomatic until stage 2 or 3. The majority of affected patients have EM, and one fourth manifest arthritis; neurologic manifestations and cardiac involvement are uncommon.

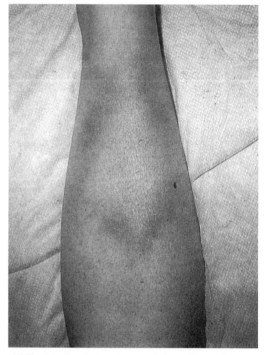

Figure 16-5 Erythema chronicum migrans. (From Habif TP: *Clinical dermatology,* ed 2, St Louis, 1990, Mosby.)

Arthritis

Arthralgia and myalgia are common features of early Lyme disease, but frank arthritis during EM is unusual. Arthritis is a well-described complication of Lyme disease and characteristically occurs months to years after *Borrelia* infection. Therefore cases of Lyme arthritis occur during every month of the year. Lyme arthritis and parvovirus B19 arthritis can occur in the absence of other symptoms such as the characteristic rash. Some suspected cases of Lyme arthritis might be caused by parvovirus B19, particularly those occurring during the parvovirus B19 season.

Arthritis in patients with chronic Lyme disease may be associated with a long-standing infiltration of the joints by *B. burgdorferi* spirochetes along with a local inflammatory response. It may not be triggered simply by the presence of circulating IgG antibodies against outer surface proteins.

Cutaneous Manifestations

Cutaneous manifestations (Figure 16-5) can be demonstrated as early EM, secondary (disseminated lesions and lymphocytoma), and late lesions (acrodermatitis chronica atrophicans). With the exception of the late lesions, cutaneous manifestations generally resolve spontaneously over weeks to months. The red papule at the site of the tick bite is most commonly located on the thigh, groin, or axilla. Facial EM is more commonly seen in children.

Several days to weeks after the onset of EM, nearly half of untreated patients develop secondary skin lesions. A rare early manifestation of Lyme disease is borrelia lymphocytomas, a tumorlike violaceous swelling or nodules at the base of the earlobe or the nipple caused by a dense lymphocytic infiltrate of the dermis. This lesion occurs at the site of a tick bite and in conjunction with other symptoms; it may be confused with lymphoma.

Acrodermatitis chronica atrophicans is a late skin manifestation of Lyme disease more prevalent in Europe than in the United States. Lesions display bluish-red discoloration, doughy swelling, and fibrotic nodules. Eventually, striking atrophy of skin and subcutaneous tissues follows. Polyneuropathy coexists in 30% to 45% of patients.

Cardiac Manifestations

Lyme carditis occurs in approximately 8% of untreated patients within 1 to 2 months (range: <1 week to 7 months) after the onset of infection, and may be the initial manifestation of Lyme disease. Cardiac features of Lyme disease usually results in a fluctuating degree of atrioventricular conduction defect (first-degree, second-degree, and complete block, as well as bundle branch and fascicular blocks) or tachyarrhythmias. Myopericarditis can occur, but symptomatic congestive heart failure is uncommon. Patients usually develop signs of light-headedness, syncope, dyspnea, palpitations, and/or chest pain. Symptoms are more common in patients with more severe degrees of heart block. The carditis usually follows a self-limited and mild course, but temporary pacing may be needed in a small percentage of patients.

Neurologic Manifestations

Neurologic abnormalities occur in approximately 15% of untreated patients. These manifestations are usually observed 2 to 8 weeks after disease onset and may include aseptic meningitis, cranial nerve palsies, peripheral radiculoneuritis, and peripheral neuropathy. The predominant symptoms of Lyme meningitis are severe headache and mild neck stiffness, which may fluctuate for weeks after a posterythema migrans latent period.

Months to years after the initial infection with *B. burgdorferi,* patients with Lyme disease may have chronic encephalopathy, polyneuropathy, or less commonly, leukoencephalitis. The appearance of mild encephalopathy has been observed to begin from 1 month to 14 years after the onset of disease. Encephalopathy is characterized by memory loss, mood changes, or sleep disturbance. In addition, increased cerebrospinal fluid protein levels and/or evidence of intrathecal production of antibody to *B. burgdorferi* may occur. Chronic neurologic manifestations can also include polyneuropathy with radicular pain or distal paresthesias, fatigue, headache, hearing loss, and verbal memory impairment. These chronic neurologic abnormalities usually improve with antibiotic therapy.

Ocular manifestations may occur in Lyme disease and include cranial nerve palsies, optic neuritis, panophthalmitis with loss of vision, and choroiditis with retinal detachment.

Pregnancy. Transplacental transmission of *B. burgdorferi* with fetal infection has been confirmed. A uniform pattern of congenital malformations has not been identified in maternal-fetal transmission of Lyme disease.

In observed cases cited, infants succumbed shortly after birth. The mothers acquired infection during the first trimester and received inadequate or no treatment.

Immunologic Manifestations

Cellular immune responses to *B. burgdorferi* antigens begin concurrently with early clinical illness. An increase in spontaneous suppressor cell activity and reduction in natural killer cell activity have been noted. Mononuclear cell antigen-specific responses develop during spirochetal dissemination, and humoral (antibody) immune responses soon follow.

Serodiagnostic tests are insensitive during the first several weeks of infection. In the United States, approximately 20% to 30% of patients have positive responses, usually of the immunoglobulin (Ig)M isotype, during this period, but by convalescence 2 to 4 weeks later, about 70% to 80% have seroreactivity even after antibiotic treatment. After about 1 month, the majority of patients with active infection have IgG antibody responses. After antibiotic treatment, antibody titers fall slowly but IgG and even IgM responses may persist for many years after treatment. Therefore, an IgM response cannot be interpreted as a manifestation of recent infection or reinfection unless the appropriate clinical characteristics are present. Antibodies formed include cryoglobulins, immune complexes, antibodies specific for *B. burgdorferi,* and anticardiolipin antibodies. Elevated titers of IgM are noted in early disease. Immunoblot analysis demonstrates that IgM antibodies form initially against the flagellar 41 KD polypeptide but react later to additional cell wall antigens. An overlapping IgG response to these antigens develops in some individuals. These antigen-specific cellular and humoral responses are neither known to eradicate infection in early disease nor to participate in disease pathogenesis.

Specific IgM or IgG antibodies against *B. burgdorferi* are usually not detectable in a patient's serum unless symptoms have been present for at least 2 to 4 weeks. In cases of Lyme arthritis, tests for serum antinuclear antibodies, rheumatoid factor, and the VDRL (Venereal Disease Research Laboratories Test) are generally negative. However, anti-*B. burgdorferi* antibodies of the IgG type should be present in the serum of patients with Lyme arthritis.

Outer surface protein A antibodies develop late in the course of human Lyme infection, and then only in a subset of patients. Recent reports suggest that a temporal association exists between the onset of chronic Lyme arthritis in 4HLA-DR4–positive patients and the development of antibodies to the outer surface protein.

Persistent organisms and spirochetal antigen deposits elicit a vigorous immune reaction as manifested by a tissue-rich plasma cell and lymphocytic exudate containing abundant T cells, predominantly of the helper subset, plus IgD-bearing B cells. *B. burgdorferi* antigens elicit a strong immune reaction that intensifies with chronicity of arthritis and stimulates macrophages to secrete interleukin-1 (IL-1). IL-1 is capable of stimulating synovial cells and fibroblasts to secrete collagenase and prostaglandin E_2, both of which are elevated in Lyme synovial fluid and can cause erosion of joint cartilage and bone.

TABLE 16-2	Various Methods of Lyme Disease Detection
Isolation	Successful cultures have been obtained from ticks, skin biopsies, ear punches, cerebrospinal fluid, blood and synovial fluid; blood is not a reliable sample for culture. Isolation of spirochetes is highly variable.
Histology	Lyme spirochetes are rarely observed in blood smears; examination of tissue is usually performed, in addition to an immunologic assay such as fluorescence microscopy. The process is labor intensive; the test is of limited value.
Serology	Not sufficiently reliable to make a definitive diagnosis of Lyme disease; only IFA and EIA test systems are FDA approved.
Antigen detection systems	Screen for antigenic products rather than for the host's immune response to the infection.

Diagnostic Evaluation

The culture of *B. burgdorferi* from specimens in Barbour-Stoenner-Kelly medium permits a definitive diagnosis. With a few exceptions, positive cultures have been obtained only early in the illness, primarily from biopsy samples of EM lesions, less often from plasma samples, and only occasionally from cerebrospinal fluid samples in patients with meningitis. Later in the infection, polymerase chain reaction (PCR) testing is superior to culture in the detection of *B. burgdorferi* in joint fluid.

In the United States, the diagnosis is usually based on the recognition of the characteristic clinical findings, a history of exposure in an area where the disease is endemic, and except in patients with EM, an antibody response to *B. burgdorferi* by enzyme-linked immunosorbent assays (ELISA) and Western blotting. More than half the time, positive test results are inconsequential because physicians feel comfortable making the diagnosis based on symptoms and patient history. The importance of testing, however, comes into play when the tell-tale "bull's eye" rash or other symptoms characteristic of Lyme disease do not occur.

In the early phase of Lyme disease, laboratory findings are nonspecific and typically may include an elevated sedimentation rate (ESR), elevated serum IgM levels, and mildly elevated hepatic transaminase (serum glutamate-pyruvate transaminase/alanine aminotransferase [SGPT]) levels. Various methods (Table 16-2) for detection of disease are available.

Much of the diagnostic process in late, disseminated disease often involves ruling out other illnesses and defining the extent of damage that might require separate evaluation and treatment. Consideration should be given to tick exposure, rashes (even atypical ones), evolution of typical symptoms in a previously asymptomatic individual, and results of tests for tick-borne pathogens. In late disease there may be repeatedly peaking IgMs; therefore a reactive IgM may not differentiate early from late disease, but it does suggest an active infection. When late cases of Lyme disease are seronegative, 36% will transiently become seropositive at the completion of successful therapy.

Lyme disease is now been diagnosed based on its relative value (Table 16-3). Lyme borreliosis is highly likely if its relative value score is 7 or above. Lyme borreliosis is possible if its relative value is between 5 and 6, and Lyme borreliosis is unlikely if its relative value is 4 or below.

Antibody Detection

Assays for the detection of antibodies to *B. burgdorferi* are the most practical means of confirming infection. At present,

TABLE 16-3	Lyme Borreliosis Diagnostic Criteria Relative Value	
Two or more systems (e.g., monoarthritis and facial palsy)		2
Erythema migrans, physician confirmed		7
Acrodermatitis chronica atrophicans, biopsy confirmed		7
Seropositivity		3
Seroconversion on paired sera		4
Tissue microscopy, silver stain		3
Tissue microscopy, monoclonal immuno-fluorescence		4
Culture positivity		4
B. burgdorferi antigen recovery		4
B. burgdorferi DNA/RNA recovery		4

From Burrascano J: *Advance topics in Lyme disease,* ed 13, May, 2000, website: www/LymeNet.org.

rapid tests usually rely on detecting antibodies produced by a patient. However, an antibody response may be delayed or may not occur. This leads to false-negative laboratory assay results. In addition, false-positive results can occur if an individual has been exposed to a related bacteria.

The most common laboratory assays for *B. burgdorferi* antibody detection include indirect fluorescent antibody (IFA) staining methods, ELISA for total Igs or IgM and IgG antibodies and PreVue *B. burgdorferi* Antibody Detection Assay for Lyme disease (Wampole Laboratories, Princeton, NJ). Immunoblotting techniques can be used along with ELISA to characterize immune response and for diagnosis.

Enzyme-linked Immunosorbent Assay

The ELISA is the standard test method; it is the most widely available and commonly performed test. The sensitivities of IFA and ELISA methods are usually low during the initial 3 weeks of infection; therefore negative results are common. The most serious disadvantages of current techniques are low sensitivity and lengthy processing time. In addition, false-positive reactions resulting from cross-reactivity can occur in tests for Lyme disease. For example, tick-borne relapsing fever spirochetes, *Borrelia hermsii*, are closely related to *B. burgdorferi*. Antibodies to *B. hermsii*, an agent that coexists with the Lyme disease spirochete in portions of the western

United States, strongly cross-react with *B. burgdorferi* in IFA staining and ELISA testing. Common antigens are shared among the *Borrelia* organisms and even with the treponemes. Serum from syphilitic patients reacts positively in assays for Lyme disease. Therefore serologic test results for antibodies to *B. burgdorferi* should be considered along with clinical data and epidemiologic information when a patient is evaluated for Lyme disease.

PreVue *B. burgdorferi* Antibody Detection Assay

PreVue *B. burgdorferi* Antibody Detection Assay (Wampole PreVue Assay for Lyme disease, Princeton, NJ) is a CLIA-waived procedure intended to be used as the first presumptive step in testing individuals suspected of having Lyme disease. Positive results must be confirmed with a Western blot test done by a laboratory. Two-stage testing is recommended by the Centers for Disease Control and Prevention. The new test uses antigenic proteins developed by recombinant DNA techniques rather than a whole cell *B. burgdorferi* preparation. Antigenic proteins developed by recombinant DNA techniques allow for more accuracy. The "false-positive" rate is similar to that of laboratory tests for Lyme disease.

Western Blot Analysis

Western blot analysis can verify reactivity of antibody to major surface or flagellar proteins of *B. burgdorferi* (Figure 16-6). Western blot is helpful in determining "borderline" negative or weakly positive results obtained from other tests, but the values are not always reliable. This procedure is more definitive in later Lyme disease when multiple antibody bands specific for *B. burgdorferi* appear. Reported results from test done by Western blots for Lyme disease in its late phase indicates reactive bands for IgM levels. 41KD bands appear the earliest but can cross-react with other spirochetes. The 18KD, 23-25KD (Osp C), 31KD (Osp A), 34KD (Osp B), 37KD, 39KD, 83KD, and 93KD bands are the most specific but appear later or may not appear at all.

Polymerase Chain Reaction

PCR can detect spirochete in the synovial fluid around the joints or in other clinical samples. PCR looks for DNA of the organism. In the past, PCR has been taken as definitive evidence that a person has an infection, but it is possible to have antigens in the presence of nonviable organism. PCR amplifies small amounts of DNA that may remain even when intact organisms are no longer present—an indicator that the organism does or did exist. The PCR technique may miss the spirochete in the blood, allowing it to move into other tissues.

PCR directly identifies the pathogen instead of measuring the host's immune response to it. PCR can detect the DNA from as few as one to five organisms, even those that are nonviable. Different specific probes have been produced, and PCR has been used to detect *B. burgdorferi* DNA in a variety of body fluids. The appeal of PCR lies in its rapid turnaround time (2 days compared with 6 to 8 weeks for culture) and the avoidance of the difficulties of identifying the organism by culture or immunohistochemistry. The procedure has very high specificity, but the sensitivity may be as low as 70%. It may be useful in diagnosing early Lyme disease when the patient is still seronegative.

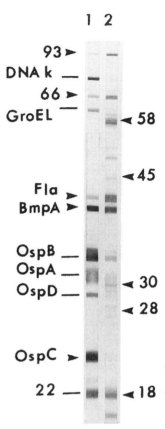

Figure 16-6   An example of immunoblot calibration. Lane 1, monoclonal antibodies defining selected antigens to *B. burgdorferi* B31 separated in a linear SDS-PAGE gel Marblot (MarDx Diagnostics, Carlsbad, Calif.). Lane 2, human serum (IgG) reactive with the 10 antigens scored in the currently recommended criteria for blot scoring; lines indicate other calibrating antibodies. Molecular masses are in kilodaltons. (From Rose NR et al: editors, *Manual of clinical laboratory immunology,* ed 5, Washington, DC, 1997, American Society for Microbiology Press, p 531.)

Other Methods Used for Antibody Detection

Spinal taps are not routinely recommended, as a negative tap does not rule out Lyme disease. Antibodies to *B. burgdorferi* can be detected in the cerebrospinal fluid in just 20% of patients with late disease. Therefore spinal taps are performed only on patients with pronounced neurologic manifestations. When spinal taps are done, the goal is to rule out other conditions, and to determine if *B. burgdorferi* antigens are present. It is especially important to look for elevated protein and mononuclear cells, which would dictate the need for more aggressive therapy, as well as the opening pressure, which can be elevated and add to headaches, especially in children.

Antigen Detection Systems. Antigen detection systems screen for antigenic products rather than for the host's immune response to the infection. Antigen detection systems could be expected to confirm both infections in patients with depressed immune systems and early infections in patients who have not yet produced a detectable antibody response. It is presumed that clearance of such antigens from hosts would be indicative of successful treatment and elimination of infecting spirochetes in patients. In addition, an antigen system can detect bacteria in the tick itself.

Two categories of procedures have been developed: T-cell proliferative assays and antibody-based antigen detection systems. T-cell proliferative assays recognize spirochetal antigens by cloned, antigen-specific cells. When T cells bind and recognize Lyme spirochetes in a specimen, T-cell division is induced. This division can be measured by counting T cells or by measuring the incorporation of labeled nutrients into the T cells. The T-cell proliferative assay may be a helpful diagnostic test in the small subset of patients with late Lyme disease who have negative or indeterminate antibody response by ELISA.

In 1993 the p39 antigen, a protein unique to *B. burgdorferi,* was first identified. A recombinant p39 antigen diagnostic test was developed, and the Food and Drug Administration (FDA) approved three p39-based test kits (one is a dipstick test kit). The tests detect antibodies to the p39 antigen, which is not found in closely related bacteria such as syphilis and tick-borne relapsing fever. Unfortunately this procedure is of limited use because the p39 antigen is rarely found in early stages of infection, but it is a highly specific marker for late Lyme disease.

Monoclonal or polyclonal antibodies also detect specific Lyme spirochete antigens. Quantities of proteins including flagellin, OspA, and OspB are detectable. Assays based on OspA and OspB, two closely related *B. burgdorferi* proteins from the outer wall of the bacteria, are available. Both of these proteins are characteristically exposed on the surface of different strains of the Lyme disease spirochete, but are not found in other species of bacterial spirochetes (e.g., syphilis). This system of antigen capture is useful for screening various fluids and tissues, including urine, blood, and cerebrospinal fluid.

Treatment and Prevention

Treatment

The factors that influence the decision about what to do after a tick bite include:
- Probability that the tick is a carrier of *B. burgdorferi*
- Length of time the tick was attached
- Chance that disease will develop without the telltale rash
- Risk and severity of short- and long-term sequelae
- Accuracy of antibody tests
- Efficacy of antibiotics at various stages of the disease
- Risk of adverse reactions to the antibiotics
- Patient's level of anxiety
- Chance that the patient will comply with follow-up monitoring
- Cost of various strategies, presence of coinfections, immune deficiencies, prior significant steroid use while infected, age, weight, gastrointestinal function, and blood levels achieved.

Antibiotics

It is unclear whether antimicrobial treatment after an *I. scapularis* tick bite will prevent Lyme disease. One study concluded that a single 200-mg dose of doxycycline given within 72 hours after an *I. scapularis* tick bite can prevent the development of Lyme disease.

Another study concluded that there is considerable impairment of health-related quality of life among patients with persistent symptoms despite previous antibiotic treatment for acute Lyme disease. In two clinical trials, however, treatment with intravenous and oral antibiotics for 90 days did not improve symptoms more than placebo.

Various types of antibiotics are in general use for *B. burgdorferi* treatment. The tetracyclines, including doxycycline and minocycline, are bacteriostatic unless given in high doses. If high blood levels are not attained, treatment failures in early and late disease are common; however, it is difficult to tolerate high doses.

Penicillins are bactericidal. As would be expected in managing an infection with a gram-negative organism such as *B. burgdorferi,* amoxicillin has been shown to be more effective than oral penicillin V. Because of its short half-life and need for high levels, amoxicillin is usually administered along with probenecid. Because of variability, blood levels are usually measured. Third-generation agents are currently the most effective of the cephalosporins because of their very low blood level counts (0.06 for ceftriaxone), and they have been shown to be effective in penicillin and tetracycline failures. Cefuroxime axetil (Ceftin), a second-generation agent, is also effective against staphylococcus and thus is useful in treating atypical EM that may represent a mixed infection containing some of the more common skin pathogens in addition to *B. burgdorferi.* Because this agent's gastrointestinal side effects and high cost, it is not used as first-line drug.

Vaccination

In 2001 the FDA reconvened to evaluate the previously approved OspA vaccine because of the significantly increasing rate of adverse reactions attributed to the vaccine. In March of 2000, research conducted showed that, human leukocyte function-associated antigen I (hLFA-1 a), which is found on many cells throughout the body, cross-reacts with the piece of the OspA used to make the current vaccine. On vaccination, a genetically vulnerable person's own OspA-primed antibodies can start an autoimmune war by attacking and binding to its own hLFA-1a.

It is estimated that roughly 30% of the population is HLS-DR4. In a recently filed lawsuit, a claim is made that anyone with this genetic marker who takes LYMErix vaccine risks contracting "degenerative, treatment-resistant Lyme arthritis." With new evidence on the danger associated with the vaccine, more research and analysis was conducted on the safety of the vaccine in humans. As of February 25, 2002, the manufacturer of LYMErix, a recombinant outer-surface protein A Lyme disease vaccine for humans, announced that the vaccine will no longer be commercially available.

Pets, especially dogs rather than cats, can become infected with Lyme disease. Effective vaccines are available (e.g., LymeVax, Wyeth Pharmaceuticals, Fort Dodge Animal Health, Overland Park, KS; Galaxy Lyme, Schering-Plough Pharmaceuticals, Kenilworth, NJ). LymeVax has been shown to maintain antibody levels for 53 weeks after vaccination in a Lyme-endemic area. According to the manufacturer, Galaxy Lyme is the only Lyme disease vaccine with isolates from two seroprotective groups (S-1-10 and C-1-11) and covers all outer surface proteins (Osp) for development of protective immunity in canines.

Preventive Practices

When hiking in the woods or mountains, picnicking at local parks, or walking in tall grass in shore areas, individuals should:

- Check daily for ticks
- Wear light-colored clothing so tick viewing is easier
- Tuck pants into socks

HUMAN EHRLICHIOSIS

Human ehrlichiosis was first described in the United States in 1986. Reporting of tick-borne illnesses has increased since then. Unlike Lyme disease, which tends to be indolent, Rocky Mountain spotted fever and ehrlichiosis can be fatal and must be recognized and treated promptly.

Etiology

Tick-borne rickettsiae of the genus *Ehrlichia* have recently been recognized as a cause of human illness in the United States. *Ehrlichia* species belong to the same family as the organism that causes Rocky Mountain spotted fever. *E. chaffeensis,* the novel etiologic agent of human monocytic ehrlichiosis in the United States, was demonstrated to cause disease in a patient from Arkansas with tick bites in 1987. Since then two more *Ehrlichia* species, *E. ewingii* and *E. phagocytophila*-like agent that differs antigenically and genetically from *E. chaffeensis* have been identified. Both of these *Ehrlichia* species have been identified as the cause of human granulocytic ehrlichiosis.

Epidemiology

Although the prevalence rates are low, human ehrlichiosis is endemic in the United States. Some fatalities have been reported. Incidence rates increase with age and are higher among men than women. Human ehrlichiosis occurs most frequently in the southern mid-Atlantic and south-central states during spring and summer.

The major vector for *E. chaffeensis* is the Lone Star tick, *Amblyomma americanum.* The principal reservoir for *E. chaffeensis* is the white-tailed deer, which hosts all stages of *A. americanum.* The primary tick vector for the agent of human granulocytic ehrlichiosis is *I. scapularis* in the eastern United States and *I. pacificus* in California. *Dermacentor variabilis* represents a second tick vector in the United States. The major reservoir for infection may be the white-footed mouse in the eastern United States. The onset of illness in spring and early summer for most cases parallels the time when the ticks, *A. americanum* and *D. variabilis,* are most active.

Signs and Symptoms

Ehrlichiosis is a general term for both human granulocytic ehrlichiosis (HGE) and human monocytic ehrlichiosis (HME). The syndrome of human ehrlichiosis is not commonly recognized by physicians, but should be considered in patients with a history of tick exposure and acute febrile flulike illness. Most patients are not suspected of having a rickettsial infection. Because ehrlichiosis can cause fatal infections in humans, early detection and treatment with tetracycline or chloramphenicol appear to offer the best chance for complete recovery.

Symptoms are nonspecific and can include fever, chills, and headache. Fever and skin rashes are the most common physical findings. In children, fever and headache are universal. Myalgias, nausea, vomiting, and anorexia are also common.

Diagnostic Evaluation

Laboratory investigations indicate that the hematologic, hepatic, and central nervous systems are commonly involved in human ehrlichiosis. Definitive diagnosis is based on inclusions in leukocytes (Figure 16-7). *Ehrlichia* species undergo three developmental stages:

1. Elementary bodies enter a leukocyte by phagocytosis and multiply rapidly
2. After 3 to 5 days, small numbers of tightly packed elementary bodies (initial bodies) are visible
3. During the next 7 to 12 days, the initial bodies develop into morula or mulberry forms

Characteristically the presence of intracytoplasmic inclusions (morula) in leukocytes of patients presenting with temperature of 38.5° C or higher can be observed when a blood smear is examined by light microscopy. Careful examination should reveal morula in 20% to 80% of acutely infected individuals. For HGE, direct observation of intraleukocytic morulae in Wright-Giemsa stained peripheral blood or buffy coat smears is a rapid and inexpensive laboratory test. In HME, intraleukocytic morula are difficult to detect in peripheral blood smears. The quantitative buffy coat method can also be used for diagnosis of either HME or HGE.

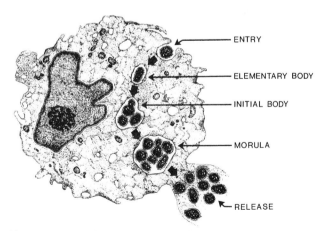

Figure 16-7 Schematic representation of the growth cycle of ehrlichiae in an infected cell. Elementary bodies (EB; individual ehrlichiae) enter the leukocyte by phagocytosis and multiply. After 3 to 5 days, small numbers of tightly packed EBs are observable and are called *initial bodies.* During the next 7 to 12 days, additional growth and replication occur, and the initial bodies develop into mature inclusions, which appear by light microscopy as mulberry or morulae forms. This morulae configuration is a hallmark of ehrlichiae infection. (From McDade J: *J Infect Dis* 161:609, 1990. The University of Chicago Press, Chicago, Ill.)

In most cases reported a lymphocytopenia is present either at diagnosis or at some time during the illness. Early in the course of antibiotic treatment (48 to 72 hours), the lymphocytopenia corrects itself and is rapidly followed by a lymphocytosis of T cells that express CD3 but are negative for CD4 and CD8. Blood smears usually become negative 24 to 48 hours after the beginning of antibiotic therapy. In addition to leukopenia, thrombocytopenia is usually evident.

In HGE the diagnosis is confirmed by seroconversion or by a single serologic titer greater than 1:80 in patients with a supporting history and clinical symptoms. Seroconversion is defined as a fourfold rise in the titer of paired acute and convalescent sera. In HME, the diagnosis is confirmed by seroconversion or by a serologic titer greater than 1:128 patients with a supporting history and clinical symptoms. Serum or cerebrospinal fluid can be analyzed for IgM and IgG antibodies to *Ehrlichia* species.

PCR-based detection of the *E. phagocytophila*-like agent of HGE represents the most sensitive and direct approach to diagnosis. PCR-based detection of *E. chaffeensis* includes amplification of sequences with 16SrDNA.

Treatment and Prevention

Both HME and HGE are treated with doxycycline. No established guidelines exist for long-term therapy. Prevention consists of reduction in the risk of exposure to ticks (see Lyme disease prevention).

BABESIOSIS
Etiology

Babesiosis is a rare, severe, and sometimes fatal tick-borne disease caused by various types of *Babesia,* a microscopic parasite that infects red blood cells (Figure 16-8). The causative organism of babesiosis was first described by Babes in 1888. In New England and the eastern United States, the disease is caused by *B. microti;* in California, it is caused by *B. equi.* In Europe, the disease is caused by *B. divergens* and *B. bovis. B. canis* has been found to be responsible for several cases in Mexico and France.

Epidemiology

B. microti is transmitted by the tick *I. scapularis* in the northeastern United States. The larvae of the tick feed mainly on the white-footed mouse *(P. leucopus).* When larvae develop into nymphs and adults, they feed on the white-tailed deer *(Odocoileus virginianus),* but may also choose a human host.

Babesiosis is seen most frequently in older individuals, splenectomized patients, or in immunocompromised individuals. In the 1970s cases of this disease have been primarily reported during spring, summer, and fall in coastal areas in the northeastern United States, especially Nantucket Island off the coast of Massachusetts and on Long Island in New York. Cases have also been reported in Wisconsin, California, Georgia, and Missouri, and in some European countries. The organism has also been transmitted via blood transfusion from asymptomatic donors.

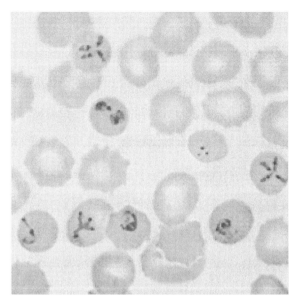

Figure 16-8   *Babesia* in red blood cells. (From Forbes BA, Sahm DF, Weissfeld AS: *Bailey & Scott's diagnostic microbiology,* ed 11, St Louis, 2002, Mosby.)

Signs and Symptoms

The incubation period is approximately 7 to 21 days. The clinical presentation is variable, ranging from asymptomatic to rapidly progressive and, sometimes, fatal. Infections caused by *B. divergens* tend to be more severe (frequently fatal if not appropriately treated) than those caused by *B. microti,* where clinical recovery usually occurs.

The disease can cause fever, fatigue, and hemolytic anemia lasting from several days to several months. It may take from 1 to 8 weeks, sometimes longer, for symptoms to appear. The disease course is characterized by high fever, massive hemolysis, hemoglobinemia, and hemoglobinuria.

Diagnostic Evaluation

Because of the hemolytic component of the disease, many patients exhibit an increased reticulocyte count, elevated lactate dehydrogenase, increased bilirubin, and decreased haptoglobin levels. Variant lymphocytes are usually present on a peripheral blood smear. The ESR is usually elevated.

Two rapid screening methods are used for the identification of *Babesia* organisms. The "gold standard" for identification of *Babesia* organisms is the visualization of the intraerythrocytic organisms in thick or thin blood films. *Babesia* organisms can be made visible by Giemsa staining of peripheral blood smears. The organisms appear as intraerythrocytic oval ring structures (1 to 3 g) with pale blue cytoplasm and one or two tiny red dots. As the *Babesia* organisms mature, they assume an ameboid morphology, and there can be multiple organisms inside the same cell.

The *Babesia* organism ring structures can be easily confused with the ring forms in malaria infections. Several features distinguish *Babesia* ring structures from malaria. *B. microti* occasionally have four to five rings per erythrocyte and sometimes form a tetrad, called a Maltese Cross. Because these organisms may be difficult to detect in peripheral blood, direct visualization lacks sensitivity, producing false-negative results with low-level parasitemia. The degree of parasitemia varies between 1% and 20% in patients with a normal, functioning spleen. It can be as high as 85% in splenectomized patients.

The Field's test is a rapid method performed with a thick peripheral blood film. Erythrocytes in the film are lysed and stained with methylene blue, azure B, and eosin. The method dehemoglobinizes and stains in less than 15 seconds.

This rapid screening method is being replaced by the quantitative buffy coat method (QBC) method. The QBC was initially developed for detection of malaria parasites, but it can be used as a screening test for babesiosis and is at least as sensitive as peripheral blood smear analysis. This method requires centrifuging the patient's blood in a microcapillary tube with a coating on its wall of acridine orange (AO) stain. AO stains nucleic acid. Denser, infected erythrocytes concentrate with the rest of the red blood cells and are detected by fluorescence microscopy.

Acute and convalescent antibody titers may be useful for diagnosis. A titer of greater than 1:256 is considered diagnostic of acute infection. Only IgG antibody determinations are performed. PCR amplification can be used for diagnosis.

Molecular diagnosis can also be useful. In some infections with intraerythrocytic parasites, the morphologic characteristics observed on microscopic examination of blood smears do not allow an unambiguous differentiation between *Babesia* and *Plasmodium* organisms. In these cases, the diagnosis can be derived from molecular techniques (e.g., PCR, using the appropriate primers, and single-step, or the more sensitive nested PCR technique). In addition, molecular approaches are valuable in investigations of new *Babesia* variants (or species) observed in recent human infections in the United States and Europe.

Treatment and Prevention

Standardized treatments for babesiosis have not been developed. However, some drugs used in the treatment of malaria have been found to be effective in some patients with babesiosis.

Antimicrobial therapy is recommended for splenectomized or immunodeficient patients, older patients, and patients with severe infections. The usual regimen consists of a combination of clindamycin and oral quinine. An alternative treatment option is oral azithromycin and oral atovaquone. Exchange transfusion has been proven effective for patients with a high level of parasites (>10%), severe disease, or massive hemolysis.

Prevention requires vigilance when in tick-infested areas (see Lyme disease prevention).

Case Study

A 42-year-old executive lived in New York City. Her company annually sponsored a Memorial Day weekend golf outing at a Long Island club. In early June she noticed a solid, bright-red spot on her left thigh. The spot was about 2 inches wide in the bright-red area with an overall diameter of about 6 inches including the surrounding pale area. The ensuing 11 months passed without further incident.

The following Memorial Day weekend, she was stung several times by bees. Both a systemic and a local reaction followed. About a week later, last year's red ring on the thigh reappeared. During this interval, she experienced fever, malaise, arthromyalgias, headache, and a stiff neck, but recovered completely.

In the fall she noticed insidiously progressive fatigue, malaise, memory deficits, irritability, and inattentiveness to the demands of her job.

She visited a physician, but no abnormalities were noted and she was referred to a Manhattan neurologist. The patient was eventually diagnosed as having Lyme disease.

Questions and Discussions

1. Did the patient's residence or travel history suggest that she might have been exposed to Lyme disease?

    Yes. Although the patient did not travel far from her urban residence, she did visit a nearby endemic area. In the United States there are three major foci of infection: the northeastern coastal states from Massachusetts to Maryland, the upper midwestern states of Minnesota and Wisconsin, and portions of four western states: California, Oregon, Nevada, and Utah. In this case, Long Island happens to be a "hot spot" for Lyme disease.

2. Why did it take so long for the patient to develop symptoms of Lyme disease?

    Lyme disease often has a prolonged latency period. It usually begins during the summer months with EM and flulike symptoms and may be accompanied by right upper-quadrant tenderness and a mild hepatitis (stage 1). This stage is followed weeks to months later by acute cardiac or neurologic disease in a minority of untreated individuals (stage 2), and is then followed by arthritis and chronic neurologic disease (stage 3) in many untreated patients weeks to years after disease onset.

Diagnosis

Lyme disease

Case Study

This 25-year-old graduate student visited his local family physician because of episodic arthromyalgias, sporadic global headaches, fatigue, irritability, and depression. Over the last several months he had become seriously dysfunctional at work and home.

His residence and travel history revealed a week-long vacation on Cape Cod last summer. He could not recall any tick bites or any skin lesions fitting the description of EM.

A laboratory test revealed a positive test, and a 4-week course of doxycycline was initiated. Two weeks later he noted significant improvement in symptoms, but 3 months later his previous symptoms recurred. His laboratory test was repeated and again was positive. A month's regimen of amoxicillin and probenecid was initiated. This time there was no improvement. No neurologic findings were apparent. His joints were painful, but no overt synovitis was present. Two months after the second course of antibiotic, his Lyme test was still positive and he was put on 2-week infusion therapy with ceftriaxone. His symptoms disappeared after this treatment.

Questions and Discussion

1. Why was the treatment regimen initially unsuccessful?

    For most patients with a positive Lyme antibody titer whose only symptoms are nonspecific myalgia or fatigue, the risks and costs of empirical parenteral antibiotic therapy exceed the benefits. Treatment usually fails because the patient is not suffering from Lyme disease.

2. Why did the patient demonstrate a positive laboratory result, even though the usual treatment regimen was unsuccessful?

    False-positive results can occur if an individual has been exposed to a related bacteria. For example, tick-borne relapsing fever spirochetes, *B. hermsii,* are closely related to *B. burgdorferi.* Antibodies to *B. hermsii,* an agent that coexists with the Lyme disease spirochete in portions of the western United States, strongly cross-react with *B. burgdorferi* in IFA staining and ELISA testing. Common antigens are shared among the *Borrelia* and even with the treponemes. Serum from syphilitic patients reacts positively in assays for Lyme disease. Therefore serologic test results for antibodies to *B. burgdorferi* should be considered along with clinical data and epidemiologic information when a patient is evaluated for Lyme disease.

Diagnosis

Lyme disease

Case Study

A 45-year old man from Upstate New York visited his physician because of a worsening headache, myalgia, arthralgia, and generalized weakness. He had been in good health until about 1 week before the appointment. A fever and myalgia began after the patient removed a small tick from his left thigh while he was on vacation in an area in which *B. burgdorferi* is endemic. In addition, the deer tick found in locale that he visited on vacation is the vector of Lyme disease, babesiosis, and most likely human granulocytic ehrlichiosis. On physical examination, the patient had a slight temperature. His thigh had a rash suggestive of EM. Laboratory results included a complete blood count and liver function tests. A

skin scraping was obtained for the purpose of culturing *B. burgdorferi.* Buffy-coat smears of peripheral blood were also requested.

The patient had a slight leukopenia, normal white blood cell differential, and a normal hemoglobin and hematocrit. His liver function tests were slightly abnormal. Wright-stained buffy coat smears revealed the presence of human granulocytic ehrlichiosis morulae. The patient was given a prescription for oral doxycycline twice daily for 14 days. Nine days after the commencement of treatment, the patient felt markedly better. Repeat laboratory tests were all within the normal reference range. His rash had resolved.

Questions and Discussion

1. Can the vector of *B. burgdorferi* and the agent of human granulocytic ehrlichiosis be the same?

    Yes. *Ixodes* ticks infected with *B. burgdorferi* and the agent of human granulocytic ehrlichiosis have been identified.

2. Is it important to determine if one or both infections are present in the same host?

    Yes. Simultaneous infection with *B. burgdorferi* and the agent of human granulocytic ehrlichiosis is important because the natural history of each of the diseases may change in the presence of the other. Another consideration by a physician is selection of antimicrobial therapy. In addition, dual infection with *B. burgdorferi* may result in more serious disease than an infection with either agent alone.

3. How can coinfection with *B. burgdorferi* and the agent of human granulocytic ehrlichiosis be demonstrated in the laboratory?

    Coinfection with *B. burgdorferi* and human granulocytic ehrlichiosis can be demonstrated by the isolation of both organisms from clinical specimens. Serologic evidence alone is insufficient. Among the many problems that exist with a dual infection, one is that human granulocytic ehrlichiosis may by itself produce false positive results on serologic tests for Lyme disease. Even with PCR testing care must be taken to avoid contamination and to use appropriately specific primers.

Diagnosis

Coinfection with *B. burgdorferi* (Lyme disease) and HGE

Case Study

This 73-year-old previously healthy man had spent the summer on Martha's Vineyard. On returning to his home in Boston after Labor Day, he began to feel unusually tired and having difficulty breathing. He also reported that his urine had become dark-brown several days after returning home.

On physical examination the patient was jaundiced, and he had an enlarged spleen. A complete blood count, urinalysis, and blood chemistries were ordered. His total white blood cell count was normal, but he had an increased percentage of segmented neutrophils. His hemoglobin, hematocrit, and platelet count were all below the normal reference range. He had hematuria and proteinuria in his urine. His liver function tests were markedly elevated. His renal function assays were also elevated. A follow-up Wright-stained peripheral blood smear revealed numerous *B. microti* organisms.

The patient was treated with quinine and the antibiotics, clindamycin and doxycycline. He also received 2 U of packed red blood cells. Six days later the patient was discharged from the hospital.

Questions and Discussion

1. Would the patient's travel history be suggestive of malaria or another blood-borne infectious disease?

    Although some of the patient's symptoms resemble malaria, it would not be associated with the area that the patient visited; however, other tick-borne illnesses (e.g., Lyme disease, babesiosis) are considerations.
2. What is the definitive diagnosis for babesiosis?

    Definitive diagnosis relies predominantly on the demonstration of intraerythrocytic ring-shaped or pleomorphic parasites in Wright-Giemsa stained blood smears.
3. What additional laboratory tests are of diagnostic value?

    PCR should be used only when blood smear results are questionable or negative in patients in whom babesiosis is strongly suspected and a travel history to a malaria-endemic area is absent. In cases of diagnostic uncertainty or suspected chronic infection, serologic studies can be conducted. The method of choice is the IFA test. Western blot assay is also available.

Diagnosis

Babesiosis

Case Study

A 35-year-old field biologist from central Missouri was positive for human immunodeficiency virus (HIV). Her work required that she spend a great deal of time in the woods in the surrounding areas. Although she was in good health despite the HIV positivity, she began having back pain fever, chills, sweats, a productive cough, and extreme tiredness before her visit to the Emergency Room.

She was admitted to the hospital because her laboratory results demonstrated severe leukopenia and thrombocytopenia. Her liver function tests were also extremely abnormal. Later on the day of admission, renal failure developed. The patient died the next day.

Questions and Discussion

1. What was the cause of death?

    The cause of death was determined to be human monocytic ehrlichiosis. The presence of inclusion, predominantly in monocytic cells, established the diagnosis.
2. What immunologic studies could be performed?

    At autopsy, tissue samples from the spleen, kidneys, lymph nodes, and bone marrow were obtained for further study. These specimens were examined immunohistologically using monoclonal and polyclonal anti-*Ehrlichia chaffeensis* antibodies. The antibodies reacted strongly with the inclusions in the tissues.
3. Is human monocytic ehrlichiosis a risk in the United States?

    Human ehrlichiosis is endemic in the United States. HME is seen in the south central and southeast United States. In contrast, HGE has been identified in the upper Midwest and northeastern United States.

Diagnosis

Human monocytic ehrlichiosis

CHAPTER HIGHLIGHTS

Lyme disease has become recognized as an important infectious disease in the United States. The infection, which is caused by the tick-borne spirochete *Borrelia burgdorferi*, has emerged as a major health hazard for humans and domestic animals. In some cases the disease may be transitory and of little consequence, but in others it may become chronic and severely disabling. Accurate diagnosis therefore is of great importance, but laboratory testing techniques still need improvement. The spirochete is transmitted by certain ixodid ticks. In the United States, the preferred host for both the larval and nymphal states of *I. scapularis* is the white-footed mouse, *P. leucopus*. White-tailed deer, which are not involved in the life cycle of the spirochete, are the preferred host for *I. scapularis* adult stage, and they seem to be critical to tick survival.

Spirochetes are transmitted from the gut of the tick to human skin at the site of a bite and then migrate outwardly into the skin. This migration causes the unique expanding skin lesion, EM. Subsequent dissemination of spirochetes to secondary sites may cause major organ system involvement in humans. In dogs, the most common symptom is arthritis.

In the United States the European rash was virtually unknown until 1969, when a case of a physician bitten by a tick while hunting in Wisconsin was reported. It was not until 1982 that Burgdorfer and Barbour isolated a previously unrecognized spirochete, now called *B. burgdorferi*, from *I. scapularis* ticks and Lyme disease became a recognized vector-borne, infectious disease. Two factors influence the chance that a bitten patient will get the disease: the likelihood that local ixodid ticks carry the Lyme spirochete, and the likelihood of infection after a bite by an infected tick. The probability of infection after an ixodid tick bite in an area of endemic disease is about 3%, but it varies in different regions from less than 1% to as high as 5%. Lyme disease now accounts for more than 95% of all reported vector-borne illness in America.

Lyme disease is considered an emerging infectious disease because of the impact of changing environmental and socioeconomic factors, such as the transformation of farmland into suburban woodlots favorable for deer and deer ticks. Although pets may represent a spirochete reservoir, it is unlikely that human beings can be infected directly by them. However, in areas of endemic Lyme disease, both adult and nymphal ticks, carried into the household by dogs and cats, may infest humans.

The basic features of the disease are similar worldwide, but there are regional variations, primarily between the illness found in America and that found in Europe and Asia. In at least 60% to 80% of patients in the United States, Lyme disease begins with a slowly expanding skin lesion, EM, which occurs at the site of the tick bite. The skin lesion is frequently accompanied by flulike symptoms.

Lyme borreliosis is a multisystem illness that primarily involves the skin, nervous system, heart, and joints. Lyme disease usually begins during the summer months with EM and flulike symptoms.

Cellular immune responses to *B. burgdorferi* antigens begin concurrently with early clinical illness. An increase in spontaneous suppressor cell activity and reduction in natural killer cell activity have been noted. Mononuclear cell antigen-specific responses develop during spirochetal dissemination, and humoral (antibody) immune responses soon follow. Serodiagnostic tests are insensitive during the first several weeks of infection. In the United States, approximately 20% to 30% of patients have positive responses, usually of the IgM isotype, during this period, but by convalescence 2 to 4 weeks later, about 70% to 80% have seroreactivity even after antibiotic treatment. After about 1 month, the majority of patients with active infection have IgG antibody responses. After antibiotic treatment, antibody titers fall slowly but IgG and even IgM responses may persist for many years after treatment. Therefore, an IgM response cannot be interpreted as a manifestation of recent infection or reinfection unless the appropriate clinical characteristics are present. Antibodies formed include cryoglobulins, immune complexes, antibodies specific for *B. burgdorferi,* and anticardiolipin antibodies. Elevated titers of IgM are noted in early disease. Immunoblot analysis demonstrates that IgM antibodies form initially against the flagellar 41 KD polypeptide but react later to additional cell wall antigens. An overlapping IgG response to these antigens develops in some individuals. These antigen-specific cellular and humoral responses are neither known to eradicate infection in early disease nor to participate in disease pathogenesis.

Specific IgM or IgG antibodies against *B. burgdorferi* are usually not detectable in a patient's serum unless symptoms have been present for at least 2 to 4 weeks. In cases of Lyme arthritis, tests for serum antinuclear antibodies, rheumatoid factor, and the VDRL (Venereal Disease Research Laboratories) Test are generally negative. However, anti-*B. burgdorferi* antibodies of the IgG type should be present in the serum of patients with Lyme arthritis.

Outer surface protein A antibodies develop late in the course of human Lyme infection, and then only in a subset of patients. The culture of *B. burgdorferi* from specimens in Barbour-Stoenner-Kelly medium permits a definitive diagnosis.

In the United States, the diagnosis is usually based on the recognition of the characteristic clinical findings, a history of exposure in an area where the disease is endemic, and except in patients with EM, an antibody response to *B. burgdorferi* by ELISA and the Western blot test. More than half the time, positive test results are inconsequential because physicians feel comfortable making the diagnosis based on symptoms and patient history. The importance of testing, however, comes into play when the telltale "bull's eye" rash or other symptoms characteristic of Lyme disease do not occur.

The most common laboratory assays for *B. burgdorferi* antibody detection include IFA staining methods, ELISA for total Igs or IgM and IgG antibodies, and PreVue *B. burgdorferi* Antibody Detection Assay. Immunoblotting techniques can be used along with ELISA to characterize immune response and for diagnosis. PreVue *B. burgdorferi* Antibody Detection Assay (Wampole PreVue Assay for Lyme disease) is a CLIA-waived procedure intended to be used as the first presumptive step in testing individuals suspected of having Lyme disease. Positive results must be confirmed with a Western blot test done by a laboratory. Two-stage testing is recommended by the Centers for Disease Control and Prevention. The new test uses antigenic proteins developed by recombinant DNA techniques rather than a whole cell *B. burgdorferi* preparation. Antigenic proteins developed by recombinant DNA techniques allow for more accuracy. The "false-positive" rate is similar to that of laboratory tests for Lyme disease. Western blot analysis can verify reactivity of antibody to major surface or flagellar proteins of *B. burgdorferi*. Western blot is helpful in determining "borderline" negative or weakly positive results obtained from other tests, but the values are not always reliable. This procedure is more definitive in later Lyme disease when multiple antibody bands specific for *B. burgdorferi* appear. PCR can detect spirochete in the synovial fluid around the joints or in other clinical samples. PCR looks for DNA of the organism. In the past, PCR has been taken as definitive evidence that a person has an infection, but it is possible to have antigens without the organism being viable. PCR amplifies small amounts of DNA that may remain even when intact organisms are no longer present—an indicator that the organism does or did exist. The PCR technique may miss the spirochete in the blood, allowing it to move into other tissues.

Antigen detection systems screen for antigenic products rather than for the host's immune response to the infection. Antigen detection systems could be expected to confirm both infections in patients with depressed immune systems and early infections in patients who have not yet produced a detectable antibody response.

Two categories of procedures have been developed: T-cell proliferative assays and antibody-based antigen detection systems. Monoclonal or polyclonal antibodies also detect specific Lyme spirochete antigens. Quantities of proteins including flagellin, OspA, and OspB are detectable. Assays based on OspA and OspB, two closely related *B. burgdorferi* proteins from the outer wall of the bacteria, are available.

Various types of antibiotics are in general use for *B. burgdorferi* treatment. As of February 25, 2002, the manufacturer of LYMErix, a recombinant outer-surface protein A Lyme disease vaccine for humans, announced that the vaccine will no longer be commercially available. Pets, especially dogs rather than cats, can become infected with Lyme disease. Effective vaccines are available for pets.

When hiking in the woods or mountains, picnicking at local parks, or walking in tall grass in shore areas, individuals should check for ticks, wear light-colored clothing so tick viewing is easier, and tuck pants into socks.

Human ehrlichiosis was first described in the United States in 1986. Tick-borne rickettsiae of the genus *Ehrlichia* have recently been recognized as a cause of human illness in the United States. *Ehrlichia chaffeensis* was demonstrated to cause disease in 1987. Since then two more *Ehrlichia* species, *E. ewingii* and *E. phagocytophilia*-like agent, have been identified. Although the prevalence rates are low, human ehrlichiosis is endemic in the United States.

Ehrlichiosis is a general term for both HGE and HME. The syndrome of human ehrlichiosis is not commonly recognized by physicians, but should be considered in patients with a history of tick exposure, and acute, febrile, flulike illness. Definitive diagnosis is based on inclusions in leukocytes.

In HGE the diagnosis is confirmed by seroconversion or by a single serologic titer greater than 1:80 in patients with a supporting history and clinical symptoms. Seroconversion is defined as a fourfold rise in the titer of paired acute and convalescent sera. In HME, the diagnosis is confirmed by seroconversion or by a serologic titer greater than 1:128 patients with a supporting history and clinical symptoms. Serum or cerebrospinal fluid can be analyzed for IgM and IgG antibodies to *Ehrlichia* organisms. PCR-based detection of the *E. phagocytophila*-like agent of HGE represents the most sensitive and direct approach to diagnosis. PCR-based detection of *E. chaffeensis* includes amplification of sequences with 16SrDNA.

Both HGE and HME are treated with doxycycline. No established guidelines exist for long-term therapy. Prevention consists of reduction in the risk of exposure to ticks (see Lyme disease prevention).

Babesiosis is a rare, severe, and sometimes fatal tickborne disease caused by various types of *Babesia*, a microscopic parasite that infects red blood cells.

B. microti is transmitted by the tick *I. scapularis* in the northeastern United States. The larvae of the tick feed mainly on the white-footed mouse *(P. leucopus)*. When larvae develop into nymphs and adults, they feed on the white-tailed deer *(O. virginianus)*, but may also choose a human host. Babesiosis is seen most frequently in older patients, splenectomized patients, or in immunocompromised individuals. Cases of this disease have been primarily reported during spring, summer, and fall in coastal areas in the northeastern United States, especially Nantucket Island off the coast of Massachusetts and on Long Island in New York. Cases have

also been reported in Wisconsin, California, Georgia, Missouri, and some European countries. The organism has also been transmitted via blood transfusion from asymptomatic donors.

The disease can cause fever, fatigue and hemolytic anemia lasting from several days to several months. It may take from one to 8 weeks, sometimes longer, for symptoms to appear.

The "gold standard" for identification of *Babesia* is the visualization of the intraerythrocytic organisms in thick or thin blood films. The Field's test is a rapid method performed with a thick peripheral blood film. Acute and convalescent antibody titers may be useful for diagnosis. A titer of greater than 1:256 is considered diagnostic of acute infection. Only IgG antibody determinations are performed. PCR amplification can be used for diagnosis.

Standardized treatments for babesiosis have not been developed. However, some drugs used in the treatment of malaria have been found to be effective in some patients with babesiosis. Prevention requires vigilance when in tick-infested areas.

REVIEW QUESTIONS

1. Common vectors of Lyme disease include all but:
   A. *I. pacificus*
   B. *I. scapularis*
   C. *I. ricinus*
   D. *D. variabilis*

2. The only continent without Lyme disease is:
   A. Asia
   B. Europe
   C. Africa
   D. Antarctica

3. The primary reservoir in nature for *B. burgdorferi* is the:
   A. white-tail deer
   B. white-footed mouse
   C. lizard
   D. meadowlark

4. The first *B. burgdorferi* antigen to elicit an antibody response is:
   A. outer surface protein A
   B. outer surface protein B
   C. flagellar 41-KD polypeptide
   D. 60-kilodalton polypeptide

5. The incidence of infection following an *I. scapularis* tick bite in an endemic area on average is:
   A. 1%
   B. 3%
   C. 5%
   D. 10%

6. Erythema migrans:
   A. occurs in all patients
   B. harbors *B. burgdorferi* in the advancing edge
   C. is easily distinguished from other erythemas
   D. is more common in the winter months

7. The predominant symptoms of Lyme meningitis are:
   A. severe headache and mild neck stiffness
   B. aseptic meningitis and double vision
   C. cranial nerve palsies and blurred vision
   D. peripheral radiculoneuritis and peripheral neuropathy

8. Cardiac involvement in Lyme disease may include:
   A. murmurs
   B. conduction abnormalities
   C. congestive heart failure
   D. vasculitis

9. Ocular involvement in Lyme disease includes all of the following except:
   A. cranial nerve palsies
   B. conjunctivitis
   C. panophthalmitis with loss of vision
   D. choroiditis with retinal detachment

10. Pregnancy in Lyme disease:
    A. does not produce high fetal mortality
    B. has been associated with transplacental infection
    C. should be terminated because of maternal risk
    D. is not associated with congenital abnormalities

11. The most useful test for distinguishing between true- and false-positive serologic tests is:
    A. enzyme-linked immunosorbent assay
    B. immunofluorescence assay
    C. polymerase chain reaction
    D. T-cell assay

12. Preventive methods include all of the following except:
    A. wearing light-colored clothes
    B. removing ticks
    C. tucking pants into socks
    D. applying insect repellent to skin and clothes

13. Lyme disease, the most common tick-borne disease in the United States, is a major health hazard for:
    A. dogs
    B. horses and cattle
    C. humans
    D. all of the above

14. Lyme disease is a _____ type of infection.
    A. bacterial
    B. parasitic
    C. viral
    D. fungal

15. The first case of Lyme disease occurred in:
    A. Connecticut
    B. Wisconsin
    C. Florida
    D. New York

Questions 16-19. Fill in the blanks, choosing from the following answers.

Possible answers for question 16.
   A. 3 days
   B. 1 week
   C. 4 weeks
   D. 3 months

Possible answers for question 17.
   A. neurologic
   B. rheumatoid
   C. cutaneous (e.g., erythema migrans)
   D. cardiac

Possible answers for question 18.
   A. hours to weeks
   B. days to weeks
   C. weeks to months
   D. weeks to years

Possible answers for question 19.
   A. arthritis
   B. Lyme carditis
   C. transplacental transmission
   D. lymphocytoma

Clinical Features of Lyme Disease

Stage	Length of Time	Common Signs and Symptoms
I	16. _____ (median)	17. _____ manifestation after infection
II	Follows a variable latent period	Target organs and systems can manifest abnormalities
III	18. _____ after infection	19. _____ , late neurologic complications

20. Unlike some procedures, polymerase chain reaction (PCR) can be used to detect Lyme disease-causing organisms in:
    A. urine
    B. cerebrospinal fluid
    C. synovial fluid
    D. blood

Questions 21 and 22. Fill in the blanks, choosing from the following answers.

Possible answers for questions 21 and 22.
   A. antibody
   B. microorganisms
   C. antigenic products
   D. the infected tick

Antigen detection systems in Lyme disease testing screen for

(21) _____ rather than for (22) _____ associated with the infection.

23. A patient who has a specific Lyme disease–associated manifestation may be treated with:
    A. vaccination
    B. interferon
    C. antibiotic
    D. analgesic

24. *Ehrlichia* species belong to the same family as the organism that causes:
    A. Lyme disease
    B. Rocky Mountain spotted fever
    C. toxoplasmosis
    D. infectious mononucleosis

25. One of the most common physical findings in adults with ehrlichiosis is:
    A. hives
    B. fever
    C. erythema migrans
    D. nausea

26. Definitive diagnosis of ehrlichiosis requires:
    A. a complete blood count
    B. detection of the presence of lymphocytopenia
    C. acute and convalescent serum antibody titers
    D. direct microscopic observation of inclusions in leukocytes

27. In human granulocytic ehrlichiosis, the diagnosis is confirmed by seroconversion or by a single serologic titer of _____ in patients with a supporting history and clinical symptoms.
    A. 1:2
    B. 1:16
    C. 1:80
    D. 1:160

28. In the eastern United States, babesiosis is caused by:
    A. *B. microti*
    B. *B. canis*
    C. *B. bovis*
    D. *B. equi*

29. Babesiosis is characterized by:
    A. fever
    B. fatigue
    C. hemolytic anemia
    D. all of the above

30. *Babesia* organisms can be found in:
    A. peripheral blood
    B. sputum
    C. synovial fluid
    D. various exudates

BIBLIOGRAPHY

Adler T: Lyme disease may not harm kids' brains, *Science News* 146:116, 1994.

Aronowitz R: Prevention of Lyme disease after tick bites, *N Engl J Med* 328(2):136, 1993.

Barenfanger J, Patel PG, Dumler JS, Walker DH: Identifying human ehrlichiosis, *Lab Med* 27:372-374, 1996.

Berger BW et al: Cultivation of *Borrelia burgdorferi* from human tick bite sites: a guide to the risk of infection, *J Am Acad Dermatol* 32(2):184-187, 1995.

Berger BW: Laboratory tests for Lyme disease, *Dermatol Clin* 12(1):19-24, 1994.

Branch DR: Some Lyme arthritis patients have genetic resistance to antibiotics, *Intern Med News Cardiol News* 27(2):5, 1994.

Brown S et al: Role of serology in the diagnosis of Lyme disease, *JAMA* 282(1):62, 1999.

Buechner SA, Rufli T, Erb P: Acrodermatitis chronica atrophicans: a chronic T-cell-mediated immune reaction against *Borrelia burgdorferi*? Clinical, histologic, and immunohistochemical study of five cases, *J Am Acad Dermatol* 28(3):399-405, 1993.

Burrascano J: *Advance topics in Lyme disease,* ed 13, May, 2000, website: www/LymeNet.org.

Caldwell CW et al: Lymphocytosis of gamma/delta T cells in human ehrlichiosis, *Am J Clin Pathol* 103(6):761-766, 1995.

Callister SM et al: Lyme disease: laboratory diagnosis and serologic testing, *Endeavour* 18(2):80-84, 1994.

Callister SM et al: Detection of borreliacidal antibodies by flow cytometry: an accurate, highly specific serodiagnostic test for Lyme disease, *Arch Intern Med* 154(14):1625-1632, 1994.

Campbell GL et al: An evaluation of media for transport of tissues infected with *Borrelia burgdorferi*, *Am J Clin Pathol* 101(2): 154-156, 1994.

Centers for Disease Control and Prevention. Lyme disease: vaccine recommendations, June 14, 2002, www.cdc.gov/ncidod/dvbid/lyme/vaccine.htm.

Chen SM et al: Identification of the antigenic constituents of *Ehrlichia chaffeensis, Am J Trop Med Hyg* 50(1):52-58, 1994.

Cimmino MA: The risk of *Borrelia burgdorferi* infection is not increased in pet owners, *JAMA* 262(21):2997, 1989.

Coon D, Versalovic J: Three tick-borne diseases in the northeastern United States: Lyme disease, babesiosis, and ehrlichiosis, *Turn-Around Times-Clinical Laboratory Reviews* (Mass Gen Hosp, Div of Lab Med) 9:5-10, 2001.

Current WL: The polymerase chain reaction assay for *Borrelia burgdorferi* in the diagnosis of Lyme disease, *Ann Intern Med* 120(6):520-521, 1994.

Dinerman H, Steere AC: Lyme disease associated with fibromyalgia, *Ann Intern Med* 117(4):281-285, 1992.

Dressler F, Yoshinari NH, Steere AC: The T-cell proliferative assay in the diagnosis of Lyme disease, *Ann Intern Med* 115(7):533-539, 1991.

Eskow E et al: Concurrent infection of the central nervous system by *Borrelia burgdorferi, Arch Neurol* 58:1357-1362, 2001.

Everett ED et al: Human ehrlichiosis in adults after tick exposure. Diagnosis using polymerase chain reaction, *Ann Intern Med* 120(9):730-735, 1994.

Fallon BA, Nields JA: Lyme disease: a neuropsychiatric illness, *Am J Psychol* 151(11):1571-1583, 1994.

FDA Consumer magazine: New vaccine targets Lyme disease, FDA 99-1304, May-June 1999.

Feder HM, Hunt MS: Pitfalls in the diagnosis and treatment of Lyme disease in children, *JAMA* 274(1):66-68, 1995.

Fichtenbaum CJ, Peterson LR, Weil GJ: Ehrlichiosis presenting as a life-threatening illness with features of the toxic shock syndrome, *Am J Med* 95(4):351-357, 1993.

Fikrig E et al: Vaccination against Lyme disease caused by diverse *Borrelia burgdorferi, J Exp Med* 181(1):215-221, 1995.

Finn AF, Dattwyler RJ: The immunology of Lyme borreliosis, *Lab Med* 21(5):305-309, 1990.

Fishbein DB, Dawson JE, Robinson L: Human ehrlichiosis in the United States, 1985 to 1990, *Ann Intern Med* 120(9):43, 1990.

Fishbein DB, Dennis DT: Tick-borne disease—a growing risk, *N Engl J Med* 333(7):452-453, 1995.

Fung B et al: Humoral immune response to outer surface protein C of *Borrelia burgdorferi* in Lyme disease: role of the immunoglobulin M response in the serodiagnosis of early infection, *Infect Immun* 62(8):3213-3221, 1994.

Gerber MA, Zalneraitis EL: Childhood neurologic disorders and Lyme disease during pregnancy, *Pediatr Neurol* 11(1):41-43, 1994.

Girouard L et al: Immune recognition of human Hsp60 by Lyme disease patient sera, *Microb Pathog* 14(4):287-297, 1993.

Goldfarb D, Sataloff RT: Lyme disease: a review for the otolaryngologist, *Ear Nose Throat J* 73(11):824-829, 1994.

Goldman DP, Artenstein AW, Bolan CD: Human ehrlichiosis: a newly recognized tick-borne disease, *Am Fam Physician* 46(1):199-208, 1992.

Habif TP: *Clinical dermatology,* ed 2, St Louis, 1990, Mosby.

Hamann-Brand A, Flondor M, Brade V: Evaluation of a passive hemagglutination assay as screening test and of a recombinant immunoblot as confirmatory test for serological diagnosis of Lyme disease, *Eur J Clin Microbiol Infect Dis* 13(7):572-575, 1994.

Harkess JR et al: Ehrlichiosis in children, *Pediatrics* 87(2):199-203, 1991.

Huppertz HI et al: Acute childhood neuroborreliosis with a selective immune response to a low molecular weight protein expressed by *Borrelia garinii, Eur J Pediatr* 153(12):898-902, 1994.

Johnston AM, Kober M, Callaway TH: Enzyme immunoassay with western blot confirmation for Lyme disease testing, *Lab Med* 23(10):663-666, 1992.

Jouben LM, Steele RJ, Bono J: Orthopaedic manifestations of Lyme disease, *Orthop Rev* 23(5):395-400, 1994.

Kaell AT et al: Positive Lyme serology in subacute bacterial endocarditis, *JAMA* 264(22):2916-2922, 1990.

Kantor FS: Disarming Lyme disease, *Sci Am* 271(3):34-39, 1994.

Karch H et al: Demonstration of *Borrelia burgdorferi* DNA in urine samples from healthy humans whose sera contain *B. burgdorferi*-specific antibodies, *J Clin Microbiol* 32(9):2312-2314, 1994.

Karma A et al: Diagnosis and clinical characteristics of ocular Lyme borreliosis, *Am J Ophthalmol* 119(2):127-135, 1995.

Kassirer JP: Is a tick's bark worse than its bite? *N Engl J Med* 327(8):562-563, 1992.

Keller D et al: Safety and immunogenicity of a recombinant outer surface protein a Lyme vaccine, *JAMA* 271(22):1764-1768, 1994.

Klempner MS et al: Two controlled trials of antibiotic treatment in patients with persistent symptoms and a history of Lyme disease, *N Engl J Med* 345(2):85-92, 2001.

Lang J: Catching the bug: how scientists found the cause of Lyme disease and why we're not out of the woods yet, *Conn Med* 53(6):357-364, 1989.

Lengl-Janssen B et al: The T helper cell response in Lyme arthritis: differential recognition of *Borrelia burgdorferi* outer surface protein A in patients with treatment-resistant or treatment-responsive Lyme arthritis, *J Exp Med* 180(6):2069-2078, 1994.

Leslie TA et al: Acrodermatitis chronica atrophicans: a case report and review of the literature, *Br J Dermatol* 131(5):687-693, 1994.

Liegner KB: Prevention of Lyme disease after tick bites, *N Engl J Med* 328(2):136, 1993.

Logigian EL, Kaplan RF, Steere AC: Chronic neurologic manifestations of Lyme disease, *N Engl J Med* 323(21):1438-1444, 1990.

Lovrich SD et al: Seroprotective groups of Lyme borreliosis spirochetes from North America and Europe, *J Infect Dis* 170(1):115-121, 1994.

Luft BJ et al: Appropriateness of parenteral antibiotic treatment for patients with presumed Lyme disease, *Ann Intern Med* 119(6):516-517, 1993.

Lyme disease knowledge, attitudes, and behaviors—Connecticut, 1992, *MMWR* 41(28):505-507, 1992.

Lyme disease surveillance—United States, 1989-1990, *MMWR* 40(25):417-421, 1991.

Lyme disease—United States, 1991-1992, *MMWR* 42(18):345-348, 1993.

Lyme disease—United States, 1993, *MMWR* 43(31):564-565, 1994.

Lyme disease—United States, 1999, *MMWR* 50(10):181-183, 2001.

Lyme disease—United States, 2000, *MMWR* 51:29-31, 2002.

Lyme disease—United States, 2001, www.lyme.org 2002.

Magid D et al: Prevention of Lyme disease after tick bites, *N Engl J Med* 327(8):534-541, 1992.

Magnarelli LA: Laboratory analyses for Lyme disease, *Conn Med* 53(6):331-334, 1989.

Marshall WF et al: Detection of *Borrelia burgdorferi* DNA in museum specimens of *Peromyscus leucopus, J Infect Dis* 170(4):1027-1032, 1994.

Masuzawa T et al: Relationship between infectivity and OspC expression in Lyme disease *Borrelia, FEMS Microbiol Lett* 123(1):319-324, 1994.

Mayo DR, Vance DW Jr: Parvovirus B19 as the cause of a syndrome resembling Lyme arthritis in adults, *N Engl J Med* 324(6):419, 1991.

Middleton DB: Tick-borne infections. What starts as a tiny bite may have a serious outcome, *Postgrad Med* 95(5):131-139, 1994.

Miller GL et al: The epidemiology of Lyme disease in the United States 1987-88, *Lab Med* 21(5):285-289, 1990.

Miller LC et al: Balance of synovial fluid IL-1 beta and IL-1 receptor antagonist and recovery from Lyme arthritis, *Lancet* 341 (8838):146-148, 1993.

Mitchell PD et al: Comparison of four immunoserologic assays for detection of antibodies to *Borrelia burgdorferi* in patients with culture-positive erythema migrans, *J Clin Microbiol* 32(8):1958-1962, 1994.

Moll-van-Charante AW, Groen J, Osterhaus AD: Risk of infections transmitted by arthropods and rodents in forestry workers, *Eur J Epidemiol* 10(3):349-351, 1994.

Montgomery RR, Nathanson MH, Malawista SE: Fc- and non-Fc-mediated phagocytosis of *Borrelia burgdorferi* by macrophages, *J Infect Dis* 170(4):890-893, 1994.

Nadelman RB et al: Prophylaxis with single-dose doxycycline for the prevention of Lyme disease after an *Ixodes scapularis* tick bite, *N Engl J Med* 345(2):79-84, 2001.

Nadelman RB et al: Simultaneous human granulocytic ehrlichiosis and Lyme borreliosis, *N Engl J Med* 337:27-30, 1997.

Nocton JJ et al: Detection of *Borrelia burgdorferi* DNA by polymerase chain reaction in synovial fluid from patients with Lyme arthritis, *N Engl J Med* 330(4):229-234, 1994.

Nohlmans MK et al: Evaluation of nine serological tests for diagnosis of Lyme borreliosis, *Eur J Clin Microbiol Infect Dis* 13(5):394-400, 1994.

Padula SJ et al: Use of recombinant OspC from *Borrelia burgdorferi* for serodiagnosis of early Lyme disease, *J Clin Microbiol* 32(7):1733-1738, 1994.

Pantanowitz L, Ballesteros E, DeGirolami P: Laboratory diagnosis of babesiosis, *Lab Med* 32:184-186, 2001.

Paparone PWV, Glenn WB: Lyme disease with concurrent ehrlichiosis, *J Am Osteopath Assoc* 94(7):568-570, 1994.

Paparone PW: Polymyalgia rheumatica or Lyme disease? How to avoid misdiagnosis in older patients, *Postgrad Med* 97(1):161-164, 167-170, 1995.

Persing DH et al: Target imbalance: disparity of *Borrelia burgdorferi* genetic material in synovial fluid from Lyme arthritis patients, *J Infect Dis* 169(3):668-677, 1994.

Rahn DW: Lyme disease—where's the bug? *N Engl J Med* 330(4):282-283, 1994.

Rathore MH: Infection due to *Ehrlichia canis* in children, *South Med J* 85(7):703-705, 1992.

Rittig MG et al: *Borrelia burgdorferi*-induced ultrastructural alterations in human phagocytes: a clue to pathogenicity? *J Pathol* 173(3):269-282, 1994.

Rose CD et al: The overdiagnosis of Lyme disease in children residing in an endemic area, *Clin Pediatr* 33(11):663-668, 1994.

Scarpa C, Trevisan G, Stinco G: Lyme borreliosis, *Dermatol Clin* 12(4):669-685, 1994.

Schering-Plough Pharmaceutical Co. Galaxy®Lyme, June 14, 2002, website: www.spah.com.

Schoen RT: Identification of Lyme disease, *Rheum Dis Clin North Am* 20(2):361-369, 1994.

Schutzer SE et al: Early and specific antibody response to OspA in Lyme disease, *J Clin Invest* 94(1):454-457, 1994.

Schwan TG, Simpson WJ: Diagnosing Lyme disease, *Ann Intern Med* 115(7):577-578, 1991.

Shadick NA et al: The long-term clinical outcomes of Lyme disease, *Ann Intern Med* 121(8):560-567, 1994.

Shadick NA et al: The cost-effectiveness of vaccination against Lyme disease, *Ann Intern Med* 161:554-561 2001.

Shanafelt MC et al: Costimulatory signals can selectively modulate cytokine production by subsets of CD4+ T cells, *J Immunol* 154(4):1684-1690, 1995.

Shapiro ED et al: Doxycycline for tick bites: not for everyone, *N Engl J Med* 345:133-134, 2001.

Shapiro ED et al: A controlled trial of antimicrobial prophylaxis for Lyme disease after deer-tick bites, *N Engl J Med* 327(25):1769-1773, 1992.

Shih CM, Spielman A, Telford SR: Short report: mode of action of protective immunity to Lyme disease spirochetes, *Am J Trop Med Hyg* 52(1):72-74, 1995.

Sindern E, Malin JP: Phenotypic analysis of cerebrospinal fluid cells over the course of Lyme meningoradiculitis, *Acta Cytol* 39(1):73-75, 1995.

Spach DH et al: Tick-borne diseases in the United States, *N Engl J Med* 329(13):936-947, 1993.

Spielman A: The emergence of Lyme disease and human babesiosis in a changing environment, *Ann NY Acad Sci* 740:146-156, 1994.

Standaert SM et al: Ehrlichiosis in golf-oriented retirement community, *N Engl J Med* 333(7):420-424, 1995.

Stark E, Wurster U: Chronic neurologic manifestations of Lyme disease, *N Engl J Med* 324(16):1137, 1991.

Steere AC: Lyme disease, *N Engl J Med* 345:115-123, 2001.

Steere AC et al: The overdiagnosis of Lyme disease, *JAMA* 269(14):1812-1816, 1993.

Steere AC: Lyme disease: a growing threat to urban populations, *Proc Natl Acad Sci USA* 91(7):2378-2383, 1994.

Steere AC: Lyme disease, *N Engl J Med* 321(9):586-596, 1989.

Stefanelli S et al: Isolation of *Borrelia burgdorferi* in Tuscany (Italy), *Microbiologica* 17(4):333-336, 1994.

Stover CK et al: Protective immunity elicited by rBCG vaccinces, *Dev Biol Stand* 82:163-170, 1994.

Szer IS, Taylor E, Steere AC: The long-term course of Lyme arthritis in children, *N Engl J Med* 325(3):159-163, 1991.

Telford SR et al: Human granulocytic ehrlichiosis in Massachusetts, *Ann Intern Med* 123(4):277-279, 1995.

The Medical Letter® on Drugs and Therapeutics, 2000, website: www.medletter.com.

Trock DH, Craft JE, Rahn DW: Clinical manifestations of Lyme disease in the United States, *Conn Med* 53(6):327-330, 1989.

Tsai TF, Bailey RE, Moore PS: National surveillance of Lyme disease, *Conn Med* 53(6):324-326, 1989.

Uhaa IJ et al: A case of human ehrlichiosis acquired in Mali: clinical and laboratory findings, *Am J Trop Med Hyg* 46(2):161-164, 1992.

van Dam AP et al: Different genospecies of *Borrelia burgdorferi* are associated with distinct clinical manifestations of Lyme borreliosis, *Clin Infect Dis* 17(4):708-717, 1993.

Verdon M et al: Recognition and management of Lyme disease, *Am Fam Physician* 56(2):427-442, 1997.

Wampole Laboratories. Wampole PreVue package insert, 2002.

Weyth Pharmaceutical Co. "LymeVax®," June 14, 2002, website: www.wyeth.com.

White DJ et al: The geographic spread and temporal increase of the Lyme disease epidemic, *JAMA* 266(9):1230-1236, 1991.

Wienecke RN et al: Molecular subtyping of *Borrelia burgdorferi* in erythema migrans and acrodermatitis chronica atrophicans, *J Invest Dermatol* 103(1):19-22, 1994.

Zbinden RD et al: Comparison of two methods for detecting intrathecal synthesis of *Borrelia burgdorferi*-specific antibodies and PCR for diagnosis of Lyme neuroborreliosis, *J Clin Microbiol* 32(7):1795-1798, 1994.

Chapter 17

Toxoplasmosis

LEARNING OBJECTIVES

At the conclusion of this chapter, the reader should be able to:
- Describe the etiology and epidemiology of toxoplasmosis.
- Explain the signs and symptoms of acquired and congenital toxoplasmosis infection.

- Discuss the immunologic manifestations and diagnostic evaluation of toxoplasmosis, including the quantitative determination of immunoglobulin M (IgM) antibodies to *Toxoplasmosis gondii*.

ETIOLOGY

Toxoplasmosis is a widespread disease in humans and animals. The microorganism *Toxoplasma gondii* causes this infection. Recently the *Toxoplasma* organism was recognized as a tissue coccidia.

EPIDEMIOLOGY

T. gondii was first discovered in a North African rodent and has been observed in numerous birds and mammals around the world, including humans. It is a parasite of cosmopolitan distribution able to develop in a wide variety of vertebrate hosts. Human infections are common in many parts of the world. For unknown reasons, the incidence rates vary from place to place. The highest recorded rate (93%) occurs in Parisian women who prefer undercooked or raw meat; a 50% rate of occurrence exists in their children.

The definitive host is the house cat and certain other Felidae (Figure 17-1). Domestic cats are a source of the disease because oocysts are often present in their feces. Accidental ingestion of oocysts by humans and animals, including the cat, produces a proliferative infection in the body tissues. Fecal contamination of food or water, soiled hands, inadequately cooked or infected meat, and raw milk can be major sources of human infection. The hazard of transfusion-transmitted toxoplasmosis has been recently recognized in connection with the use of leukocyte concentrates. Patients at risk are those receiving immunosuppressive agents or corticosteroids.

All mammals, including humans, can transmit the infection transplacentally. Transplacental transmission usually takes place in the course of an acute but inapparent or undiagnosed maternal infection. New evidence indicates that the number of infants born in the United States each year with congenital *T. gondii* infection is considerably higher than the 3000 previously estimated. It is estimated that 6 out of every 1000 pregnant women in the United States will acquire primary infection with *Toxoplasma* during a 9-month gestation. Approximately 45% of the women who acquire the infection for the first time and who are not treated will give birth to congenitally infected infants. Consequently, the expected incidence of congenital toxoplasmosis is 2.7 per 1000 live births.

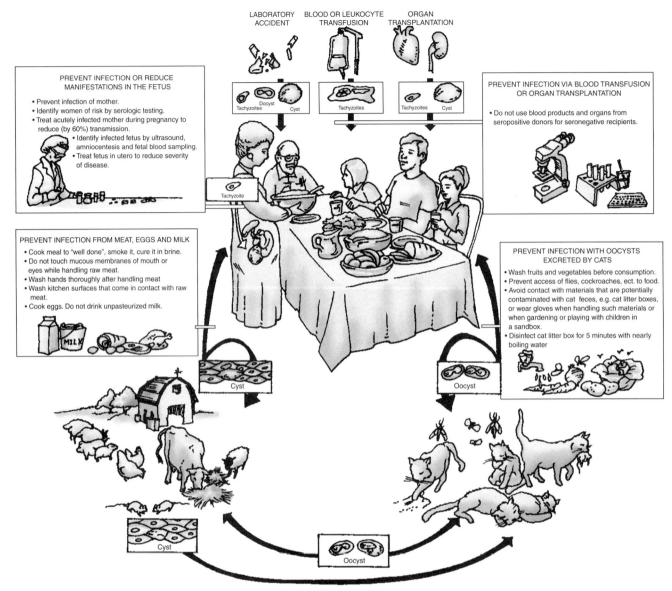

LABORATORY
ACCIDENT

BLOOD OR LEUKOCYTE
TRANSFUSION

ORGAN
TRANSPLANTATION

PREVENT INFECTION OR REDUCE MANIFESTATIONS IN THE FETUS
• Prevent infection of mother.
• Identify women of risk by serologic testing.
• Treat acutely infected mother during pregnancy to reduce (by 60%) transmission.
  • Identify infected fetus by ultrasound, amniocentesis and fetal blood sampling.
  • Treat fetus in utero to reduce severity of disease.

Tachyzoites   Docyst   Cyst   Tachyzoites   Tachyzoites   Cyst

Tachyzoite

PREVENT INFECTION VIA BLOOD TRANSFUSION OR ORGAN TRANSPLANTATION
• Do not use blood products and organs from seropositive donors for seronegative recipients.

PREVENT INFECTION FROM MEAT, EGGS AND MILK
• Cook meal to "well done", smoke it, cure it in brine.
• Do not touch mucous membranes of mouth or eyes while handling raw meat.
• Wash hands thoroughly after handling meat
• Wash kitchen surfaces that come in contact with raw meat.
• Cook eggs. Do not drink unpasteurized milk.

PREVENT INFECTION WITH OOCYSTS EXCRETED BY CATS
• Wash fruits and vegetables before consumption.
• Prevent access of flies, cockroaches, ect. to food.
• Avoid contact with materials that are potentially contaminated with cat feces, e.g. cat litter boxes, or wear gloves when handling such materials or when gardening or playing with children in a sandbox.
• Disinfect cat litter box for 5 minutes with nearly boiling water

Cyst   Oocyst

Cyst   Oocyst

Figure 17-1 Life cycle of *Toxoplasma gondii.* (Redrawn from Krugman S et al: *Infectious diseases of children,* ed 9, St Louis, 1992, Mosby.)

| Box 17-1 | **Methods for Prevention of Congenital Toxoplasmosis** |

Avoid touching mucous membranes of the mouth and eye while handling raw meat.

Wash hands thoroughly after handling raw meat.

Wash kitchen surfaces that come in contact with raw meat.

Cook meat to >18.8° C; smoke it or cure it in brine.

Wash fruits and vegetables before consumption.

Prevent access of flies, cockroaches, and other insects to fruits and vegetables.

Avoid contact with or wear gloves when handling materials that are potentially contaminated with cat feces (e.g., cat litter boxes), or when gardening.

It is recommended that all pregnant women be tested for toxoplasmosis immunity. If a patient is susceptible, screening should be repeated during pregnancy and at delivery. Prevention of infection in pregnant women should be practiced to avert congenital toxoplasmosis (Box 17-1). To further prevent infection of the fetus, women at risk should be identified by serologic testing, and drug therapy should be provided to pregnant women suffering from primary infections. Treatment consists of a combination of drugs (pyrimethamine and sulfadiazine). These drugs, with leucovorin to counter the side effects, can be administered orally from midpregnancy to delivery. The newborn is treated with the same drugs for the first 2 weeks postpartum.

Seroprevalence (antibody to *T. gondii*) varies considerably in the general population. It ranges from 96% in Western Europe to 10% to 40% in the United States. Of those patients

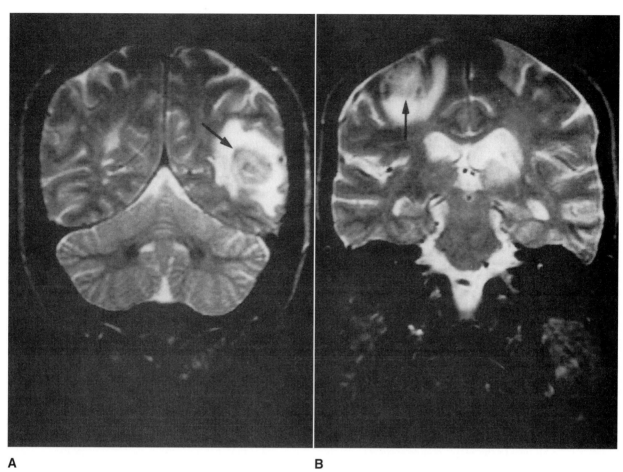

A   B

Figure 17-2   A and **B** Toxoplasmosis encephalitis. The *arrows* indicate areas infected with toxoplasmosis in MRI brain scans of patients with AIDS.

with acquired immunodeficiency syndrome (AIDS) who are seropositive for *T. gondii,* approximately 25% to 50% will develop toxoplasmic encephalitis. In areas with a lower seroprevalence such as the United States, the percentage of patients with AIDS who develop toxoplasmic encephalitis is lower (5% to 10%).

SIGNS AND SYMPTOMS

In adults and children other than newborns, the disease is usually asymptomatic. A generalized infection probably occurs. Although spontaneous recovery follows acute febrile disease, the organism can localize and multiply in any organ of the body or the circulatory systems. Toxoplasmosis encephalitis (Figure 17-2) in patients with AIDS may result in death even when treated. Persons at risk can be identified by screening patients positive for human immunodeficiency virus (HIV) for antibody to *T. gondii.*

Acquired Infection

When symptoms are seen, they are frequently mild. The disease can simulate infectious mononucleosis, with chills, fever, headache, lymphadenopathy, and extreme fatigue. Primary infection may be promoted by immunosuppression.

A chronic form of toxoplasmic lymphadenopathy exists. *T. gondii* presents a special problem in immunosuppressed or otherwise compromised hosts. In such patients some have developed reactivation of a latent toxoplasmosis. The types of cases in which this has been observed include Hodgkin's and non-Hodgkin's lymphoma, as well as in recipients of organ transplants.

Reactivation of cerebral toxoplasmosis is not uncommon in patients with AIDS; in these patients toxoplasmosis encephalitis is almost always a reactivation of a preexisting latent infection, most often occurring when the total CD4 count falls below 100 X 10^9/L. The possible reasons that some *T. gondii*-seropositive, HIV-infected persons develop toxoplasmic encephalitis include genetic susceptibility in the human immune response to *T. gondii,* subtle differences in the degree and type of immunocompromise of individual patients infected with HIV, differences in the virulence of individual strains of *T. gondii,* possible recurrent infections with different strains of *T. gondii,* and variation in the prevalence and type of coinfections with other opportunistic pathogens.

Congenital Infection

Congenital toxoplasmosis can result in central nervous system malformation or prenatal mortality. In infants who are serologically positive at birth, many fail to display neurologic, ophthalmic, or generalized illness at birth. In as many as 75% of the cases of congenitally infected newborns not serologically diagnosed at birth, the disease remains dormant, only to be discovered when other symptoms such as chorioretinitis, unilateral blindness, or severe neurologic sequelae become apparent.

IMMUNOLOGIC MANIFESTATIONS

Because *T. gondii* is difficult to culture, diagnosis must be supported by serologic methods. Both clinical and laboratory findings in this disease resemble infectious mononucleosis. An increased number of variant lymphocytes can be seen on a peripheral blood smear.

The diagnosis is established by serologically demonstrating marked elevations of toxoplasma antibodies. Antibodies are demonstrable within the first 2 weeks after infection, rising to high levels early in the infection, then falling slightly but persisting at an elevated level for many months before declining to low levels after many years.

Levels of IgM- and IgG-specific antibodies to *T. gondii* can be determined serologically. The presence of IgM to *T. gondii* in an adult is indicative of an active infection. In the newborn, detection of IgM also suggests an active infection because IgM antibodies are not able to cross the placenta; therefore they are of fetal origin.

DIAGNOSTIC EVALUATION

Detection of *T. gondii* in the blood could represent a major advance in the diagnosis of toxoplasmosis in patients with AIDS. A new cell culture method for the growth of *T. gondii* has been developed using a monocyte cell culture. After 4 days, parasites in the culture are revealed by immunofluorescence with an anti-P30 monoclonal antibody. A quantitative and qualitative analysis by cytofluorometry can then be performed on the cultured cells.

The enzyme-linked immunosorbent assay (ELISA) is considered by many to be the method of choice for detection of IgM antibodies in toxoplasmosis. The most common diagnostic testing methods for *T. gondii* include:
- Indirect fluorescent antibody (IFA)
- ELISA
- Polymerase chain reaction (PCR)

For the detection of IgM antibodies to *T. gondii*, indirect immunofluorescence (Figure 17-3) and enzyme-linked immunoassays have been developed. Indirect qualitative enzyme immunoassay for IgM or IgG, IgM (capture), microparticle enzyme immunoassay using the AxSYM System, and chemiluminescent immunoassay are available methods of antibody detection.

The presence of *Toxoplasma* IgM antibody in adults is indicative of active toxoplasmosis infection. In newborns, detection of IgM antibodies also suggests active infection because the antibodies are not transported across the placenta and indicate fetal origin. *Toxoplasma* infection acquired in utero can cause severe central nervous system and ocular abnormalities in the newborn. Any positive IgM antibody levels in prenatal screening should be confirmed with amniocentesis and PCR testing for *T. gondii*.

Serial samples for detection of specific IgG and IgM by ELISA offer the best chance of early diagnosis and recognition of remote infection. Specific IgM levels demonstrated by the ELISA method usually are elevated for 4 to 8 months (may persist for up to 12 months postinfection), compared to IFA titers, which have usually fallen by the second to fourth month. IgM measured by EIA for *Toxoplasma*-specific IgM is positive in about 75% of infants with proven congenital infection, compared to 25% positivity with IgM evaluation by IFA methodology. In the measurement of IgG antibody, seroconversion between acute and convalescent sera is considered strong evidence of current or recent infection. The best evidence for infection is a significant change on two appropriately timed (acute and convalescent) specimens with both as

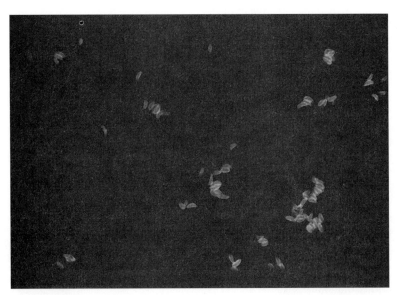

Figure 17-3   Indirect fluorescent antibody test for *Toxoplasma gondii* antibodies. *Toxoplasma* organisms affixed to the slide bind specific antibodies in the patient's serum. Antihuman antibody conjugated with fluorescein binds in turn to the bound patient's antibodies, causing the organisms to fluoresce. (From Baron EJ, Peterson LR, Finegold SM: *Bailey and Scott's diagnostic microbiology,* ed 9, St Louis, 1994, Mosby.)

says being done in the same laboratory at the same time. The Centers for Disease Control and Prevention suggest that any confirmed equivocal or positive results should be retested using a different assay.

PCR can be used to detect the presence or absence of *T. gondii* DNA in fresh or frozen biopsy tissue, cerebrospinal fluid, amniotic fluid, serum, or plasma. A negative result does not rule out the presence of PCR inhibitors in the specimen or *T. gondii* DNA concentrations that are below the level of detection by the assay.

 ## Quantitative Determination of IgM Antibodies to Toxoplasma Gondii*

Principle

Soluble antigens from *T. gondii* (RH strain) are attached to wells of microplates. Test specimens are diluted in a diluent containing an absorbent that removes any interfering rheumatoid factor. Diluted test specimens are added to the coated wells and incubated. If antibodies to *T. gondii* are present in the specimen, they will bind to the antigen-coated well during incubation. After being washed to remove unbound material, antibodies to human IgM labeled with alkaline phosphatase (conjugate) are added. The conjugate binds to any IgM antibodies bound to *Toxoplasma* antigens. The well is washed to remove unbound conjugate and incubated with p-nitrophenyl phosphate. The p-nitrophenyl phosphate is hydrolyzed by alkaline phosphatase to form p-nitrophenol, a yellow end product. The intensity of the absorbance is proportional to the amount of *Toxoplasma* IgM-specific antibody present in the specimen.

Specimen Collection and Preparation

No special preparation of the patient is required before specimen collection. The patient must be positively identified when the specimen is collected, and the specimen is to be labeled at the bedside. Specimen labels must include the patient's full name, the date the specimen is collected, the patient's hospital identification number, and the phlebotomist's initials.

Blood should be drawn by an aseptic technique. A minimum of 2 ml of clotted blood (red top evacuated tube) or anticoagulated blood (lavender top evacuated tube) is required. The specimen should be centrifuged promptly and an aliquot of serum or plasma removed.

Specimens should be stored in a refrigerator at 2° to 6° C or frozen (–20° C) if kept for more than 7 days. Specimens containing visible particulate matter should be clarified by centrifugation before testing. Serum sample should not be heat-inactivated, as this may cause false-positive results.

Reagents, Supplies, and Equipment

Kit reagents are available commercially from Sigma Chemical Co, St Louis, MO.

---

*Sigma Diagnostics, Sigma Chemical Co, St Louis, MO.

NOTE: Store reagents at 2° to 6° C. The reagents are stable until the expiration date on the label.

1. Kit Components:
1. Antigen wells. Microplate wells coated with *T. gondii*. Store antigen wells with dessicant in the reusable plastic bag and reseal the bag after opening.
2. Holder for wells.
3. Sample diluent. This is a buffered protein solution containing surfactant and blue dye, pH 7.5. It contains absorbent (heat-aggregated human IgG) and 0.1% sodium azide as a preservative.
4. Calibrator. This human serum contains IgM antibodies to *T. gondii*. It also contains 0.1% odium azide as a preservative.
5. Conjugate. The conjugate contains goat antibodies to human IgM labeled with calf alkaline phosphatase. It contains a pink dye and 0.02% sodium azide as a preservative.
6. Substrate. The substrate contains p-nitrophenyl phosphate, disodium, hexahydrate 1 mg/ml, pH 9.6. The substrate may turn slightly yellow on storage. Do not use if absorbance of the undiluted substrate is greater than 0.4 at 405 nm when measured against water using a microplate reader or a spectrophotometer with a 1-cm lightpath.
7. Wash concentrate. This is a buffer solution concentrate with surfactant. It contains 0.1% sodium azide as a preservative. The wash solution is prepared by adding the contents of the wash concentrate bottle to 1 liter of deionized water. Mix well.
8. Stop solution. This is an alkaline solution, pH 12.0. Store at room temperature. Reagent is stable until expiration date on the label.

   WARNING: Stop if solution causes irritation. Avoid contact with eyes, skin, and clothing. Avoid breathing vapor. Wash thoroughly after handling.

   NOTE: Do not interchange reagents from different lots.

Additional Required Equipment and Supplies

1. Spectrophotometer that accommodates a 1-μL volume or microplate reader capable of accurately measuring absorbance at 405 nm
2. Pipetting device for the accurate delivery of 5-μL, 100-μL, and 200-μL volumes
3. Timer
4. 1-L measuring cylinder
5. Squeeze bottle for dispensing wash solution
6. Dilution plates or tubes
7. Test tubes or cuvettes, 1.0-μL

Quality Control

Positive control: Human serum containing IgM antibodies to *T. gondii*. Content (expected range, expressed as % of calibrator) indicated on the label. It also contains 0.1% sodium azide.

Negative control: Human serum containing no detectable antibodies to *T. gondii*. It also contains 0.1% sodium azide.

CAUTION: Because the antigen wells and control and calibrator sera are derived from human sources, they should be handled in the same manner as clinical serum specimens (see Universal Blood and Body Fluid Precautions in Chapter 6).

WARNING: The reagents and controls contain sodium azide as a preservative. Sodium azide may react with lead and copper plumbing to form highly explosive metal azides. On disposal, flush with a large volume of water to prevent azide buildup. Sodium azide is also toxic. Care should be taken to avoid ingestion.

Procedure

1. Dilute the calibrator, positive and negative controls, and test samples by combining 5 μL of the respective sera with 200 μL of sample diluent in labeled tubes or dilution plates.
2. Place the desired number of antigen wells in the holder.
3. Using a clean pipette tip for each specimen, mix the samples and diluent by drawing up and expelling two or three times. Transfer 100 μL of each diluted specimen to the appropriate antigen well.
4. Include one well that contains only 100 μL of sample diluent. This serves as the reagent blank and is used to zero the photometer.
5. Allow the plate to stand at room temperature (18° to 26° C) for 30 ± 2 minutes.
6. Shake out or aspirate contents of wells. Wash wells by filling them with wash solution from a squeeze bottle and shaking out or aspirating. Wash three times. Drain wells on paper towel to remove excess fluid.

   NOTE: Thorough washing is necessary to achieve accurate results. Avoid bubbles.
7. Place 2 drops (or 100 μL) conjugate into each well, including the reagent blank well.
8. Allow to stand at room temperature (18° to 26° C) for 30 ± 2 minutes.
9. Wash wells by repeating step 6.
10. Place 2 drops (or 100 μL) of substrate into each well, including the reagent blank well.
11. Allow to stand at room temperature (18° to 26° C) for 30 ± 2 minutes.
12. Place 2 drops (or 100 μL of stop solution) into each well.
13. Read and record absorbance of each test at 405 nm within 2 hours after the reaction has been stopped.

Microplate reader. Set absorbance at 405 nm to zero with water as reference. Read and record absorbance of reagent blank (A blank). Then set absorbance to zero with the reagent blank as a reference. Read and record the absorbance of samples (A sample) and calibrator (A calibrator).

Spectrophotometer. Completely remove contents of each well and transfer to cuvette or test tube. Add 800 μL of deionized water to each sample and mix. Set absorbance at 405 nm to zero with water as a reference. Read and record the absorbance of each sample including the reagent blank. Subtract the absorbance of the reagent blank from the absorbance of each specimen.

Calculation

$$\text{Antibody concentration as percent of calibrator} = \frac{\text{A sample} \times 100}{\text{A calibrator}}$$

Example:

ABSORBANCE MEASURED USING A MICROPLATE READER

A sample = 0.597
A calibrator = 0.842

Antibody concentration as percent of calibrator =

$$\frac{0.597 \times 100}{0.842} = 72$$

ABSORBANCE MEASURED USING A SPECTROPHOTOMETER

A blank = 0.006
A sample = 0.242
A calibrator = 0.332
A sample − A blank = 0.242 − 0.006 = 0.236
A calibrator − A blank = 0.332 − 0.006 = 0.326
Antibody concentration as percent of calibrator =

$$\frac{0.236 \times 100}{0.326} = 72$$

Reporting Results

Reference ranges should be established by each laboratory to reflect the characteristics of the populations of the area in which it is located.

> 40% = Positive for IgM antibodies to *T. gondii*.

Procedure Notes

Specimens giving absorbance values above that of the calibrator should be diluted appropriately and reassayed. The value obtained should be multiplied by the dilution factor.

Sources of Error

False-positive results can be caused by the presence of rheumatoid factor in the specimen. In this procedure the sample diluent contains heat-aggregated IgG sufficient to neutralize the immunoglobulin activity of up to 348 IU/mL of IgM rheumatoid factor.

False-negative results have been reported in assays detecting IgM antibodies as a result of the competition between specific IgG antibodies and low levels of specific IgM antibodies. In addition, specimens taken from patients early in the course of infection may contain no detectable level of IgM-specific antibody to *T. gondii*.

Clinical Applications

Demonstration of *Toxoplasma* IgM antibody is indicative of a recent or current acute infection in adults or children and a congenital infection in the newborn. *Toxoplasma* IgM antibodies should be absent in noninfected individuals.

Limitations

Detection of *Toxoplasma*-specific IgM is reliable except when the specimen is collected too early (an increase is sometimes apparent within 1 month) or too late (more than 4 to 8 months after infection).

An additional limitation is that the detection of IgM antibodies to *T. gondii* is designed to serve as an aid to definitive diagnosis. Clinical considerations should be integrated with serologic findings.

Case Study

History and Physical Examination

A 24-year-old woman with a history of AIDS presents for evaluation of left-sided weakness. She has also been experiencing headaches and seizures, and others have observed an alteration in her mental status.

Her medical history is notable for an episode of *Pneumocystis carinii* pneumonia, primary syphilis treated with penicillin 5 years ago, and occasional thrush. She takes zidovudine and monthly aerosolized pentamidine for pneumocystis prophylaxis. An urgent CT scan of the head shows two 1-cm lesions in the right basal ganglia with enhancement seen with intravenous contrast media.

Laboratory Data

CD4 cell count: 50 × 109/L.
RPR: positive at 1:2
Toxoplasmosis IgG: positive
Toxoplasmosis IgM: negative

Questions and Discussion

1. What is the most common cause of lesions in the brain?

   Cerebral toxoplasmosis is the most common cause of central nervous system mass lesions in patients with AIDS. In these patients, lesions occur in approximately one third of those who are seropositive for *T. gondii*. Other conditions that may produce CNS mass lesions in patients with AIDS include CNS lymphoma, progressive multifocal leukoencephalopathy, and, more rarely, bacterial and fungal brain abscesses.

2. What is the source of this infection?

   Disease is believed to occur from the reactivation of a prior infection. Initially, in cases of toxoplasmosis, accidental ingestion of oocysts by humans and animals, including cats, produces a proliferative infection in the body tissues. Fecal contamination of food or water, soiled hands, inadequately cooked or infected meat, and raw milk can be major sources of human infection. The hazard of transfusion-transmitted toxoplasmosis has been recently recognized in connection with the use of leukocyte concentrates. Patients at risk are those who are receiving immunosuppressive agents or corticosteroids.

3. Is this a newly acquired infection?

   In these cases, serologic studies usually show a positive IgG and a negative IgM that indicate that the initial infection took place in the past.

The diagnosis is established by serologically demonstrating marked elevations of *Toxoplasma* antibodies. Antibodies are demonstrable within the first 2 weeks after infection, rising to high levels early in the infection, and falling slightly, but persisting, at an elevated level for many months before declining to low levels after many years.

Levels of IgM- and IgG-specific antibodies to *T. gondii* can be determined serologically. The presence of IgM to *T. gondii* in an adult is indicative of an active infection. In the newborn, detection of IgM also suggests an active infection because IgM antibodies are able to cross the placenta; therefore they are of fetal origin.

4. How can the patient be treated?

   Lifelong therapy is needed because of the tendency for this infection to recur in those with prior disease.

5. Should pregnant women be tested for this microorganism?

   It is recommended that all pregnant women be tested for toxoplasmosis immunity. If a patient is susceptible, screening should be repeated during pregnancy and at delivery. Prevention of infection in pregnant women should be practiced in order to avert congenital toxoplasmosis. To further prevent infection of the fetus, women who are at risk should be identified by serologic testing, and drug therapy should be provided to pregnant women suffering from primary infections. Treatment consists of a combination of drugs (pyrimethamine and sulfadiazine). These drugs, with leucovorin to counter the side effects, can be administered orally from mid-pregnancy to delivery. The newborn is treated with the same drugs for the first 2 weeks postpartum.

Diagnosis

Toxoplasmosis

CHAPTER HIGHLIGHTS

Toxoplasmosis is a widespread disease in humans and animals. The microorganism *T. gondii* causes this infection. It is a parasite of cosmopolitan distribution, with the definitive host being the house cat and certain other Felidae. Domestic cats may be a source of the disease because oocysts are often present in their feces. Accidental ingestion of oocysts by humans and animals, including the cat, produces a proliferative infection in the body tissues. Fecal contamination of food or water, soiled hands, inadequately cooked or infected meat, and raw milk can be important sources of human infection. All mammals, including humans, can transmit the infection transplacentally, which usually occurs in the course of an acute but inapparent or undiagnosed maternal infection.

In adults and children other than newborns the disease is usually asymptomatic. A generalized infection probably occurs. Although spontaneous recovery follows acute febrile disease, the organism can localize and multiply in any organ of the body or the circulatory system. In acquired infection, when symptoms are seen, they are frequently mild. Disease conditions may simulate infectious mononucleosis. In contrast, congenital toxoplasmosis can result in central nervous system malformation or prenatal mortality. Because *T. gondii* is difficult to culture, diagnosis must be supported by serologic methods. Levels of IgM- and IgG-specific antibodies to *T. gondii* can be determined serologically. The presence of IgM to *T. gondii* in an adult is indicative of an active infection. In the newborn, detection of IgM also suggests an active infection because IgM antibodies are able to cross the placenta; therefore they are of fetal origin. The enzyme-linked immunosorbent assay is considered by many to be the method of choice for detection of IgM antibodies in toxoplasmosis. Serologic testing methods for *T. gondii* antibody can include IFA, ELISA, chemiluminescent immunoassay, and PCR.

REVIEW QUESTIONS

1. Toxoplasmosis is a _____ infection.
   A. bacterial
   B. mycotic
   C. parasitic
   D. viral

2. The definitive host of *T. gondii* is the _____.
   A. horse
   B. pig
   C. dog
   D. house cat

3. All of the following are specific methods for preventing congenital toxoplasmosis except:
   A. avoid touching mucous membranes while handling raw meat
   B. wash hands thoroughly after handling raw meat
   C. eliminate food contamination by flies, cockroaches, and other insects
   D. dispose of fecally contaminated cat litter into plastic garbage bags

4. The presence of IgM to *T. gondii* in an adult is indicative of:
   A. carrier state
   B. active infection
   C. chronic infection
   D. latent disease

5. All of the following characteristics are correct regarding toxoplasmosis except:
   A. it is recognized as a tissue coccidia
   B. domestic dogs are a source of the disease
   C. it can be transmitted by infected blood
   D. it can be transmitted transplacentally

6. Toxoplasmosis is a serious health threat to:
   A. AIDS patients
   B. adults
   C. children more than 2 years old
   D. elderly patients

7. Congenital toxoplasmosis can cause:
   A. congenital heart disease
   B. central nervous system malformation
   C. urinary tract infections
   D. muscular disorders

8. Antibodies to *T. gondii* are demonstrable _____ after infection.
   A. 3 to 5 days
   B. within 10 days
   C. within 2 weeks
   D. within 4 weeks

9. The method of choice for detecting IgM antibodies in toxoplasmosis is:
   A. enzyme-linked immunosorbent assay (ELISA)
   B. indirect fluorescent antibody (IFA)
   C. indirect hemagglutination (IHA)
   D. complement fixation

BIBLIOGRAPHY

ARUP Reference Test Guide, 2002, website:www.aruplab.com.
Beaman MH, Luft BJ, Remington JS: Prophylaxis for toxoplasmosis in AIDS, *Ann Intern Med* 117(2):163-164, 1992.
Bruce-Chwatt LJ: Transfusion associated parasitic infections. In Bruce-Chwatt LJ: *Infection, immunity, and blood transfusion,* New York, 1985, Alan R Liss.
Forbes BA, Sahm DF, Weissfeld AS: *Bailey and Scott's diagnostic microbiology,* ed 11, St Louis, 2002, Mosby.
Franco EL, Walls KW, Sulzer AJ: Reverse enzyme immunoassay for detection of specified anti-toxoplasma immunoglobulin M antibodies, *J Clin Microbiol* 13:859, 1981.
Krogstasd DJ et al: Blood and tissue protozoa. In Lennette EH et al, editors: *Manual of clinical microbiology,* ed 4, Washington, DC, 1985, American Society of Microbiology.
Markell EK et al: *Medical parasitology,* ed 6, pp 112-117, Philadelphia, 1986, WB Saunders.
SIA Toxoplasma IgM product literature, St Louis, 1988, Sigma Chemical.
Tirard V et al: Diagnosis of toxoplasmosis in patients with AIDS by isolation of the parasite from the blood, *N Engl J Med* 324(9):634, 1991.
Turgeon ML: *Clinical hematology,* ed 3, Philadelphia, 1999, Lippincott Williams & Wilkins.
Turgeon ML: *Fundamentals of immunohematology,* ed 2, Baltimore, 1995, Williams & Wilkins.
Walls KW: Serodiagnostic tests for parasitic diseases. In Lennette EH et al, editors: *Manual of clinical microbiology,* ed 4, Washington, DC, 1985, American Society of Microbiology.
Wilson CB, Remington JJ: What can be done to prevent toxoplasmosis? *Am J Obstet Gynecol* 138:357-363, 1980.

Chapter 18

Cytomegalovirus

LEARNING OBJECTIVES

At the conclusion of this chapter, the reader should be able to:
- Discuss the etiology and epidemiology of acquired, latent, and congenital cytomegalovirus (CMV) infection.
- Explain the signs and symptoms of acquired and congenital CMV infections.
- Describe the immunologic manifestations of CMV.

- Name and explain the serologic markers and diagnostic evaluation of CMV.
- Discuss the principles and applications of the passive latex agglutination and quantitative determination of immunoglobulin M (IgM) antibody.

ETIOLOGY

CMV is a ubiquitous human viral pathogen. The first descriptive report of histologic changes characteristic of the changes now associated with CMV infection was originally published in 1904 when protozoan-like cells in the lungs, kidneys, and liver of a syphilitic fetus were seen. However, it was not until 1956 and 1957 that the CMV was isolated in the laboratory (Figure 18-1). In 1966 the actual isolation of the virus after transfusion, as well as the observation of elevated antibody titers, was noted.

Human CMV is classified as a member of the herpes family of viruses. There are presently five recognized human herpes viruses: herpes simplex I, herpes simplex II, varicella-zoster virus, Epstein-Barr virus, and CMV. All of the herpes viruses are relatively large, enveloped DNA viruses that undergo a replicative cycle involving DNA expression and nucleocapsid assembly within the nucleus. The viral structure gains an envelope when the virus buds through the nuclear membrane, which in turn is altered to contain specific viral proteins.

Although the herpes family produces diverse clinical diseases, the viruses share the basic characteristics of being cell associated. The requirements for cell association vary, but all five herpes family viruses may spread from cell to cell, presumably via intercellular bridges and in the presence of antibody in the extracellular phase. CMV spreads to the lymphoid tissues and proceeds to circulate to systemic lymph nodes. The virus finally comes to rest in the epithelial cells of many tissues. This common characteristic may play a role in the ability of these viruses to produce subclinical infections that can be reactivated under appropriate stimuli.

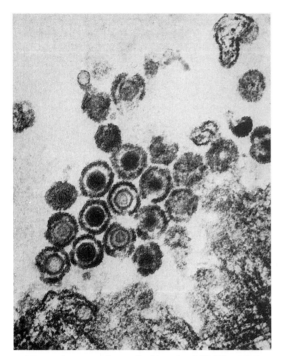

Figure 18-1 A group of negatively stained CMV particles propagated in human lung fibroblasts. The typical hexagonal capsid (actually icosahedral in three dimensions) of a herpesvirus can be seen, surrounded by a tegument and double-layered envelope (×155.000). (From Krugman S et al: Courtesy Janet D. Smith, PhD: *Infectious diseases of children,* ed 8, St Louis, 1985, Mosby.)

EPIDEMIOLOGY

CMV infection is endemic worldwide. Dissemination of the virus may be by oral, respiratory, or venereal routes. It may also be transmitted parenterally by organ transplantation or via the transfusion of fresh blood. Transmission of CMV appears to require intimate contact with secretions or excretions (primarily urine, respiratory, and genital secretions, tears, and feces of infected persons). Infection of a child by the mother is possible via intrauterine means and at birth. The most likely mode of acquisition is via a venereal route through contact with infectious virus in body secretions.

The incidence of demonstrable antibody to CMV ranges from 21% to 34% in persons between the ages of 6 and 22 years. For this reason, CMV is a major health risk because a large proportion of women, particularly white women, entering their childbearing years lack antibody to CMV; however, the prevalence of CMV seropositivity increases steadily with age. In fact, 90% of the urban adult population is infected with CMV. Infection is common around the globe and in all socioeconomic classes. Those at the greatest risk of infection are fetuses and immunocompromised persons.

The virus can be present in urine, saliva, feces, breast milk, blood, cervical secretions, virus-infected grafts from a donor, semen, vaginal fluid, and respiratory droplets. The virus may be shed without any signs or symptoms. This poses a serious threat, as intimate contact is favorable for transmission. It has been recognized for more than 15 years that transfusion of blood from healthy asymptomatic blood donors is occasionally followed by active CMV infection in the recipient. There is strong evidence to incriminate peripheral blood leukocytes and transplanted tissues as sources of CMV.

Acquired Infection

Although fatal infections have been reported in children with leukemia and premature infants of less than 1200-g birth weight, the incidence of primary infections during childhood is low. The rate of exposure to the virus, however, may be accelerated during the first years of life in toddlers and children in daycare centers. During adolescence the infection rate rises significantly. By adulthood most individuals have experienced asymptomatic contact with CMV. Because CMV can persist in a latent state, active infections may develop under a variety of conditions (e.g., pregnancy; immunosuppression; after organ, bone, or stem cell transplantation). Active CMV infection is a major cause of morbidity and often mortality in patients with acquired immunodeficiency syndrome.

Of patients who are immunosuppressed, only seronegative patients appear to be at a significant risk of developing CMV infection. Patients at the highest risk of mortality from CMV infections are allograft transplant seronegative patients who receive tissue from a seropositive donor. The great majority of infections in allograft recipients are transmitted by a donor kidney or arise from the reactivation of the recipient's latent virus. One drug, valacyclovir hydrochloride (Valtrex), has been shown to prevent CMV infection after transplantation. Avoiding CMV infection reduces the risk of injury to the donor tissue, which in turn could lead to rejection.

Transmission of CMV by transfusion of blood or blood components containing white cells is assuming increased importance in patients with severely impaired immunity who require supportive therapy. Low-birth-weight neonates are also at high risk for CMV infection through transfusion of CMV-infected blood products. In these patients, effective donor screening, leukocyte-depleted blood products, and immune globulin containing passively acquired CMV antibodies are all methods of prevention.

Health care professionals are one of the groups becoming increasingly concerned about the risks associated with exposure to CMV. Nosocomial transmission from patients to health care workers has not been documented, but observance of good personal hygiene and hand washing offer the best measures for preventing transmission.

Latent Infection

Persistent infections characterized by periods of reactivation are frequently termed latent infections, although this condition has not been clearly defined for CMV. True viral latency is defined by the presence of the genetic information in an unexpressed state in the host cell. An operational definition of latency can include the conditions of a dynamic relationship between the virus and the host, along with evidence of latency and reactivation of a latent infection. As with any herpes virus, reactivation is possible at any time, but it is rarely manifested in immunocompetent individuals.

Evidence that CMV produces latent infections in humans is circumstantial and indirect. The mechanism of latency and identity of the host cells that harbor the latent virus remains undocumented. Leukocytes from the peripheral blood of patients with active CMV infections have been cultured with the subsequent recovery of CMV, but attempts to recover the virus from the leukocytes of healthy donors have remained unsuccessful, with the exception of one report. In animal models the virus is present and recoverable from neutrophilic leukocytes in active infections, but it is also believed that splenic B lymphocytes, and possibly monocytes, may harbor latent infections. Additionally, salivary gland, heart, and prostate tissue may be sites of latent infections. In fact, in relationship to the heart, latent infection may prove to be a causative factor in atherosclerosis. The types of cells and the mechanism of latency remain to be demonstrated in humans. The estimated CMV carrier rate among blood donors, which is defined as the number of seroconversions (patients changing from being negative for antibodies to the virus to being positive for these viral antibodies) per 100 units of blood transfused, ranges from 1% to 12%.

Congenital Infection

Primary and recurrent maternal CMV infection can be transmitted in utero. Congenital CMV infection is the most common intrauterine infection, affecting from 0.4% to 2.3% of all live births in the United States. The presence of maternal antibody to CMV before conception provides substantial protection against damaging congenital CMV infection in the newborn.

Primary maternal infection during pregnancy, occurring in 1% to 3% of women in the United States, is associated with more severe sequelae of congenital CMV infection. Infected infants can become severely ill, and death may result in premature infants. Most newborns infected with CMV survive, but they may be mentally retarded or suffer from other health problems.

SIGNS AND SYMPTOMS

Acquired Infection

Acquired CMV infection is usually asymptomatic and can persist in the host as a chronic or latent infection. The incubation period is believed to be between 3 and 12 weeks.

In the majority of patients, CMV infection is asymptomatic. Occasionally a self-limited, heterophile-negative, mononucleosis-like syndrome results. CMV hepatitis can occur as well.

Symptoms include a sore throat and fever, swollen glands, chills, profound malaise, and myalgia. Lymphadenopathy and splenomegaly may be observed. Infections occurring in healthy immunocompetent individuals usually result in seroconversion. Virus may be excreted in the urine during both primary and recurrent CMV infection (Figure 18-2); it can persist sporadically for months or years. Persons experiencing acquired infection, reinfection with the same or different strains of CMV, or reactivation of a latent infection can excrete the virus in titers as high as 10^6 infective units/mL in the urine and/or saliva for weeks or months.

Normal adults and children usually experience CMV infection without serious complications. Infrequent complications of CMV infection in previously healthy individuals, however, include interstitial pneumonitis, hepatitis, Guillain-

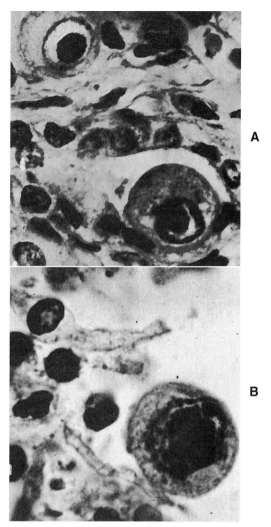

Figure 18-2 CMV infection of kidney. **A,** Section showing two huge nuclear inclusions in tubular epithelium. **B,** Diagnostic cell in hematoxylin and eosin-stained urinary sediment *(lower right)*. Compare with normal-appearing tubular epithelial cell *(upper left)*. (From Kissane JM: *Anderson's pathology*, ed 9, St Louis, 1990, Mosby.)

Barré syndrome, meningoencephalitis, myocarditis, thrombocytopenia, and hemolytic anemia.

CMV infection, however, can be life threatening in immunosuppressed patients. Infections in these patients may result in disseminated multisystem involvement including pneumonitis, hepatitis, gastrointestinal ulceration, arthralgias, meningoencephalitis, and retinitis. Retinitis and encephalitis are common manifestation of disseminated CMV. Ulcerative damage of tissues (e.g., esophagus) is another demonstration of the cytopathic effect of CMV. Interstitial pneumonitis, frequently associated with CMV infection, is a major cause of death after allogeneic bone marrow transplantation. In premature infants, acquired CMV infection can result in atypical lymphocytosis, hepatosplenomegaly, pneumonia, or death.

Transfusion-acquired CMV infections may cause not only mononucleosis-like syndrome but hepatitis and an increase in rejection of transplanted organs. Three types of CMV infections are possible in blood transfusion recipients:

- Primary infection occurs when a previously unexposed (seronegative) recipient is transfused with blood from

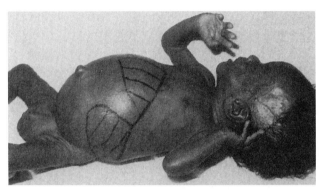

Figure 18-3   A 4-month-old child with symptomatic congenital infection manifesting severe failure to thrive, hepatitis with hepatosplenomegaly, bilateral inguinal hernias, and micropenis. (From Krugman S et al: *Infectious diseases of children,* ed 9, St Louis, 1992, Mosby.)

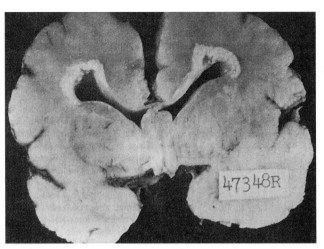

Figure 18-4   Brain of an infant with congenital CMV infection. Note extensive periventricular necrosis and calcification. (From Krugman S et al: *Infectious diseases of children,* ed 9, St Louis, 1992, Mosby.)

an actively or latently infected donor. This type of infection is accompanied by the presence of virus in the blood and urine, an immediate antibody response, and eventual seroconversion. Primary infections may be symptomatic, but the great majority is not.

- Reactivated infections can be manifested when a seropositive recipient is transfused with blood from either a CMV antibody-positive or negative donor. Donor leukocytes are thought to trigger an allograft reaction, which in turn reactivates the recipient's latent infection. Such infections may be accompanied by significant increases in CMV-specific antibody. Some reactivated infections exhibit viral shedding as their only manifestation. Reactivated infections are largely asymptomatic.

- Reinfection by a strain of CMV in the donor's blood that is different from the one originally infecting the recipient can occur. A significant antibody response is observed in this situation, and viral shedding occurs. Although it is difficult to differentiate a reactivated infection if both the patient and the donor are CMV antibody-positive before transfusion, reinfections can be documented if isolates can be obtained from both donor and recipient.

Congenital Infection

The classic congenital CMV syndrome is manifested by a high incidence of neurologic symptoms, as well as neuromuscular disorders, jaundice, hepatomegaly, and splenomegaly (Figure 18-3). Petechia is the most commonly noted clinical sign. It is observed in about 50% of infants infected with CMV.

Congenitally infected newborns, especially those who acquire CMV during a maternal primary infection, are more prone to develop severe cytomegalic inclusion disease (CID). The severe form of CID may be fatal or can cause permanent neurologic sequelae such as intracranial calcifications (Figure 18-4), mental retardation, deafness, vision defects, microcephaly, and motor dysfunction. Psychomotor retardation is seen in 51% to 75% of survivors. Hearing loss is observed in 21% to 50% of cases, and visual impairment

in 20% of cases. Infants without symptoms at birth may develop hearing impairment and neurologic impairment at a later date.

IMMUNOLOGIC MANIFESTATIONS

Alterations in the Immune System

CMV infection is known to alter the immune system, as well as to produce overt manifestations of infection. Infection interferes with immune responsiveness in both normal and immunocompromised individuals. This diminished responsiveness results in a decreased proliferative response to the CMV antigen, which persists for several months. In patients with CMV mononucleosis-like syndrome, alterations of T-lymphocyte subsets result, producing an increase in the absolute number of CD8+ lymphocytes and a decrease in CD4+ lymphocytes. These subset abnormalities persist for months.

Questions have been raised regarding CMV as a potentially oncogenic virus because viral antigens and/or nucleic acid have been found in human malignancies, which include adenocarcinoma of the colon, carcinoma of the cervix, cancer of the prostate, and Kaposi's sarcoma. CMV does have transforming properties in vitro. Although considerable circumstantial evidence exists linking CMV to human malignancies (especially Kaposi's sarcoma), a direct cause-and-effect relationship has not been established.

Serologic Markers

In cells infected by CMV, several antigens appear at varying times after infection. Before replication of viral DNA takes place, immediate-early antigens and early antigens are present in the nuclei of infected cells. Immediate-early antigens appear within 1 hour of cellular infection, and early antigens are present within 24 hours. At about 72 hours after infection, or the end of the viral replication cycle, late antigens are demonstrable in the nucleus and cytoplasm of infected cells.

The immune antibody response to these various antigens differs in incidence and significance. The presence of antibodies against immediate-early and early antigens is associated with active infection of either a primary or reactivated nature.

Antibody to early antigen undergoes a relatively rapid decline after recovery but can persist for up to 250 days, and it may identify patients with recent, as well as active, infections. The presence of antibody to early antigen is strongly associated with viral shedding. Antibodies to late antigens persist in high titer long after the recovery from an active infection.

The incidence of viral exposure and subsequent antibody formation (seropositivity) varies greatly depending on the socioeconomic status and living conditions of the population surveyed. The prevalence of CMV antibody varies with age and geographic location but ranges from 40% to 100%.

The incidence of antibodies against CMV-induced immediate-early antigens, early antigens, and late antigens was studied in a population of healthy blood donors. Antibodies to immediate-early antigens were found in 9.6%, antibodies to early antigens in 10.2%, and antibodies to late antigens in 76% of the donors. The incidence of antibodies to CMV-induced immediate-early and early antigens increased with age and was higher in females than males. In another study 51% of donors were seronegative for CMV antibodies. The highest percentage of seronegative findings (60%) was among donors who were 18 to 35 years old. This age-group represented 57% of the donors. If donors with viremia are a source of transfusion-acquired CMV in high-risk patients, then screening blood for early antigen antibodies is warranted.

The characteristic antibody responses associated with infection are:

- Primary infection, demonstrated by a transient virus-specific IgM antibody response and eventual seroconversion to produce IgG antibodies to the virus.
- Reactivation of latent infection in seropositive (IgG) individuals, which may be accompanied by significant increases in IgG antibodies to the virus but which elicit no detectable IgM response.
- Reinfection by a strain of CMV different from the original infecting strain. A significant IgG antibody response is demonstrated. Whether an IgM response occurs is unknown.

Vaccine development is important in the prevention of congenital CMV. Clinical research continues on live attenuated CMV vaccine; however, an alternative may be to use a subunit vaccine against the surface glycoproteins of the virus. This method should entail less risk of reactivation or oncogenicity.

DIAGNOSTIC EVALUATION

In CMV infection hematologic examination of the blood usually reveals a characteristic leukocytosis. A slight lymphocytosis with more than 20% variant lymphocytes is common. CMV infection should be viewed as a possibility if:

- The patient has mononucleosis-like symptoms but exhibits a negative Epstein-Barr virus test result, and
- Manifests hepatitis symptoms but does not demonstrate any positive results when tested for common hepatitis viruses

TABLE 18-1 Methods of Testing for Cytomegalovirus

Method	Constituent Tested
Complement fixation	Antibody
Latex particle agglutination	Antibody
Anticomplement immuno-fluorescence	IgG antibody
Indirect fluorescent antibody	IgM antibody
Enzyme immunoassay	IgG and IgM antibody
Direct electron microscopy	Antigen
Enzyme immunoassay	Antigen
Nucleic acid probe	CMV mRNA
In situ hybridization	cDNA probe

In afflicted infants the most common laboratory abnormality is a low platelet count (thrombocytopenia). Clinical chemistry assays may demonstrate abnormal liver function tests. Another assessment of the presence of infection is the demonstration of inclusion bodies in leukocytes in urinary sediment.

A definitive diagnosis can be made only by viewing intranuclear inclusion in enlarged epithelial cells of various tissues (e.g., lung, and by isolating the CMV from urine, throat swabs, or blood samples). Demonstration of CMV-specific IgM or increasing CMV-specific IgG antibody titers (Table 18-1) is also conclusive evidence of infection. Methods for measuring CMV IgM antibodies include indirect immunofluorescence or indirect and reverse enzyme-linked immunosorbent assay (ELISA) tests. Virus detection in urine by electron microscopy is reliable if positive, but a negative result does not rule out CMV infection. Human CMV is indistinguishable by negative-staining electron microscopy from its close relatives, herpes simplex and varicella, which is the cause of chickenpox. Viral culture is the method of choice for confirming CMV infection. Early detection of CMV in viral cultures is done routinely by direct fluorescent antibody (DFA) examination, and demonstration of CMV in bronchoalveolar lavage specimens by DFA. More rapid methods are needed.

Serologic methods to detect the presence of IgM antibodies can aid in the diagnosis of primary infection. Detection of CMV-specific IgM can represent primary infection or rare reactivation of infection. False-positive results, however, can occur because of the presence of other antibodies such as rheumatoid factor. Although tests for heterophil, Epstein-Barr virus, and *Toxoplasma* antibodies are generally negative, elevated concentrations (titers) of several antibodies may occur. These include antinuclear antibody (ANA), rheumatoid factor antibodies (RA), and nonspecific cold agglutinins. The inability to demonstrate IgM in a blood specimen can result from the presence of a large amount of virus-specific IgG. Lack of a CMV-specific IgM response is especially common in congenital infections, of which 50% are CMV–IgM negative by immunofluorescent antibody (IFA) (up to 89% positive by radioimmunoassay and 69% positive by enzyme immunoassay [EIA]) even in the presence of virus excretion in the urine.

Detection of significant increases in CMV-specific IgG antibody by methods such as complement fixation (CF), anticomplement immunofluorescence (ACIF), and EIA suggest, but do not prove, recent infection or reactivation of latent infection. The EIA method for IgM and IgG antibodies to CMV has replaced CF, ACIF, and IFA. Latex particle agglutination and indirect hemagglutination are useful screening methods to obtain seronegative donors.

Newer CMV detection methods are being explored. CMV antigen detection in urine by EIA and cDNA is being developed. RNA transcript of CMV DNA is detectable in peripheral blood mononuclear cells of seropositive individuals by in situ hybridization (ISH) with cDNA of CMV. The ISH technique, which is more sensitive than dot-blot hybridization (Northern blot), promises to be a new early detection method for CMV expression. Quantitative evaluation of CMV DNA in the blood may be possible by using polymerase chain reaction technique. Nucleic acid sequence based amplification (Cytomegalovirus [CMV] pp67 mRNA by Organon Teknika, Durham, NC) is a currently available method.

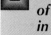

Passive Latex Agglutination for Detection of Antibodies to Cytomegalovirus in Human Serum

Principle

In this procedure latex particles previously sensitized with CMV viral antigen are mixed with serum. If antibody to CMV is present, the agglutinated particles will be macroscopically visible. In the absence of specific antibody or in the event of low antibody concentration, the latex particles will not agglutinate in the reaction mixture and the particles will appear smooth and evenly dispersed. The absence of CMV antibodies suggests that a person has not been exposed to this virus. The presence of CMV antibodies, however, is indicative of previous exposure to the virus. Although recurrent infection is possible, it may not be as severe as in primary infection. Because CMV is a blood-borne pathogen, infection with this virus is of greatest concern to newborn infants in need of transfusion and to immunosuppressed allograft recipients.

Specimen Collection and Preparation

No special preparation of the patient is required before specimen collection. The patient must be positively identified when the specimen is collected, and the specimen is to be labeled at the bedside. Specimen labels must include the patient's full name, the date the specimen is collected, the patient's hospital identification number, and the phlebotomist's initials.

Blood should be drawn by an aseptic technique. A minimum of 2 mL of clotted blood (red top evacuated tube) or anticoagulated blood (lavender top evacuated tube) is required. The specimen should be centrifuged promptly and an aliquot of serum or plasma removed. Plasma specimens containing EDTA or heparin as an anticoagulant can be used for qualitative or quantitative testing using the same technique as for serum samples. Plasma specimens containing CPDA-1 as an anticoagulant can also be used for qualitative or quantitative testing after a 1% dilution is made with the buffer.

Serum or plasma specimens may be stored for up to 1 week at 2° to 8° C or frozen at –18° C or lower if longer storage is required. Serum specimens with obvious microbial contamination should not be used for testing. The presence of mild lipimea or hemolysis will not affect the test.

Testing of CPDA-1 plasma specimens from platelet units stored at 22° C for 5 days and from red cell units prepared for transfusion stored at 2° to 6° C for 14 days has been successful.

Reagents, Supplies, and Equipment

The following reagents and equipment are supplied with the CMV Scan Kit (Becton Dickinson, Cockeysville, Md):

1. Kit components
   a. Latex antigen: CMV antigen-coated latex particles prepared from disrupted CMV judged to be inactivated by bioassay procedures. This preparation contains 0.02% gentamicin and 0.02% sodium azide. Refrigerate at 2° to 8° C to store and return to refrigerator when not in use. Do not freeze or use beyond expiration date on the label.
   b. Dilution buffer: phosphate-buffered saline solution, pH 7.4, containing bovine serum albumin with 0.02% sodium azide. Refrigerate at 2° to 8° C to store and return to refrigerator when not in use. Do not freeze or use beyond expiration date on the label.
   c. Test cards. These cards must be flat for proper reactions. If necessary, flatten cards by bowing back in a direction opposite to that of the curl. Care should be taken not to put fingerprints on the test areas, as this may result in an oily deposit and improper test results. Use each card once and discard. Store the cards in their original packaging in a dry area at room temperature.
   d. Plastic stirrers
   e. Dispensing needle, 21-gauge, green hub. On completion of daily tests, remove the needle from the dispensing bottle and recap the bottle. Rinse the needle with distilled water to maintain a clear passage and accurate drop delivery. Do not wipe the dispensing needle because it is silicone coated and wiping can remove the silicone.

Additional Required Equipment and Supplies

1. Centrifuge
2. Rotator with humidifying cover. The recommended rotation speed is 100 rpm, but rotation between 95 and 110 rpm does not significantly affect the results obtained. The rotator should circumscribe a circle approximately 2 cm in diameter in the horizontal plane. A moistened humidifier cover must be used to prevent drying of test specimens during rotation.
3. High-intensity incandescent lamp
4. Micropipettors, 25 µL delivery

5. Vortex mixer
6. General equipment necessary for preparation, storage, and handling of serologic specimens

Quality Control

High-reactive control: serum (human serum) with 0.1% sodium azide. This control should demonstrate agglutination when tested.

Allow-reactive control: serum (human serum) with 0.1% sodium azide. This control should demonstrate agglutination when tested.

Nonreactive control: serum (human serum) with 0.1% sodium azide. This control should demonstrate no agglutination when tested.

NOTE: If controls do not produce appropriate reactions, the test results are invalid (see procedure notes).

CAUTION: Because the control serum is derived from human sources, it should be handled in the same manner as clinical serum specimens (see Universal Blood and Body Fluid Precautions in Chapter 6).

WARNING: The latex reagent, controls, and buffer contain sodium azide as a preservative. Sodium azide may react with lead and copper plumbing to form highly explosive metal azides. On disposal, flush with a large volume of water to prevent azide buildup. Sodium azide is toxic if inhaled.

Procedure

Preliminary Preparation

1. Allow the reagents to come to room temperature before testing.
   NOTE: Do not mix reagents from different kit lot numbers and avoid microbial contamination of reagents.
2. The latex reagent should be mixed for 5 to 10 seconds (use the highest speed setting for variable speed mixers). Vortexing is necessary at the beginning of each batch of specimens even if more than one batch is tested per day.
3. Remove the cap from the latex reagent and attach the green hub needle to the tapered fitting.
4. Label each circle of the card with the appropriate identification of patient sera and controls.

Procedure

1. (Qualitative method) Using a micropipettor, place 25 μL of each specimen (patient, high-reactive control, and negative reactive control) on the appropriately labeled, separate circles, using a new tip each time.
   Optional: Quantitative Method
   a. Using a micropipettor, place 25 μL of the negative control onto circle number 1 in the row marked nonreactive control. This control requires no dilution.
   b. Move to a new row. With a micropipettor, place 25 μL of dilution buffer in circle numbers 2 through 7. Leave circle number 1 empty.
   c. Pipette 25 μL of high-reactive control onto circle number 1.
   d. Using the same micropipettor and tip, add an additional 25 μL of high-reactive control directly into the buffer in circle number 2. Mix the serum and buffer by drawing the constituents up and down with the micropipettor 7 times. The serum in this circle (circle number 2) is now a 1:2 dilution.
   e. Using the same micropipettor and tip, transfer 25 μL of the 1:2 dilution directly into the buffer in circle number 3. Mix as in step d. Continue this method of preparing serial twofold dilutions to circle number 7.
   f. Withdraw 25 μL of serum-buffer dilution from circle number 7 and discard. The dilution in circle number 7 is now 1:64.
      NOTE: If further dilutions are required, continue the process described in steps b through e. To continue the dilutions, 25 μL of the serum-buffer in circle number 7 is transferred to the next row of circles. When the final desired dilution is prepared, discard 25 μL of the serum-buffer dilution from the last circle.
   g. Repeat steps a through f for the low-reactive control and each patient specimen.
2. Using a new plastic stirrer for each circle, spread the serum to fill the entire circle.
3. Hold the bottle cap over the tip of the needle and gently invert the latex reagent dispensing bottle several times. While holding the bottle in an inverted, vertical position, dispense several drops of the latex reagent into the bottle cap until a drop of uniform size has been formed. This predropped reagent may be recovered after testing by aspirating it back into the bottle.
4. Dispense one free-falling drop (approximately 15 μL) of latex reagent onto each circle containing the serum.
   NOTE: To ensure proper drop delivery when dispensing latex antigen, the dispensing bottle must be inverted vertically.
5. Hand rotate the card (back and forth) three or four times to distribute the latex antigen throughout each circle. Avoid cross-contamination with adjacent circles.
6. Place the card on a rotator and mix for 8 minutes under a moistened humidifying cover.
7. Immediately after rotation, read the card macroscopically in the wet state. To help differentiate weak agglutination from no agglutination, a brief hand rotation of the card (3 or 4 back-and-forth motions) must be made after mechanical rotation. Results should be read under a high-intensity incandescent lamp. Fluorescent light is generally insufficient to distinguish minimally reactive results.

Reporting Results

Qualitative Method

Positive (reactive): any agglutination of the latex reagent.
Negative (nonreactive): suspension remains evenly dispersed with no agglutination.

Quantitative Method

Report reactivity in terms of the highest dilution showing any agglutination of the latex reagent. Serum showing no agglutination at any dilution is reported as nonreactive.

TABLE 18-2	Serum Dilutions						
	Undiluted	**1:2**	**1:4**	**1:8**	**1:16**	**1:32**	**1:64**
High-reactive control	R	R	R	R	R	R	R
Low-reactive control	R	R	R	R	N	N	N
Nonreactive control	N						
Patient 1	R	R	N	N	N	N	N
Patient 2	R	R	R	R	R	R	N

R = reactive
N = nonreactive
Report as:
High-reactive control = positive, ≥1:64 dilution
Low-reactive control = positive, 1:8 dilution
Nonreactive control = negative
Patient 1 = positive, 1:2 dilution
Patient 2 = positive, 1:32 dilution

Reference range: The incidence of CMV infection depends on geographic and socioeconomic factors and the age of the patient. Serologic studies indicate that 25% to 50% of the American population demonstrate CMV antibodies present by the age of 15 years. In adult populations the incidence of antibodies to CMV has been reported between 15% and 70%.

Procedure Notes

Procedure can be performed qualitatively on undiluted serum to determine presence of antibodies to CMV. Quantitative procedures using serial twofold dilutions can be performed to determine the titer of CMV antibody.

The control serum must react appropriately. Examples of appropriate reactions are presented in Table 18-2.

Sources of Error

Incorrect test results may be caused by a variety of factors. Specimens that are incorrectly collected or stored can produce errors in the test results. The use of components or procedures other than those previously described may also lead to erroneous results.

Clinical Applications

The absence of CMV antibodies suggests that a patient has not been previously exposed to CMV; however, in the early stages of a primary infection, antibodies may not be detectable. The presence of CMV antibodies in qualitative testing on a single acute or convalescent-phase specimen is an indication of previous exposure to the virus but does not indicate immunity to subsequent reinfection.

When paired specimens are tested simultaneously, the absence of a fourfold titer rise does not definitively rule out the possibility of exposure and infection. Demonstration of seroconversion in quantitative testing (or a fourfold or greater rise in antibody titer) on paired specimens collected at least 2 weeks apart may suggest recent infection. Conversion from seronegativity to positivity or a change in antibody titer between paired

specimens may occasionally be caused by influenza A or *Mycoplasma pneumoniae* infections, suggesting stress reactivation of CMV antibody.

Clinically the selection of CMV seronegative blood donors or organs by screening with a serologic test for antibody has been reported to be effective in reducing the occurrence of CMV infection in CMV seronegative recipients. The most suitable candidates for seronegative blood for transfusion are newborn and unborn infants and immunocompromised organ-transplant recipients.

Limitations

Several limitations are inherent in CMV antibody detection. These limitations include:
1. Patients with acute infection may not have detectable antibody.
2. Seroconversion may indicate recent infection, but an increase in antibody titer by this method does not differentiate between a primary and secondary antibody response.
3. The timing of antibody response during a primary infection may differ slightly. The pattern of antibody response during a primary CMV infection has not been demonstrated.
4. Test results from neonates should be interpreted with caution because the presence of CMV antibody is usually the result of passive transfer from the mother to the fetus.
5. Although the CMV latex procedure will detect IgM and IgG antibodies, detection of IgA and IgE antibodies has not yet been demonstrated.
6. A negative CMV test result may be useful in excluding possible infection, but the diagnosis of an actual CMV infection should be documented by demonstrating the presence of the virus directly or by viral culture.

Package insert CMV Scan, Becton Dickinson Microbiology Systems, Cockeysville, Md.

Quantitative Determination of IgM Antibodies to Cytomegalovirus in Human Serum

Principle

The CMV IgM assay is an indirect enzyme-labeled immunosorbent assay for determination of IgM antibodies to CMV using antigen-coated microwells as a solid phase. CMV antigens are attached to wells of microplates. Test samples are diluted in sample diluent containing an absorbent that removes any CMV-specific IgG and IgM rheumatoid factor, which can interfere with the test. Diluted test samples are added to the coated wells and incubated. During incubation, antibodies to CMV present in the sample will bind to the antigen-coated well. After being washed to remove unbound material, antibodies to human IgM labeled with alkaline phosphatase (conjugate) are added. The conjugate binds to any IgM antibodies bound to CMV antigens. The well is washed to remove unbound conjugate and incubated with p-nitrophenyl phosphate. The p-nitrophenyl phosphate is hydrolyzed by alkaline phosphatase to form p-nitrophenol, a yellow end product with absorbance maximum at 405 nm. The intensity of the absorbance at 405 nm is proportional to the amount of IgM antibody to CMV present in the sample. The serologic detection of IgM antibodies to CMV is a clinically useful aid in the diagnosis of primary CMV infection.

Specimen Collection and Preparation

No special preparation of the patient is required before specimen collection. The patient must be positively identified when the specimen is collected, and the specimen is to be labeled at the bedside. Specimen labels must include the patient's full name, the date the specimen is collected, the patient's hospital identification number, and the phlebotomist's initials.

Blood should be drawn by an aseptic technique. Serum or plasma can be used. A minimum of 2 mL of clotted blood (red top evacuated tube) or anticoagulated blood (lavender top evacuated tube) is required. The specimen should be centrifuged promptly and an aliquot of serum removed. Lipemia, hemolysis, or contamination with bacteria render a specimen unsuitable for testing. Although icteric and turbid specimens have given valid results, fresh non-heat-inactivated serum is recommended for use in the test.

If the test cannot be performed immediately, the specimen should be refrigerated (2° to 8° C). If the specimen must be kept for more than 7 days, it should be frozen at −18° C or below. Frozen serum should be thawed rapidly at 37° C.

Specimens containing visible particulate matter should be clarified by centrifugation before testing. The test specimens should not be heat inactivated, as this may cause false-positive results.

Reagents, Supplies, and Equipment

Kit reagents available commercially in the SIA CMV IgM Procedure*

*SIA CMV IgM Product Brochure, Sigma Chemical Co, St Louis, MO.

NOTE: Store reagents at 2° to 6° C. The reagents are stable until the expiration date on the label.
1. Kit components
   a. Antigen wells: microplate wells coated with CMV antigen (strain AD 169). Store these antigen wells with desiccant in the reusable plastic bag and carefully reseal the bag after opening.
   b. Holder for wells
   c. Sample diluent. This is a buffered protein solution containing surfactant and blue dye, pH 7.5. It contains absorbent (heat-aggregated human IgG) and 0.1% sodium azide as a preservative.
   d. Calibrator. This is human serum containing IgM antibodies to CMV at 100 arbitrary units (AU/mL). It contains 0.1% sodium azide as a preservative.
   e. Conjugate. This component contains goat antibodies to human IgM labeled with calf alkaline phosphatase. It contains a pink dye and 0.02% sodium azide as a preservative.
   f. Substrate. The substrate contains p-nitrophenyl phosphate, disodium, hexahydrate 1 mg/mL, pH 9.6. This solution may develop a slight yellow color on storage. Do not use if the absorbance of the undiluted substrate is greater than 0.4 at 405 nm when measured against water using a microplate reader or a spectrophotometer with a 1-cm lightpath.
   g. Wash concentrate. This is a buffer solution concentrate with surfactant. It contains 0.1% sodium azide as a preservative. The wash solution is prepared by adding the contents of the wash concentrate bottle to 1 liter of deionized water. Mix well.
   h. Stop solution. An alkaline solution, pH 12.0. Store at room temperature. This reagent is stable until the expiration date on the label.
      WARNING: Stop solution causes irritation. Avoid contact with eyes, skin, and clothing. Avoid breathing vapor. Wash hands thoroughly after handling.
NOTE: Do not interchange reagents from different lots.
WARNING: The reagents and controls contain sodium azide as a preservative. Sodium azide may react with lead and copper plumbing to form highly explosive metal azides. On disposal, flush with a large volume of water to prevent azide buildup. Sodium azide is also toxic. Take care to avoid ingestion.

Additional Required Equipment and Supplies

1. Spectrophotometer that accommodates a 1-mL volume, or microplate reader capable of accurately measuring absorbance at 405 nm
2. Pipette tips (10 μL, 100 μL, and 200 μL) or pipette, or
3. Timer
4. 1-liter measuring cylinder
5. Squeeze bottle for dispensing wash solution
6. Dilution plates or tubes
7. Test tubes or cuvettes, 1 μL

Quality Control

Positive Control

This is a human serum containing IgM antibodies to CMV. Content (expected range, expressed as percent of calibrator) indicated on the label. It contains 0.1% sodium azide.

Negative Control

This is a human serum containing no detectable antibodies to CMV. It contains 0.1% sodium azide. The negative control should be less than 30% of the calibrator.

NOTE: If these requirements are not satisfied, the results may be inaccurate and the assay should be repeated.

CAUTION: Because the antigen wells and control and calibrator sera are derived from human sources, they should be handled in the same manner as clinical serum specimens (see Universal Blood and Body Fluid Precautions in Chapter 6).

Procedure

1. Dilute calibrator, positive and negative controls, and test specimens by combining 10 μL of each with 200 μL of sample diluent in labeled tubes or dilution plates.
2. Place the desired number of antigen wells in the holder.
3. Using a pipette tip, mix the samples and diluent by drawing up and expelling two or three times. Transfer 100 μL of each diluted specimen to the appropriate antigen well.
4. Include one well that contains only 100 μL sample diluent. This serves as the reagent blank and is used to zero the photometer.
5. Allow the plate to stand at room temperature (18° to 26° C) for 30 ± 2 minutes.
6. Shake out or aspirate contents of wells. Wash the wells by filling them with wash solution from a squeeze bottle and shaking out or aspirating. Wash three times. Drain the wells on a paper towel to remove excess fluid.

    NOTE: Thorough washing is necessary to achieve accurate results. Avoid bubbles.
7. Place 2 drops (or 100 μL) conjugate in each well, including the reagent blank well.
8. Allow to stand at room temperature (18° to 26° C) for 30 minutes ± 2 minutes.
9. Wash wells by repeating step 6.
10. Place 2 drops (or 100 μL) substrate into each well, including the reagent blank well.
11. Allow to stand at room temperature (18° to 26° C) for 30 minute ± 2 minutes.
12. Place 2 drops (or 100 μL) stop solution into each well.
13. Read and record absorbance of each test at 405 nm within 2 hours after the reaction has been stopped.

Microplate Reader

Set absorbance at 405 nm to zero with water as reference. Read and record absorbance of reagent blank (A blank). Then set absorbance to zero with the reagent blank as a reference. Read and record absorbance of samples (A sample) and calibrator (A calibrator).

Spectrophotometer

Completely remove contents of each well and transfer to cuvette or test tube. Add 800 mL of deionized water to each sample and mix. Set absorbance at 405 nm to zero with water as a reference. Read and record the absorbance of each sample including the reagent blank. Subtract the absorbance of the reagent blank for the absorbance of each sample.

Calculation

CMV IgM antibody concentration as percent of

$$\text{calibrator} = \frac{\text{A sample} \times 100}{\text{A calibrator}}$$

Example:
ABSORBANCE MEASURED USING A MICROPLATE READER

$$\text{A sample} = 0.413$$
$$\text{A calibrator} = 0.571$$

Antibody concentration as percent of
$$\text{calibrator} = \frac{0.413}{0.571} \times 100 = 72$$

ABSORBANCE MEASURED USING A SPECTROPHOTOMETER

$$\text{A blank} = 0.009$$
$$\text{A sample} = 0.083$$
$$\text{A calibrator} = 0.115$$
$$\text{A sample} - \text{A blank} = 0.083 - 0.009 = 0.074$$
$$\text{A calibrator} - \text{A blank} = 0.115 - 0.009 = 0.106$$

Antibody concentration as percent of
$$\text{calibrator} = \frac{0.074}{0.106} \times 100 = 70$$

Reporting Results

± 30% of calibrator: positive for IgM antibody to CMV and indicates the probability of current or recurrent infection
<30% of calibrator: negative for IgM antibody to CMV.

Procedure Notes

Specimens giving absorbance values above that of the calibrator should be diluted appropriately and reassayed. The value obtained should be multiplied by the dilution factor.

If cord blood is tested, contamination with maternal blood should be avoided. A follow-up specimen directly from the newborn should be tested to confirm positive IgM antibody results.

Sources of Error

False-negative and false-positive test results may occur in IgM assays for a variety of reasons.

The reasons for false-negative results include:
- A low level of specific IgM antibodies is known to produce false-negative reactions. If the specimen

is obtained too early in the development of the infection, it may contain no detectable IgM antibody by serum assay. To avoid this situation, a subsequent specimen should be obtained 7 to 14 days later for retesting.

- In many IgM assays, interference by competitive antigen-specific IgG can result in false-negative reactions. High levels of CMV-specific IgG may be present in the serum of congenitally infected newborn infants because of the presence of maternal IgG. However, in this procedure comparative testing before and after removal of IgG has no significant effect on the CMV IgM assay results.

The reasons for false-positive results include:

- Interference by IgM rheumatoid factor can produce false-positive results. Thus IgM assays must be designed to eliminate these interfering substances. In the SIA method, the sample diluent contains heat-aggregated IgG sufficient to neutralize the immunologic activity of up to 348 IU/mL of IgM rheumatoid factor.
- Interference by specific IgG antibody can produce false-positive results. Serum containing very high levels of antibody to DNA (>2000 IU/mL) (e.g., patients with systemic lupus erythematosus) may yield false-positive results in the CMV IgM SIA test.

Viral infections have also been reported to elicit heterotypic CMV IgM responses. Approximately 30% of sera from patients with heterophil (antibody-positive) mononucleosis show heterotypic CMV IgM responses. In addition, varicella-zoster virus has been reported to cause heterotypic CMV IgM response.

Clinical Applications

The presence of IgM antibodies to CMV is, in general, indicative of primary CMV infection. Specific IgM antibody, however, has been reported in reactivations and reinfections. IgM antibody may persist for as long as 9 months in immunocompetent individuals and for longer periods in immunosuppressed patients.

IgM responses vary among individuals. Of infants congenitally infected with CMV, 10% to 30% fail to develop IgM antibody responses. Approximately 27% of adults with primary CMV infection may not demonstrate an IgM response. In pregnant women the presence or absence of CMV IgG or IgM response is of limited value in predicting congenital CMV infection. However, the presence of CMV-specific IgM antibody in the circulation of the newborn is indicative of infection.

Limitations

The detection of IgM is of limited value in determining the timing of primary infection. In addition, testing results should serve only as an aid to diagnosis and should not be interpreted as diagnostic in themselves.

Treatment

The drugs ganciclovir and foscarnet can be used to treat CMV infection.

Case Study

History and Physical Examination

A 35-year-old man has recently been the recipient of a kidney transplant. He had been feeling well until 2 weeks ago, when he experienced a sore throat, fever, chills, profound malaise, and myalgia. Lymphadenopathy and splenomegaly may be observed. His medications include cyclosporine.

Questions and Discussion

1. Could this patient be suffering from an infectious disease?

   Yes, this patient could be suffering from a CMV infection. CMV infection is endemic worldwide. Dissemination of the virus may be by oral, respiratory, or venereal routes. It may also be transmitted parenterally by organ transplantation or via the transfusion of fresh blood.

   It has been recognized for more than 15 years that transfusion of blood from healthy asymptomatic blood donors is occasionally followed by active CMV infection in the recipient. There is strong evidence to incriminate peripheral blood leukocytes and transplanted tissues as sources of CMV.

2. Why would this patient be susceptible to an opportunistic infection?

   By adulthood most individuals have experienced asymptomatic contact with CMV. Because CMV can persist latently, active infections may develop under a variety of conditions, such as pregnancy or immunosuppression, or subsequent to organ or bone marrow transplantation. Of patients who are immunosuppressed, only seronegative patients appear to be at a significant risk of developing CMV infection. Patients at the highest risk of mortality from CMV infections are allograft transplant seronegative patients who receive tissue from a seropositive donor. The great majority of infections in allograft recipients are transmitted by the donor kidney or arise from the reactivation of the recipient's latent virus.

   CMV infection can be life threatening in immunosuppressed patients. Infections in these patients may result in disseminated multisystem involvement, including pneumonitis, hepatitis, gastrointestinal ulceration, arthralgias, meningoencephalitis, and retinitis. Interstitial pneumonitis, frequently associated with CMV infection, is a major cause of death after allogeneic bone marrow transplantation.

3. How could an infection of this type be potentially eliminated?

   Transmission of CMV by transfusion of blood or blood components containing white cells is receiving more critical attention, particularly as it affects patients with severely impaired immunity who require supportive therapy. In these patients, methods of prevention include effective donor screening, leukocyte-depleted blood products, and immune globulin containing passively acquired CMV antibodies.

4. Are health care workers at risk for infections of this type?

Yes, health care professionals are one of the groups becoming increasingly concerned about the risks associated with exposure to CMV. Nosocomial transmission from patients to health care workers has not been documented, but observance of good personal hygiene and hand washing offers the best measures for preventing transmission.

5. Can congenital infections of this type occur?

Primary, as well as recurrent maternal, CMV infection can be transmitted in utero. Congenital CMV infection is the most common intrauterine infection, affecting from 0.4% to 2.3% of all live births. The presence of maternal antibody to CMV before conception provides substantial protection against damaging congenital CMV infection in the newborn.

Primary maternal infection during pregnancy is associated with more severe sequelae of congenital CMV infection. The majority of CMV-infected newborns are asymptomatic, but 1% manifest damage caused by CMV. Infected infants can become severely ill, and death may result in premature infants. In premature infants, acquired CMV infection can result in atypical lymphocytosis, hepatosplenomegaly, pneumonia, or death.

Congenitally infected newborns, especially those who acquire CMV during a maternal primary infection, are more prone to develop severe CID. The severe form of CID may be fatal or can cause permanent neurologic sequelae, such as intracranial calcifications, mental retardation, deafness, vision defects, microcephaly, and motor dysfunction. Psychomotor retardation is seen in 51% to 75% of survivors. Hearing loss is observed in 21% to 50% of cases, and visual impairment in 20% of cases. Infants without symptoms at birth may develop hearing and neurologic impairment at a later date.

6. How can this disease be diagnosed?

A definitive diagnosis can be made only by isolating the CMV from urine or blood samples or by the demonstration of CMV-specific IgM or increasing CMV-specific IgG antibody titers. Methods for measuring CMV IgM antibodies include indirect immunofluorescence or indirect and reverse ELISA tests. Virus detection in urine by electron microscopy is reliable if positive; however, a negative result does not rule out CMV infection. Human CMV is indistinguishable by negative staining electron-microscopy from its close relatives, herpes simplex and varicella (the cause of chickenpox). Viral culture is the method of choice for confirming CMV infection. Early detection of CMV in viral cultures is done routinely by DFA examination; demonstration of CMV by DFA examination of bronchoalveolar lavage specimens is possible.

Serologic methods to detect the presence of IgM antibodies can aid in the diagnosis of primary infection. Detection of CMV-specific IgM can represent primary infection or rare reactivation of infection. False-positive results, however, can occur because of the presence of other antibodies, such as rheumatoid factor. Although tests for heterophil, Epstein-Barr virus, and toxoplasma antibodies are generally negative, elevated concentrations (titers) of several antibodies may occur. These include ANA, RA, and nonspecific cold agglutinins. The inability to demonstrate IgM in a blood specimen can result from the presence of a large amount of virus-specific IgG. Lack of a CMV-specific IgM response is especially common in congenital infections. Detection of significant increases in CMV-specific IgG antibody by methods such as CF, ACIF, and EIA suggest, but do not prove, recent infection or reactivation of latent infection. The EIA method for IgM and IgG antibodies to CMV has replaced CF, ACIF, and IFA. Latex particle agglutination and indirect hemagglutination are useful screening methods to obtain seronegative donors.

Newer CMV detection methods include CMV antigen detection in urine by EIA; in addition, a detection method using cDNA is being developed. RNA transcript of CMV DNA is detectable in peripheral blood mononuclear cells of seropositive individuals by ISH with cDNA of CMV. The ISH technique, which is more sensitive than dot-blot hybridization (Northern blot), promises to be a new early detection method for CMV expression.

Diagnosis

Cytomegalovirus

CHAPTER HIGHLIGHTS

CMV is a ubiquitous human viral pathogen. Human CMV is classified as a member of the herpes family of viruses. All of the herpes viruses are relatively large, enveloped DNA viruses that undergo a replicative cycle involving DNA expression and nucleocapsid assembly within the nucleus. Although the herpes family produces diverse clinical diseases, the viruses share the basic characteristics of being cell associated. These characteristics may play a role in the ability of the virus to produce subclinical infections that can be reactivated under appropriate stimuli. Dissemination of the virus may occur by oral, respiratory, or venereal routes. It may also be transmitted parenterally by organ transplantation or by transfusion of fresh blood.

The incidence of primary infections during childhood is low. Of patients who are immunosuppressed, only seronegative patients appear to be at a significant risk of developing CMV infection. Patients at the highest risk of mortality from CMV infections are allograft transplant seronegative patients who receive tissue from a seropositive donor. Most infections in allograft recipients are transmitted by the donor kidney or arise from the reactivation of the recipient's latent virus.

Transmission of CMV by transfusion of blood or blood components containing white cells is assuming increasing importance in patients with severely impaired immunity who require supportive therapy. Low-birth-weight neonates are also at high risk for CMV infection through transfusion of

CMV-infected blood products. Persistent infections characterized by periods of reactivation of CMV are frequently termed latent infections, although this condition has not been clearly defined for CMV.

CMV is considered to be one of the most important causes of congenital viral infections in the United States because primary and recurrent maternal CMV infection can be transmitted in utero. Acquired CMV infection is usually asymptomatic and can persist in the host as a chronic or latent infection. In most patients, CMV infection is asymptomatic. Occasionally a self-limited, heterophil-negative, mononucleosis-like syndrome results. CMV infection is known to alter the immune system and produce overt manifestations of infection. Infection interferes with immune responsiveness in both normal and immunocompromised individuals. This diminished responsiveness results in a decreased proliferative response to the CMV antigen, which persists for several months. In patients with CMV mononucleosis-like syndrome, alterations of T-lymphocyte subsets result, producing an increase in the absolute number of suppressor (CD) lymphocytes, and a decrease in helper (CD) lymphocytes. These subset abnormalities persist for months. In addition, questions have been raised regarding CMV as a potentially oncogenic virus because viral antigens and/or nucleic acid have been found in some human malignancies.

In cells infected by CMV, several antigens appear at varying time intervals after infection. Before replication of viral DNA takes place, immediate-early antigens and early antigens are present in the nuclei of infected cells. Immediate-early antigens appear within 1 hour of cellular infection, and early antigens are present within 24 hours. At about 72 hours postinfection or at the end of the viral replication cycle, late antigens are demonstrable in the nucleus and cytoplasm of infected cells. The immune antibody response to these various antigens differs in incidence and significance. The presence of antibodies against immediate-early and early antigens is associated with active infection of either a primary or reactivated nature. The characteristic antibody responses associated with infection are as follows: primary infection, which is demonstrated by a transient virus-specific IgM antibody response and eventual seroconversion to produce IgG antibodies to the virus; reactivation of latent CMV infection in seropositive (IgG) individuals, which may be accompanied by significant increases in IgG antibodies to the virus but elicits no detectable IgM response; and reinfection by a strain of CMV that is different from the original infecting strain in which a significant IgG antibody response is demonstrated but in which it is unknown whether an IgM response occurs.

Serologic methods to detect the presence of IgM antibodies can aid in the diagnosis of primary infection. Detection of CMV-specific IgM can represent primary infection or rare reactivation of infection. Detection of significant increases in CMV-specific IgG antibody by methods such as CF, ACIF, and EIA suggest, but do not prove, recent infection or reactivation of latent infection. The EIA method for IgM and IgG antibodies to CMV has replaced CF, ACIF, and IFA. Latex particle agglutination and indirect hemagglutination are useful screening methods to obtain seronegative blood donors. Newer CMV detection methods are being explored. CMV antigen detection in urine by EIA and cDNA is being developed. RNA transcript of CMV DNA is detectable in peripheral blood mononuclear cells of seropositive individuals by ISH with cDNA of CMV. The ISH technique, which is more sensitive than dot-blot hybridization (Northern blot), promises to be a new early detection method for CMV expression.

REVIEW QUESTIONS

1. All of the following descriptive characteristics are true of cytomegalovirus except that it is:
   A. a herpes family virus
   B. a DNA virus
   C. a cell-associated virus
   D. epidemic worldwide

2. Because CMV can persist latently, an active infection may develop as a result of all of the following conditions except:
   A. pregnancy
   B. immunosuppression therapy
   C. organ or bone marrow transplantation
   D. transfusion of leukocyte-poor blood

3. CMV is recognized as the cause of congenital viral infection in _____% of all live births:
   A. 0.1 to 0.4
   B. 0.5 to 2.4
   C. 2.5 to 4.9
   D. 5.0 to 9.9

4. Transfusion-acquired CMV infection can cause:
   A. mononucleosis-like syndrome
   B. hepatitis
   C. rejection of a transplanted organ
   D. all of the above

Match the three types of CMV infection with their appropriate description.

5. _____ Primary infection

6. _____ Reactivated infection

7. _____ Reinfection
   A. a significant antibody response and viral shedding caused by a different strain of virus
   B. when a seronegative recipient is transfused with blood from an actively or latently infected donor
   C. when a seropositive recipient is transfused with blood from either a CMV antibody-positive or negative donor

Match the following serologic markers of CMV infection.

8. _____ Early antigens

9. _____ Immediate-early antigens

10. _____ Late antigens
    A. appear at about 72 hours postinfection or at the end of the viral replication cycle
    B. appear within 1 hour of cellular infection
    C. present within 24 hours

11. Antibodies to immediate-early and early antigens are associated with:
    A. primary active infection
    B. reactivated active infection
    C. latent infection
    D. increasing age and gender of the patient

Match the following.

12. _____ Primary infection

13. _____ Reactivation of latent infection in seropositive IgG patient

14. _____ Reinfection with a strain of CMV different from the original strain
    A. IgG but IgM response unknown
    B. specific IgM antibody response
    C. IgG (no detectable IgM)

Match the following.

15. _____ Latex particle agglutination

16. _____ Indirect fluorescent antibody

17. _____ Enzyme immunoassay
    A. antibody
    B. IgM
    C. IgG and IgM antibody

18. All of the herpes family of viruses share the characteristic of being _____ viruses.
    A. RNA
    B. small
    C. cell-associated
    D. nonenveloped

19. The most likely mode of CMV acquisition is:
    A. transplantation
    B. blood transfusion
    C. venereal route
    D. respiratory infection

20. Of patients who are immunosuppressed, only _____ appear to be at a significant risk of acquiring CMV infection.
    A. transplant patients
    B. seronegative patients
    C. seropositive patients
    D. health care workers

21. All of the following are methods for prevention of CMV except:
    A. effective donor screening
    B. leukocyte-depleted blood products
    C. immune globulin with CMV antibodies
    D. transfusion of fresh blood

Questions 22-25. Indicate true statements with the letter "A," and false statements with the letter "B."

22. _____ Primary and recurrent maternal CMV infections can be transmitted in utero.

23. _____ CMV is the most common intrauterine infection.

24. _____ Few CMV-infected newborns are asymptomatic.

25. _____ Normal adults and children usually experience CMV infection without serious complications.

Questions 26 and 27. Fill in the blanks below, choosing from the following answers:

Possible answers for question 26.
    A. 1
    B. 24
    C. 48
    D. 72

Possible answers for question 27.
    A. nucleus and nucleoli
    B. nucleus and cytoplasm
    C. nucleus only
    D. cytoplasm only

At about (26) _____ hour(s) after infection, or the end of the viral replication cycle, late antigens are demonstrable

in the (27) _____ of infected cells.

BIBLIOGRAPHY

Adler SP: Transfusion-associated cytomegalovirus infections, *Rev Infect Dis* 5:977-993, 1983.

Bailey TC et al: Ganciclovir for cytomegalovirus after heart transplantation, *N Engl J Med* 327(12):891, 1992.

Betts RF: The relationship of epidemiology and treatment factors to infection and allograft survival in renal transplantation. In Platkin SA et al, editors: *CMV pathogenesis and prevention of human infection,* New York, 1984, Alan R Liss.

Bowden R et al: Cytomegalovirus immune globulin and seronegative blood products to prevent primary cytomegalovirus infection after marrow transplantation, *N Engl J Med* 314:1006-1010, 1986.

Brady MT: Cytomegalovirus infections: occupational risk for health professionals, *Am J Infect Control* 14(5):197-203, 1986.

Brennan D: Dancing partners: cytomegalovirus and allograft injury, XVIII International Congress of the Transplantation Society, Aug. 27, 2000, Rome, Italy.

Demmler GJ et al: Enzyme-linked immunosorbent assay for the detection of IgM-class antibodies to cytomegalovirus, *J Infect Dis* 153:1152-1155, 1986.

Dobbins JG, Stewart JA: Surveillance of congenital cytomegalovirus disease, 1990-1991, *MMWR* 41(55-2):35-44, 433-434, 1992.

Feng CS et al: A comparison of four commercial test kits for detection of cytomegalovirus antibodies in blood donors, *Transfusion* 26(2):203, 1986.

Fiesthumel S et al: Cytomegalovirus (CMV) infection in blood donors: correlation of serologic markers with viral shedding, *Transfusion* 26(6):554, 1986 (abstract).

Fowler KB et al: The outcome of congenital cytomegalovirus infection in relation to maternal antibody status, *N Engl J Med* 326(10):663-667, 1992.

Nightingale SL: CMV-IGIV approved, *JAMA* 264(2):168, 1990.

Package insert CMV Scan, Becton Dickinson Microbiology Systems, Cockeysville, Md.

Schrier RD, Nelson JA, Nelson MB: Detection of human cytomegalovirus in peripheral blood lymphocytes in a natural infection, *Science* 230:1048-1051, 1985.

Schuster V et al: Detection of human cytomegalovirus in urine by DNA-DNA and RNA-DNA hybridization, *J Infect Dis* 154:309-314, 1986.

Sia IG et al: Evaluation of the COBAS AMPLICOR CMV MONITOR test for detection of viral DNA in specimens taken from patients after liver transplantation, *J Clin Microbiol* 38(2):600-606, 2000.

SIA CMV IgM Product Brochure, Sigma Chemical Co, St Louis, Mo.

Taswell HF et al: Comparison of three methods for detecting antibody to cytomegalovirus, *Transfusion* 26(3):285-289, 1986.

Turgeon ML: *Clinical hematology,* ed 3, Philadelphia, 1999, Lippincott Williams & Wilkins.

Turgeon ML: *Fundamentals of immunohematology,* ed 2, Baltimore, 1995, Williams & Wilkins.

Yow MD, Demmler GJ: Congenital cytomegalovirus disease—20 years is long enough, *N Engl J Med* 326(10):702-703, 1992.

Chapter 19

Infectious Mononucleosis

LEARNING OBJECTIVES

At the conclusion of this chapter, the reader should be able to:
- Describe the etiology, epidemiology, and signs and symptoms of infectious mononucleosis.
- Explain the immunologic manifestations of infectious mononucleosis, including heterophil antibodies.

- Discuss the elements of EBV serology and the diagnostic clinical applications of the presence of each component.
- Compare the serologic procedures and clinical applications of the Paul-Bunnell, Davidsohn differential, and agglutination techniques.

ETIOLOGY

The Epstein-Barr virus (EBV) was first discovered in 1964 as the cause of infectious mononucleosis. This disorder is usually an acute, benign, and self-limiting lymphoproliferative condition. EBV is also the cause of Burkett's lymphoma (a malignant tumor of the lymphoid tissue occurring mainly in African children), nasopharyngeal carcinoma, and neoplasms of the thymus, parotid gland, and supraglottic larynx. EBV is an important factor in the development of nasopharyngeal carcinoma, an epithelial cancer. Although nasopharyngeal carcinoma is rare in North American and European Caucasians, it is among the most common cancers in southern China and parts of southeast Asia. Genetics and environmental factors appear to contribute to the elevated risk of nasopharyngeal carcinoma among the Chinese.

EBV infections can result in complications involving the cardiac, ocular, respiratory, hematologic, digestive, renal, and neurologic systems. EBV-associated neurologic syndromes include Bell's palsy, Guillain-Barré syndrome, meningoencephalitis, Reye's syndrome, myelitis, cranial nerve neuritis, and psychotic disorders. Respiratory paralysis caused by bulbar involvement can be fatal.

EPIDEMIOLOGY

EBV is widely disseminated. It is estimated that 95% of the world's population is exposed to the virus, which makes it the most ubiquitous virus known to humans. EBV is a human herpes DNA virus. In infectious mononucleosis the virus infects B lymphocytes, but the variant lymphocytes produced in response to and seen in microscopic examination of the peripheral blood have T-cell characteristics. A young child recently died from sporadic fatal infectious mononucleosis involving monoclonal proliferation of cytotoxic T cells containing the EBV genome. One of the habitats of the persisting viral genome in hosts with a latent infection is the B lymphocytes of the lymphoreticular system and in epithelial cells of the oropharynx.

Although EBV appears to be transmitted primarily by close contact with infectious oral-pharyngeal secretions, the virus has been reported to be transmitted by blood transfusion and transplacental routes. Under ordinary conditions, transmission of the virus through transfusion or transplacental exposure is unlikely. In addition, EBV-associated posttransplantation lymphoproliferative disease develops in 1% to 10% of organ transplant recipients.

The frequency of seronegative patients is nearly 100% in early infancy but declines with increasing age, more or less rapidly, depending on socioeconomic conditions, to less than 10% in young adults. After primary exposure, a person is considered to be immune and generally no longer susceptible to overt reinfection. In Western society primary exposure to EBV occurs in two waves. Approximately half of the population is exposed to the virus before the age of 5 years; a second wave of seroconversion occurs during late adolescence (15 to 24 years). Approximately 90% of adult patients demonstrate antibodies to the virus.

Individuals at risk include those who lack antibodies to the virus. EBV is only a minor problem for immunocompetent persons, but it can become a major one for immunologically compromised patients. Blood transfusion from an immune donor to a nonimmune recipient may produce a primary infection in the recipient known as infectious mononucleosis postperfusion syndrome. Infectious mononucleosis or infectious mononucleosis-like illness after blood transfusion often may be the result of a concomitant cytomegalovirus (CMV) infection rather than the EBV. In addition, the association with EBV appears to be a specific finding in malignant lymphoma developing after severe immunosuppression, such as that induced by treatment with cyclosporine.

A low percentage of patients experience symptomatic reactivation. Reactivation of latent infection has been implicated in a persistent illness referred to as the EBV-associated fatigue syndrome, but this phenomenon is not universally accepted.

Clinically apparent infectious mononucleosis has an estimated frequency of 45:100,000 in adolescents. In immunosuppressed patients the incidence of EBV infection ranges from 35% to 47%. As occurs with other herpes viruses, there is a carrier state after primary infection.

SIGNS AND SYMPTOMS

The majority of individuals experience seroconversion without any significant clinical signs and symptoms of disease. Immunocompetent persons maintain EBV as a chronic latent infection. In children less than 5 years old, infection is either asymptomatic or frequently characterized by mild, poorly defined signs and symptoms. Although anyone can suffer from this viral disorder, it is typically manifested in young adults.

The incubation period of infectious mononucleosis is from 10 to 50 days; once fully developed, it lasts for 1 to 4 weeks. Clinical manifestations include extreme fatigue, malaise, sore throat, fever, and cervical lymphadenopathy. Splenomegaly occurs in about 50% of cases. Jaundice is infrequent, although the most common complication is hepatitis. A smaller percentage of patients develop hepatomegaly or splenomegaly

and hepatomegaly. Because abnormal liver function is more marked with EBV-induced infectious mononucleosis than in CMV-associated mononucleosis, EBV must be considered in the differential diagnosis of hepatitis. A significant number of cases of infectious mononucleosis do not manifest classic signs and symptoms.

IMMUNOLOGIC MANIFESTATIONS

Heterophil Antibodies

Heterophil antibodies are composed of a broad class of antibodies. These antibodies are stimulated by one antigen and react with an entirely unrelated surface antigen present on cells from different mammalian species. Heterophil antibodies may be present in normal individuals in low concentrations (titers), but a titer of 1:56 or greater is clinically significant in suspected cases of infectious mononucleosis.

The immunoglobulin M (IgM) type of heterophil antibody usually appears during the acute phase of infectious mononucleosis, but the antigen that stimulates its production remains unknown. IgM heterophil antibody is characterized by the following features:
- Reacts with horse, ox, and sheep erythrocytes
- Absorbed by beef erythrocytes
- Not absorbed by guinea pig kidney cells
- Does not react with EBV-specific antigens

Paul and Bunnell first associated infectious mononucleosis with sheep cell agglutination and developed a test for the infectious mononucleosis heterophil. Davidsohn modified the original Paul-Bunnell test, introducing a differential adsorption aspect to remove the cross-reacting Forssman and serum sickness heterophil antibodies. Since then the Davidsohn test has become the classic laboratory reference test for the diagnosis of infectious mononucleosis; however, this test is time consuming and cumbersome.

Rapid slide tests based on the principle of agglutination of horse erythrocytes are now available. The use of horse erythrocytes appears to increase the sensitivity of the test.

Epstein-Barr Virus Serology

Within the adult population, 10% to 20% of individuals with acute infectious mononucleosis do not produce infectious mononucleosis heterophil antibody. The pediatric population is of particular concern because more than 50% of children less than 4 years old with infectious mononucleosis are heterophil negative. In diagnostically inconclusive cases of infectious mononucleosis, a more definitive assessment of immune status may be obtained through an EBV serologic panel. Candidates for EBV serology include those who do not exhibit classic symptoms of infectious mononucleosis, who are heterophil negative, or who are immunosuppressed.

EBV-infected B lymphocytes express a variety of "new" antigens encoded by the virus. Infection with EBV results in the expression of viral capsid antigen (VCA), early antigen (EA), and nuclear antigen (NA), with corresponding antibody responses. Assays for IgM and IgG antibodies to these EBV antigens are available. EBV-specific serologic studies (Figure 19-1 and Table 19-1) are beneficial in defining immune sta-

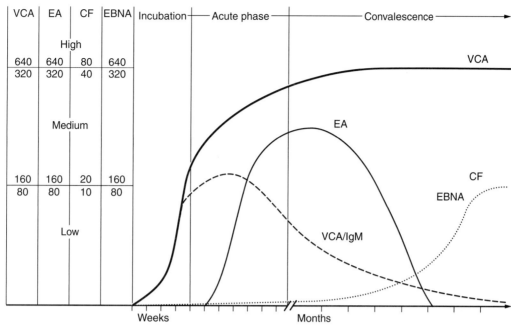

Figure 19-1   EBV antibody response during the course of infectious mononucleosis. *EA*, Early antigen; *VCA*, viral capsid antigen; *EBNA*, EB nuclear antigen; *CF*, complement fixation test. (Redrawn from Krugman S et al: *Infectious diseases of children*, ed 9, St Louis, 1992, Mosby.)

TABLE 19-1	Characteristic Antibody Formation in Infectious Mononucleosis					
	VCA IgM	**VCA IgG**	**EA-D**	**EA-R**	**EBNA IgG**	**Heterophil**
No previous exposure	–	–	–	–	–	–
Recent (acute) infection	+	+	+/–	–	–	+
Past infection (convalescent) period	–	+	–	–	+	–
Reactivation of latent infection	+/–	+	+/–	+/–	+	+/–

EA-D, Early antigen (diffuse); *EA-R*, early antigen (restricted); *EBNA*, Epstein-Barr nuclear antigen; *VCA*, viral capsid antigen.

tus, and their time of appearance may be indicative of the stage of disease. This can provide important information for both the diagnosis and management of EBV-associated disease. Patients with nasopharyngeal carcinoma have elevated titers of IgA antibodies to EBV replicative antigens, including VCA. These antibodies, which frequently precede the appearance of the tumor, serve as a prognostic indicator of remission and relapse.

Viral Capsid Antigen

VCA is produced by infected B cells and can be found in the cytoplasm. Anti-VCA IgM is usually detectable early in the course of infection, but it is low in concentration and disappears within 2 to 4 months. Anti-VCA IgG is usually detectable within 4 to 7 days after the onset of signs and symptoms and persists for an extended period, perhaps lifelong.

Early Antigen

EA is a complex of two components, early antigen-n-diffuse (EA-D), which is found in both the nucleus and the cyto-

plasm of the B cells, and early antigen-restricted (EA-R), which is usually found as a mass only in the cytoplasm.

Anti-EA-D of the IgG type is highly indicative of acute infection, but it is not detectable in 10% to 20% of patients with infectious mononucleosis. EA-D disappears in about 3 months; however, a rise in titer is demonstrated during reactivation of a latent EBV infection.

Anti-EA-R IgG is not usually found in young adults during the acute phase, but it is sometimes demonstrated in the serum of very young children during the acute phase. Anti-EA-R IgG appears transiently in the later convalescent phase. In general, anti-EA-D and anti-EA-R IgG are not consistent indicators of the disease stage.

Epstein-Barr Nuclear Antigen

Epstein-Barr nuclear antigen (EBNA) is found in the nucleus of all EBV-infected cells. Although the synthesis of NA precedes EA synthesis during the infection of B cells, EBV-NA does not become available for antibody stimulation until after the incubation period of infectious mononucleosis, when activated T lymphocytes destroy the EBV genome-carrying

TABLE 19-2	Characteristic Diagnostic Profile of Epstein-Barr Virus
Susceptibility	If the patient is seronegative (lacks antibody to VCA
Primary Infection	Antibody (IgM) to viral capsid antigen is present; EBNA is absent
	A high or rising titer of antibody (IgG) to VCA and no evidence of antibody to EBNA after at least 4 weeks of symptoms
Reactivation	If antibody to EBNA and an elevation of antibodies to EA are present, the patient may be suffering from reactivation
Past Infection	Antibodies to VCA and EBNA are present

VCA, Viral capsid antigen; *EBNA*, Epstein-Barr nuclear antigen; *EA*, early antigen.

B cells. As a result, antibodies to NA are absent or barely detectable during acute infectious mononucleosis.

Anti-EBNA IgG does not appear until a patient has entered the convalescent period. EBV-NA antibodies are almost always present in sera containing IgG antibodies to VCA of EBV unless the patient is in the early acute phase of infectious mononucleosis. Patients with severe immunologic defects or immunosuppressive disease may not have EBV-NA antibodies, even if antibodies to VCA are present.

Under normal conditions antibody titers to NA gradually increase through convalescence and reach a plateau between 3 and 12 months postinfection. The antibody titer remains at a moderate, measurable level indefinitely because of the persistent viral carrier state established after primary EBV infection. Most healthy individuals with previous exposure to EBV have antibody titers to EBV-NA that range from 1:10 to 1:160. In EBV-associated malignancies, the levels of EBNA antibody are usually high in patients with nasopharyngeal carcinoma and can range from barely detectable to very high in patients with Burkitt's lymphoma.

Test results of antibodies to EBV-NA should be evaluated in relationship to patient symptoms, clinical history, and antibody response patterns to EBV-VCA and EA to establish a diagnosis (Table 19-2). The antibody profile can be especially useful. For example, a patient with an infectious mononucleosis-like illness caused by reactivation of a persistent EBV infection resulting from an immunosuppressive malignancy or non-malignant disease can demonstrate high titers of both IgM and IgG VCA antibodies. If the antibody to EBV-NA is also elevated, however, a diagnosis of primary EBV infection can be excluded.

Additional Testing

A test commonly used in the EBV serology is based on immunofluorescence. Antigen substrate slides containing EBV-infected B cells are incubated with the patient's serum. The presence of specific antibody is detected by the addition of fluorescein-conjugated antihuman IgG or IgM. The disadvantages of this type of testing are that it is time consuming, difficult to interpret, and prone to interference from other serum components such as rheumatoid factor.

Enzyme-linked immunosorbent assay testing may be used to detect antibodies to EBNA. This method of testing uses a synthetic peptide antigen to determine relative amounts of IgM and IgG antibodies in patient serum or plasma. The sensitivity of this form of assay is approximately 98.9%, with a specificity of 99.0%.

Diagnostic Evaluation

In addition to clinical signs and symptoms, laboratory testing is necessary to establish or confirm the diagnosis of infectious mononucleosis.

Hematologic studies reveal a leukocyte count ranging from 10 to 20 × 10/L in about two thirds of patients; about 10% of the patients with this disorder demonstrate leukopenia. A differential leukocyte count may initially disclose a neutrophilia, although mononuclear cells usually predominate as the disorder develops. Typical relative lymphocyte counts range from 60% to 90% with 5% to 30% variant lymphocytes. These variant lymphocytes exhibit diverse morphologic features and persist for 1 to 2 months and as long as 4 to 6 months (Figure 19-2).

If the classic signs and symptoms of infectious mononucleosis are absent, a diagnosis of infectious mononucleosis is more difficult to make. A definite diagnosis of infectious mononucleosis can be established by serologic antibody testing. The antibodies present in infectious mononucleosis are heterophil and EBV antibodies.

■ *Paul-Bunnell Screening Test*

Principle

The Paul-Bunnell test is a hemagglutination test designed to detect heterophil antibodies in patient serum when mixed with antigen-bearing sheep erythrocytes. Dilutions of inactivated patient serum are mixed with sheep erythrocytes, incubated, centrifuged, and macroscopically examined for agglutination. Positive reactions are preliminarily associated with the manifestation of infectious mononucleosis.

Specimen Collection and Preparation

No special preparation of the patient is required before specimen collection. The patient must be positively identified when the specimen is collected. The specimen should be labeled at the bedside and include the patient's full name, date the specimen is collected, patient's hospital identification number, and phlebotomist's initials. Blood should be drawn by an aseptic technique. The required specimen is a minimum of 2 mL of clotted blood (red top evacuated tube). The presence of hemolysis makes the specimen unsuitable for testing.

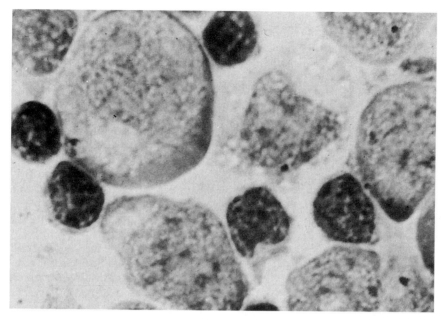

Figure 19-2 Lymph node imprint, infectious mononucleosis. (Wright's stain; ×1200; courtesy Dr. JC Sieracki.) (From Miale JB: *Hematology,* ed 6, St Louis, 1982, Mosby.)

Centrifuge the tube of blood and remove an aliquot of clear serum. Inactivate the serum at 56° C for 30 minutes before testing.

Reagents, Supplies, and Equipment

2% suspension of washed sheep cells in normal saline (prepared by pipetting 0.2 mL of packed erythrocytes into 9.8 mL of saline)
0.9% sodium chloride (normal physiologic saline)
12 × 75-mm test tubes
NOTE: The cell should be no more than 1 week old.
Graduated serologic pipettes
Centrifuge
37° C incubator (optional)

Quality Control

A known positive control should be run concurrently.

Procedure

1. Label two sets of test tubes. Each set should consist of 10 tubes.
2. Pipette 0.5 mL of saline into tube 1 and 0.25 mL of saline into each of the remaining nine tubes.
3. To the first set of tubes, add 0.1 mL of patient's inactivated serum to the first tube; mix and transfer 0.25 mL of the dilution to the second tube; mix and transfer 0.25 mL of the dilution to the third tube. Repeat this process to tube 10. Discard 0.25 mL from the final tube, tube 10.
4. To the second set of tubes, add 0.1 mL of the control serum and proceed to dilute it as in step 3.
5. Add 0.1 mL of 2% sheep cells to each tube.
6. Gently shake the tubes until mixed.

7. Incubate the tubes at 37° C for 1 hour or overnight at room temperature.
8. Centrifuge the tubes for 1 minute at 1500 rpm.
9. Gently shake each tube and examine macroscopically for agglutination.
10. Record the results.

Reporting Results

A titer of greater than 1:56 is considered to be a positive presumptive test.

Procedure Notes

The antigens on sheep erythrocytes are associated with infectious mononucleosis, serum sickness, and the Forssman antigen.

Sources of Error

False-positive reactions have been observed in conditions such as hepatitis infection and Hodgkin's disease. An improperly inactivated serum will produce hemolysis.

Clinical Applications

The Paul-Bunnell test is a useful screening test for the presence of heterophil antibodies because it is simple and inexpensive. Although the specificity of the heterophil assay is rated as good, negative results are demonstrated in individuals who do not produce infectious mononucleosis heterophil antibody. If negative results are displayed, however, EBV serology may be indicated.

Limitations

The test is only indicative of the presence or absence of heterophil antibodies. Demonstrating agglutination by using sheep erythrocytes does not make a distinction between antibodies associated with infectious mononucleosis, serum sickness, or the Forssman antigen.

Heterophil antibody assay lacks sensitivity as a diagnostic criterion for infectious mononucleosis. Sheep erythrocytes are less sensitive than erythrocytes from other species such as the horse. A patient may take as long as 3 months to develop a detectable heterophil titer.

References

Paul JR, Bunnell WW: The presence of heterophile antibodies in infectious mononucleosis, *Am J Med Sci* 183:90-104, 1932.

Sumaya CV: Infectious mononucleosis and other EBV infections: diagnostic factors, *Lab Manage* 24:37-45, 1986.

 Davidsohn Differential Test

Principle

This classic test distinguishes between the heterophil antibodies that agglutinate the antigen-bearing erythrocytes of sheep. The differential nature of the test is predicated on the fact that sheep and beef (ox) erythrocytes bear some common antigens not present on the kidney cells of the guinea pig. Exposure of patient serum both to guinea pig cells, which are rich in Forssman antigen, and beef erythrocytes, which are poor in Forssman antigen, produces differential absorption. Any absorbed antibodies are removed by centrifugation, and the supernatant fluid is tested with sheep erythrocytes. This test classically differentiates the heterophil types of antibody associated with infectious mononucleosis, serum sickness, or Forssman antigen.

Specimen Collection and Preparation

No special preparation of the patient is required before specimen collection. The patient must be positively identified when the specimen is collected. The specimen should be labeled at the bedside and include the patient's full name, the date the specimen is collected, the patient's hospital identification number, and the phlebotomist's initials.

Blood should be drawn by an aseptic technique. The required specimen is a minimum of 2 mL of clotted blood (red top evacuated tube). The presence of hemolysis makes the specimen unsuitable for testing.

Centrifuge the tube of blood and remove an aliquot of clear serum. Inactivate the serum at 56° C for 30 minutes before testing.

Reagents, Supplies, and Equipment

0.9% sodium chloride (normal physiologic saline)
2% suspension of washed sheep cells in normal saline (prepared by pipetting 0.2 mL of packed erythrocytes into 9.8 mL of saline)

12 × 75-mm test tubes
NOTE: The cell should be no more than 1 week old.
20% beef erythrocytes
20% suspension of guinea pig kidney cells
NOTE: Sheep, beef, and guinea pig kidney cells are commercially available from Baltimore Biological Laboratories, Cockeysville, MD.
12 × 75-mm test tubes
2 conical centrifuge tubes
Graduated serologic pipettes
Test tube racks

Quality Control

A known positive control should be run concurrently.

Procedure

Preliminary Specimen Preparation

1. Pipette 1 mL of beef cells into an appropriately labeled conical centrifuge tube.
2. Pipette 1 mL of guinea pig cells into an appropriately labeled conical centrifuge tube.
3. Pipette 0.25 mL of inactivated patient serum into each tube and shake.
4. Incubate the tubes at room temperature for 5 minutes. Shake the tubes periodically to resuspend the cells.
5. Centrifuge for 10 minutes at 1500 rpm.

Procedure

1. Label two sets of test tubes: beef 1-8 and guinea pig 1-8.
2. Pipette 0.25 mL of saline into each test tube.
3. Carefully pipette 0.25 mL of clear supernatant from the beef erythrocyte conical centrifuge tube to the first tube of the beef set of test tubes.
4. Carefully pipette 0.25 mL of clear supernatant from the guinea pig conical centrifuge tube to the first tube of the guinea pig set of test tubes.
5. Mix the contents of the first beef tube and transfer 0.25 mL of the dilution to the next tube. Continue to mix and transfer 0.25 mL until the last tube, tube 8, is reached. Discard 0.25 mL from the last tube.
6. Mix the contents of the first guinea pig tube and transfer 0.25 mL of the dilution to the next tube. Continue to mix and transfer 0.25 mL until the last tube, tube 8, is reached. Discard 0.25 mL from the last tube.
7. Pipette 0.1 mL of sheep erythrocytes into each tube.
8. Shake gently until the cells are well mixed.
9. Incubate at room temperature for 2 hours.
10. Gently shake each tube and examine macroscopically for agglutination. Record the results.

Reporting Results

Agglutination patterns are presented next. If the pattern of reactivity demonstrates reduced titers with either beef or guinea pig cells, the antibody source can be attributed to one of the heterophil antibody types.

Differential Absorption Patterns

Type of heterophil antibody	Yes
Absorbed by guinea pig kidney cells	No
Absorbed by beef erythrocytes	No
Forssman	Yes
infectious mononucleosis	Yes (partially)
Serum sickness	Yes (completely)

Procedure Notes

The Davidsohn differential is performed only if the preliminary Paul-Bunnell test is positive in a titer of 1:56 or above. Serum sickness occurs as the result of sensitization to animal serum, usually horse serum.

Sources of Error

Incorrect pipetting or the use of noninactivated serum can contribute to errors.

Clinical Applications

The Davidsohn differential can distinguish between three types of heterophil antibodies.

Limitations

The test is time consuming.

References

Davidsohn I: Serologic diagnosis of infectious mononucleosis, *JAMA* 108:289, 1937.

 MonoSlide Test

Principle

This procedure is based on agglutination of horse erythrocytes by heterophil antibody present in infectious mononucleosis. Because horse red cells exhibit antigens directed against both Forssman and infectious mononucleosis antibodies, a differential absorption of the patient's serum is necessary to distinguish the specific heterophil antibody from those of the Forssman type. The basic principle of the absorption steps in this procedure is comparable to those originally described by Davidsohn in his sheep agglutinin test. Serum or plasma are absorbed with both guinea pig kidney and beef erythrocyte stroma. Guinea pig kidney contains only the Forssman antigen, and beef erythrocytes contain only the antigen associated with infectious mononucleosis. Guinea pig kidney will absorb only heterophil antibodies of the Forssman type, and beef erythrocytes will absorb only the heterophil antibody of infectious mononucleosis. Agglutination of horse red blood cells by the absorbed patient specimen is indicative of a positive reaction for heterophil antibody.

BBLMonoSlide Test uses a disposable card, guinea pig kidney antigen for absorption, and specially treated horse erythrocytes (color-enhanced) to increase specificity and sensitivity and to enhance readability. No special equipment is required to read the BBLMonoSlide Test.

Specimen Collection and Preparation

No special preparation of the patient is required before specimen collection. The patient must be positively identified when the specimen is collected. The specimen should be labeled at the bedside and include the patient's full name, date the specimen is collected, patient's hospital identification number, and phlebotomist's initials. Blood should be drawn by an aseptic technique. The required specimen is a minimum of 2 mL of whole blood. Serum or plasma mixed with anticoagulants including EDTA, sodium oxalate, potassium oxalate, sodium citrate, acid-citrate-dextrose (ACD) solution, or heparin may be used.

Centrifuge the tube of blood and remove an aliquot of serum. Serum or plasma samples should be clear and particle-free. The presence of hemolysis makes the specimen unsuitable for testing. Inactivation of the serum is not necessary; however, inactivated serum may be used. Before testing, serum or plasma may be stored at 2° to 8° C for several days after collection. If prolonged storage is desired, the serum or plasma may be frozen.

Reagents, Supplies, and Equipment

All of the following required materials are provided in the BBLMonoSlide Test kit:

1. Reagent A: guinea pig antigen. A suspension of guinea pig kidney antigen preserved with 0.1% sodium azide. Store at 2° to 8° C. Do not freeze. If properly stored, the reagent is stable until the expiration date.

2. Reagent B: horse erythrocytes. A suspension of stabilized horse red blood cells preserved with 0.1% sodium azide. Store at 2° to 8° C. Do not freeze. If properly stored, the reagent is stable until the expiration date. Hemolysis will indicate that the cells are deteriorating, but proper reactivity may be verified by use of the positive control serum.

   WARNING: The reagents and controls contain sodium azide as a preservative. Sodium azide may react with lead and copper plumbing to form highly explosive metal azides. On disposal, flush with a large volume of water to prevent azide buildup.

3. Test cards (must be stored flat in the original package in a dry area at room temperature) and test disposables.

Additional Required Equipment

Stopwatch or laboratory timer
Test tubes (13 × 75 mm)
0.85% sodium chloride solution
Transfer pipettes for dilutions
Laboratory equipment used for preparation, storage, and handling of serologic specimens.

Quality Control

Positive control serum (human): a human serum containing the heterophil antibody of infectious mononucleosis, preserved with 0.1% sodium azide.

Negative control serum (human): a human serum not containing the heterophil antibody of infectious mononucleosis, preserved with 0.1% sodium azide. The control sera should be checked when the kit arrives and periodically during the dating period.

CAUTION: Because the control sera are derived from human sources, they should be handled in the same manner as clinical serum specimens (see Universal Blood and Body Fluid Precautions in Chapter 6).

Procedure

NOTE: All of the reagent cells should be shaken well to provide a homogeneous suspension before testing. Reagents should be kept at room temperature.

Qualitative Method

1. Place the slide on a flat surface under a direct light source.
2. Put 1 drop of thoroughly mixed guinea pig antigen (reagent A) in the left side of the test circle on the card.
3. Put 1 drop of thoroughly mixed horse erythrocytes (reagent B) in the circle to the right side of the test circle on the card.
4. Using a disposable plastic pipette, add 1 drop of the patient serum or plasma reagent A on the left side of the test circle.
5. Invert the pipette and use the paddle end to thoroughly mix (10 to 15 circular strokes) reagent A (clear liquid) and sample (patient or control). Gradually mix this solution into reagent B (reddish-brown liquid, covering entire test circle).
6. Rock the card by hand slowly and gently for 1 minute—about 13 to 16 rocks/min.
7. Immediately observe for agglutination.

Reporting Results

Qualitative Method

Positive: a positive infectious mononucleosis reaction will have dark clumps against a blue-green background, distributed uniformly throughout the test circle.

Negative: a negative reaction will have no agglutination but may have fine granularity against a brown/tan background. Peripheral color development associated with fine granularity should be interpreted as negative (e.g., a giant blue-green color halo on the periphery of the test circle should not be interpreted as a positive result).

Procedure Notes

If a positive qualitative result is demonstrated, a titration procedure may be performed to provide a quantitative indication of the level of heterophil antibody.

Titration Procedure for Semiquantitative Method

1. Serial dilutions of serum (see Appendix A) can be prepared by pipetting 0.5 mL of 0.85% saline into each of the desired number of tubes. Pipette 0.5 mL of patient serum into the first tube, mix, and transfer 0.5 mL of the diluted serum to the second tube. Repeat this process until the final tube is reached. Discard 0.5 mL of the diluted serum from the last tube.

Tube	Dilution
1	1:2
2	1:4
3	1:8
4	1:16
5	1:32
6	1:64

2. Place a titration slide on a flat surface under a direct light source. Treat each of the dilutions as if it were individual sera and follow the steps for the qualitative procedure for each of the appropriately labeled circles.
3. The highest dilution in which visible agglutination occurs is the end point. If agglutination is present in all of the dilutions, extend the serial dilutions. Record the titration value.
4. A quantitative result can be approximated by multiplying the reciprocal of the highest dilution in which agglutination occurs (end point) by 28.

Although the titration value is not indicative of the severity of the disease, sequential examinations may provide information of value to the clinician.

Sources of Error

For accurate results, only clear, particle-free serum or plasma specimens should be used.

False-positive results can be caused by:
1. Observing agglutination after the observation time.
2. Misinterpreting agglutination.
3. Simultaneous occurrence of infectious mononucleosis and hepatitis has been reported.

A result interpreted as false-positive may be caused by residual heterophil antibody present after clinical symptoms have subsided.

Clinical Applications

Infectious diseases such as influenza, rubella, and hepatitis may cause clinical symptoms that mimic infectious mononucleosis and present problems in diagnosis. Although the final diagnosis of infectious mononucleosis depends on clinical, hematologic, and serologic findings, a positive test result is indicative of the presence of the heterophil antibody specific for infectious mononucleosis.

Limitations

Diagnosis of infectious mononucleosis should be based on the results of all clinical and laboratory findings. Some segments of the population do not produce detectable heterophil antibody (e.g., approximately 50% of children less than 4 years old, and 10% of adolescents). Detectable levels of heterophile antibody may persist for months, and more rarely for years, in some individuals.

Procedure Notes

Other forms of rapid testing include Wampole Laboratories, Wampole Colorcard Mono and Mono-plus.

References

BD BBLMonoSlide product insert, 2002.

Case Study

History and Physical Examination

A female college freshman reports to the infirmary, complaining of extreme fatigue, frequent headaches, and a sore throat. A routine physical examination by the college physician shows that the patient has swollen lymph nodes (lymphadenopathy), redness of the throat, and a slightly enlarged spleen. A complete blood count (CBC), urinalysis, and mononucleosis screening test are ordered.

Laboratory Data

CBC
> Hemoglobin and microhematocrit: within normal range
> Total leukocyte count: elevated (13.5×10^9/L)
> Leukocyte differential: elevated lymphocytes (56%)
> Many variant forms of lymphocytes (25%)

Urinalysis: normal
Mononucleosis screening test: negative

Follow-Up

The physician prescribes bed rest and medication for the patient's headache. A follow-up appointment is scheduled for 10 days later.

Questions and Discussion

1. What is this patient's absolute lymphocyte count? Is this considered normal?

   The patient's absolute lymphocyte count = 7.83×10^9/L.

   This represents an increase; hence, a lymphocytosis is present. Lymphocytosis associated with infectious mononucleosis results from preferential infection of B cells by EBV. This infection results in a short burst of B-cell proliferation and mobilization, which produces the transient rise in the number of B cells with the variant lymphocyte structure. The altered membrane of the B cells further induces a prolonged proliferation response in T cells.

2. What is the most probable diagnosis of this disorder?

   The age and physical findings in this patient are highly suggestive of infectious mononucleosis. The laboratory findings of an increase in variant lymphocytes further support the suspected diagnosis of mononucleosis. However, the absence of a positive heterophil screening test precludes a definitive diagnosis of infectious mononucleosis.

3. If repeat testing is performed on the patient after 10 days, could any of the results vary?

   The heterophil antibody test usually becomes positive within 3 weeks after the initial symptoms.

4. Discuss the antibodies that could occur in this patient's condition.

   Heterophil antibodies are the antibodies normally encountered in infectious mononucleosis. Rare cases of infectious mononucleosis have been described as heterophil-negative. The clinical manifestations of infectious mononucleosis are present in these patients, but the heterophil test result remains negative for weeks after the onset. An Epstein-Barr antibody test may be helpful in distinguishing these cases from syndromes caused by other agents, such as CMV or toxoplasmosis. Occasionally unusual antibodies occur in cases of infectious mononucleosis. Some of them may produce false-positive results for ANA, rheumatoid factor, and syphilis.

   Anti-i can also be encountered in acquired hemolytic anemia, subsequent to infectious mononucleosis.

   Heterophil antibodies make up a broad class of antibody. They are stimulated by one antigen and react with an entirely unrelated surface antigen present on cells from different mammalian species. Heterophil antibodies may be present in normal individuals in low concentrations (titers), but a titer of 56 or greater is clinically significant in suspected infectious mononucleosis.

   The IgM type of heterophil antibody usually appears during the acute phase of infectious mononucleosis, but the antigen that stimulates its production remains unknown. IgM heterophil antibody is characterized by these features. First, it reacts with horse, ox, and sheep erythrocytes and is absorbed by beef erythrocytes. It is not absorbed by guinea pig kidney cells, however, and it does not react with EBV-specific antigens.

5. What type of antigens could be tested for in the blood?

   EBV-infected B lymphocytes express a variety of "new" antigens encoded by the virus. Infection with EBV results in the expression of VCA, EA, and NA, with corresponding antibody responses. Assays for IgM and IgG antibodies to these EBV antigens are available. EBV-specific serologic studies (see Table 19-1) are beneficial in defining immune status; the time of appearance for IgM and IgG antibodies may be indicative of the stage of disease. This can provide important information for both the diagnosis and management of EBV-associated disease.

Diagnosis

Infectious mononucleosis

CHAPTER HIGHLIGHTS

The EBV was first discovered in 1964 as the cause of infectious mononucleosis. This disorder is usually an acute, benign, and self-limiting lymphoproliferative condition. EBV is also the cause of Burkett's lymphoma (a malignant tumor of the lymphoid tissue occurring mainly in African children), nasopharyngeal carcinoma, and neoplasms of the thymus, parotid gland, and supraglottic larynx.

EBV is widely disseminated. It is estimated that 95% of the world's population is exposed to the virus, which makes it the most ubiquitous virus known to humans. EBV is a human herpes DNA virus. In infectious mononucleosis the virus infects B lymphocytes. Although EBV appears to be transmitted primarily by close contact with infectious oral-pharyngeal secretions, the virus has been reported to be transmitted by blood transfusion and transplacental routes. Under ordinary conditions, transmission of the virus by transfusion or transplacental exposure is unlikely. The frequency of seronegative patients is nearly 100% in early infancy but declines with increasing age, more or less rapidly, depending on socioeconomic conditions, to less than 10% in young adults. After primary exposure, a person is considered to be immune and generally no longer susceptible to overt reinfection. In Western society primary exposure to EBV occurs in two waves among children and adolescents. EBV is only a minor problem for immunocompetent persons, but it can become a major one for immunologically compromised individuals.

The antibodies present in infectious mononucleosis are heterophil and EBV antibodies. Heterophil antibodies male up a broad class of antibodies. They are defined as antibodies that are stimulated by one antigen and react with an entirely unrelated surface antigen present on cells from different mammalian species. The IgM type of heterophil antibody usually appears during the acute phase of infectious mononucleosis, but the antigen that stimulates its production remains unknown. EBV-infected B lymphocytes express a variety of "new" antigens encoded by the virus. Infection with EBV results in the expression of viral capsid antigen (VCA), early antigen (EA), and nuclear antigen (NA), with corresponding antibody responses. Assays for IgM and IgG antibodies to these EBV antigens are available. EBV-specific serologic studies are beneficial in defining immune status, and their time of appearance may be indicative of the stage of disease. This can provide important information for both the diagnosis and management of EBV-associated disease.

REVIEW QUESTIONS

1. The Epstein-Barr virus can cause all the following except:
   A. infectious mononucleosis
   B. Burkitt's lymphoma
   C. nasopharyngeal carcinoma
   D. neoplasms of the bone marrow

2. The primary mode of EBV transmission is:
   A. exposure to blood
   B. exposure to oral-pharyngeal secretions
   C. congenital transmission
   D. fecal contamination of drinking water

3. IgM heterophil antibody is characterized by all the following features except:
   A. reacts with horse, ox, and sheep RBC
   B. absorbed by beef erythrocytes
   C. absorbed by guinea pig kidney cells
   D. does not react with EBV-specific antigens

4. Characteristics of EBV-infected lymphocytes include all the following except:
   A. B type
   B. express viral capsid antigen
   C. express early antigen
   D. express the EBV genome

5. Which of the following stages of infectious mononucleosis infection is characterized by antibody to EBNA?
   A. recent (acute) infection
   B. past infection (convalescent) period
   C. reactivation of latent infection
   D. both B and C

6. Heterophil antibody can be found in patients with:
   A. recent (acute) infection
   B. past infection (convalescent) period
   C. reactivation of latent infection
   D. both A and C

7. It is estimated that _____% of the world's population is exposed to the Epstein-Barr virus (EBV).
   A. 25
   B. 50
   C. 75
   D. 95

8. Infectious mononucleosis postperfusion syndrome is a primary infection resulting from a blood transfusion from a(an) _____ to a(an) _____ recipient.
   A. immune-nonimmune
   B. nonimmune-immune
   C. infected-nonimmune
   D. infected-immune

9. In infectious mononucleosis, there is no _____ state.
   A. acute
   B. latent
   C. carrier
   D. reactivation

10. The incubation period of infectious mononucleosis is _____ days.
    A. 2-4
    B. 10-15
    C. 10-50
    D. 51-90

11. The use of horse erythrocytes in rapid slide tests for infectious mononucleosis increases the _____ of the test.
    A. cost
    B. sensitivity
    C. specificity
    D. availability

12. Epstein-Barr virus-infected B lymphocytes express a variety of "new antigens." These antigens include all of the following except:
    A. viral capsid antigen (VCA)
    B. early antigen (EA)
    C. cytoplasmic antigen (CA)
    D. nuclear antigen (NA)

13. Anti-EBNA IgG does not appear until a patient has entered:
    A. the initial phase of infection
    B. the primary infection phase
    C. the convalescent period
    D. reactivation of the infectious stage

Questions 14-16. Match each procedure to the appropriate description.

14. _____ Paul-Bunnell screening test
15. _____ Davidsohn differential test
16. _____ Monospot

A. distinguishes between heterophil antibodies; uses beef erythrocytes, guinea pig kidney cells, and sheep erythrocytes
B. detects heterophil antibodies and uses horse erythrocytes
C. detects heterophil antibodies and uses sheep erythrocytes

BIBLIOGRAPHY

Akashi K et al: Severe infectious mononucleosis-like syndrome and primary human herpesvirus 6 infection in an adult, *N Engl J Med* 329(3):168-172, 1993.

Andiman W: Use of cloned probes to detect Epstein-Barr viral DNA in tissues of patients with neoplastic and lymphoproliferative diseases, *J Infect Dis* 148:967-977, 1983.

Bush JL, Radich PC: The Epstein-Barr virus receptor, *Lab Med* 20(5):318-322, 1989.

Chretien JH et al: Predictors of the duration of infectious mononucleosis, *South Med J* 70:437-439, 1977.

Cohen JI: Epstein-Barr virus and the immune system, *JAMA* 278(6):510-514, 1997.

Davidsohn I: Serologic diagnosis of infectious mononucleosis, *JAMA* 108:289, 1937.

Evans AS, Niederman JC: Epstein-Barr virus. In Evans AS, editor: *Viral infections of human epidemiology and control,* ed 2, New York, 1982, Plenum Medical.

Fleisher GR: Epstein-Barr virus. In Belshe M, editor: *Textbook of human virology,* Littleton, Mass, 1984, PSG Publishing.

Gallo D, Walen KH, Riggs JL: Improved immunofluorescence antigens for detection of immunoglobulin M antibodies to Epstein-Barr viral capsid antigen and antibodies to Epstein-Barr virus nuclear antigen, *J Clin Microbiol* 15:243-248, 1982.

Geltosky JE et al: Use of a synthetic peptide-based ELISA for the diagnosis of infectious mononucleosis and other diseases, *J Clin Lab Anal* 1:153-162, 1987.

Henle W, Henle G: *Epstein-Barr virus and blood transfusions, Infection, immunity, and blood transfusion,* New York, 1985, Alan R Liss.

Henle W, Henle G: Epstein-Barr virus and infectious mononucleosis. In Glaser R, Gotlieb-Stematksy T, editors: *Human herpesvirus infections: clinical aspects,* New York, 1982, Marcel Dekker.

Henle W, Henle G: Epstein-Barr virus and infectious mononucleosis, *N Engl J Med* 288:263-264, 1973.

Henle W et al: Antibodies to early antigens induced by Epstein-Barr virus in infectious mononucleosis, *J Infect Dis* 124:8-67, 1971.

Horwitz CA et al: Heterophil-negative infectious mononucleosis and mononucleosis-like illnesses: laboratory confirmation in 43 cases, *Am J Med* 63:947-957, 1977.

Horwitz CA et al: Long-term serological follow-up of patients for Epstein-Barr virus after recovery from infectious mononucleosis, *J Infect Dis* 151:1150-1153, 1985.

Lennette ET, Henle W: Epstein-Barr virus infections: clinical and serologic features, *Lab Management* 25:23-28, 1987.

Leyvraz S et al: Association of Epstein-Barr virus with thymic carcinoma, *N Engl J Med* 312:1296-1299, 1985.

Mandell GE, editor: *Principles and practices of infectious disease,* ed 3, New York, 1994, John Wiley & Sons.

Mori JA et al: Monoclonal proliferation of T cells containing Epstein-Barr virus in fatal mononucleosis, *N Engl J Med* 327(1):58, 1992.

Monospot Product Brochures, May 1984, Ortho Diagnostics, Raritan, NJ.

Papadopoulos EB et al: Infusion of donor leukocytes to treat Epstein-Barr virus-associated lymphoproliferative disorders after allogeneic bone marrow transplantation, *N Engl J Med* 330(17):1185-1196, 1994.

Pathmanathan R et al: Clonal proliferation of cells infected with Epstein-Barr virus in preinvasive lesions related to nasopharyngeal carcinoma, *N Engl J Med* 333(11):693-698, 1995.

Paul JR, Bunnell WW: The presence of heterophile antibodies in infectious mononucleosis, *Am J Med Sci* 183:90-104, 1932.

Randhawa PS et al: Expression of Epstein-Barr virus-encoded small RNA (by The EBER-1 gene) in liver specimens from transplant recipients with post-transplantation lymphoproliferative disease, *N Engl J Med* 327(24):1710-1714, 1992.

Ray CG, Hicks MJ, Minnich LL: Viruses, rickettsia, and chlamydia. In Henry JB, editor: *Clinical diagnosis and management by laboratory methods,* ed 18, Philadelphia, 1991, WB Saunders.

Schmitz H: Acute Epstein-Barr virus infections in children, *Med Microbiol Immunol* 158:58-63, 1972.

Smith RS et al: A synthetic peptide for detecting antibodies to Epstein-Barr virus nuclear antigen in sera from patients with infectious mononucleosis, *J Infect Dis* 154:885-889, 1986.

Sumaya CV, Ench Y: Epstein-Barr virus infectious mononucleosis in children. I. Clinical and general laboratory findings, *Pediatrics* 75:1003-1010, 1985.

Sumaya CV, Ench Y: Epstein-Barr virus infectious mononucleosis in children. II. Heterophil antibody and viral-specific responses, *Pediatrics* 75:1011-1019, 1985.

Sumaya CV: Epstein-Barr virus serologic testing: diagnostic indications and interpretations, *Pediatr Infect Dis* 5:337-342, 1986.

Sumaya CV: Infectious mononucleosis and other EBV infections: diagnostic factors, *Lab Management* 24:37-45, 1986.

Sumaya CV: Serological testing for Epstein-Barr virus–development in interpretation, *J Infect Dis* 151:984-987, 1985.

Turgeon ML: *Fundamentals of immunohematology,* ed 2, Baltimore, 1995, Williams & Wilkins.

Turgeon ML: Leukocytes: *Clinical hematology,* ed 3, Philadelphia, 1999, Lippincott Williams & Wilkins.

Zilmans et al: Epstein-Barr virus-associated lymphoma in a patient treated with cyclosporine, *N Engl J Med* 326(20):1362, 1992.

Chapter 20

Viral Hepatitis

LEARNING OBJECTIVES

At the conclusion of this chapter, the reader should be able to:
- Name the various forms of primary infectious hepatitis.

- Compare the etiology, epidemiology, signs and symptoms, laboratory evaluation, and prevention of hepatitis.
- Analyze representative case studies.

GENERAL CHARACTERISTICS OF HEPATITIS

Etiology

Viral hepatitis is the most common liver disease worldwide. Approximately one half of the population of Western society has serologic evidence of prior infection with viral hepatitis. The viral agents of acute hepatitis can be divided into two major groups:
- Primary hepatitis viruses: A, B, C, D, E, and G
- Secondary hepatitis viruses: Epstein-Barr virus (EBV), cytomegalovirus (CMV), herpesvirus, and others

Incidence

Primary hepatitis viruses account for approximately 95% of the cases of hepatitis. These viruses are classified as primary hepatitis viruses because they attack primarily the liver and have little direct effect on other organ systems. The secondary viruses involve the liver secondarily in the course of systemic infection of another body system. The viruses for types A, B, C, D, E, and G, as well as secondary viruses, (e.g., EBV and CMV) have been isolated and identified.

Signs and Symptoms

As a clinical disease hepatitis can occur in acute or chronic forms. The signs and symptoms of hepatitis are extremely variable. It can be mild, transient, and completely asymptomatic, or it can be severe, prolonged, and ultimately fatal. Many fatalities are attributed to hepatocellular carcinoma in which hepatitis B and C are the primary causes. The course of viral hepatitis can take one of four forms (Table 20-1).

TABLE 20-1 Forms of Hepatitis	
Form	**Characteristics**
Acute hepatitis	Typical form with associated jaundice
	Four phases: *incubation, preicteric, icteric,* and *convalescence*
	Incubation period, from the time of exposure and the first day of symptoms, ranges from a few days to many months.
	Average length of time is 75 days (range of 40-180 days) in hepatitis B.
Fulminant acute hepatitis	Rare form of hepatitis associated with hepatic failure.
Subclinical hepatitis without jaundice	Probably accounts for persons with demonstrable antibodies in their serum but no reported history of hepatitis
Chronic hepatitis	Accompanied by hepatic inflammation and necrosis that lasts for at least 6 months
	Occurs in about 10% of patients with HBV

HEPATITIS A VIRUS

Etiology

The hepatitis A virus (HAV) is a small, RNA-containing picornavirus (Figure 20-1) and the only hepatitis virus that has been successfully grown in culture. The structure is a simple nonenveloped virus with a nucleocapsid designated as the hepatitis A antigen (HA Ag). Inside the capsid is a sin-

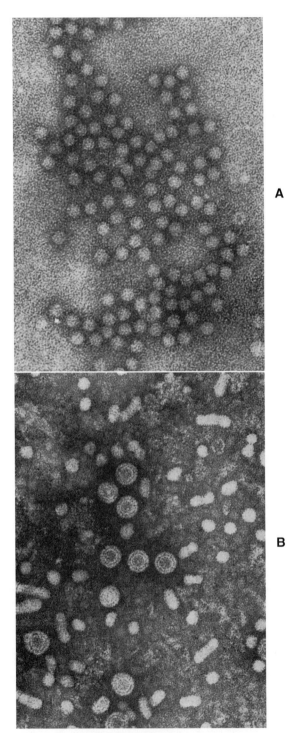

A

B

Figure 20-1   Electron micrographs of type A and type B hepatitis viruses. (From Krugman S et al: *Infectious diseases of children,* ed 9, St Louis, 1992, Mosby.)

gle molecule of single-stranded RNA. The RNA has a positive polarity and that proteins are translated directly from the RNA. Replication of HAV appears to be limited to the cytoplasm of the hepatocyte.

The highest titers of HAV are detected in acute-phase stool samples. Human infectivity of saliva and urine from patients with acute hepatitis A does not pose a significant risk. Sexual contact has been suggested as a possible mode of transmission.

Epidemiology

HAV was formerly called infectious hepatitis or short-incubation hepatitis. In developing countries, hepatitis A is primarily a disease of young children; the prevalence of infection, as measured by the presence of antibody (immunoglobulin G [IgG] anti-HAV), approaches 100% at or shortly after 5 years of age. In the United States, HAV is the cause of 32% of the acute cases of hepatitis. In developed countries, the prevalence of infection is low in all age groups; only minimal increases are seen with increasing age, due in large part to hepatitis A infections acquired by adults during travel to HAV endemic, developing areas.

In intermediate nations, including the United States, the prevalence of HAV is decreasing. The cumulative number of reported cases of HAV in the United States in 2000 was 13,397; in 2001 the cumulative number of reported cases was 10,777. The overall rate of hepatitis A reported during 1999 was the lowest ever recorded. Because hepatitis A rates tend to vary from year to year and from region to region, however, it is important to monitor the incidence to determine if low rates are sustained over time. In the United States about 33% of the population has evidence of past infection with HAV.

Susceptibility to infection is independent of sex and race. Crowded, unsanitary conditions are a definite risk factor. The hepatitis A virus is transmitted almost exclusively by a fecal-oral route during the early phase of acute illness because the virus is shed in feces for up to 4 weeks after becoming infected. Large outbreaks are usually traceable to a common source such as an infected food handler, a contaminated water supply, or the consumption of raw shellfish. Institutions and daycare centers are known to be favorable sources for transmission as well.

HAV infection is noted for occurring in isolated outbreaks or as an epidemic, but it also may occur sporadically. Although HA is very rarely a transfusion-acquired hepatitis because of its transient nature, an outbreak of HAV infection that occurred in 52 patients with hemophilia in Italy was documented to have been acquired through infusion of contaminated factor VIII concentrate. This concentrate had been treated by a virucidal method (solvent-detergent) that ineffectively inactivates nonenveloped viruses.

Improvements in socioeconomic and sanitary conditions and declining family size may be responsible for a declining frequency of infection. The incidence of HAV infection is not increasing among health care workers or in dialysis patients. Maternal-neonatal transmission of HAV is not recognized as an epidemiological entity. Person-to-person contact, usually among children and young adults, remains at the root of HAV infection.

Signs and Symptoms

Nonimmune adult patients infected with HAV can develop clinical symptoms within 2 to 6 weeks after exposure (average about 4 weeks); however, hepatitis A is often a subclinical disease, with many patients being anicteric. In clinically apparent cases, elevated serum liver function test enzymes and bilirubin levels are exhibited, with jaundice developing several days later. Viremia and fecal shedding of virus disappear at the onset of jaundice. Atypical presentations include prolonged intrahepatic cholestasis, a relapsing course, and extrahepatic immune complex deposition, all of which resolve spontaneously.

Complete clinical recovery (Figure 20-2) is anticipated in virtually all patients. Hepatitis A rarely causes fulminant hepatitis, and it does not progress to chronic liver disease. Unusual clinical variants of hepatitis A include cholestatic hepatitis, relapsing hepatitis, and protracted hepatitis. In cholestatic hepatitis, the serum bilirubin may be dramatically elevated (levels may exceed 20 mg/dL), and jaundice persists for many weeks to months before resolution. In relapsing and protracted hepatitis, complete resolution is anticipated. Chronic carrier state (persistent infection) and chronic hepatitis (chronic liver disease) do not occur as long-term sequelae of hepatitis A. Very rarely, injection with HAV may cause fulminant hepatitis, with a fatality rate of about 0.1%. Fulminant hepatitis is the most likely complication that arises from coinfection with other hepatitis viruses.

Immunologic Manifestations

Shortly after the onset of fecal shedding, an IgM antibody is detectable in serum, followed within a few days by the appearance of an IgG antibody. IgM anti-HA is almost always detectable in patients with acute HAV. IgG anti-HAV, a manifestation of immunity, peaks after the acute illness and remains detectable indefinitely, perhaps lifelong.

The finding of IgM anti-HAV in a patient with acute viral hepatitis is highly diagnostic of acute HAV. Demonstration of IgG anti-HAV indicates previous infection. The presence

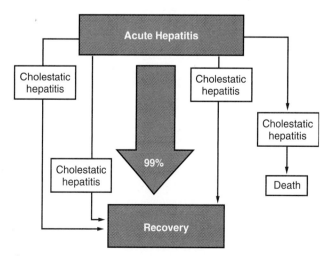

Figure 20-2   Clinical sequelae of hepatitis A. (Redrawn from Gollan JL: Viral hepatitis. In *International Review of Internal Medicine,* Boston, 1995, Brigham and Women's Hospital, Harvard University Medical School, pp 781-792.)

of IgG anti-HAV protects against subsequent infection with HAV, but it is not protective against hepatitis B virus (HBV) or other viruses.

Diagnostic Evaluation

Testing methods for HA include:
- Hepatitis A antibodies (total) enzyme immunoassay (microparticle enzyme immunoassay [EIA])
- Hepatitis A antibody, IgM antibody

The short period of viremia makes detection difficult. Specific IgM antibody usually appears about 4 weeks after infection and may persist for up to 4 months after the onset of clinical symptoms. The presence of IgG or total (IgM and IgG) antibody indicates past infection or immunization and associated immunity. The total assay detects IgM and IgG antibodies but does not differentiate between them. The hepatitis A antibody, IgM assay is appropriate when acute hepatitis A infection is suspected. Specific IgG antibody apparently protects an individual from symptomatic infection, but specific IgM may increase with reinfection. In the acute phase of HAV liver function tests (e.g., alanine aminotransferase [ALT]) will be elevated and may aid in establishing the diagnosis.

Prevention and Treatment

The first effective control measures to prevent enterically transmitted viral hepatitis resulted from research conducted during World War II. In 1945 it was demonstrated that infectious virus could be transmitted by contaminated drinking water, that treatment of the water by filtration and chlorination made it safe to drink, and that gamma globulin derived from convalescent-phase serum from patients with hepatitis could protect adults from clinical hepatitis. For 50 years refinements in the preparation of food and water and the establishment of standards for the preparation and use of immune globulin constituted the methods of prevention of hepatitis A infection. If a person has had close personal contact with a person with hepatitis A, passive immunization with immune globulin should be administered intramuscularly.

A safe, highly immunogenic, formalin-inactivated, single dose vaccine is available (0.6 mL, 25 HAV units) for the prevention of hepatitis A infection (Box 20-1). Larger than standard doses may be required in older or heavier individuals. HAV vaccine should be targeted at high-risk groups (e.g., staff in child care centers, food handlers, international travelers including military personnel, homosexual men, and institutionalized patients).

Universal childhood vaccination may prove to be the most cost-effective method of protecting large populations both nationally and globally. Routine childhood hepatitis A vaccination is recommended in states where the average annual hepatitis A rate from 1987 to 1997 was 20 cases/100,000 population (i.e., twice the national average). Routine childhood vaccination should be considered in states where the average rate from 1987 to 1997 was at least 10 cases/100,000 population, but <20/100,000 population.

In May 2001, the U.S. Food and Drug Administration (FDA) approved a new combination vaccine that protects individuals 18 years of age and older against diseases caused

---

Box 20-1   Hepatitis Vaccine Q&A

HEPATITIS A

1. Who should get hepatitis A vaccine?
   Individuals in any of the following risk groups should receive hepatitis a vaccine:
   - Individuals traveling to or living in areas where hepatitis A is endemic; regions with low rates of infection include the United States and Canada, western Europe, Australia and New Zealand, and Japan
   - Homosexual men who are sexually active
   - IV drug abusers
   - Individuals with chronic liver disease (e.g., hepatitis B or hepatitis C)
   - Children in certain high-risk groups (e.g., daycare centers)

2. At what time before anticipated exposure should the vaccine be administered?
   Hepatitis A vaccine must be given at least 1 month before exposure is expected. Travelers with less than a month before a trip to an endemic area can receive vaccine and immune globulin (injected at separate anatomic sites).

3. How long does a vaccination last?
   It appears that healthy individuals who receive at least two doses of vaccine are protected for at least 5 years and probably much longer (20 years).

4. If you are unvaccinated and experience an unusual exposure, what can be done to prevent transmission?
   Immune globulin 0.02 mL/kg should be given to all close personal contacts including sexual partners and members of the household. Health care workers without unusual exposure to feces or blood do not generally need immune globulin.

HEPATITIS B

1. After hepatitis B vaccination, when should retesting take place?
   Antibody levels to the hepatitis B surface antigen should be checked 2 months after the last dose of vaccine.

2. Do you need to be tested periodically to see if you are still protected?
   Routine testing for antibody to hepatitis B surface antigen is not recommended unless there is a high risk of exposure. When three doses of recombinant HBV vaccine are given to healthy adults, 95% develop effective antibody levels. HBV infection is very rare and almost never symptomatic in persons who previously responded to vaccine.

3. When should a booster dose of HBV vaccine be given?
   For health care workers with normal immune status who have demonstrated an anti-HBs response following vaccination, booster doses of vaccine are not recommended nor is periodic anti-HBs testing.

Source: Modified from Johns Hopkins, Department of Infectious Diseases, 2002.

---

by HAV and HBV. The vaccine, called Twinrix (GlaxoSmithKline Beecham, Philadelphia, PA), combines two already approved vaccines, Havrix (Hepatitis A Vaccine, Inactivated) and Engerix-B (Hepatitis B Vaccine [Recombinant]) so that people at high risk for exposure to both viruses can be immunized against both at the same time. Areas with a high rate of both HAV and HBV include Africa, parts of South

America, and most of the Middle East, and South and Southeast Asia. Clinical trials of Twinrix, given in a 3-dose series at ages 0, 1 month, and 6 months, showed that the combination vaccine was as safe and effective as the already licensed separate HAV and HBV vaccines.

HEPATITIS B

Etiology

HBV is the classic example of a virus acquired through blood transfusion. In part, this observation led to the name "serum hepatitis" by which HBV was previously known. Hepatitis B (see Figure 20-1) serves as a model when transfusion-transmitted viral infections are considered.

The Australia antigen, now called hepatitis B surface antigen (HBsAg), was discovered in 1966. This discovery and its subsequent association with HBV permitted characterization of the biochemical and epidemiologic characterization of HBV infection.

HBV is a complex DNA virus that belongs to a new class called the HepadnaVirus. The intact virus is a double-shelled particle referred to as the Dane particle (Figure 20-3). It has an outer surface structure, HBsAg, and an inner core component, the hepatitis B core antigen (HBcAg). Inside this core is the viral genome, a single molecule of partially double-stranded deoxyribonucleic acid (DNA).

The unique structure of the DNA of HBV is one of the distinguishing characteristics of the HepadnaVirus. The DNA is circular and double stranded, but one of the strands is incomplete, leaving a single-stranded or gap region that accounts for 10% to 50% of the total length of the molecule. The other DNA strand is nicked (the 3' and 5' ends are not joined). The entire DNA molecule is small, and all the genetic information for producing both the surface and core antigens is on the complete strand. In addition to the DNA configuration, the core of the virus also contains an enzyme that is a DNA-dependent DNA polymerase. This polymerase acts to complete the single-stranded region of the DNA. During the disease process, the viral DNA of HBV is actually incorporated into the host's DNA.

Epidemiology

HBV infection was previously called serum hepatitis or long incubation hepatitis. The cumulative number of reported cases of HBV in the United States in 2000 was 8036; in 2001 the cumulative number of reported cases was 6718. Reported cases of acute hepatitis B have decreased >60% in the United States in the past decade; however, the rate of HBV infection among infants and young children is underestimated because most cases are asymptomatic.

In the past, HBV infection was one of the most frequent clinical infections transmitted by blood transfusion. Today the incidence of HBV infection is increasingly rare posttransfusion (estimated 0.3% to 0.9%). The incidence of transfusion-acquired HBV has been severely reduced since high-risk donor groups (e.g., paid donors, prison inmates, military recruits) have been eliminated as major sources of donated blood, and because specific serologic screening procedures have been instituted. This shift to an all-voluntary donor supply

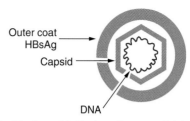

Figure 20-3 The hepatitis B virus (Dane particle). (From Bauer JD: *Clinical laboratory methods,* ed 9, St Louis, 1982, Mosby.)

probably accounts for a 50% to 60% reduction of transfusion-related hepatitis. The overall incidence of HBV, however, is high among patients who have received multiple transfusions or blood components prepared from multiple donor plasma pools, hemodialysis patients, drug addicts, and medical personnel.

Persons at risk of exposure to HBV, including those mentioned previously, include members of the following groups: heterosexual men and women, homosexual men with multiple partners, household contacts and sexual partners of HBV carriers, infants born to HBV-infected mothers, patients and staff in custodial institutions for the developmentally disabled, recipients of certain plasma-derived products (including patients with congenital coagulation defects), health and public safety workers who may be in contact with infected blood, and persons born in areas of high HBV endemicity and their children.

HBV does not seem capable of penetrating through the skin or mucous membranes; therefore some break in these barriers is required for disease transmission. Transmission of HBV occurs via percutaneous or permucosal routes, and infective blood or body fluids can be introduced at birth, through sexual contact, or by contaminated needles. Infection can also occur in settings of continuous close personal contact.

HBV is largely a disease spread by the parenteral route through blood transfusion, needlestick accidents, and contaminated needles, although the virus can be transmitted in the absence of obvious parenteral exposure. About half the patients with acute type B hepatitis have a history of parenteral exposure. Inapparent parenteral exposure involves close intimate or sexual contact with an infectious individual. Transmission between siblings and other household contacts readily occurs through transmission from skin lesions such as eczema or impetigo, sharing of potentially blood-contaminated objects such as toothbrushes and razor blades, and occasionally through bites. HBV has been found in saliva, semen, breast milk, tears, sweat, and other biologic fluids of HBV carriers. Urine and wound exudate are capable of harboring HBV. Stool is not considered to be infectious.

Signs and Symptoms

Infection with hepatitis B virus causes a broad spectrum of liver disease (Figure 20-4), ranging from subclinical infection to acute, self-limited hepatitis and fatal, fulminant hepatitis. Exposure to HBV, particularly when it occurs early in life, may also cause an asymptomatic carrier state that can progress to chronic active hepatitis, cirrhosis of the liver, and eventually hepatocellular carcinoma.

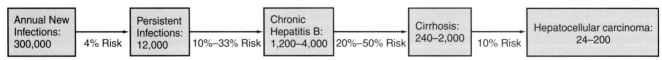

Figure 20-4 Progression to chronic liver disease in hepatitis B infection. (Redrawn from Gollan JL: Viral hepatitis. In *International Review of Internal Medicine,* Boston, 1995, Brigham and Women's Hospital, Harvard University Medical School, pp 781-792.)

TABLE 20-2	Serologic Markers for Hepatitis B Virus (HBV) Infection					
	Early (Asymptomatic)	Acute or Chronic	Low-Level Carrier	Immediate Recovery	Long After Infection	Immunized With HB$_s$AG
HB$_s$AG	+	+	−	−	−	−
Anti-HBs	−	±	−	−	±	+
Anti-HBc	−	+	+	+	±	−
Anti-HBc (IgM)	−	+	−	+	−	−

(Modified from Hoofnagle JH: Type A and type B hepatitis, *Lab Med* 14(11):713, 183.)

A number of factors, for example, the dose of the agent and an individual's immunologic host response ability, influence the clinical course of the infection. Extrahepatic manifestations, reflecting an immune-complex mediate serum sickness-like syndrome, are seen in fewer than 10% of patients with acute hepatitis B. Extrahepatic manifestations include rash, glomerulonephritis, vasculitis, arthritis, and angioneurotic edema. Manifestations such as vasculitis, glomerulonephritis, arthritis, and dermatitis are mediated by circulating immune complex deposition (HBV antigen-antibody) in blood vessels.

HBV infection in the adolescent or adult usually results in complete recovery. In fewer than 1% of patients with acute hepatitis B, fulminant disease develops; this complication is often fatal, but liver transplantation has dramatically increased survival. In about 5% to 10% of individuals with HBV, especially patients with immunodeficiencies (e.g., acquired immunodeficiency syndrome), the disease will progress to a chronic state.

Persistent infection is the usual consequence of HBV infection acquired at an early age. Persistent infection is signaled by the prolonged presence of HBsAg. Some individuals with chronic HBV infection are asymptomatic carriers, whereas others have clinical, laboratory, and/or histologic evidence of chronic hepatitis that may be associated with the development of postnecrotic cirrhosis. Persistent HBV infection is believed to be a precursor of primary hepatocellular carcinoma.

Asymptomatic Infection

The most frequent clinical response to HBV is an asymptomatic or subclinical infection. In patients developing clinical symptoms of transfusion-associated hepatitis B, jaundice, and abnormal serum enzymes, transaminase (ALT/serum glutamate-pyruvate transaminase [SGPT]) levels can be manifested from a few weeks to up to 6 months after a single transfusion episode. However, there is rarely any doubt about the diagnosis in patients with a classic serologic response associated with HBV, even in the absence of significant symptoms. Diagnosis is more difficult in asymptomatic patients with negative HBV serology who develop a mild elevation of serum enzyme (transaminase) levels a few weeks after a transfusion. Elevated enzyme levels may persist for 1 or 2 weeks.

Laboratory Assays of Immunologic Manifestations

Laboratory diagnosis and monitoring of both acute and chronic hepatitis B infections (see following discussion) involve the use of several of the following tests (Table 20-2):

1. HBsAg
2. Hepatitis Be antigen (HBeAg)
3. Hepatitis B core antibody, total or IgM (anti-HBc)
4. Hepatitis Be antibody (anti-HBe)
5. Hepatitis B surface antibody (anti-HBs)
6. Hepatitis B viral DNA by polymerase chain reaction (PCR) (qualitative and quantitative)

These procedures may be performed by enzyme immunoassay, microparticle enzyme immunoassay, PCR, or hybridization/chemiluminescent detection assay.

Hepatitis B Surface Antigen

The initial detectable marker found in serum during the incubation period of HBV infection is HBsAg. HBsAg usually becomes detectable 2 weeks to 2 months before clinical symptoms, and as little as 2 weeks after infection. This marker is usually present for 2 to 3 months. This procedure screens for the presence of the major coat-protein of the virus (HBsAg) in serum and is considered to be the most reliable method of choice for preventing the transmission of HBV via blood. The presence of HBsAg indicates active HBV infection, either acute or chronic.

The titer of HBsAg rises and generally peaks at or shortly after the onset of elevated serum enzymes, for example,

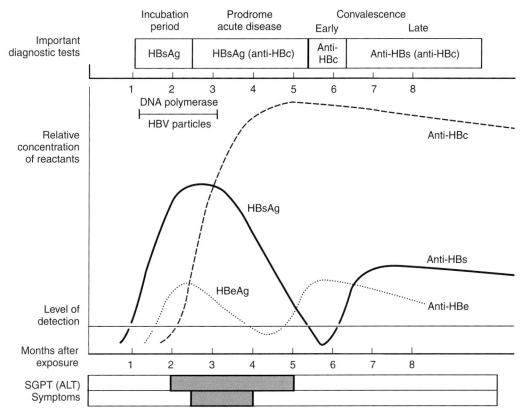

Figure 20-5   Serologic and clinical patterns observed during acute hepatitis B viral infection. (Redrawn from Hollinger FB, Dreesman GR. In Rose RN, Friedman H, editors: *Manual of clinical immunology,* ed 2, Washington, DC, 1980, American Society for Microbiology.)

ALT/SGPT. Clinical improvement of the patient's condition and a decrease in serum enzyme concentrations are paralleled by a fall in the titer of HBsAg, which subsequently disappears. There is, however, variability in the duration of HBsAg positivity and in the relationship between clinical recovery and the disappearance of HBsAg (Figure 20-5). About 5% of positive HBsAgs are false positive.

Among persons infected with HBV with detectable HBsAg in their serum, not all of the HBsAg represents complete Dane particles. HbsAg-positive serum also contains two other viruslike structures, which are incomplete spherical and tubular forms consisting entirely of HBsAg and devoid of any HBcAg, DNA, or DNA polymerase. The incomplete HBsAg particles can be present in serum in extremely high concentrations and form the bulk of the circulating HBsAg.

Test protocols for HBsAg are EIA or microparticle enzyme immunoassay. One of the most popular methods is the Ayszyme II EIA (Enzyme Immuno Assay) procedure.

Hepatitis Be Antigen

A hepatitis B-related antigen, the HBeAg, is found in the serum of some HbsAg-positive patients. HBV DNA and DNA polymerase will appear along with HBeAg. These are all indicative of active viral replication. HBeAg is rarely found in the absence of HBsAg. HBeAg appears to be associated with the HBV core; however, the relationship between HBeAg and the structure of HBV is unclear. HBeAg appears to be a reliable marker for the presence of high levels of virus and a high degree of infectivity.

Hepatitis B Core Antibody

During the course of most HBV infections, HBsAg forms immune complexes with the antibodies produced as part of the recovery process. Because the HBsAg contained in these complexes is usually undetectable, HBsAg disappears from the serum of up to 50% of symptomatic patients. During this phase an indicator of a recent hepatitis B infection is anti-HBc, the antibody to the core antigen. The time between the disappearance of detectable HBsAg and the appearance of detectable antibody to HBsAg (anti-HBs) is called the anticore window or hidden antigen phase of HBV infection. This window phase may last for a few weeks, several months, or a year; during this time anti-HBc may be the only serologic marker. Anti-HBc occurs in 3% to 5% of persons. Of 100 anti-HBc-positive persons, 97 will have anti-HBs, 2 will have HBsAg, and 1 may have only anti-HBc.

Testing for antibody to the core of the virus (anti-HBc) may provide some additional advantage, as it may lead to the identification of a person recently recovered from a HBV infection who may still be infectious. EIA or microparticle immunoassay are the methods of choice.

An Anti-HBc Test is the Corzyme (Abbott Laboratories, Abbott Park, IL) EIA Test. The most recent assay to be developed is the test for IgM antibody to hepatitis B core antigen (anti-HBc IgM). This test is considered a reliable marker during the so-called core window period, diagnostic of acute infection, when most other markers may be absent. The IgM anti-HBc titer rises rapidly in the acute phase and becomes negative in most patients in 3 to 9 months, although it may persist for many years.

Antibodies to HBeAg and HBsAg

Antibodies to HBeAg (anti-HBe) and HBsAg (anti-HBs) develop during convalescence and recovery from HBV infection. The development of anti-HBe in a case of acute hepatitis is the first serologic evidence of the convalescent phase. Antibody to HBsAg (anti-HBs), unlike anti-HBc and anti-HBe, does not arise during the acute disease; it is manifested during convalescence. Anti-HBs is a serologic marker of recovery and immunity. Anti-HBs is probably the major protective antibody in this disease. Thus hepatitis B immune globulin is so named because it contains high levels of anti-HBs.

The first diagnostic antihepatitis B surface (anti-HBs) antigen assay on a random access system has been recently introduced by Ortho-Clinical Diagnostics (Raritan, NJ).

Hepatitis B Viral DNA

The newest tests in the assessment of HBV infections are the qualitative and quantitative measures of HBV DNA by molecular methods (e.g., PCR). In the qualitative assay, a highly conserved region of the surface gene of HBV is detected at a level as low as 1.5×10^4 copies of the viral genome per milliliter. This assay may be of value in confirming HBV infection in patients with questionable results. A less sensitive, quantitative assay that uses an RNA probe is available for monitoring therapeutic responsiveness in chronically infected patients.

Diagnostic Evaluation

Appropriate diagnostic procedures should be ordered depending on clinical factors such as patient history, signs and symptoms being evaluated, or in cases of donated blood. The various components of HBV infection can be measured by laboratory assay (Box 20-2).

Interrelationship of Test Results

If HBsAg is negative and anti-HBc is positive, the anti-HBs will confirm previous HBV infection or immunity. The presence of anti-HBc IgM in the absence of HBsAg in the serum indicates a recent HBV infection. An absence of IgM anti-HBc in the presence of HBsAg and HBeAg suggests high infectivity in chronic HBV disease; the presence of anti-HBe in this situation indicates low infectivity.

A vaccine-type response includes test results negative for anti-HBc and positive for anti-HBs. In evaluation of individuals before vaccination, positive results for both anti-HBc and anti-HBs should be required as proof of immunity, especially if the result for anti-HBs displays a low positive reaction. Because there is a positive relationship between the amount of HBsAg present and a positive reaction for HBeAg, testing for HBeAg is usually not necessary except in pregnant women. In these cases a positive HBsAg during pregnancy results in an 80% to 90% risk of infection in the newborn in the absence of prophylaxis.

Differentiating Acute and Chronic Hepatitis and the Chronic Carrier State

Acute HBV Infection

In an individual who is HBsAg positive, the differential diagnosis should include acute hepatitis B, reactivation of chronic HBV infection, an HBeAg seroconversion to anti-HBe flare, superinfection by other hepatitis viruses, and liver injury resulting from other causes such as drug-induced, alcoholic, or ischemic hepatitis. Accurate diagnosis requires testing for serologic markers and sequential studies.

The first antibody to appear during an acute HBV infection is antibody to hepatitis B core antigen (anti-HBc). Anti-HBc becomes measurable shortly after HBsAg is detected and reaches peak levels within several weeks of the onset of infection. It persists long after the disappearance of HBsAg. Initially the predominant Ig class of anti-HBc is IgM. Early after the development of serologic tests for HBV markers, when tests for anti-HBs were less sensitive than current ones, a "window" period between the loss of HBsAg and the appearance of anti-HBs was recognized. During this infrequently encountered "window," or when levels of HBsAg do not reach detection thresholds, the detection of IgM anti-HBc is the sole marker of acute HBV infection. Over several weeks to months the titer of IgM anti-HBc falls and tends to become undetectable after 6 months. Total anti-HBc reactivity declines at a considerably slower rate; the predominant immunoglobulin form of anti-HBc during the late recovery phase is of the IgG class. This IgG anti-HBc persists in slowly declining titers for many years to decades after acute infection.

Within a few days to a week or two of the appearance of HBsAg, hepatitis Be antigen (HBeAg) also becomes detectable in the circulation of acutely infected individuals. HBeAg, a nonstructural nucleocapsid protein, is a marker of HBV replication; its presence is correlated with the presence of complete HBV particles and HBV DNA in the circulation. In acute HBV infection, patients are most infectious during that period in which HBeAg can be detected. In self-limited HBV infection, HBeAg disappears before HBsAg disappears. With the disappearance of HBeAg, its corresponding antibody, anti-HBe, becomes detectable and persists for a prolonged period.

HBV DNA, and possibly HBV virions, may persist in circulating immune complexes. The viral genome can remain in an active form in peripheral blood mononuclear cells for more than 5 years after complete clinical and serologic recovery from acute viral hepatitis B.

Chronic Infection

HBV leads to chronic infection, and these patients have been shown to have the viral DNA actually incorporated

---

Box 20-2	**Enzyme Immunoassay Measurement of Hepatitis B Virus Serologic Markers**

HBsAg
Total anti-HBs
Total anti-HBc
IgM anti-HBc
HBeAg
Anti-HBe

into the DNA of their liver cells. This integration may be an important factor in the eventual development of liver cell cancer, hepatocellular carcinoma, a well-known long-term outcome of chronic HBV infection. A viral protein called HBX may also have a role in the development of hepatocellular carcinoma.

The hepatitis B virus is not directly cytopathic, and the hepatocellular necrosis that evolves is a result of the host immune response to the viral antigens of the replicating virus present in infected hepatocytes. Cytotoxic T cells recognized both histocompatibility and hepatitis B core antigenic receptors on the liver cell membrane surface. T-cell attachment to the receptors, together with natural killer cells, results in hepatocellular necrosis; in the setting of an effective immune response, HBV replication ceases.

Studies, mainly of peripheral blood mononuclear cells, have revealed that patients with acute HBV produce vigorous T-cell responses against multiple HBV antigenic determinants located on the viral core, envelope, and polymerase proteins, whereas patients with chronic infection have a very weak or undetectable cellular immune response. These findings suggest that a prompt, vigorous, and broad-based cellular immune response results in clearance of the virus from the liver, whereas a qualitatively or quantitatively less efficient or restricted immune response may permit the persistence of virus and the development of ongoing, immunologically mediated liver cell injury. In addition to a patient's immune response, viral factors (the HBV genome) may also be important in determining the course of HBV infection.

Chronic HBV occurs in two phases: a more infectious replicative phase (high levels of circulating virions, HBV DNA, HBeAg) and a minimally infectious nonreplicative phase (few virions, circulating spherical and tubular forms of HBsAg, undetectable HBV DNA and HBeAg, but circulating anti-HBe and integrated HBV DNA in hepatocytes). In patients with chronic HBV infection, HBsAg remains detectable for more than 6 months, and in rare cases HBsAg persists for decades. Spontaneous HBsAg clearance in chronic infection is unusual. Clearance of the virus results in complete clinical and histologic recovery, ultimately leaving the patient with a serologic pattern characterized by hepatitis B core antibody (IgG anti-HBc) and anti-HBs, the latter conferring immunity.

Individuals in whom tests for HBsAg remain positive and who are asymptomatic are labeled HbsAg carriers. Other chronically infected HbsAg-positive individuals may have clinical or laboratory evidence of chronic liver disease. Anti-HBc is present in all chronic HBV infections. In most chronically infected patients, IgM anti-HBc is a minor fraction of total anti-HBc reactivity. In all patients with HBV infection, HBeAg can be detected during the early phase of infection, but in contrast to the situation with acute self-limited HBV infection, HBeAg may remain detectable in chronically infected individuals for many months to years. In these patients, HBV DNA is also readily detected in the circulation. The presence of circulating HBV DNA is highly correlated with the presence of whole virus replication and hence with the potential infectivity of the patient. HBV DNA is also detectable in the hepatocytes of individuals with chronic HBV infection. For a variable but generally prolonged period, this hepatic HBV DNA is present in a free, episomal replicating form. In some patients, HBV DNA becomes integrated into

the genome of the host hepatocyte. Viral replication may diminish spontaneously over time or after treatment, signaled by the decline or disappearance of serum HBV DNA, loss of HBeAg, and the appearance of anti-HBe in the circulation as detected by commercial assays. Research suggests that both anti-HBe and anti-HBs may be present early in chronic hepatitis B complexed to HBeAg and HBsAg. In 10% to 40% of patients with chronic HBV infection, anti-HBs is detected concurrently with HBsAg. Its presence does not signal reduced infectivity or imminent clearance of HBsAg.

Carrier State

It is estimated that there are 400 to 500 million HBV carriers in the world today. In the United States, between 50,000 and 100,000 people acquire HBV infection each year, even though a highly effective vaccine is available. Approximately 5% to 10% of infected patients become long-term carriers of the virus. Immunocompromised patients, including those with human immunodeficiency virus (HIV) infection, are at increased risk for chronic HBV infection.

Age at the time of acquisition of HBV infection is a major determinant of chronicity, as reflected by the development of the HBsAg carrier state. As many as 90% of infected neonates become carriers. The rate falls progressively with increasing age at the time of infection, so that only 1% to 10% of newly infected adults fail to clear HBsAg. Another important risk factor for chronicity is the presence of intrinsic or iatrogenic immunosuppression. Immunosuppressed individuals are at increased risk of becoming carriers after HBV infection. Gender is a determinant of chronicity. Women are more likely than men to clear HBsAg. As a consequence, men predominate in all populations of HBsAg carriers.

The prevalence of the HBsAg carrier state varies widely throughout the globe. In the United States, as in many Western nations, carriers account for approximately 0.2% of the general population. However, among certain groups (e.g., homosexual men and intravenous drug abusers) within the general population, carrier rates 4 to 10 times greater have been identified. Carrier rates as high as 25% have been recognized among Alaskan natives in some Alaskan villages.

Perinatal transmission continues to occur. This rate should be reduced significantly by the implementation of routine screening of all pregnant women for HBsAg followed by vaccination of their newborn. Hepatitis B vaccination is gradually being incorporated into routine infant immunization programs. A multivalent triple antigen-HBV vaccine has been developed that will have wide practical application.

Carriers can be divided into two categories based on differing infectivity, depending on the presence in their serum of another antigen, hepatitis Be antigen (HBeAg), or its antibody (anti-HBe). The types of carrier states include:

- The more commonly identified carriers have anti-HBe in their serum and are at a later stage of infection.
- Anti-HBe carriers are less infectious but may transmit infection through blood transfusion.
- HBsAg positive carriers will become anti-HBe positive carriers at a rate of about 5% to 10% per year.
- All HbsAg-positive individuals must be excluded from giving blood for transfusion.
- About 1 in 4 carriers has HBeAg in their serum. It is likely that these individuals have recently become carriers and that their blood is highly infectious.

Prevention and Treatment

The most important factors in preventing transfusion-acquired HBV are donor interviewing, screening of donor blood, the use of hepatitis-free products when possible, or the appropriate use of blood and blood components. In addition, the avoidance of high-risk blood components such as untreated Factor VIII prepared from multiple donor pools reduces the incidence of HBV.

Elimination of high-risk donors has accounted for at least a 50% reduction in the incidence of hepatitis, and routine testing of donated blood for HBsAg has further reduced the incidence by another 20% to 30%. Testing for anti-HBc will detect almost 100% of HbsAg-positive persons, the rare asymptomatic donor in the core window, and the large number of donors who have had subclinical hepatitis B infections and are now immune.

The use of recombinant vaccine against hepatitis B licensed in 1982 is warranted for high-risk persons, including medical personnel (Box 20-1 and Table 20-3). HBV vaccine is administered in three doses within a span of 7 months. It has been demonstrated to be about 80% to 95% effective. The vaccine is now included in the childhood vaccination schedule. Hepatitis B vaccine is also a vaccine against cancer (hepatocellular carcinoma). Vaccination offers a new approach to preventing transfusion-acquired HBV and the dependent hepatitis D virus (HDV) in patients who are likely to need ongoing transfusion therapy, such as nonimmune patients with hemophilia, sickle cell anemia, or aplastic anemia.

In cases of accidental needlestick exposure or exposure of mucous membranes or open cuts to HbsAg-positive blood, hepatitis B immune globulin (HBIG) should be administered within 24 hours of exposure and again 25 to 30 days later to nonimmunized patients. Infants born to mothers with acute hepatitis B in the third trimester or with HBsAg at the time of delivery should be given HBIG as soon as possible and no later than 24 hours after birth. Persons who are either HBsAg positive or who have anti-HBs need not be given HBIG unless the HBV titer is shown to be low or unknown.

Current FDA-approved drug treatment protocols for HBV consist of administration of Intron A (interferon [IFN]-alpha-2b, Schering-Plough, Kenilwood, NJ), and is an antiretroviral nucleoside analog, LAMIVUDINE (3TC, Epivir, GlaxoSmithKline, Philadelphia, PA). Many other drugs are in preclinical, clinical phase I, or clinical phase II trials. BayHep B (Bayer Corp. U.S., Pittsburgh, PA) and Nabi-Hb (Nabi Corp., Boca Raton, FL) are FDA-approved HBV immunoglobulin therapies. Liver transplantation is also used in some severe cases of liver disease caused by HBV, although the new organ usually becomes infected with HBV.

HEPATITIS D

Etiology

The HDV, initially called the delta agent and then called the hepatitis delta virus, was first described in 1977 as a pathogen that superinfects some patients already infected with HBV. Persons with acute or chronic HBV infection as demonstrated by serum HBsAg can be infected with HDV. HBV is required as a "helper" to initiate infection.

HDV is a replication defective or incomplete RNA virus that is unable by itself to cause infection. HDV consists of a single-stranded, circular RNA coated in HBsAg. HDV is interesting because it can force the host's RNA polymerase to transcribe the virus' RNA genome.

Epidemiology

Hepatitis D was originally described in Italy and appears to be most common in southern European countries. It also appears to be endemic among Indian tribes living in the Amazon basin. In the United States, northern Europe, and Asia, infection is uncommon. In the United States hepatitis D is seen predominantly in IV drug users and their sexual partners, but it has been reported in homosexual men and men with hemophilia. Hepatitis D is a relatively uncommon disease in this country, accounting for approximately 6% of all cases of chronic viral hepatitis. According to the Centers for Disease Control and Prevention (CDC), there are approximately 70,000 people with chronic HDV infection in the United States.

Hepatitis D is a severe and rapidly progressive liver disease for which no therapy has proved effective. Patients with this form of hepatitis are significantly more likely to have cirrhosis and liver failure and to require liver transplantation than are patients with HBV infection alone. Chronic HDV infection is responsible for more than 1000 deaths each year in the United States. The mortality rate can be up to 20% of infected patients.

HDV is spread chiefly by direct contact of HBsAg carriers with HDV/HBV-infected individuals. Family members and intimate contacts of infected individuals are at greatest risk. IV drug abusers and individuals with multiple sex partners are two other high-risk groups. Maternal-neonatal transmission is uncommon.

HDV can be acquired either as a coprimary infection (coinfection) with HBV (e.g., after inoculation with blood or secretions containing both agents), or as a superinfection in persons with established HBV infection (HBsAg carriers or patients with chronic hepatitis B). A superinfection can make an HBV infection worse by transforming a mild infection into a persistent infection 80% of the time. In contrast, coinfection rarely leads to a chronic condition. Although HDV is dependent on HBV for its expression and pathogenicity, replication of HDV appears to be independent of the presence of its associated hepadnavirus.

Signs and Symptoms

Hepatitis D infection may be benign and brief, but fulminant hepatitis and chronic hepatitis are being attributed with increasing frequency to HDV. Chronic HDV infection is associated with increased hepatic damage and a more severe clinical course than is expected from chronic HBV infection alone. The occurrence of sequential attacks of HBV in the same patient is probably attributable in most cases to HDV infection superimposed on a previous acute HBV infection.

Infection with HDV agent can occur in several conditions, and the symptoms would be typical of either acute or chronic hepatitis. These situations are:

- Acute hepatitis D with a concurrent acute hepatitis B (coinfection)

TABLE 20-3 — Hepatitis B Prevention Mandates*

State	Hep B Prenatal Screening Law?	Hep B Childhood Vaccination Law?	Hep B Daycare Law, Year in Effect	Hep B Elementary School Law, Year in Effect	Hep B Middle School Law, Year in Effect
Alabama					
Alaska		Yes	2001	2001	2001
Arizona		Yes	1997	1997	2000
Arkansas	Yes	Yes	2000	2000	2000
California	Yes	Yes	1997	1997	1999
Colorado		Yes	1997	1997	1997
Connecticut		Yes	1995	1996	2000
Delaware		Yes	1999	1999	1999
Dist of Columbia		Yes	1997	1997	1997
Florida	Yes	Yes		1998	1997
Georgia		Yes	1997	1997	
Hawaii	Yes	Yes	1998	1998	7/2002
Idaho		Yes	1995	1995	Children born after 11/22/1991
Illinois	Yes	Yes	1997		1997
Indiana		Yes		1999	
Iowa		Yes		1999	
Kansas	Yes				
Kentucky	Yes	Yes	1998	1998	2001
Louisiana	Yes	Yes	1998	1998	
Maine					
Maryland		Yes	1995	2001	
Massachusetts	Yes	Yes	1992	1996	1999
Michigan	Yes	Yes	1997	2001	1/2003
Minnesota		Yes		2000	2001
Mississippi		Yes		1999	
Missouri	Yes	Yes	1995	1997	1999
Montana	Yes				
Nebraska		Yes		1999	2000
Nevada	Yes	Yes		7/2002	
New Hampshire		Yes	1996	1996	Children born after 1/1/1993
New Jersey		Yes		2001	2001
New Mexico		Yes	2000	9/2002	1999
New York	Yes	Yes	1995	1998	2000
North Carolina	Yes	Yes	1994	1999	2005-2006
North Dakota	Yes	Yes		2000	
Ohio		Yes	1999	1999	
Oklahoma		Yes	1999	1997	1997
Oregon		Yes	1998	1998	2000
Pennsylvania		Yes	1994	1997	2002
Rhode Island		Yes	1998	1999	2000
South Carolina		Yes	1994	1998	1998
South Dakota					
Tennessee	Yes	Yes	1998	1999	7/2002
Texas	Yes	Yes	1998	1998	2000
Utah		Yes		1999	
Vermont		Yes			1999
Virginia	Yes	Yes	1994	1994	2001
Washington		Yes	1997	1997	
West Virginia	Yes				
Wisconsin		Yes	1997	1997	1997
Wyoming		Yes	1999	1999	1998

*An empty box in this table indicates a NO answer.

Source: Immunization Action Coalition, June 10, 2002, website: www.immunize.org.

Effective July 2002, some temporary deviation from the required mandates has been authorized by states experiencing a shortage of vaccine.

- Acute hepatitis D in a chronic HBsAg carrier
- Chronic hepatitis D in a chronic HBsAg carrier

Immunologic Manifestations

HDV probably partially suppresses HBV replication. Hepatitis D infection is diagnosed by the appearance of HDV antigen in serum or by development of IgM or IgG HDV antibodies that appear sequentially in a time frame similar to that described for hepatitis A or B antibodies. The presence of HBsAg will be present as well.

Coinfection with HBV

In patients with acute, self-limited HDV coinfection with HBV, various serologic responses indicative of HDV infection have been identified. Early detection of serum HDV RNA and HDV antigen (HDAg) may be detected, concurrent with the detection of HBsAg. HDAg disappears as HBsAg disappears, and seroconversion to anti-hepatitis D (anti-HD) (initially IgM and later IgG class) follows. The IgM reactivity usually appears several days to a few weeks after the onset of illness, whereas IgG anti-HD appears in the convalescent phase. In about 60% of coinfections, HDAg is not detected by anti-HD; but patients can manifest both IgM and IgG antibodies. IgM anti-HD in self-limited coinfections is usually transient; IgG anti-HD often disappears as well but occasionally persists in declining titer for many months and may remain detectable for as long as 1 to 2 years after the disappearance of HBsAg. In a small number of patients, the early appearance of isolated IgM anti-HD, or appearance during convalescence of isolated IgG anti-HD, may be the only detectable markers of HDV infection.

Superinfection of HBV Carrier

HDV superinfection of HBV (HBsAg) carriers causes the appearance of HDV antigen (HDAg) and HDV RNA, a simultaneous reduction in HBV replication, and a consequent diminution in the titer of circulating HBsAg. Termination of the HBsAg carrier state appears to be an infrequent consequence of HDV inhibition of HBV replication. More often than not, HDV infection becomes chronic, and HDAg and HDV RNA may remain detectable at low levels in the serum; in persistent HDV infection large quantities of HDAg can be detected in hepatocytes. High titers of IgM and IgG anti-HD are maintained in persistent HDV infection, reflecting progressive HDV-induced chronic liver disease.

Diagnostic Evaluation

HDV appears in the circulating blood as a particle with a core of delta antigen and a surface component of HBsAg. A person with hepatitis D will have detectable antigen in the liver and antibody in the serum. Test methodologies for HDV include:
- Total antibody by EIA
- IgM assay by radioimmunoassay (RIA)
- Antigen detection by double immunodiffusion (DIF)
- HDV RNA hybridization
- Reverse transcription PCR

In addition, HDV antigen can be demonstrated in liver biopsies by DIF and immunoperoxidase, and in serum by cloned DNA (cDNA). The importance of detection of anti-

bodies to HDV is largely prognostic. Detection of IgG anti-HDV in the presence of IgM anti-HBc antibody strongly suggests simultaneous infection (coinfection). Detection of IgM anti-HDV in a patient with chronic HBV infection is evidence of HDV superinfection.

Screening for total HDV antibodies in serum is important in the identification of a subpopulation of apparently healthy HBsAg carriers whose risk of serious liver damage is fourfold higher than that of anti-HDV negative carriers. The combined presence of total anti-HDV antibody and abnormal liver function tests in a symptom-free carrier suggests parenchymal damage and is considered an indication for liver biopsy. Hepatic lesions in anti-HDV-positive carriers often consist of chronic active hepatitis or advanced cirrhosis. A positive test result for IgM anti-HDV increases the likelihood of occult active HBV infection.

HEPATITIS C

Etiology

Until recently hepatitis C was referred to as non-A, non-B (NANB) hepatitis, a term introduced in the 1970s. This form of hepatitis was regarded as a diagnosis of exclusion because of the absence of specific serologic markers and unknown viral origin. The hepatitis C virus (HCV) has now been identified and immunologic assays developed for its detection. No homology exists between type A and B hepatitis viruses, or the delta agent, and HCV.

Viral Characteristics

HCV is a small, enveloped, single-stranded RNA virus. Because the virus mutates rapidly, changes in the envelope protein may help it evade the immune system.

There are six known major genotypes and more than 50 subtypes of HCV. The different genotypes have different geographic distributions; genotypes 1a and 1b are the most common genotypes in the United States. But the HCV genotype does not appear to make a difference in terms of the severity of the disease. Knowing the genotype-specific antibodies of HCV is useful to physicians in making recommendations and counseling patients regarding therapy. Patients with genotypes 2 and 3 are more likely to respond to IFN-alpha treatment.

Epidemiology

In the past hepatitis C was considered a disease limited to transfusion recipients. HCV is now recognized in many other epidemiologic settings and as a major cause of chronic hepatitis worldwide. The cumulative number of reported cases of HCV in the United States in 2000 was 3197; in 2001 the cumulative number of reported cases was 3227. However, the number of cases reported to the National Notifiable Disease Surveillance System are considered unreliable because of the lack of a serologic marker for acute infection, and the inability of most health departments to determine if a positive laboratory result for HCV represents acute infection, chronic infection, repeated testing of a person previously reported, or a false-positive result. Almost 3 million Americans are in-

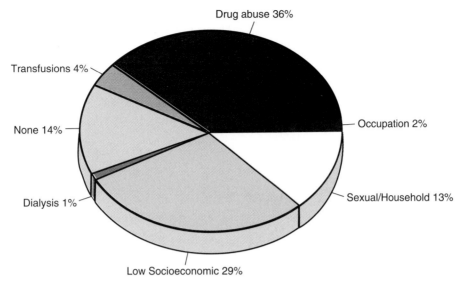

Figure 20-6 Risk factors associated with reported cases of acute hepatitis C, United States, 1990. (Redrawn from Gollan JL: Viral hepatitis. In *International Review of Internal Medicine,* Boston, 1995, Brigham and Women's Hospital, Harvard University Medical School, pp 781-792.)

TABLE 20-4	Characteristics of Viral Hepatitis			
	Type A Travelers	**Type B Hospital Personnel**	**Delta**	**Type C Posttransfusion**
Agent	Hepatitis A RNA	Hepatitis B DNA	Delta agent RNA	Hepatitis C (one agent recently identified) DNA
Antigens	HA Ag	HBsAg, HBcAg, HBeAg	Delta	HCV
Antibodies	Anti-HAV	Anti-HBs, anti-HBc, anti-HBe	Antidelta	Anti-HCV
Epidemiology	Fecal-oral	Parenteral	Parenteral	Parenteral and nonparenteral
Incubation period (in days)	15-45	40-180	30-50	15-150

fected with HCV, and many of them do not even know they have it. In the United States the current mortality figures may triple in the 10 years.

Almost 4 million Americans, or 1.8% of the U.S. population, have tested positive for HCV. Demonstration of antibody to HCV (anti-HCV) indicates ongoing or previous infection with the virus. Hepatitis C is one of the most important causes of chronic liver disease in the United States. The majority of patients infected with HCV develop chronic hepatitis and an estimated 8000 to 10,000 deaths occur in the United States as a result of the disease.

Hepatitis C (Table 20-4) is mainly transmitted parenterally and is associated with the form of hepatitis that develops posttransfusion or as sporadic (community-acquired) hepatitis occurring primarily in developed countries. Hepatitis C is prevalent in the United States and Western Europe and resembles type B hepatitis (HBV) in terms of transmission characteristics.

In the United States parenterally transmitted HCV accounts for 20% to 40% of cases of acute viral hepatitis (Figure 20-6). Most cases (50% to 70%) of acute hepatitis C evolve into chronic hepatitis, and about 20% progress to cirrhosis, which in turn carries an increased risk for hepatocellular carcinoma. An estimated 3.5 million people in the United States have chronic hepatitis C. Each year 8000 to 10,000 chronically infected patients die of liver-related complications, and 1000 undergo liver transplantation (Figure 20-7).

HCV Transmission

HCV is spread primarily by percutaneous contact with infected blood or blood products. Today injectable drug abuse is the most common risk factor for contracting the disease; however, occupational needlestick injuries, infants born to HCV-infected mothers, individuals with multiple sexual partners, and recipients of unscreened donor blood can contribute to contracting HCV.

Although the majority of hepatitis C patients are injectable drug abusers, many patients acquire HCV without any known exposure to blood or drug abuse. Sporadic or community-acquired infections without a known source of infection occurs in about 10% of acute hepatitis C cases and in 30% of chronic hepatitis C cases.

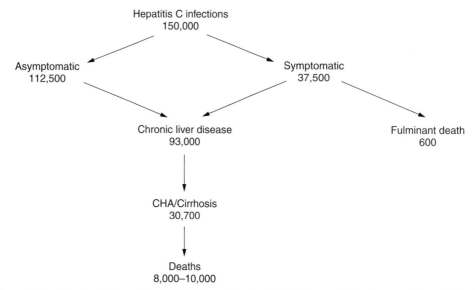

Figure 20-7 Acute and chronic hepatitis C disease burden, United States, 1990 estimates. (From Gollan JL: Viral hepatitis. In *International Review of Internal Medicine,* Boston, 1995, Brigham and Women's Hospital, Harvard University Medical School, pp 781-792.)

Posttransfusion Hepatitis

After the introduction of serologic testing in the screening of blood donors, the rate of posttransfusion hepatitis C decreased from 33% to approximately 15%. Before laboratory screening, the transfusion of infected blood or blood components such as Factors VIII or IX composed a clearly documented route of transmission of HCV. The incidence of posttransfusion hepatitis C declined in the 1980s for two major reasons. Dialysis patients now require fewer blood transfusions because recombinant erythropoietin (EPO) is used to stimulate the patient's own bone marrow to produce red blood cells. The second major reason is the effort to replace the pool of high-risk, paid donors.

Parenteral and Occupational Sources of Exposure

Although hepatitis C is traditionally associated with a history of blood transfusion, parenteral transmission of HCV is more likely to occur from other types of parenteral exposure than transfusions. The most prevalent type of parenteral exposure has been observed in IV drug abusers. A total of 42% of patients identified with hepatitis C had a history of IV drug abuse.

Accidental needlesticks also are a clearly documented route of hepatitis transmission (Figure 20-8). The Occupational Safety and Health Administration estimate that the general risk to health care workers of occupational transmission of HCV is 20 to 40 times higher than the risk of contracting human immunodeficiency virus (HIV). The CDC more conservatively estimates that the average risk of HCV transmission after a needlestick injury is six times greater than HIV transmission. Because of these grim statistics, occupationally acquired HCV infection is a growing concern for health care providers.

A person with a high level of circulating HCV may be capable of transmitting the virus by exposing others percutaneously or mucosally to small amounts of blood or other body fluids. A person with a low level of circulating HCV

Hepatitis C infection after accidental needlestick injury	
Donor source	Hepatitis
• Anti-HCV positive	0-10%
• HBsAg positive	7-30%

Figure 20-8 Hepatitis C infection after accidental needlestick injury. (Redrawn from Hernandez ME, et al: Risk of needlestick injuries in the transmission of hepatitis C in hospital personnel, *J Hepatol* 16:56-58, 1992; Mitsui T et al: Hepatitis C infection in medical personnel after needlestick accident, *J Hepatol* 16:1109-1114, 1992.)

may be capable of transmitting the virus only by exposing others percutaneously to a large volume of blood. The threshold concentration of virus needed to transmit or cause infection is uncertain.

Sexual Transmission

Sexual transmission is believed to occur, but it is infrequent. Spouses of patients with HCV viremia and chronic liver disease have an increased risk of acquiring HCV proportional to the duration of marriage.

Other Sources of Transmission

Mother-to-infant transmission has been documented. HCV is vertically transmitted from mother to infant, and the risk of transmission is correlated with the level of HCV RNA in the mother. Personal contact is thought to be a route of infection, but it has not been conclusively demonstrated, and the actual risk for such transmission is unknown.

Between 25% and 50% of sporadic community-acquired cases of hepatitis in the United States are of the HCV type and are unrelated to parenteral exposure. Some of these cases

Interval from post-transfusion hepatitis to liver disease	
• Liver disease	Years (mean ± SD)
• Chronic hepatitis	10 ±11.3
• Cirrhosis	21.2 ±9.6
• HCC	29 ± 13.2

Figure 20-9 Hepatitis C infection: natural history. (Redrawn from Gollan JL: Viral hepatitis. In *International Review of Internal Medicine,* Boston, 1995, Brigham and Women's Hospital, Harvard University Medical School, pp 781-792.)

are believed to result from heterosexual transmission, but in approximately 40% of cases, the route of infection cannot be identified. Therefore transmission can occur by unapparent as well as apparent parenteral routes, and this form of hepatitis cannot be distinguished from other types of viral hepatitis solely by epidemiologic characteristics.

In addition, liver disease can occur among the recipients of organs from donors with antibodies to HCV. Nearly all the recipients of organs from anti-HCV positive donors become infected with HCV. The current tests for anti-HCV antibodies may underestimate the incidence of transmission and the prevalence of HCV infection among immunosuppressed organ recipients. If the medical condition of the potential recipient is so serious that other options no longer exist, however, the use of an organ from an anti-HCV seropositive donor should be considered.

Prognosis

The natural history and outcome of HCV infection are beginning to be understood (Figure 20-9). Several strains of HCV exist; the genotype of HCV may influence the clinical course of HCV, as well as the response to IFN treatment.

It is believed that about 50% of patients with acute hepatitis C will continue to have elevated serum ALT levels more than 6 months after the onset of illness. These patients usually have persistent HCV RNA detected in their serum, as well as evidence of chronic hepatitis on liver biopsy. Viremia as detected by the HCV RNA assay may persist for months to years in patients in whom serum ALT levels return to normal, and liver biopsy may reveal chronic hepatitis. Chronic hepatitis C appears to be a slowly progressive and often silent disease. In addition, HCV may be associated with hepatocellular carcinoma predominantly, if not exclusively, in the setting of cirrhosis.

Clinical Signs and Symptoms

Although the clinical characteristics of the acute disease of both types of hepatitis C are basically indistinguishable, the chronic consequences are markedly different. The signs and symptoms of hepatitis C are extremely variable. It can be mild, transient, and completely asymptomatic, or it can be severe, prolonged, and ultimately fatal.

The diagnosis of hepatitis C was previously a diagnosis of exclusion. If viral hepatitis was suspected, the other primary causes such as HAV and HBV, secondary causes such as EBV, as well as the other causes of liver inflammation were excluded before hepatitis C was considered.

Hepatitis C more closely resembles HBV than HAV in regard to transmission and clinical features. Hepatitis C, like HBV, can be acute, ranging from mild anicteric illness to fulminant disease. A fulminant course with a rapidly fatal outcome is rare. Most frequently the patient is only mildly symptomatic and nonicteric; less than 25% of patients develop jaundice. Transfusion-associated hepatitis C can be divided into short and long incubation types. Incubation periods for the short duration type range from 1 or 2 to 5 weeks; the longer duration type ranges from 7 to 12 weeks to 6 months or longer.

Hepatitis C is characterized by ALT levels in the 200 to 800 range and marked fluctuations with rapid rises and falls and intervening periods of normalcy. Mean ALT and bilirubin levels of patients with hepatitis C, however, are significantly lower than those of patients with HBV, and the extensive overlap of the ranges of elevation precludes identification of the type of viral hepatitis by the use of these assays.

The diagnosis of hepatitis C has a guarded prognosis. Although hepatitis C was initially thought to be a relatively benign disease, there is increasing evidence of progression to cirrhosis in about 20% of patients, liver failure, and even hepatoma. The hepatic damage is due both to the cytopathic effect of the virus and the inflammatory changes secondary to immune activation. Up to 60% of patients with posttransfusion hepatitis C develop chronic liver disease based on biopsy analysis, and up to 20% of these patients develop cirrhosis.

Posttransfusion hepatitis C affects men and women equally, but it has been documented that 75% of patients developing chronic hepatitis were men. Patients with parenterally acquired (nontransfusion) hepatitis C, including those who have no identifiable source, have the same clinical characteristics and develop chronic liver disease with the same frequency.

Extrahepatic immunologic abnormalities have been shown to occur frequently in patients with chronic HCV infection. HCV infection has been linked with a number of extrahepatic conditions, including Sjögren's syndrome, cryoglobulinemia, urticaria, erythema nodosum, vasculitis, glomerulonephritis, and peripheral neuropathy. HCV now appears to cause those cases of mixed cryoglobulinemia previously considered essential.

Laboratory Testing

Three major types of assays are available for HCV testing:
1. EIA
2. Western blot or RIA
3. PCR amplification

Enzyme Immunoassay

The first-generation of enzyme-linked immunosorbent assay (ELISA) procedures appeared on the market in 1990. This generation contained a single HCV recombinant antigen (c100-3). The procedure was used for testing donated blood to reduce the incidence of posttransfusion NANB hepatitis C. In 1992, a second-generation ELISA was developed that contained recombinant antigens from the virus' nonstructural region (c100-3 and c33c) and an antigen (c22-3) from the core viral protein. This assay was more sensitive than its predecessor and became widely used as a clinical diagnostic method. More recently, a third-generation ELISA that has even greater sensitivity and that contains three recombinant antigens (c22-3, c200, and NS5) has been approved by the FDA for screening donated blood.

Western Blot Assay

Western blot or recombinant immunoblot assay (RIBA) can be used to confirm anti-HCV reactivity. Three successive generations of recombinant immunoblot have evolved since 1990, with each providing incrementally improved specificity. In this procedure, serum is incubated on nitrocellulose strips on which four recombinant viral proteins are blotted. Color changes indicate that antibodies are adhering to the proteins. An immunoblot is considered positive if two or more proteins react. The assay is considered indeterminate if only one positive band is detected.

In some clinical situations, confirmatory testing by immunoblotting is helpful (e.g., a positive anti-HCV detected by EIA but a negative for HCV RNA). The positive EIA anti-HCV reactivity could represent:
- False-positive reaction
- Recovery from hepatitis C
- A viral infection with levels of virus too low to be detected.

If the immunoblot test for anti-HCV is positive, the patient has most likely recovered from hepatitis C and has persistent antibody without virus. If the immunoblot test is negative, the EIA result was probably false positive.

Immunoblot tests are used routinely in blood banks when an anti-HCV-positive sample is found by EIA. Immunoblot assays are highly specific and valuable in verifying anti-HCV reactivity. Indeterminate tests require further follow-up testing, including attempts to confirm the specificity by repeat testing for HCV RNA.

The current third-generation RIBA uses three recombinant antigens (c33c, c100-3, and NS5) and one synthetic peptide from the core region. Because the RIBA is based on the same recombinant antigens and synthetic peptides as the ELISA, it is licensed as an additional, more specific test.

PCR Amplification

PCR amplification can detect low levels of HCV RNA in serum. Testing for HCV RNA is a reliable way of demonstrating that hepatitis C infection is present and is the most specific test for infection. Testing for HCV RNA by PCR is particularly useful when:
- Aminotransferases are normal or only slightly elevated
- Anti-HCV is not present
- Several causes of liver disease are possible

The best confirmatory assay to confirm a diagnosis of hepatitis C is to test for HCV RNA using a PCR assay. In addition, HCV RNA testing is of value when EIA tests for anti-HCV are unreliable (e.g., immunocompromised patients who may not produce a high enough antibody titer for detection with EIA). Immunosuppressed or immunocompetent patients pose diagnostic problems because of their inability to produce anti-HCV. HCV RNA testing may be required for patients who are:
- Immunosuppressed (e.g., recipients of a solid-organ transplant)

- On dialysis because of chronic renal failure
- Taking corticosteroids
- Have agammaglobulinemia

Patients exhibiting anti-HCV who have another form of liver disease (e.g., alcoholism or an autoimmune disorder) can be difficult to diagnose. In these situations the anti-HCV may represent a false-positive reaction, previous HCV infection, or mild hepatitis C occurring concurrently with another hepatic abnormality. In these cases, HCV RNA testing can help to confirm that hepatitis C is contributing to the liver problem.

HCV RNA Titers in Serum

Several methods are available for measuring the titer or level of virus in serum, which is an indirect assessment of viral load. These methods include a quantitative PCR and a branched DNA test. Because these assays are not standardized, different laboratories can provide different results on the same specimen. In addition, serum levels of HCV RNA can vary spontaneously by threefold to tenfold over time. With these limitations in mind, however, carefully performed quantitative assays provide important insights into the nature of hepatitis C.

The utility of determining the viral load does not correlate with the severity of the hepatitis or with a poor prognosis, but viral load does correlate with the likelihood of a response to antiviral therapy. Monitoring viral load during the early phases of treatment may provide early information on the likelihood of a response Rates of response to a course of IFN-alpha and ribavirin are higher in patients with low levels of HCV RNA. The usual definition of a low level of HCV RNA is below 2 million copies per milliliter.

A new procedure for HCV was introduced in 2001 by Quest Diagnostics, Inc, Teterboro, NJ. This assay, HEPTI-MAX, is an ultrasensitive hepatitis C quantitative test that detects levels of HCV based on an innovative application of transcription-mediated amplification technology. Because this technology can detect minute quantities of HCV, physicians can monitor HCV infection better, demonstrate posttreatment resolution, and detect relapses with greater sensitivity.

Surrogate Testing

In the past the absence of a specific HCV serologic marker was compensated for by the use of surrogate testing. Blood donor screening was instituted to eliminate those donors who might transmit hepatitis C. Surrogate procedures consisted of the transaminase enzyme, ALT or SGPT, and anti-HBc tests.

Acute Hepatitis C

The signs and symptoms of acute hepatitis C infection usually include jaundice, fatigue, and nausea. Laboratory manifestations include a significant increase in ALT (usually greater than 10-fold elevation), and presence of anti-HCV or de novo development of anti-HCV.

Demonstration of HCV antibodies can be problematic because anti-HCV is not always present when the patient presents to the physician with symptoms. In 30% to 40% of patients, anti-HCV is not detected until 2 to 8 weeks after onset of symptoms. Acute hepatitis C can also be diagnosed by testing for HCV RNA. HCV RNA appears to be the earliest detectable marker of acute HCV infection, preceding the appearance of anti-HCV by several weeks. The current generation ELISA for antibodies to recombinant HCV antigens becomes positive earlier and is more sensitive than preceding generation assays. Another approach is to repeat the anti-HCV testing 1 month after onset of illness.

HCV viremia may persist despite the normalization of serum ALT levels. Intracytoplasmic HCV antigen has been found in the hepatocytes of acutely infected chimpanzees, and by analogy is presumed to be present in acute hepatitis C in human beings. HCV antigens were not detected in hepatocyte nuclei, in Kupffer or sinusoidal lining cells, in bile duct epithelium, or in blood vessels.

Chronic Hepatitis C

Chronic hepatitis C varies greatly in its course and outcome. At one end of the spectrum are asymptomatic patients who generally have a favorable prognosis; at the other end of the spectrum are patients with severe hepatitis C who have symptoms, HCV RNA present in their serum, and elevated serum liver. These patients typically develop cirrhosis and end-stage liver disease.

Episodic fluctuations in the serum levels of ALT appear to be a feature of chronic hepatitis C. This pattern, presumably reflecting waves of hepatocellular inflammation and necrosis, may last for months to years. Such episodes of disease activity may be related to the emergence of HCV neutralization escape mutants, but other ill-defined mechanisms also may play a role. HCV RNA is detected in the serum by PCR in virtually all patients with chronic hepatitis C. HCV replication may be increased in advanced liver disease and may play a role in the progression of disease.

At least 20% of patients with chronic hepatitis C develop cirrhosis, a process that takes 10 to 20 years. After 20 to 40 years, a smaller percentage of patients with chronic disease develop liver cancer. Liver failure from chronic hepatitis C is one of the most common reasons for liver transplants in the United States.

Chronic hepatitis C is diagnosed when anti-HCV is present and serum aminotransferase levels remain elevated for more than 6 months. Testing for HCV RNA by PCR confirms the diagnosis and documents that viremia is present. Most patients with chronic infection will have the viral genome detectable in serum by PCR.

Approximately one third of those infected with HCV manifest anti-HCV antibodies within several weeks; others may take months or, less commonly, some individuals may take as long as a year to express antibodies. The current test antigen represents only 12% of the encoding capacity of the virus. Although they are good markers for chronic viremia, present assays are not comprehensive enough to detect all stages of infection. Therefore a reactive test implies infection with HCV but not infectivity or immunity.

Treatment and Prevention

Treatment

The main goal of treatment of chronic hepatitis C is to eliminate detectable viral RNA from the blood. Lack of detectable hepatitis C virus RNA from blood 6 months after completing therapy is known as a sustained response and has a very favorable prognosis that may be equivalent to a cure. There may be other more subtle benefits of treatment, such as slowing the progression of fibrosis in patients who do not achieve a sustained response.

All current treatment protocols for hepatitis C are based on the use of various preparations of IFN-alpha, a naturally occurring glycoprotein that is secreted by cells in response to viral infections. It exerts its effects by binding to a membrane receptor which initiates a series of intracellular signaling events that ultimately leads to enhanced expression of certain genes. This leads to enhancement and induction of certain cellular activities including augmentation of target cell killing by lymphocytes and inhibition of virus replication in infected cells.

IFN-alpha-2a (Roferon-A; Hoffmann-La Roche, Basel, Switzerland), IFN-alpha-2b (Intron-A; Schering-Plough, Kenilworth, NJ) and IFN-alfacon-1 (Infergen; Intermune) are all approved in the United States for the treatment of adults with chronic hepatitis C as single agents. Treatment is administered for 6 months to 2 years. Treatment with IFN alone leads to a sustained response in less than 15% of subjects. Because of this low response rate, these IFNs alone are rarely used for the treatment of patients with chronic hepatitis C.

More recently peginterferon alpha, sometimes called pegylated IFN, has been available for the treatment of chronic hepatitis C. There are two preparations of peginterferon alpha: peginterferon alpha-2b (Peg-Intron; Schering-Plough) and peginterferon alpha-2a (Pegasys; Hoffmann-La Roche). With peginterferon alpha-2a alone, approximately 30% to 40% of patients achieve a sustained response to treatment for 24 to 48 weeks. The addition of ribavirin to IFN-alpha is superior to IFN-alpha alone in the treatment of chronic hepatitis C.

Ribavirin is a synthetic nucleoside that has activity against a broad spectrum of viruses. The FDA did not approve ribavirin alone for hepatitis C, but the FDA did approve IFN-alpha-2b plus ribavirin (1998) for the treatment of individuals with chronic hepatitis C who "relapsed" after previous IFN-alpha therapy. "Relapsers" were defined as patients who had normal serum ALT activities at the end of up to 18 months IFN-alpha therapy with abnormal ALT activities within 1 year after the end of the most recent course of therapy. Most recently, the FDA has approved the combination of peginterferon alpha plus ribavirin for the treatment of chronic hepatitis C. For eligible patients with chronic hepatitis C, a peginterferon alpha plus ribavirin is likely to be the best treatment option. Clinical trials have shown that the sustained response rate is approximately 50% of patients given this combination for 24 to 48 weeks.

Most studies indicate that genotypes 1a and 1b are more resistant to treatment with any IFN-alpha-based therapy than non-type-1 genotypes. For this reason, some doctors may prescribe longer durations of treatment for patients infected with viral genotypes 1a or 1b. The best available current treatment for chronic hepatitis C of peginterferon alpha plus ribavirin leads to an overall sustained response rate in more than 50% of all patients. The sustained response rates are even better for individuals infected with non-type-1 genotypes of the hepatitis C virus.

Several drugs known as "immune modifiers" or "immunomodulators" that alter the immune response are being tested in clinical trials for chronic hepatitis C. Some are being studied along with IFN-alpha. These drugs alter the inflammatory response against liver cells infected with the virus; however, their mechanisms of action are poorly understood. Compounds of this type that are currently being tested in humans include thymosin-alpha-1 (Zadaxin, Sci-Clone Pharmaceuticals, San Mateo, CA) and histamine dihydrochloride (Ceplene, Maxim Pharmaceuticals, San Diego).

New medications and approaches to treatment are needed. Most promising for the immediate future are newer forms of long-acting IFNs. In addition, molecular approaches to treating hepatitis C are promising. Molecular therapies consist of using ribozymes, enzymes that break down specific viral RNA molecules, and antisense oligonucleotides, small complementary segments of DNA that bind to viral RNA and inhibit viral replication.

Therapeutic vaccines are also being developed to enhance the immune response against the HCV. In contrast to a preventive vaccine, which is likely to be a very long way off for hepatitis C, a therapeutic vaccine is administered to already infected individuals to stimulate the immune system to fight the infection. Several therapeutic vaccines are in preclinical development for hepatitis C. The most promising of these are DNA vaccines involving injection of DNA copies of the HCV RNA genome, which are taken up by certain immune system cells. These cells theoretically then express viral proteins, stimulating an immune response against the virus.

Who Should or Should Not Be Treated?

Patients with anti-HCV, HCV RNA, elevated serum ALT levels, and evidence of chronic hepatitis on liver biopsy, and with no contraindications, should be offered therapy with a combination of IFN-alpha and ribavirin. The National Institutes of Health Consensus Development Conference Panel recommended that therapy for hepatitis C be limited to those patients who have histologic evidence of progressive disease without signs of decompensation. Their present recommendation is that all patients with fibrosis or moderate to severe degrees of inflammation and necrosis on liver biopsy be treated and that patients with less severe histologic disease be managed on an individual basis. Patient selection should not be based on the presence or absence of symptoms, the mode of acquisition, the genotype of HCV RNA, or serum HCV RNA levels.

IFN and combination therapy have not been shown to improve survival or the ultimate outcome in patients with preexisting cirrhosis. The benefit of treatment in patients over 60 years old has not been well documented. The role of IFN therapy in children with hepatitis C remains uncertain.

Prevention

Preventive practices among health care workers to avoid needlestick injuries should be exercised. Recent investigations have shown that removal of blood from donors with anti-HBcAg from the blood supply and the use of third-generation anti-HCV testing have reduced the incidence of posttransfusion hepatitis C.

Vaccines and Ig products do not exist for prevention or treatment of hepatitis C. Development of preventive strategies appears unlikely in the near future because these products would require antibodies to all the genotypes and variants of hepatitis C; however, some type of vaccine may eventually be developed.

HEPATITIS E

Etiology

The precise classification of this RNA-containing hepatitis E (HEV) virus remains uncertain.

Epidemiology

Only a few cases have been reported, and none have originated in the United States. All have been seen in travelers returning from the Indian subcontinent, northern Africa, the Far East, portions of the Newly Independent States (the former Soviet Union), and Mexico.

HEV is transmitted by the fecal-oral route. Infection is usually the result of poor sanitation conditions. HEV is responsible for large water-borne outbreaks of hepatitis in the developing world and is the most common cause of sporadic hepatitis in young adults in developing nations. Clinically apparent disease frequently is found in patients between 15 and 40 years old.

The HEV infection rate among household contacts of infected patients appears to be low. The seroprevalence of HEV in blood donors is approximately 2%.

Viruslike particles have been observed in the stool from patients with HEV infection. In addition, serologic tests (IgM and IgG anti-HEV) have been developed now that the HEV genome has been cloned and sequenced.

Signs and Symptoms

The incubation period of hepatitis E ranges from 2 to 9 weeks, with an average of 6 weeks. The symptoms of HEV infection are similar to those of other forms of viral hepatitis. HEV particles may appear in feces, inconstantly, during prodromal symptoms of hepatitis E. Fecal HEV shedding occurs predominantly during the first week after the onset of jaundice and has not been identified in stool samples obtained 8 to 15 days after the onset of jaundice. Viremia may occur during the period of fecal HEV shedding.

No form of chronic liver disease has been attributable to infection by HEV. Although most acute infections are self-limited and mild, in pregnant women about 10% to 20% of HEV infections result in fulminant hepatitis, especially in the third trimester of pregnancy.

Immunologic Manifestations

A short-lived IgM anti-HEV has been found in acute-phase sera. IgG anti-HEV appears and replaces IgM anti-HEV about 2 to 4 weeks after symptoms subside. The duration of detectable IgG anti-HEV remains uncertain.

Diagnostic Evaluation

Specific serologic tests for IgM and IgG anti-HEV are available. HEV can be diagnosed by performing immunoelectron microscopy on a stool specimen. Serum ALT and aspartate aminotransferase assay levels, if elevated, are indicative of the acute phase of the infection.

Prevention and Treatment

Standard gamma globulin preparations have not been shown to be effective in the prevention of viral E hepatitis. No effective vaccine has been developed. Treatment of HEV is usually supportive care.

HEPATITIS G

Etiology

Hepatitis G virus (HGV) is an RNA virus. HGV is similar to the previously identified GB-C virus and distantly related to the hepatitis C (HCV), GB-B, and GB-A viruses. In 1995 and 1996, two independent groups discovered and sequenced an agent with limited homology to HCV. These agents were named GBV-C/HGV, respectively. They have 96% amino acid identity and represent variants of HGV.

Epidemiology

HGV is a blood-borne agent. Transfusion recipients and IV drug abusers are at risk of infection. The virus frequently occurs as a coinfection with HCV. Prevalence patterns of GBV-C/ HGV suggest that the virus is transmitted sexually.

HGV infection is common (1% to 2% of U.S. blood donors have HGV RNA detectable in their serum). It is estimated to produce 900 to 2000 infections per year, most of which may be asymptomatic. Chronic infection develops in 90% to 100% of infected persons. Chronic disease is rare or may not occur at all.

Signs and Symptoms

Chronic HGV infection does not appear to commonly cause important liver disease and does not alter the course of chronic HCV infection. The vast majority of cases of acute non-A-E hepatitis have no evidence of HGV infection. The role of HGV (also known as GB-C) in human hepatitis remains unclear.

HGV may not be a significant cause of acute or chronic liver disease. In all, 15% of children with chronic hepatitis C or hepatitis B are infected with HGV. In these cases, HGV coinfection does not appear to cause more severe liver disease.

HGV has not been proven to cause fulminant hepatitis. In fact, recent studies suggest that the virus may not even replicate in the liver. The role of HGV in acute and chronic hepatitis remains to be fully defined.

Diagnostic Evaluation

A cDNA expression library was constructed from the plasma of a patient with chronic hepatitis C. Immunoscreening of the expression library with the patient's serum identified several HCV sequences and several other sequences that were unique. From these unique sequences, an anchored PCR method was used to amplify overlapping clones for the entire viral genome. The virus was termed the hepatitis G virus.

Prevention

Confirmation of disease association, establishment of routes of transmission, and the development of serologic screening assays are necessary before prevention measures can be considered.

TRANFUSION-TRANSMITTED VIRUS

Etiology

The newest member of the infectious hepatitis family is the transfusion-transmitted virus (TTV). TTV is an unenveloped, single-stranded DNA virus with 3739 nucleotides. Two genetic groups have been identified, differing by 30% in nucleotide sequences. This virus was discovered in 1997 through the use of cloning and DNA sequence analysis by a group of Japanese scientists. This novel, single-stranded linear DNA virus has been designated TT-virus or TTV after the initials of the first patient (TT) from whom the virus was isolated.

The most remarkable feature of TTV is the extraordinarily high prevalence of chronic viremia in apparently healthy people, up to nearly 100% in some countries.

Epidemiology

The virus has been associated with posttransfusion hepatitis of unknown etiology (non-A-G). The prevalence in the global population, particularly the United States, United Kingdom, Japan, Germany, and Thailand can reach 100% in healthy people.

There is evidence that TTV may be transmitted not only by parenteral exposure to blood, but by a fecal-oral route and transmitted from mother to child.

Signs and Symptoms

Although TTV is similar to HGV, it may be an example of a human virus with no clear disease association. This hypothesis is supported by the fact that the high prevalence of active TTV infection in the general population, both in the United Kingdom and in Japan, is not comparable to the rate of significant liver damage.

As with HGV, the pathogenicity of TTV has not been proven.

Case Study

History and Physical Examination

Several workers at a local fast-food restaurant call in sick and report to the local ambulatory clinic for treatment. All of them complain of extreme fatigue. In addition, another 26-year-old food handler, who returned from visiting his relatives in Costa Rica a month ago, is sick. Within the last week or two he has had no energy and just doesn't feel well. When he recently visited a physician at a local ambulatory clinic, he was slightly jaundiced.

Laboratory Data

The results of the 26-year-old food handler's tests were:
   Complete blood count: normal
   Serum bilirubin: slightly elevated

Questions and Discussion

1. What types of additional laboratory tests could be of value in determining the 26-year-old's source of illness?
   Because of this patient's recent travel history, hepatitis A should be considered as the possible cause of the jaundice and abnormal bilirubin. Hepatitis A infections can be acquired by adults during travel to endemic, developing areas. A viral stool culture could be of value. If this patient is suffering from hepatitis A, the highest titers of HAV are detected in acute phase stool samples. Serologic tests may also be of value.

2. What are the immunologic manifestations?
   Shortly after the onset of fecal shedding, an IgM antibody is detectable in serum followed within a few days by the appearance of an IgG antibody. IgM anti-HA is almost always detectable in patients with acute HAV. IgG anti-HA peaks after the acute illness and remains detectable indefinitely, perhaps lifelong. The finding of IgM anti-HA in a patient with acute viral hepatitis is highly diagnostic of acute HAV. Demonstration of IgG anti-HA indicates previous infection. The presence of IgG anti-HA protects against subsequent infection with HAV, but it is not protective against HBV or other viruses.

3. What is the prognosis in this disease?
   Complete clinical recovery is anticipated in virtually all patients; however, rare instances of fulminant and even fatal disease have been documented. Unusual clinical variants of hepatitis A include cholestatic hepatitis, relapsing hepatitis, and protracted hepatitis. In cholestatic hepatitis, the serum bilirubin may be dramatically elevated (>20 mg/dL), and jaundice persists for many weeks to months before resolution. In relapsing and protracted hepatitis, complete resolution is anticipated. A chronic carrier state (persistent infection) and chronic hepatitis (chronic liver disease) do not occur as long-term sequelae of hep-atitis A.

4. What are the methods of prevention and prophylaxis?
   Careful hand washing when preparing food is essential. In addition, after close personal contact with a person with hepatitis A, unvaccinated individuals should receive immune globulin intramuscularly. Unvaccinated persons who travel to or remain in an endemic area for more than 3 months should receive immune globulin injections every 5 months. The availability of a hepatitis A vaccine should be taken advantage of by persons who are at risk of contracting the disease.

5. Because of this patient's occupation, could particular infectious diseases be of concern?
   HAV is transmitted by a fecal-oral route during the early phase of acute illness. Large outbreaks are usually traceable to a common source such as an infected food handler or contaminated water supply.

HAV is noted for occurring in isolated outbreaks or as an epidemic, but it also may occur sporadically.

Diagnosis

Hepatitis A infection

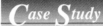

History and Physical Examination

This 30-year-old phlebotomist presented with fever, persistent fatigue, and joint pain. She reports that a needle in a plastic garbage bag nicked her finger about 2 months ago. Her physical examination is within normal limits.

Laboratory Data

Her laboratory data, however, revealed an elevated serum enzyme (ALT) level and an elevated total bilirubin. Additional laboratory data included a positive HBsAg and a positive IgM anti-HBc. Her IgM anti-HAV and anti-HCV tests were negative.

Questions and Discussion

1. Does this patient suffer from a form of infectious hepatitis? If yes, what type?
   Yes, the patient's history and laboratory results support a working diagnosis of infectious hepatitis, probably type B.

2. Can any further tests be done to confirm the diagnosis?
   Additional tests can include HBeAg testing.

3. What is the patient's prognosis?
   Treatment with IFN-alpha is effective in about 50% of patients with HBV. However, this patient could become a carrier of HBV and could eventually develop hepatocellular carcinoma.

Diagnosis

Hepatitis B infection

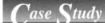

History and Physical Examination

This 75-year-old Caucasian woman had an 18-month history of right-side abdominal pain and progressive fatigue. Her other medical problems include insulin-dependent diabetes mellitus and hypertension.
   She reported no history of blood transfusion, IV drug abuse, or excessive alcohol use. She has no family history of liver disease. Her physical examination showed no cutaneous stigmata of chronic liver disease, hepatosplenomegaly, or ascites. Her daily medications include Humulin U-100 insulin and a medication for her high blood pressure.

Laboratory Data

Her abnormal laboratory values included elevated liver serum enzymes (ALT) and total bilirubin. She also exhibited hypergammaglobulinemia. Other relevant findings include a negative HBsAg, positive anti-HCV antibody (by recombinant immunoblot assay), and positive HCV RNA (by PCR technique).

Questions and Discussion

1. Does this patient suffer from a form of infectious hepatitis? If yes, what type?

   This patient demonstrates the clinical and laboratory findings that support a diagnosis of hepatitis C.

2. Can any further tests be done to confirm the diagnosis?

   Radiologic studies including abdominal ultrasound, CT scan, and an upper gastrointestinal series were performed. The results of all of these tests were unremarkable. In addition, a liver biopsy specimen showed features of moderately severe chronic hepatitis.

3. What is the patient's prognosis?

   The patient was treated with steroids (prednisone) and azathioprine. She responded clinically and biochemically. Her liver enzymes returned to normal 8 months after therapy began. A liver biopsy specimen obtained 3 years after treatment showed marked improvement. In addition, her hypergammaglobulinemia resolved. However, the patient remains positive for HCV RNA.

Case Study

History and Physical Examination

A 45-year-old previously healthy medical technologist visited her primary care physician because of increasing fatigue and loss of appetite. She has had a monogamous sexual relationship with her husband for 25 years.

Laboratory Data

After an initial workup for chronic fatigue, including a risk factor history that revealed several needlesticks on the job, she was found to be anti-HCV positive by both EIA and RIBA, and to have an abnormal liver function profile.

Questions and Discussion

1. What is the probable source of the HCV infection?

   The CDC cited that HCV infection is a rapidly growing concern among health care providers. CDC estimates that the average risk of HCV transmission to a health care worker after a needlestick is 1.8% or six times greater than HIV transmission.

2. What steps should be taken after exposure?

   HCV prevention and postexposure evaluation are not set in stone. Testing for HCV in the source patient depends on cost and how quickly an exposed worker wants to know his or her status. At least 15% of people with HCV do not have the virus circulating in their bodies. PCR in addition to an anti-HCV test would tell if the patient has circulating antibodies. If the PCR is negative, the risk of transmission in a worker would be virtually nonexistent.

   Follow-up strategies include counseling. Many health care providers discourage pregnancy or breastfeeding.

3. What behavioral changes are necessary now that the patient knows that she suffers from HCV infection?

   Condoms may be suggested, although the risk of sexually transmitted HCV is low. In addition, only a few cases of provider-to-patient transmission of HCV have been noted.

Diagnosis

Hepatitis C infection

CHAPTER HIGHLIGHTS

Viral hepatitis is the most common liver disease worldwide. Approximately one half of the population of Western society has serologic evidence of prior infection with viral hepatitis. Viral agents of acute hepatitis can be divided into primary hepatitis viruses: A, B, C, D, E, and G, as well as secondary hepatitis viruses including Epstein-Barr virus, CMV, herpesvirus, and others.

Primary hepatitis viruses account for approximately 95% of the cases of hepatitis. As a clinical disease hepatitis can occur in acute or chronic forms. The signs and symptoms of hepatitis are extremely variable. It can be mild, transient, and completely asymptomatic, or it can be severe, prolonged, and ultimately fatal. Many fatalities are attributed to hepatocellular carcinoma in which hepatitis B and C are the primary causes.

The HAV was formerly called infectious hepatitis or short-incubation hepatitis. In developing countries, hepatitis A is primarily a disease of young children; the prevalence of infection, as measured by the presence of antibody (IgG anti-HAV), approaches 100% at or shortly after 5 years of age. In the United States, HAV is the cause of 32% of the acute cases of hepatitis. The hepatitis A virus is transmitted almost exclusively by a fecal-oral route during the early phase of acute illness because the virus is shed in feces for up to 4 weeks after infection occurs. The incidence of HAV is not increased among health care workers or in dialysis patients. Maternal-neonatal transmission of HAV is not recognized as an epidemiologic entity. Person-to-person contact, usually among children and young adults, remains at the root of HAV infection. A safe, highly immunogenic, formalin-inactivated, single dose vaccine is available (0.6 mL, 25 HAV units) for the prevention of hepatitis A infection.

HBV is the classic example of a virus acquired through blood transfusion. HBV infection was previously called serum hepatitis or long incubation hepatitis. Reported cases of acute hepatitis B have decreased >60% in the

United States in the last decade. HBV is largely a disease spread by the parenteral route through blood transfusion, needlestick accidents, and contaminated needles, although the virus can be transmitted in the absence of obvious parenteral exposure. HBV has been found in saliva, semen, breast milk, tears, sweat, and other biologic fluids of HBV carriers. Urine and wound exudate have been found to be capable of harboring HBV. Stool is not considered to be infectious. Several serologic markers for HBV infection have been defined: HBsAg, HBeAg, anti-HBc, anti-HBe, anti-HBs, and DNA analysis. The most important factors in preventing transfusion-acquired HBV are donor interviewing, screening of donor blood, the use of hepatitis-free products when possible, and the appropriate use of blood and blood components. In addition, avoidance of high-risk blood components such as untreated Factor VIII prepared from multiple donor pools reduces the incidence of HBV.

The HDV, initially called the *delta agent* and then called the *hepatitis delta virus,* was first described in 1977 as a pathogen that superinfects some patients already infected with HBV. Persons with acute or chronic HBV infection as demonstrated by serum HBsAg can be infected with HDV. HBV is required as a "helper" to initiate infection.

In the past, hepatitis C was referred to as non-A, non-B (NANB) hepatitis, a term introduced in the 1970s. This form of hepatitis was regarded as a diagnosis of exclusion because of the absence of specific serologic markers and unknown viral origin. HCV has now been identified and immunologic assays developed for its detection. Hepatitis C is mainly transmitted parenterally and is associated with the form of hepatitis that develops after transfusion or as sporadic (community-acquired) hepatitis occurring primarily in developed countries. Hepatitis C is prevalent in the United States and Western Europe and resembles HBV in terms of transmission characteristics. Because the RIBA is based on the same recombinant antigens and synthetic peptides as the ELISA, it is licensed as an additional, more specific test. Preventive practices among health care workers to avoid needlestick injuries should be exercised. Recent investigations have shown that removal of blood from donors with anti-HBcAg from the blood supply and the use of third-generation anti-HCV testing have reduced the incidence of posttransfusion hepatitis C. Vaccines and Ig products do not exist for prevention or treatment of hepatitis C.

HEV is transmitted by the fecal-oral route. Infection is usually due to poor sanitation conditions. No form of chronic liver disease has been attributable to infection by HEV. Although most acute infections are self-limited and mild, in pregnant women about 10% to 20% of HEV infections result in fulminant hepatitis, especially in the third trimester of pregnancy. Standard gamma globulin preparations have not been shown to be effective in the prevention of viral E hepatitis. No effective vaccine has been developed. Treatment of HEV is usually supportive care.

Hepatitis G is a blood-borne agent. Transfusion recipients and IV drug abusers are at risk of infection. The virus frequently occurs as a coinfection with HCV. HGV is estimated to produce 900 to 2000 infections per year; most of them may be asymptomatic. Chronic disease is rare or may not occur at all.

TTV is the newest member of the infectious hepatitis family. This virus was discovered in 1997 through the use of cloning and DNA sequence analysis by a group of Japanese scientists. The most remarkable feature of TTV is the extraordinarily high prevalence of chronic viremia in apparently healthy people, up to nearly 100% in some countries. As with HGV, the pathogenicity of TTV has not been proven.

REVIEW QUESTIONS

Questions 1-4. Match each of the following forms of hepatitis with its representative description.

1. _____ acute hepatitis

2. _____ fulminant acute hepatitis

3. _____ subclinical hepatitis without jaundice

4. _____ chronic hepatitis

   A. this rare form is associated with hepatic failure
   B. typical form of hepatitis with associated jaundice
   C. probably accounts for persons with serum antibodies but no history of hepatitis
   D. accompanied by hepatic inflammation and necrosis

Questions 5-8. Match (use an answer only once).

5. _____ hepatitis A

6. _____ hepatitis B

7. _____ delta hepatitis

8. _____ hepatitis C

   A. intact virus is the Dane particle
   B. transmission by both parenteral and nonparenteral routes
   C. requires HBV as a helper
   D. most common form of hepatitis

Questions 9-12. Match (use an answer only once).

9. _____ hepatitis A

10. _____ hepatitis B

11. _____ delta agent

12. _____ hepatitis C

   A. should receive Ig intramuscularly after exposure
   B. defective or incomplete RNA virus
   C. has an epidemiology similar to HA virus
   D. previously called Australian antigen

Questions 13-17. Match.

13. _____ HBsAg

14. _____ HBeAg

15. _____ anti-HBc

16. _____ anti-HBe

17. _____ anti-HBs

    A. indicator of recent HBV infection may be only sero-logic marker during the window phase
    B. found in the serum of some patients who are HBsAg positive; marker for level of virus, infectivity
    C. a serologic marker of recovery and immunity
    D. initial detectable marker found in serum during incubator period of HBV infection
    E. in the case of acute hepatitis is the first serologic evidence of the convalescent phase

18. Hepatitis B accounts for less than approximately

_____% of cases of transfusion-acquired hepatitis.

    A. 5
    B. 10
    C. 25
    D. 75

19. Hepatitis C previously accounted for approximately

_____% of cases of transfusion-acquired hepatitis.

    A. 10
    B. 20
    C. 40
    D. 60

Questions 20-22. Match the following average incubation times (in days) with the appropriate form of hepatitis.

20. _____ hepatitis A

21. _____ hepatitis B

22. _____ hepatitis C

    A. 5
    B. 25
    C. 50
    D. 75
    E. 150

23. Which form of hepatitis does not have a chronic form of the disease?
    A. hepatitis A
    B. hepatitis B
    C. hepatitis C

24. Another name for hepatitis B infection is:
    A. infectious hepatitis
    B. serum hepatitis
    C. Australia antigen
    D. Dane particle

25. The most frequent clinical response to hepatitis B virus is:
    A. jaundice within 75 days
    B. asymptomatic infection
    C. subclinical infection
    D. both B and C

26. The first laboratory screening test of donor blood was for the detection of:
    A. HBc
    B. HBsAg
    C. HBe
    D. Anti-HBe

27. Which surface marker is a reliable marker for the presence of high levels of hepatitis B virus (HBV) and a high degree of infectivity?
    A. HBeAg
    B. HBsAg
    C. HBcAg
    D. anti-HBsAg

28. The serologic marker during the "window period" of type B hepatitis is:
    A. anti-HBs
    B. anti-HBc
    C. anti-HBe
    D. HBsAg

29. Which of the following is a characteristic of the delta agent?
    A. a DNA virus
    B. usually replicates only in hepatitis B virus-infected hosts
    C. infects patients who are HBcAg positive
    D. frequently found in the United States

30. Which of the following viruses is rarely implicated in transfusion-associated hepatitis?
    A. hepatitis A
    B. hepatitis B
    C. hepatitis C
    D. cytomegalovirus

31. Posttransfusion hepatitis is most frequently due to:
    A. delta agent
    B. hepatitis C
    C. hepatitis A
    D. hepatitis B

32. The specific diagnostic test for hepatitis C is:
    A. absence of anti-HAV and anti-HBsAg
    B. an increase in serum ALT
    C. detection of non-A, non-B antibodies
    D. anti-HCV

Serologic Markers for Hepatitis B Virus Infection

	Early (Asymptomatic)	Acute/Chronic	Low-Level Carrier	Immunity With HBs/Ag
HBsAg	37. _____	38. _____	−	−
Anti-HBs	−	1+	−	+
Anti-HBc	−	39. _____	40. _____	41. _____
Anti-HBc (IgM)	−	+	−	42. _____

33. Surrogate testing for hepatitis C consisted of:
    A. HBsAg and ALT
    B. anti-HBc and ALT
    C. HBsAg and anti-HBc
    D. anti-HBs and anti-HBc

34. Primary hepatitis viruses are given this name because:
    A. they primarily attack a variety of body systems
    B. they primarily attack the liver
    C. they primarily attack the skin
    D. they primarily attack the nervous system

35. Hepatitis A has all of the following characteristics except:
    A. a DNA virus
    B. short-incubation hepatitis
    C. crowded, unsanitary conditions as a risk factor
    D. very rare occurrence of transfusion acquisition

36. The Australia antigen is now called:
    A. Dane particle
    B. long incubation hepatitis
    C. hepatitis B surface antigen (HBsAg)
    D. hepatitis B core antigen (HBcAg)

Questions 37-42. Fill in the table above, using A, B, or C, as indicated.
    A. positive (+)
    B. negative (−)
    C. questionable (±)

Question 43-45. Identify the serologic markers in the figure below, choosing from the following answers.

Possible answers for questions 43-45.
    A. HBsAg
    B. anti-HBc
    C. HBeAg
    D. anti-HBs

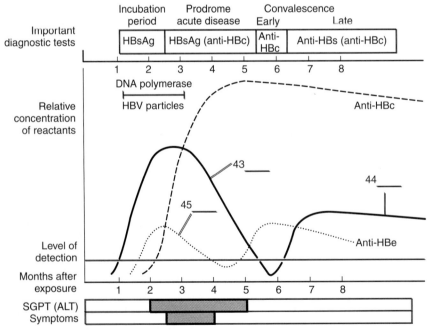

(Redrawn from Hollinger FB, Dreesman GR. In Rose RN, Friedman H, editors: *Manual of clinical immunology,* ed 2, Washington, DC, 1980, American Society for Microbiology.)

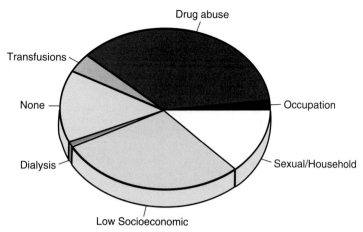

Drug abuse

Transfusions

None

Dialysis

Occupation

Sexual/Household

Low Socioeconomic

(Redrawn from Gollan JL: Viral hepatitis. In *International Review of Internal Medicine,* Boston, 1995, Brigham and Women's Hospital, Harvard University Medical School, pp 781-792.)

46. Which category in the figure above has the highest incidence of acute hepatitis C?
   A. low socioeconomic status
   B. dialysis
   C. transfusion
   D. drug abuse

47. Which category has the lowest incidence of acute hepatitis C?
   A. sexual/household
   B. dialysis
   C. drug abuse
   D. transfusion

Questions 48-51. Match each form of hepatitis to the appropriate mode of transmission. (You may use an answer more than once.)

48. _____ Hepatitis A   A. fecal-oral

49. _____ Hepatitis B   B. parenteral

50. _____ Hepatitis C   C. parenteral and
                               nonparenteral
51. _____ Hepatitis E

52. The mean length of time from posttransfusion hepatitis

   to chronic hepatitis is _____ years.
   A. 2
   B. 4
   C. 8
   D. 10

53. The mean length of time from posttransfusion hepatitis

   to cirrhosis is _____ years.
   A. 4.8
   B. 8.9
   C. 21.2
   D. 35.4

BIBLIOGRAPHY

Aikawa T, Sugai Y, Okamoto H: Hepatitis G infection in drug abusers with chronic hepatitis C (letter), *N Engl J Med* 334:195-196, 1996.

Akahane Y et al: Hepatitis C virus infection in spouses of patients with type C chronic liver disease, *Ann Intern Med* 120(9):748-752, 1994.

Alter HJ et al: The incidence of transfusion-associated hepatitis G virus infection and its relation to liver disease, *N Engl J Med* 336:747-754, 1997.

Alter HJ: The cloning and clinical implications of HGV and HGBV-C, *N Engl J Med* 334:1536-1537, 1996.

Alter MJ et al: Acute non-A-E hepatitis in the United States and the role of hepatitis G virus infection, *N Engl J Med* 336:741-746, 1997.

Alter MJ et al: The natural history of community-acquired hepatitis C in the United States, *N Engl J Med* 327(27):1899-1905, 1992.

Alter MJ: Transmission of hepatitis C virus—route, dose, and titer, *N Engl J Med* 330(11):784-785, 1994.

Anonymous. Focus: Markers on Hepatitis, *ADVANCE Administrators Lab,* vol 83, October, 2001.

Anonymous: The changing landscape of HIV-hepatitis C virus and HIV coinfection. HIV/AIDS treatment updates, Medscape 2000, website: www.medscape.com.

Bader TF et al: Hepatitis E in a U.S. traveler to Mexico, *N Engl J Med* 325(23):1660, 1991.

Bean P: The use of alternative medicine in the treatment of hepatitis C, *Am Clin Lab* 21(4):19-21, 2002.

Bean P: New strategies in the treatment of hepatitis C, *Am Clin Lab* 21(3):18-20, 2002.

Bendinelli M et al: Molecular properties, biology, and clinical implications of TT virus, a recently identified widespread infectious agent of humans, *Clin Microbiol Rev* 14:98-113, 2001.

Bronowicki J et al: Patient-to-patient transmission of hepatitis C virus during colonoscopy, *N Engl J Med* 337(4):237-240, 1997.

Bruno R et al: Challenges for hepatitis C patients coinfected with HIV, *Am Clin Lab* 21(4):26-29, 2002.

Chokephaibulkit K, Painter P, Patamasucon P: Overview of hepatitis C, *Lab Med* 23(12):798-806, 1992.

Davis GL et al: Treatment of chronic hepatitis C with recombinant interferon alpha, *N Engl J Med* 321(22):1501-1506, 1989.

de Lamballerie X, Charrel RN, Bussol B: Hepatitis GB virus C in patients on hemodialysis, *N Engl J Med* 334:1549, 1996.

DiBisceglie AM: Hepatitis G virus infection: a work in progress, *Ann Intern Med* 125:772-773, 1996.

DiBisceglie AM: Interferon therapy for chronic viral hepatitis, *N Engl J Med* 330(2):137-138, 1994.

Division of Infectious Diseases: Hepatitis, 2002, website: http://hopkins-id.edu/diseases/hepatitis.html.

Donahue JG et al: The declining risk of post-transfusion hepatitis C virus infection, *N Engl J Med* 327(6):369-373, 1992.

Dula WF, Anderson SM: Diagnosis and monitoring of hepatitis C infection, *ADVANCE Administrators Lab* 7(6):65-69, 1998.

Egan BM, Nordbo SA: Transmission of HCV by organ transplantation, *N Engl J Med* 326(6):410-411, 1992.

Farci P et al: Treatment of chronic hepatitis D with interferon alfa-2a, *N Engl J Med* 330(2):88-94, 1994.

Fried MW et al: Hepatitis G virus co-infection in liver transplantation recipients with chronic hepatitis C and nonviral chronic liver disease, *Hepatology* 25:1271-1275, 1997.

Ghuman HK, Tribhuwan SR: Acute delta hepatitis without hepatitis B surface antigen detectable in the blood, *J Infect* 25(3):317-319, 1992.

Gibb DM et al: Mother-to-child transmission of hepatitis C virus, *Hosp Physician* (review) 36(11):16, 2000.

Gindler J et al: Successful immunization for children and adults, *Patient Care* 31np(15):124, 1997.

Gollan JL: Viral hepatitis. In *International Review of Internal Medicine,* Boston, 1995, Brigham and Women's Hospital, Harvard University Medical School, pp 781-792.

Gudima, S et al: Origin of hepatitis delta virus mRNA, *J Virol* 74(16):7204-7210, 2000.

Gretch DR et al: Assessment of hepatitis C viremia using molecular amplification technologies: correlations and clinical implications, *Ann Intern Med* 123(5):321-336, 1995.

Heathcote EJ et al: Peginterferon alfa-2a in patients with chronic hepatitis C and cirrhosis, *N Engl J Med* 343:1673-1680, 2000.

Holst B, Ritter D: Managing viral hepatitis: a practical approach, *Clin Rev* 11(1):51-62, 2001.

Ince N, Wands J: The increasing incidence of hepatocellular carcinoma (editorial), *N Engl J Med* 340(10): 798-799, 1999.

Itoh K et al: Infection by an uneveloped DNA virus associated with non-A to –G hepatitis in Japanese blood donors with or without elevated ALT levels, *Transfusion* 39(5):522-527, 1999.

Jandreski MA: Hepatitis testing, *Clin Lab News* 24:10-12, 1999.

Kangxian J et al: Epidemiological survey and follow-up of transfusion-transmitted virus after an outbreak of enterically transmitted infection, *J Viral Hepat* 7(4):309, 2000.

Kew M: Viral hepatitis: diagnosis, therapy, and prevention (book review), *N Engl J Med* 341(10):770, 1999.

Kleinman S, Busch M, Holland P: Post-transfusion hepatitis C virus infection, *N Engl J Med* 327(22):1601, 1992.

Koff R: The case for routine childhood vaccination against hepatitis A (editorial), *N Engl J Med* 340(8):644-645, 1999.

Lara CR et al: Detection of hepatitis C virus RNA in persons with and without known risk factors for blood-borne viral infections in Sweden and Honduras, *J Clin Microbiol* 36(1):255-257, 1998.

Lee WM: Hepatitis B virus infection, *N Engl J Med* 337(24):1733-1743, 1997.

Linnen J et al: Molecular cloning and disease association of hepatitis G virus: a transfusion-transmissible agent, *Science* 271:505-508, 1996.

Lopez-Alcorocho JM et al: Detection of hepatitis GB virus type C RNA in serum and liver from children with chronic viral hepatitis B and C, *Hepatology* 25:1258-1260, 1997.

Lucey M: Hepatitis B virus infection, American Association for the Study of Liver Disease, 51st Annual Meeting and Postgraduate Course, Day 1, Oct 27, 2000.

Mannucci PM et al: Transmission of hepatitis A to patients with hemophilia by Factor VIII concentrates treated with organic solvent and detergent to inactivate viruses, *Ann Intern Med* 120(1):1-7, 1994.

Marcus DL, Lordi PF Jr: Transmission of hepatitis B virus associated with a finger-stick device, *N Engl J Med* 328(13):969-970, 1993.

Martinot M et al: Influence of hepatitis G virus infection on the severity of liver disease and response to interferon-alpha in patients with chronic hepatitis C, *Ann Intern Med* 126:874-881, 1997.

Masuko K et al: Infection with hepatitis GB virus C in patients on maintenance hemodialysis, *N Engl J Med* 334:1485-1490, 1996.

Mauser-Bunschoten EP: Transmission of hepatitis C virus in spouses, *Ann Intern Med* 122(2):154, 1995.

McHutchison JG et al: Interferon alfa-2b alone or in combination with ribavirin as initial treatment for chronic hepatitis, *N Engl J Med* 339(21):1485-1492, 1998.

MEDLINE plus Health Information, 2002, webwite: www.nlm.nih.gov.

Modahl LE, Lai MM: Hepatitis delta virus: the molecular basis of laboratory diagnosis, *Crit Rev Clin Lab Sci* 37(1):45-92, 2000.

Misiani R et al: Hepatitis C virus infection in patients with essential mixed cryoglobulinemia, *Ann Intern Med* 117(7):573-577, 1992.

Moradpour D, Wands JR: Understanding hepatitis B virus infection, *N Engl J Med* 332(16):1092-1093, 1995.

Morbidity and Mortality Weekly Report. Provisional cases of selected notifiable disease, United States, week ending December 29, 2001, website: www.cdc.gov/nnwr.

Morbidity and Mortality Weekly Report: Deaths and hospitalizations from chronic liver disease; Morbidity and Mortality Weekly Report: Hepatitis B and injecting-drug use among American Indians—Montana, 1989-1990, *MMWR* 41(1):13-14, 1992.

Morbidity and Mortality Weekly Report: Public health service interagency guidelines for screening donors of blood, plasma, organs, tissues, and semen for evidence of hepatitis B and hepatitis C, *MMWR* 40(RR-4):1-17, 1991.

Morbidity and Mortality Weekly Report. Severe isoniazid-associated hepatitis—New York, 1991-1993, *MMWR* 42(28):546-547, 1993.

National Institutes of Health: Chronic hepatitis C: current disease management, NIH Publication No. 99-4230, May, 1999.

Nousbaum JB et al: Hepatitis C virus type 1b (II) infection in France and Italy, *Ann Intern Med* 122(3):161-168, 1995.

Ohto H et al: Transmission of hepatitis C virus from mothers to infants, *N Engl J Med* 330(11):744-750, 1994.

Osmond DH et al: Risk factors for hepatitis C virus seropositivity in heterosexual couples, *JAMA* 269(3):361-365, 1993.

Pereira BJG et al: Prevalence of hepatitis C virus RNA in organ donors positive for hepatitis C antibody and in the recipients of their organs, *N Engl J Med* 327(13):910-915, 1992.

Pessoa MG et al: Hepatitis G virus in patients with cryptogenic liver disease undergoing liver transplantation, *Hepatology* 25:1266-1270, 1997.

Reshef RR, Sbeit W, Tur-Kaspa W: Lamivudine in the treatment of acute hepatitis B, *N Engl J Med* 343(15):1123-1124, 2000.

Robbins S et al: *Pathologic basis of disease,* ed 6, Philadelphia, 1999, WB Saunders.

Roth D et al: Detection of hepatitis C virus infection among cadaver organ donors: evidence for low transmission of disease, *Ann Intern Med* 117(6):470-475, 1992.

Sainato D: Viral testing in hepatitis, *Clin Lab News* 24:12-15, 1999.

Sato S et al: Hepatitis B virus strains with mutations in the core in patients with fulminant hepatitis, *Ann Intern Med* 122(4):241-248, 1995.

Sandler SG: Gains and strains of HCV diagnosis, *CAP TODAY* 16:22-28, 2001.

Sebastian J, Conrad A: Blood screening, *Adv Hepatitis* 10(10):30-35, 2001.

Seeff LB, Alter HJ: Spousal transmission of the hepatitis C virus, *Ann Intern Med* 120(9):807-809, 1994.

Sherker AH: Clinical news and views on hepatitis. Hepatitis G, 1998, website: www.hepnet.com.

Shier NJ et al: Contamination of a finger-stick device, *N Engl J Med* 328(13):969-970, 1993.

Simons JN et al: Identification of two flavivirus-like genomes in the GB hepatitis agent, *Proc Natl Acad Sci USA* 92:3401-3405, 1995.

Simons JN et al: Isolation of novel virus-like sequences associated with human hepatitis, *Nat Med* 1:564-569, 1995.

Stevens CE et al: Epidemiology of hepatitis C virus, *JAMA* 263(1):49-53, 1990.

Tanaka E et al: Effect of hepatitis G virus infection on chronic hepatitis C, *Ann Intern Med* 125:740-743, 1996.

Tedeschim V, Seeff LB: Diagnostic tests for hepatitis C: where are we now? *Ann Intern Med* 123(5):383-384, 1995.

Terrault N, Wright T: Interferon and hepatitis C, *N Engl J Med* 332(22):1509-1511, 1995.

Thursz MR et al: Association between an MHC class II allele and clearance of hepatitis B virus in The Gambia, *N Engl J Med* 332(16):1065-1069, 1995.

Toonisi TS: Children with chronic active hepatitis: a 10-year study, *Lab Med* 23(9):603-612, 1992.

Toyoda H et al: TT virus genotype changes frequently in multiply transfused patients with hemophilia but rarely in patients with chronic hepatitis C and in healthy subjects, *Transfusion* 41(9):1130-1135, 2001.

Turgeon ML: Hepatitis C: what's new? *ADVANCE Medical Lab Professionals* 12(23):24, 2001.

Van Der Poel CL et al: Infectivity of blood seropositive for hepatitis C virus antibodies, *Lancet* 335:558-560, 1990.

Villeneuve, JP et al: Lamivudine treatment for decompensated cirrhosis resulting from chronic hepatitis B, *Hepatology* 31(1):207-210, 2000.

Wang, JT et al: Incidence and clinical presentation of posttransfusion TT virus infection in prospectively followed transfusion recipients: emphasis on its relevance to hepatitis, *Transfusion* 40(5):596-599, 2000.

Weikersheimer P: Is hepatitis C virus targeted lookback effective? *Lab Med* 31(11):600-604, 2000.

Worman HJ: Hepatitis C: current treatment, 2002, website: http://cpmcnet.columbia.edu.

Worman HJ: New and future treatment of chronic hepatitis C, Viewpoints Newsletter, Spring/Summer 2001 ed. of the American Liver Foundation, Greater NY Chapters, website: http://cpmcnet.columbia.edu 2002.

Wong JB et al: Cost-effectiveness of interferon-alpha-2b treatment for hepatitis Be antigen-positive chronic hepatitis B, *Ann Intern Med* 122(9):664-675, 1995.

Yoshiba M, Okamoto H, Mishiro S: Detection of the GBV-C hepatitis virus genome in serum from patients with fulminant hepatitis of unknown aetiology, *Lancet* 346:1131-1132, 1995.

Zeuzem S et al: Peginterferon alfa-2a in patients with chronic hepatitis C, *N Engl J Med* 343:1666-1672, 2000.

Chapter 21

Rubella Infection

LEARNING OBJECTIVES

At the conclusion of this chapter, the reader should be able to:
- Describe the etiology and epidemiology of rubella infection.
- Explain the signs and symptoms of acquired and congenital infection.
- Compare the immunologic manifestations of acquired and congenital rubella infection.

- Explain the diagnostic evaluation of rubella, including hemagglutination inhibition, passive latex agglutination, and semiquantitative immunoassay for immunoglobulin (Ig)G.
- Analyze a representative case study.

ETIOLOGY

The rubella virus was first isolated in 1962. Acquired rubella, also known as German, or 3-day, measles, is caused by an enveloped, single-stranded RNA virus of the Togaviridae family. Because the virus is endemic to humans, the disease is highly contagious and transmitted through respiratory secretions. Before widespread rubella immunization, this viral infection occurred most commonly in childhood, although it also affected adults.

EPIDEMIOLOGY

Three strains of live attenuated rubella vaccine virus were developed and first licensed for use in the United States in 1969. Before widespread rubella immunization in the United

States and Canada, rubella infections occurred in epidemic proportion at 6- to 9-year intervals. In 1964 more than 20,000 cases of congenital rubella syndrome and an unknown number of stillbirths occurred in the United States as the result of an epidemic that year. As of August 23, 1989, the Chicago Department of Health reported 1123 confirmed cases of measles in a measles outbreak in that city. Of these cases, 78% occurred in preschool-age children, with African-Americans and Hispanics accounting for 94% of the cases. In countries where vaccination is uncommon, the incidence of rubella infection is high and epidemics are frequent. Because vaccination programs have prevented the rubella epidemics that once gave people naturally acquired immunity, individuals who have not been vaccinated have a higher level of susceptibility to rubella infection. Since 1983 the number of reported measles cases increased annually until 1986, then decreased in 1987 and 1988 (a provisional total of 3411 cases in 1988). In 1988 the age distribution of cases was similar to that in previous years. Primarily two types of outbreaks have occurred in the United States in the recent past: those among highly vaccinated school-age children and those among unvaccinated preschool-age children. The epidemiology of measles points to two major impediments to measles elimination—unvaccinated preschool-age children, a factor that allows large outbreaks such as the Chicago epidemic in inner-city areas, and vaccine failures, which account for outbreaks in highly vaccinated school-age populations. On American college and university campuses the susceptibility to rubella infection among students is estimated to be as high as 20%. There have been six documented rubella outbreaks on college campuses since 1983; however, the actual number of outbreaks among college students is suspected to be much higher. Many incidences have been either unrecognized or unreported because many cases of rubella infection are mild or subclinical.

Contracting the infection or vaccinating against rubella are the only routes to developing immunity. Individuals should be immune to rubella if they have a dated record of rubella vaccination on or after their first birthday or if they have demonstrable rubella antibody. Even when antibody titers fall to relatively low levels, previous infection or successful vaccination appears to confer permanent immunity to rubella except in cases of congenital rubella. The only proof of immunity is a positive serologic screening test for rubella antibody. History of rubella infection, even if verified by a physician, is not acceptable evidence of immunity.

It is critical to continue to determine the rubella immune status of women of childbearing age and to vaccinate those who are not immune. Individuals requiring rubella immune status determination include those belonging to the following groups:

- Preschool- and school-age children
- All females at or just before childbearing age
- Women about to be married
- Married women. If the woman is not rubella-immune, she should be vaccinated and advised not to become pregnant for 3 months because there is a remote possibility that the vaccination could lead to an infected fetus.
- Pregnant women. A positive test confirms immunity, but to rule out any possibility of unsuspected current infection, an IgM screening procedure may also be ordered. If the patient is not rubella immune, she should be cautioned to avoid exposure to rubella infection. Vaccination is contraindicated in pregnant women; however, a woman should be vaccinated immediately after termination of the pregnancy.
- Health care personnel. Both men and women should be vaccinated to prevent possible spread of nosocomial infection to pregnant patients.

Adverse reactions to rubella vaccine have been reported. The Institute of Medicine determined that a causal relationship exists between rubella vaccine and acute arthritis in adult women. Weak but consistent evidence exists for a causal relationship between rubella vaccine and chronic arthritis in adult women. Incidence rates are estimated to average 13% to 15% among adult women after vaccination. Much lower levels of arthritic adverse reaction were noted among children, adolescents, and adult men. Reliable estimates of excess risk of chronic arthritis after rubella vaccination are not available.

SIGNS AND SYMPTOMS

A diagnosis of acquired rubella is not based solely on clinical manifestation. The signs and symptoms of rubella vary widely from person to person and may not be recognized in some cases, especially if the characteristic rash is light or absent, as it may be in a substantial number of cases. Rubella infection may resemble other disorders such as infectious mononucleosis and drug-induced rashes.

Acquired Infection

The incubation period of acquired rubella infection varies from 10 to 21 days, and 12 to 14 days is typical. Infected persons are usually contagious for 12 to 15 days, beginning 5 to 7 days before the appearance (if present) of a rash. Acute rubella infection lasts from 3 to 5 days and generally requires little treatment. Permanent effects are extremely rare in acquired infections.

The clinical presentation of acquired rubella is usually mild. The clinical manifestation of infection usually begins with a prodromal period of catarrhal symptoms, followed by involvement of the retroauricular, posterior cervical, and post-occipital lymph nodes, and finally by the emergence of a maculopapular rash on the face and then on the neck and trunk (Figures 21-1 and 21-2). A fever of less than 34.4° C is usually present. In older children and adults, self-limiting arthralgia and arthritis are common.

Congenital Infection

Although rubella infection is usually a mild, self-limiting disease with only rare complications in children and adults, rubella infections in pregnant women, especially those infected in their first trimester of pregnancy, can have devastating effects on the fetus (Figure 21-3). In utero infection can result in fetal death or manifestation of rubella syndrome. This syndrome represents a spectrum of congenital defects. Some 10% to 20% of newborn infants infected in utero fail to survive past the first 18 months of life.

The point in the gestation cycle at which maternal rubella infection occurs greatly influences the severity of congenital rubella syndrome (Table 21-1), and the extent of congenital anomalies varies from one infant to another. Some infants manifest nearly all the defects associated with rubella, whereas others exhibit few, if any, consequences of infection. Clinical evidence of congenital rubella infection may not be recognized for months or even years after birth.

Rubella syndrome encompasses a number of congenital anomalies. In addition to stillbirth, fetal abnormalities associated with maternal rubella infection include encephalitis, hepatomegaly, bone defects, mental retardation, cataracts, thrombocytopenic purpura, cardiovascular defects, splenomegaly, and microcephaly. Severely afflicted children are likely to have multiple defects in different organ systems. In neonates with congenital rubella syndrome, low birth weight and failure to thrive are common.

Rubella immunity develops in almost all children who have had congenital rubella. In late childhood, however, about one third of these patients lose antibody and become

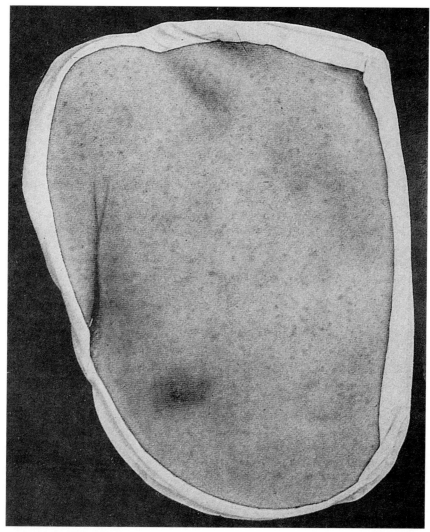

Figure 21-1   Rubella. (From Habif TP: *Clinical dermatology,* St Louis, 1985, Mosby.)

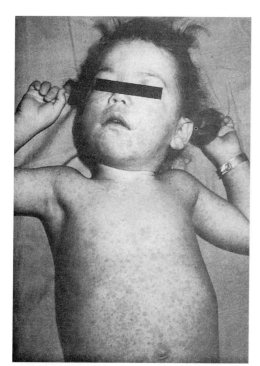

Figure 21-2   Rubella rash. (From Krugman S et al: *Infectious diseases of children,* ed 8, St Louis, 1985, Mosby.)

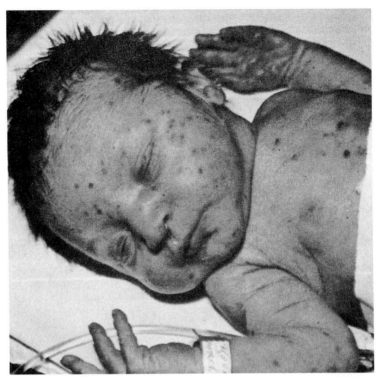

Figure 21-3 Congenital malformations of rubella. (From Krugman S et al: *Infectious diseases of children,* ed 8, St Louis, 1985, Mosby.)

TABLE 21-1	Manifestation of Anomalies in Maternal Rubella	
Period of Gestation	**Risk of Anomaly**
Prospective Studies	
First trimester	Approximately 25%
Second trimester	
First month	<1%
Second month	25% or >
Third month	10% or >
Serologically Confirmed Cases of Maternal Infection	
Before 11 weeks	90%
11-12 weeks	33%
13-14	11%
15-16	24%
After 16 weeks	0%

susceptible to acquired rubella. If acquired rubella occurs, it follows a typically benign course. Children afflicted with congenital rubella should be screened for rubella immunity in late childhood and vaccinated if necessary.

IMMUNOLOGIC MANIFESTATIONS

Acquired Infection

In a patient suffering from a primary rubella infection, the appearance of both IgG and IgM antibodies is associated with the appearance of clinical signs and symptoms when present.

IgM antibodies become detectable a few days after the onset of signs and symptoms and reach peak levels at 7 to 10 days. These antibodies persist but rapidly diminish in concentration over the next 4 to 5 weeks until antibody is no longer clinically detectable. The presence of IgM antibody in a single specimen suggests that the patient has recently experienced a rubella infection. In most cases the infection probably occurred within the preceding month.

Production of IgG is also associated with the appearance of clinical signs and symptoms. Antibody levels increase rapidly for the next 7 to 21 days, then level off or even decrease in strength. IgG antibodies, however, remain present and protective indefinitely. Detection of IgG antibody is a useful indicator of rubella infection only in cases where the acute and convalescent blood specimens are drawn several weeks apart. Optimum timing for paired testing for the diagnosis of a recent infection is 2 or more weeks apart, with the first (acute) specimen taken before or at the time signs and symptoms appear, or within 2 weeks of exposure.

Paired specimen testing may demonstrate that the antibody levels are the same. In these cases the patient was either previously immunized or the acute sample was taken after the antibody had already reached maximum levels. Demonstration of an unequivocal increase in IgG antibody concentration between the acute and convalescent specimens is suggestive of either a recent primary infection or a secondary (anamnestic) antibody response to rubella in an immune individual. In cases of an anamnestic response, IgM antibodies are not demonstrable, but IgG production begins quickly. No other signs or symptoms of disease are exhibited.

If both IgM and IgG test results are negative, the patient has never suffered from rubella infection or been vaccinated. Such patients are susceptible to infection. If no IgM is

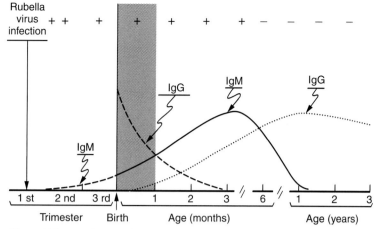

Figure 21-4 Natural history of congenital rubella. Pattern of virus excretion and antibody response. (Redrawn from Krugman S et al: *Infectious diseases of children,* ed 9, St Louis, 1992, Mosby.)

demonstrable but IgG is present in paired specimens, the patient is immune. In evaluation of the immune status of patients, IgG antibodies present in a dilution of 1:8 or greater indicate past infection with rubella virus and clinical protection against future rubella infection. The clinical significance of lower levels is not currently known. Titers of 1:16, 1:64, 1:512, or greater may be found in both acute and past infections; however, to diagnose acute infections would require an IgM antibody titer on the same specimen or a paired specimen comparison. It should be noted that IgM also appears for a transient period after vaccination.

Congenital Rubella Syndrome

Because IgG antibody is capable of crossing the placental barrier, there is no way of distinguishing between IgG antibody of fetal origin and IgG antibody of maternal origin in a neonatal blood specimen (Figure 21-4).

Testing for IgM antibody is invaluable in the diagnosis of congenital rubella syndrome in the neonate. IgM does not cross an intact placental barrier; therefore demonstration of IgM in a single neonatal specimen is diagnostic of congenital rubella syndrome. In the newborn, serologic confirmation of rubella infection can be made by testing for IgM antibody for at least the first 6 months of life. This is especially useful in instances when clinical evidence of congenital rubella is slow in emerging or is of uncertain origin.

DIAGNOSTIC EVALUATION

Physicians apply the results of rubella testing independently, frequently without the benefit of clinical signs and symptoms. Historically, hemagglutination inhibition (HAI) antibody testing has been the most frequently used method of screening for the presence of rubella antibodies. Within the past few years, the HAI test has been challenged by a number of assays that are more convenient as the screening method of choice for the determination of rubella immune (IgG) status. In some cases, such as pregnant women, it also may be necessary to determine if a recent infection has been experienced. The assays for determination of immune status and evidence of recent infection are presented in Table 21-2.

TABLE 21-2	Diagnostic Tests for Immune Status Serodiagnosis		
Method		**Immunity**	**Serodiagnosis**
Hemagglutination inhibition		Yes	Yes*
Passive hemagglutination		Yes	No
Fluorescent immunoassay		Yes	Yes*
Latex agglutination		Yes	No
Radioimmunoassay		Yes	No
Enzyme immunoassay		No	Yes
Enzyme immunoassay		Yes	Yes*

*Serodiagnosis may not differentiate between primary infection and reinfection. An IgM-specific procedure must be used.

Hemagglutination Inhibition

Despite wide acceptance and use of these other assays, HAI testing continues to be the reference method for detection and quantitation of rubella antibody. Rubella methods vary in sensitivity and specificity when samples with antibody levels near the breakpoint of immune versus nonimmune are analyzed. A gray area exists around the cutoff point of any test, but marginal results may be encountered with some methods. False-negative results with some methodologies are most frequently seen when HAI titers are at or near the cutoff antibody level of 1:8. It is important that the method used for screening demonstrates sensitivity, specificity, and reproducibility of ≥95% based on an assay of 200 or more serum samples compared with HAI. A disadvantage of HAI, however, is that although the procedure detects a combination of IgM and IgG antibodies, it does not distinguish between them. If IgG is separated from IgM, this procedure can be used as a differential method. Separation of IgM can be by sucrose density gradient fractions, protein A-Sepharose, or an affinity column.

Other Methods

Latex procedures provide more rapid and convenient alternatives to HAI. If more quantitative results are desired, enzyme immunoassay (EIA) and fluorescent immunoassay (FIA) appear to be as reliable as HAI. Widespread use of EIA for assessment of immune status (IgG) and recent infection (IgM) should soon result in simplification of rubella serology.

EIA can be used to measure total antibody, IgG, or IgM. IgM antibodies can be detected by EIA in 100% of patients between days 11 and 25 after onset of signs and symptoms of acquired infection, in 60% to 80% of persons at days 15 to 25 after vaccination, and in 90% to 97% of infants with congenital rubella between 2 weeks and 3 months after birth. The rubella-specific IgM often persists for 20 to 30 days after acute infection or vaccination and also in infants with congenital rubella. Persons with infectious mononucleosis sometimes have rubella-specific IgM in low concentrations. Cross-reactions of rubella IgM-positive sera can result from parvovirus IgM. Occasionally, pregnant women will demonstrate IgM antibodies not only to rubella but also to cytomegalovirus, varicella-zoster virus, and measles virus. In these cases diagnosis of rubella can be made only by assessment of rubella-specific IgG antibodies by HAI and/or EIA procedures supported by a detailed clinical history. Rubella-specific IgG is regularly detected by EIA only at more than 15 to 25 days after infection and at more than 25 to 50 days after vaccination.

Passive hemagglutination (PHA) methods are not licensed for serodiagnosis of recent rubella infection. PHA is faster and less complex than HAI. In PHA, erythrocytes are coated with rubella antigen. In the presence of rubella antibody, agglutination occurs.

■ *Passive Latex Agglutination Test*

Principle

Latex particles are sensitized with solubilized rubella virus antigens from disrupted virions judged to be inactivated. When the latex reagent is mixed with serum containing rubella antibodies on a dark surface, the antigen-antibody complex will form visible clumps. In the absence of antibody or if the concentration is insufficient to react, the latex particles will remain smooth and evenly dispersed. If a qualitative procedure is performed, the presence of rubella antibodies is an indication of previous infection, and presumptive immunity can be used to evaluate the immune status of that individual with regard to resistance or susceptibility to primary rubella infection.

Specimen Collection and Preparation

The protocol for specimen collection will vary depending on the testing objectives. Single specimens are required for qualitative antibody-level determinations. In suspected clinical infections or exposure, two specimens for quantitative testing should be obtained. The first should be collected within 3 days of the onset of rash or at the time of exposure and tested on arrival in the laboratory. This specimen should be frozen and stored until the second specimen is collected 7 to 21 days after the onset of the rash or at least 30 days after exposure if no clinical symptoms occur. Both specimens should be tested simultaneously.

No special preparation of the patient is required before specimen collection. The patient must be positively identified when the specimen is collected, and the specimen is to be labeled at the bedside. Specimen labels must include the patient's full name, the date the specimen is collected, the patient's hospital identification number, and the phlebotomist's initials.

Blood should be drawn by an aseptic technique. A minimum of 2 mL of clotted blood (red top evacuated tube) is required. The specimen should be centrifuged promptly and an aliquot of serum removed. Specimens may be stored up to 48 hours at 2° to 8° C. Specimens should be frozen if longer storage is required. Do not heat-inactivate the serum. The presence of particulate matter, lipemia, or hemolysis does not affect the test.

Reagents, Supplies, and Equipment

WARNING: The latex reagent, buffer, and controls contain sodium azide as a preservative. Sodium azide may react with lead and copper plumbing to form highly explosive metal azides. On disposal, flush with a large volume of water to prevent azide buildup.

1. The following reagents and supplies are provided in the Rubrascan kit (Becton Dickinson Microbiology Systems, Cockeysville, Md):
   a. Latex antigen. This reagent contains 0.02% gentamicin and 0.2% sodium azide. Store at 2° to 8° C and return to refrigeration when not in use. *Do not freeze.*
   b. Card dilution buffer: phosphate-buffered saline solution containing bovine serum albumin with 0.02% sodium azide. Store at 2° to 8° C and return to refrigeration when not in use. *Do not freeze.*
   c. Test cards. Cards must be flat for proper reactions. If necessary, flatten cards by bowing back in a direction opposite to that of the curl. Care should be taken not to finger-mark the test areas, as this may result in an oily deposit and improper test results. Use each card once and discard. Store cards in the original package in a dry area at room temperature.
   d. Plastic stirrers
   e. Dispensing needle (21-gauge, green hub). On completion of daily tests, remove the needle from the dispensing bottle and recap the bottle. Rinse the needle with distilled water to maintain clear passage and accurate drop delivery. Do not wipe the dispensing needle because it is coated with silicone.
2. Centrifuge
3. Rotator. The recommended rotation speed is 100 rpm, but rotation between 95 and 110 rpm does not significantly affect the results obtained. The rotator should circumscribe a circle approximately 2 cm in diameter in the horizontal plane. A moistened humidifying cover should be used to prevent drying of test specimens during rotation.

4. Humidifying cover
5. High-intensity incandescent lamp
6. Micropipettors: 25 μL and 100 μL
7. Other equipment and glassware for preparation, storage, and handling of serologic specimens

Quality Control

The following controls are provided in the Rubrascan kit (Becton Dickinson Microbiology System, Cockeysville, Md):

1. Low-reactive control with 0.1% sodium azide. This control is used for both the qualitative and the quantitative assay.
2. Nonreactive control with 0.1% sodium azide. This control is used for both the qualitative and quantitative assay.
3. High-reactive control with 0.1% sodium azide. This control is used in the quantitative assay only.

Each of these controls must be tested with each series of unknown patient specimens.

CAUTION: Because the control sera are derived from human sources, they should be handled in the same manner as clinical serum specimens (see Universal Blood and Body Fluid Precautions in Chapter 6).

Procedure

NOTE: The test area, reagents, specimens, and test components must be at 23° to 29° C before testing. Do not mix reagents from different lot numbers. The dispensing bottle must be held vertically.

Qualitative Testing

1. Remove the cap from the bottle of latex agglutination and attach the green hub needle to the tapered fitting.
2. Mark the card to identify the low-reactive and nonreactive controls and all samples.

With Undiluted Specimens

a. With a micropipettor, place 25 μL of low-reactive control on the appropriately marked circle.
b. With the same micropipettor and a clean tip each time, repeat the procedure in step A, using the nonreactive control and each specimen to be tested.

Alternate Procedure: 1:10 Specimen Dilution

a. Using the micropipettor, add 100 μL of buffer to the appropriate squares for each control and specimen to be tested. These squares will be used to prepare the 1:5 dilution in step C below.
b. Using the micropipettor, add 25 μL of buffer to the appropriate squares for each control and specimen to be tested. These squares will be used to prepare the 1:10 dilution in step D.
c. With the micropipette and a clean tip, pipette 25 μL flow reactive control directly into the buffer in the appropriately labeled circle and mix the serum and buffer by drawing up and down with the micropipette 12 times. Caution

should be exercised to avoid the formation of bubbles. The serum in this circle is now a 1:5 dilution.

d. Using the same micropipette and tip, transfer 25 μL of the 1:5 dilution from the circle and place directly into the buffer in the corresponding numbered circle and mix by drawing up and down with the micropipette six times. Withdraw 25 μL from the circle and discard. The serum in this circle is now a 1:10 dilution.

e. Repeat the procedure in step C for the nonreactive control and for each specimen to be tested.

3. Using a new plastic stirrer for each circle, spread each of the specimens to be tested (either 25 μL of serum of 25 μL of 1:10 diluted serum) to fill the entire circle.

4. Place the bottle cap over the tip of the needle and gently invert the bottle of latex reagent several times to mix.

5. While holding the latex reagent bottle in a vertical position, dispense several drops of antigen into the bottle cap until a drop of uniform size has been formed. Dispense one free-falling drop of antigen (approximately 15 μL) on each circle containing diluted serum. Care must be taken to avoid contamination of the bottle tip. The predropped antigen can be recovered from the bottle cap and reused.

6. Place the card on a rotator and rotate for 8 minutes under a moistened humidifying cover.

7. Immediately after mechanical rotation, read the card macroscopically in the wet state with the aid of a high-intensity incandescent lamp. A brief hand rotation of the card (three or four back-and-forth motions) must be made after mechanical rotation to help differentiate weak agglutination from no agglutination. Fluorescent lighting is generally insufficient to distinguish minimally reactive results. The use of magnification in reading test results is not recommended.

8. The reactive control should exhibit agglutination; the nonreactive control should demonstrate no agglutination.

Reporting Results

A positive reaction demonstrates agglutination.
A negative reaction demonstrates no agglutination.

Procedure Notes

A single specimen can be used to estimate the immune status of the individual because any detectable antibody is indicative of immunity and protection against subsequent viral infection. The alternate procedure using specimens diluted 1:10 should be used when data at a sensitivity level approximating that expected with hemagglutination inhibition methods are needed. Optimal sensitivity can be ensured by screening all serum samples undiluted and repeating negative specimens at a 1:10 dilution.

NOTE: The National Committee for Clinical Laboratory Standards (NCCLS) advised that the specimen should not be frozen in a frost-free freezer because the freeze-thaw cycle may be detrimental to serum proteins. The guidelines of this agency further suggest that frozen specimens be retained for at least 1 year for later follow-up examination, especially for women of childbearing age who are inadvertently exposed to the virus.

The acute-phase specimen should be collected as nearly as possible to the time of exposure, and no later than 3 days after the onset of rash. The convalescent-phase specimen should be taken 7 to 21 days after the onset of the rash or at least 30 days after exposure if no clinical symptoms appear because of a possible inapparent infection. Both specimens should be tested simultaneously.

Sources of Error

False-negative results may occur in the following conditions:

1. Reduction in the degree of agglutination has been reported with rare high-titered specimens when the test is performed undiluted.
2. In undiluted specimens, strong reactivity may cause the center of the test circle to appear clear because agglutinated latex has migrated to the periphery.
3. If only a 1:10 dilution is used, the procedure may fail to detect a low-level antibody that might have otherwise been detected with an undiluted specimen.
4. The absence of a fourfold titer rise does not necessarily rule out the possibility of exposure and infection. If the first (acute-phase) sample is taken too late or the second (convalescent-phase) sample is taken too soon, seroconversion or a fourfold rise in titer characteristic of recent infection may not be seen.

Clinical Applications

The presence of antibodies in a single patient specimen is an indication of previous exposure and immunity to rubella virus. Demonstration of any detectable antibody is indicative of immunity and protection against subsequent viral infection; however, a test configuration using an undiluted specimen may be preferred.

Demonstration of seroconversion, or a fourfold or greater rise in antibody titer with properly collected paired specimens, is diagnostic of a recent or current infection with rubella virus. Seroconversion means a positive test result of 1:5 or greater after an initial nonreactive result of less than 1:5.

Limitations

A single specimen determines immunity; it is not a serodiagnosis of infection/reinfection.

The qualitative card test is designed to detect the presence of rubella antibody. At a single dilution, the qualitative protocol will perform satisfactorily with both acute-phase and convalescent-phase antibodies; however, in cases where the presence or absence of a fourfold titer rise in paired specimens must be demonstrated, the quantitative protocol is required.

References

Rubrascan Product Brochure, Becton Dickinson Microbiology Systems, Cockeysville, Md, 1988.

Skendzel LP: New guidelines and standards for rubella antibody testing from NCCLS and CAP, *Lab Med* 18(7):461, 1987.

 ## Semiquantitative Immunoassay for Determination of IgG Antibodies to Rubella Virus*

Principle

The following procedure is an indirect enzyme-labeled immunosorbent assay using microwells as a solid phase. Rubella antigen is attached to wells of microplates. Diluted test samples are added to the coated wells and incubated. During incubation, antibodies to rubella present in the specimen will bind to the antigen-coated well. After they are washed to remove unbound material, antibodies to human IgG labeled with alkaline phosphatase (conjugate) are added. The conjugate binds to any rubella antibody bound to rubella antigen. The well is washed to remove unbound conjugate and incubated with p-nitrophenyl phosphate. The p-nitrophenyl phosphate is hydrolyzed by alkaline phosphatase to form p-nitrophenol, a yellow end product with absorbance maximum at 405 nm. The intensity of absorbance at 405 nm is proportional to the amount of IgG antibodies to rubella present in the specimen. The clinical application of this procedure is to determine the rubella immune status and susceptibility to rubella infection in individuals.

Specimen Collection and Preparation

No special preparation of the patient is required before specimen collection. The patient must be positively identified when the specimen is collected, and the specimen is to be labeled at the bedside. Specimen labels must include the patient's full name, the date the specimen is collected, the patient's hospital identification number, and the phlebotomist's initials.

Blood should be drawn by an aseptic technique. A minimum of 2 mL of clotted blood (red top evacuated tube) is required. The specimen should be centrifuged promptly and an aliquot of serum removed.

If the test cannot be performed immediately, the specimen should be refrigerated at 2° to 8° C for no longer than 72 hours. If additional delay occurs, the serum should be frozen at −20° C or below. Frozen serum should be thawed rapidly at 37° C. Specimens containing visible particulate matter should be clarified by centrifugation before testing. The serum sample should not be heat-inactivated before testing.

The NCCLS advises that the specimen should not be frozen in a frost-free freezer because the freeze-thaw cy-

_____
*Sigma Chemical Co, St Louis, Mo.

cle may be detrimental to serum proteins. The guidelines of this agency further suggest that frozen specimens be retained for at least 1 year for later follow-up evaluation, especially for women of childbearing age inadvertently exposed to the virus.

Reagents, Supplies, and Equipment*

NOTE: Store reagents at 2° to 6° C. The reagents are stable until the expiration date on the label.
1. Antigen wells: microplate wells coated with rubella antigen (Gilchrist strain). Store antigen wells with desiccant in the reusable plastic bag. Reseal the bag after opening.
2. Holder for wells
3. Sample diluent: buffered protein solution containing surfactant and blue dye, pH 7.5; contains 0.1% sodium azide as a preservative
4. Calibrator: human serum containing antibodies to rubella at 100 AU/mL. This constituent contains 0.1% sodium azide as a preservative.
5. Conjugate: goat antibodies to human IgG labeled with calf alkaline phosphatase. This solution contains a pink dye and 0.02% sodium azide as a preservative.
6. Substrate: contains p-nitrophenyl phosphate, disodium, hexahydrate 1 mg/mL, pH 9.6. The substrate may turn slightly yellow during storage. Do not use if absorbance of the undiluted substrate is greater than 0.4 at 405 nm when measured against water using a microplate reader or a spectrophotometer with a 1-cm lightpath.
7. Wash concentrate: buffer solution concentrate with surfactant. This solution contains 0.1% sodium azide as a preservative. The wash solution is prepared by adding the contents of wash concentrate bottle to 1 L of deionized water. Mix well. Wash solution may be stored at room temperature (18° to 26° C).
8. Stop solution. This is an alkaline solution, pH 12.0. Store at room temperature. Reagent is stable until expiration date on the label.

WARNING: Stop solution causes irritation. Avoid contact with eyes, skin, and clothing. Avoid breathing vapor. Wash thoroughly after handling.

NOTE: Do not interchange reagents from different lots.

WARNING: Sample diluent, calibrator, controls, and buffer contain 0.1% sodium azide as a preservative. Sodium azide may react with lead and copper plumbing to form highly explosive metal azides. On disposal, flush with a large volume of water to prevent azide buildup. Sodium azide is also toxic. Care should be taken to avoid ingestion.

Wells contain rubella antigen (Gilchrist strain) and have been tested for noninfectivity. No method, however, can ensure that all infectious agents are absent. Use Universal Precautions when handling this material.

*SIA rubella kit reagents available commercially from Sigma Chemical Co, St Louis, Mo.

Additional Required Supplies and Equipment:

1. Spectrophotometer or microplate reader capable of accurately measuring absorbance at 405 nm
2. Pipetting device for the accurate delivery of volumes required for the assay
3. Timer
4. 1-L measuring cylinder
5. Squeeze bottle for dispensing wash solution
6. Dilution plates or tubes
7. Test tubes or cuvettes, 1 mL

Quality Control
Positive Control

Human serum containing antibodies to rubella. Content (expected range, expressed as percentage of calibrator) indicated on the label. This serum contains 0.1% sodium azide. The assay value of the positive control should be within the range shown on the label.

Negative Control

Human serum containing no detectable rubella antibodies. This serum contains 0.1% sodium azide. The negative control should be less than 15% of the calibrator. If this requirement is not satisfied, test results may be inaccurate and the assay should be repeated.

CAUTION: Because the antigen wells and control and calibrator sera are derived from human sources, the specimen should be handled in the same manner as clinical serum specimens (see Universal Blood and Body Fluid Precautions in Chapter 6).

Procedure

1. Dilute calibrator, positive and negative controls, and test samples by combining 5 μL of each with 200 μL of sample diluent in labeled tubes or dilution plates.
2. Place the desired number of antigen wells in holder.
3. Using a pipette tip, mix the samples and diluent by drawing up and expelling two or three times. Transfer 100 μL of each diluted sample to the appropriate antigen well.
4. Include one well that contains only 100 μL of sample diluent. This serves as the reagent blank and is used to zero the photometer.
5. Allow the plate to stand at room temperature (18° to 26° C) for 30 ± 2 minutes.
6. Shake out or aspirate contents of wells. Wash wells by filling them with wash solution from a squeeze bottle and shaking out or aspirating. Wash three times. Drain wells on paper towels to remove excess fluid.
   NOTE: Thorough washing is necessary to achieve accurate results. Avoid bubbles.
7. Place 2 drops (or 100 μL) of conjugate into each well, including the reagent blank well.
8. Allow to stand at room temperature (18° to 26° C) for 30 minutes ± 2 minutes.
9. Wash wells by repeating step 6.

10. Place 2 drops (or 100 μL) of substrate into each well, including the reagent blank well.
11. Allow to stand at room temperature (18° to 26° C) for 30 minutes ± 2 minutes.
12. Place 2 drops (or 100 μL) of stop solution into each well.
13. Read and record absorbance of each test at 405 nm within 2 hours after reaction has been stopped:

Microplate Reader

Set absorbance at 405 nm to zero with water as reference. Read and record absorbance of reagent blank (A blank). Then set absorbance to zero with a reagent blank as a reference. Read and record absorbance of samples (A sample) and calibrator (A calibrator).

Spectrophotometer

Completely remove contents of each well and transfer to cuvette or test tube. Add 800 μL of deionized water to each sample and mix. Set absorbance at 405 nm to zero with water as a reference. Read and record the absorbance of each sample, including the reagent blank. Subtract the absorbance of the reagent blank for absorbance of each sample.

Calculation

Concentration of IgG antibodies to rubella in sample is calculated as follows:

Antibody concentration as percent of calibrator =

$$\frac{A \text{ sample}}{A \text{ calibrator}} \times 100$$

Example:
ABSORBANCE MEASURED USING A MICROPLATE READER
A sample = 0.840
A calibrator = 1.543
ANTIBODY CONCENTRATION AS PERCENT OF CALIBRATOR

$$\frac{0.8402}{1.5430} \times 100 = 54$$

ABSORBANCE MEASURED USING A SPECTROPHOTOMETER
A blank = 0.006
A sample = 0.357
A calibrator = 0.659
A sample − A blank is 0.357 − 0.006 = 0.351
A calibrator − A blank is 0.659 − 0.006 = 0.653
Antibody concentration as percent of calibrator =

$$\frac{0.3510}{0.653} \times 100 = 54$$

Reporting Results

It is recommended that each laboratory establish an expected reference range characteristic of the local population.
Positive (immune) = ≥15% of calibrator
Negative (nonimmune) = <15% of calibrator

Procedure Notes

Absorbance values will vary with temperature of room and incubation time. The absorbance value of the reagent blank when read against water at 405 nm should be less than 0.4 using a microplate reader or less than 0.09 using a spectrophotometer with a 1-cm lightpath. The absorbance value of the calibrator should be greater than or equal to 0.5 using a microplate reader when the assay is performed at 22° C.

Specimens giving absorbance values above that of the calibrator should be diluted appropriately with sample diluent and reassayed. The obtained value should be multiplied by the dilution factor.

Sources of Error

Inappropriately collected specimens can fail to detect IgG antibodies.

Clinical Applications

Determination of the presence of IgG antibodies establishes the immune status of a patient.

Limitations

The results obtained with the assay should serve only as an aid to diagnosis and should not be interpreted as diagnostic.

References

Horvath LM, LeBar WD: A comparison of methods for the determination of rubella antibody, *Am Clin Products Rev.* April 1987, pp 18-19.
Skendzel LP: New guidelines and standards for rubella antibody testing from NCCLS and CAP, *Lab Med* 18(7):461, 1987.
SIA Rubella Product Brochure, St Louis, MO 1988, Sigma Chemical Co.

Case Study

History and Physical Examination

A 20-year-old college junior comes to the student health office because she has been exposed to rubella during a recent outbreak at the college. She has been immunized as a child.

Laboratory Data

Hemagglutination inhibition test for rubella: negative
Pregnancy test: positive
Ultrasonography shows the fetus is in the eighth week of development.

Questions and Discussion

1. Is this woman susceptible to rubella infection?
   Yes, this woman is susceptible to rubella. She has no serologic evidence of antibody formation in response to viral antigen stimulation. The only proof of

immunity is a positive serologic screening test for rubella antibody. History of rubella infection, even if verified by a physician, is not acceptable evidence of immunity.

In case of a negative result, the hemagglutination inhibition test should be repeated in 3 weeks. If the antibody or HA titer has risen, infection has occurred.

2. Is the fetus at risk of a congenital defect?

Brief exposure to a person with rubella infection will not always mean that the infection will be transmitted. However, rubella infections in pregnant women, especially those infected in their first trimester of pregnancy, can have devastating effects on the fetus. In utero infection can result in fetal death or manifestation of rubella syndrome. This syndrome represents a spectrum of congenital defects. Approximately 10% to 20% of newborn infants infected in utero fail to survive past the first 18 months of life.

The point in the gestation cycle at which maternal rubella infection occurs greatly influences the severity of congenital rubella syndrome, and the extent of congenital anomalies varies from one infant to another. Some infants manifest nearly all the defects associated with rubella, whereas others exhibit few, if any, consequences of infection. Clinical evidence of congenital rubella infection may not be recognized for months, or even years, after birth.

Rubella syndrome encompasses a number of congenital anomalies. In addition to stillbirth, fetal abnormalities associated with maternal rubella infection include encephalitis, hepatomegaly, bone defects, mental retardation, cataracts, thrombocytopenic purpura, cardiovascular defects, splenomegaly, and microcephaly. Severely afflicted children are likely to have multiple defects in different organ systems. In neonates with congenital rubella syndrome, low birth weight and failure to thrive are common.

3. Is there any treatment for the infection?

Acyclovir, a commonly used antiviral medication that inhibits DNA synthesis, has no effect on rubella virus because rubella is an RNA virus. In addition, human immune serum globulin may hide infection without protecting the fetus. It should not be given unless it is known at the outset that the mother will refuse abortion even if infection occurs. In this circumstance, human immune serum globulin probably offers some protection against infection of the fetus.

Rubella vaccination is not effective if transmission has occurred because then it is too late to prevent natural infection from the contact. The live vaccine virus theoretically could infect the fetus and cause congenital anomalies, but this situation is infrequent. In addition, inadvertent vaccination during pregnancy does not necessitate the termination of pregnancy.

Rubella immunity develops in almost all children who have had congenital rubella. In late childhood, however, about one third of these patients lose anti-

body and become susceptible to acquired rubella. If acquired rubella occurs, it follows a typically benign course. Children who are afflicted with congenital rubella should be screened for rubella immunity in late childhood and vaccinated, if necessary.

4. What are the immunologic manifestations of infection?

In a patient suffering from a primary rubella infection, the appearance of both IgG and IgM antibodies is associated with the appearance of clinical signs and symptoms. IgM antibodies become detectable a few days after the onset of signs and symptoms and reach peak levels at 7 to 10 days. These antibodies persist but rapidly diminish in concentration over the next 4 to 5 weeks, until the antibody is no longer clinically detectable. The presence of IgM antibody in a single specimen suggests that the patient has recently experienced a rubella infection. In most cases, the infection probably occurred within the preceding month.

Production of IgG is also associated with the appearance of clinical signs and symptoms. Antibody levels increase rapidly for the next 7 to 21 days, then level off or even decrease in strength. IgG antibodies, however, remain present and protective indefinitely. Detection of IgG antibody is a useful indicator of rubella infection only in cases where blood specimens are drawn several weeks apart (during the acute and convalescent periods). Optimum timing for paired testing for the diagnosis of a recent infection is 2 or more weeks apart, with the first (acute) specimen taken before or at the time signs and symptoms appear, or within 2 weeks of exposure.

Paired specimen testing may demonstrate that the antibody levels are the same. In these cases, the patient was either previously immunized or the acute sample was taken after the antibody had already reached maximum levels. Demonstration of an unequivocal increase in IgG antibody concentration between specimens taken during the acute and convalescent periods suggests one of two possibilities: either a recent primary infection or a secondary (anamnestic) antibody response to rubella in an immune individual. In cases of an anamnestic response, IgM antibodies are not demonstrable, but IgG production begins quickly. No other signs or symptoms of disease are exhibited.

If both IgM and IgG test results are negative, the patient has never suffered from rubella infection or been vaccinated. Such patients are susceptible to infection. If no IgM is demonstrable but IgG is present in paired specimens, the patient is immune. In evaluation of the immune status of patients, IgG antibodies present in a dilution of 1:8 or greater indicate past infection with rubella virus and clinical protection against future rubella infection. The clinical significance of lower levels is not currently known. Titers of 1:16, 1:64, 1:512 or greater may be found in both acute and past infections; however, to diagnose acute infections would require an IgM antibody titer on the same specimen or a paired specimen comparison. It should be noted that IgM also appears after vaccination for a transient period.

Because IgG antibody is capable of crossing the placental barrier, there is no way of distinguishing between IgG antibody of fetal origin and IgG antibody of maternal origin in a neonatal blood specimen. By contrast, testing for IgM antibody is invaluable in the diagnosis of congenital rubella syndrome in the neonate. IgM does not cross an intact placental barrier; therefore, demonstration of IgM in a single neonatal specimen is diagnostic of congenital rubella syndrome. In the newborn, serologic confirmation of rubella infection can be made by testing for IgM antibody for at least the first 6 months of life. This is especially useful in instances where clinical evidence of congenital rubella is slow in emerging or is of uncertain origin.

Diagnosis
Rubella

CHAPTER HIGHLIGHTS

Acquired rubella, also know as German or 3-day measles, is caused by an enveloped, single-stranded RNA virus of the Togaviridae family. Because the virus is endemic to humans, the disease is highly contagious and transmitted through respiratory secretions. Contracting the infection or vaccinating against rubella are the only routes to developing immunity. It is critical, however, to continue to determine the rubella immune status of women of childbearing age and to vaccinate those who are not immune. A diagnosis of acquired rubella is not based solely on clinical manifestation. The signs and symptoms of rubella vary widely from person to person and may not be recognized in some cases. Although rubella infection is usually a mild, self-limiting disease with only rare complications in children and adults, rubella infections in pregnant women, especially those infected in their first trimester of pregnancy, can have devastating effects on the fetus. In utero infection can result in fetal death or manifestation of rubella syndrome. This syndrome represents a spectrum of congenital defects.

In a patient suffering from a primary rubella infection, the appearance of both IgG and IgM antibodies is associated with the appearance of clinical signs and symptoms when present. IgM antibodies become detectable a few days after the onset of signs and symptoms and reach peak levels at 7 to 10 days. These antibodies persist but rapidly diminish in concentration over the next 4 to 5 weeks until antibody is no longer clinically detectable. The presence of IgM antibody in a single specimen suggests that the patient has recently experienced a rubella infection. Demonstration of an unequivocal increase in IgG antibody concentration between the acute and convalescent specimens is suggestive of either a recent primary infection or an anamnestic antibody response to rubella in an immune individual. If both IgM and IgG test results are negative, the patient has never suffered from rubella infection or been vaccinated. Such patients are susceptible to infection. If no IgM is demonstrable but IgG is present in paired specimens, the patient is immune.

Testing for IgM antibody is invaluable in the diagnosis of congenital rubella syndrome in the neonate. IgM does not cross an intact placental barrier; therefore demonstration of IgM in a single neonatal specimen is diagnostic of congenital rubella syndrome. In the newborn, serologic confirmation of rubella infection can be made by testing for IgM antibody for at least the first 6 months of life. This is especially useful in instances where clinical evidence of congenital rubella is slow in emerging or is of uncertain origin.

Historically, HAI antibody testing has been the most frequently used method of screening for the presence of rubella antibodies. Within the past few years, the HAI test has been challenged by a number of assays that are more convenient as the screening method of choice for the determination of rubella immune (IgG) status. In some cases, such as in pregnant women, it also may be necessary to determine if a recent infection has been experienced.

Despite wide acceptance and use of these other assays, HAI testing continues to be the reference method for detection and quantitation of rubella antibody. Latex procedures provide more rapid and convenient alternative to HAI. If more quantitative results are desired, EIA and FIA appear to be as reliable as HAI. Widespread use of EIA for assessment of immune status (IgG) and recent infection (IgM) should soon result in simplification of rubella serology. EIA can be used to measure total antibody, IgG, or IgM. PHA methods are not licensed for serodiagnosis of recent rubella infection. PHA is faster and less complex than HAI. In PHA, erythrocytes are coated with rubella antigen. In the presence of rubella antibody, agglutination occurs.

REVIEW QUESTIONS

1. All of the following groups of individuals should receive rubella vaccinations except:
   A. school-age children
   B. women of childbearing age
   C. pregnant women
   D. health care personnel

2. The greatest risk of the manifestation of anomalies in maternal rubella is _____ of gestation.
   A. during the first month
   B. during the first trimester
   C. during the third month
   D. during the fourth or fifth month

3. In a patient suffering from a primary rubella infection, the appearance of _____ antibodies is associated with the clinical signs and symptoms when present.
   A. IgG
   B. IgM
   C. IgD
   D. both A and B

4. Testing for _____ antibody is invaluable in the diagnosis of congenital rubella syndrome.
   A. IgM
   B. IgG
   C. IgD
   D. IgE

5. The reference method for detection and quantitation of rubella antibody is:
   A. latex agglutination
   B. hemagglutination inhibition
   C. passive hemagglutination
   D. enzyme immunoassay

6. Before the licensing of rubella vaccine in the United States in 1969, epidemics occurred at _____ year intervals.
   A. 2-3
   B. 5-7
   C. 6-9
   D. 10-20

7. Acute rubella infection lasts from _____ days.
   A. 1-2
   B. 2-4
   C. 3-5
   D. 7-10

8. IgM antibodies to rubella virus reach peak levels at _____ days.
   A. 2-4
   B. 3-5
   C. 5-7
   D. 7-10

9. IgG antibodies to rubella virus increase rapidly for _____ days after the acquisition of infection.
   A. 2-8
   B. 3-10
   C. 5-15
   D. 7-21

Questions 10-15. Indicate "yes" answers with the letter "A," and "no" answers with the letter "B."

Diagnostic Tests for Immune Status/Serodiagnosis

Method	Immunity	Serodiagnosis
Hemagglutination	10. _____	Yes
Passive hemagglutination	Yes	11. _____
FIA	Yes	Yes
Latex agglutination	12. _____	13. _____
Radioimmunoassay	14. _____	15. _____
EIA-IgM	No	Yes
EIA-IgG	Yes	Yes

16. What percentage of serologically confirmed cases of maternal infection occur before 11 weeks of gestation?
   A. 11%
   B. 24%
   C. 33%
   D. 90%

BIBLIOGRAPHY

Bellamy K et al: IgM antibody capture enzyme linked immunosorbent assay for detecting rubella specific IgM, *J Clin Pathol* 38:1150-1154, 1985.

Chernesky MA, Mahoney JB: Rubella virus. In Rose NR, Friedman H, Fahey HJL, editors: *Manual of clinical laboratory immunology,* ed 3, Washington, DC, 1986, American Society of Microbiology.

Enders G, Knotek F, Pacher U: Comparison of various serological methods and diagnostic kits for the detection of acute, recent, and previous rubella infection, vaccination, and congenital infections, *J Med Virol* 16:219-232, 1985.

Fennes FJ, White DO: *Medical virology,* ed 2, New York, 1976, Academic Press.

Herrmann KL: Rubella virus. In Lennette EH et al, editors: *Manual of clinical microbiology,* ed 4, Washington, DC, 1985, American Society of Microbiology.

Horvath LM, LeBar WD: A comparison of methods for the determination of rubella antibody, *Am Clin Products Rev,* April 1987, pp 18-19.

Howson CP, Fineberg HV: Adverse events following pertussis and rubella vaccines, *JAMA* 267(3):392-396, 1992.

Kurtz JB, Anderson MJ: Cross-reactions in rubella and parvovirus specific IgM tests, *Lancet* 2:1356, 1985.

MMWR: Measles—United States, 1988, *JAMA* 262:13, 1989.

MMWR: Measles outbreak—Chicago, 1989, *JAMA* 262:12, 1989.

Morgan-Capner P, Tedder RS, Mace JE: Reactivity for rubella-specific IgM in sera from patients with infectious mononucleosis, *Lancet* 1:589, 1983.

Sever JL: *Laboratory advances in rubella diagnosis,* North Chicago, Ill, 1983, Abbott Laboratories.

Skendzel LP: New guidelines and standards for rubella antibody testing from NCCLS and CAP, *Lab Med* 18(7):461-462, 1987.

Chapter 22

Acquired Immunodeficiency Syndrome

LEARNING OBJECTIVES

At the conclusion of this chapter, the reader should be able to:
- Describe the etiology and viral characteristics of human immunodeficiency virus (HIV-1).
- Explain the epidemiology including modes of transmission and prevention of HIV-1.
- Discuss the signs and symptoms of various stages and the classification of HIV infection.
- Describe the immunologic manifestations and cellular abnormalities of HIV-1 infection.
- Explain the serologic markers and diagnostic evaluation of HIV.
- Analyze a representative HIV-1 case study.

ETIOLOGY

Introduction

Human immunodeficiency virus (HIV-1) is the predominant virus responsible for acquired immunodeficiency syndrome (AIDS).

In 1983 researchers at the Pasteur Institute in Paris isolated a retrovirus, lymphadenopathy-associated virus (LAV), from a homosexual man with lymphadenopathy. Concur-rently, an American research team headed by Dr. Robert Gallo isolated the same class of virus, which they labeled human T-lymphotropic retrovirus (HTLV) type III. In 1984, the Gallo team was able to demonstrate conclusively through virologic and epidemiologic evidence that HTLV-III was the cause of AIDS. When it was demonstrated that LAV and HTLV-III were the same virus, an international commission changed both names of the virus to HIV to eliminate confusion caused by the two names and to acknowledge that the virus is the cause of AIDS.

Viral Characteristics

Viral Structure

Human immunodeficiency virus is a member of the family Retroviridae, a type D retrovirus that belongs to the lentivirus subfamily. Included in this family are oncoviruses (e.g., HTLV-I and –II) that primarily induce proliferation of infected cells and formation of tumors. Since the discovery of this virus, much has been learned about the impact of the virus on human cells. Two distinct HIV viruses, types 1 and 2 (HIV-1 and HIV-2) cause AIDS. HIV-1 is divided into nine subtypes, Group M (subtypes A-H), Group N, and Group O; HIV-2 is divided into two subtypes (Groups A and B).

HIV-1 virus is composed of a lipid membrane, structural proteins, and glycoproteins that protrude. The viral genome consists of three important structural components: pol, gag, and env. These components code for various products (Table 22-1). Long terminal redundancies border these three components. HIV-2 has a different envelope and slightly different core proteins.

HIV-infected cells can be examined with an electron microscope. The virus may appear as buds of the cell membrane particles. The virion has a double membrane envelope and electron-dense laminar crescent or semicircular cores. An intermediate, less electron-dense layer lies between the envelope and core. In a free extracellular mature virion, the core appears as a bar-shaped nucleoid structure in cross section. This structure appears circular and is frequently located eccentrically. It is composed of structural proteins and glycoproteins that occupy the core and envelope regions of the particle. The virion structure consists of knoblike structures composed of a protein called gp120, which is anchored to another protein called gp41. Each knob includes three sets of these protein molecules. The core of the virus includes a protein called p25 or p24. After human exposure, these viral components and others may induce an antibody response important in serodiagnosis (Table 22-2). Retroviruses contain a single positive-stranded RNA with the virus' genetic information and a special enzyme called reverse transcriptase in their core. Reverse transcriptase enables the virus to convert viral RNA into DNA. This reverses the normal process of transcription where DNA is converted to RNA, hence the term *retrovirus.*

The genomes of all known retroviruses are organized in a similar way. In the provirus, which is formed when complementary DNA synthesis is completed from the retroviral RNA template, viral core and envelope proteins and the enzyme reverse transcriptase are encoded by the gag, env, and pol genes, respectively, whereas viral gene expression is regulated by tat, trs, sor, and 3'orf gene products. The gag gene encodes a

polyprotein found at high levels in infected cells and is subsequently cleaved to form p17 and p24, both of which are viral particle associated. The pol gene encodes for reverse transcriptase, endonuclease, and protease activities. The sor gene stands for small open-reading frame. The sor gene product is a protein that induces antibody production in the natural course of infection. The tat gene represents a small open-reading frame; the protein product has not been identified to date.

The env gene encodes for a polyprotein that contains numerous glycosylation sites. The glycoprotein form, gp160, is found on infected cells but is deficient on viral particles. gp160, however, gives rise to two glycoproteins, gp120 and gp41, which are associated with the viral envelope. The encoding genes and gene products, or antigens, of the AIDS virus that may induce an antibody response after human exposure are presented in Table 22-3. Long terminal redundancies, or LTRs, which exist at each end of the proviral genome, play an important role in the control of viral gene expression and the integration of the provirus into the DNA of the hosts. Although a structural similarity exists between the genomes of HIV-1 and HIV-2 (HTLV-IV), the nucleotide sequence homology is limited. There is a nucleotide sequence homology of only 60% between the gag genes and 30% to 40% between the remainder of the genes of HIV-1 and HIV-2.

TABLE 22-2   HIV Proteins of Serodiagnostic Importance

Virus	Protein	Location	Gene
HIV-1	gp41	Envelope (transmembrane protein)	env
	gp160/120	Envelope (external protein)	env
	p24	Core (major structural protein)	gag
HIV-2	gp34	Envelope (transmembrane protein)	env
	gp140	Envelope (external protein)	env
	P26	Core (major structural protein)	gag

TABLE 22-3   Encoding Genes and Antigens of AIDS Virus

Encoding Gene	Antigen
gag	p55
gag	p24
gag	p17
pol	p66
pol	p51
sor	p24
env	gp160
env	gp120
env	gp41
3'orf	p27

TABLE 22-1   Viral Genome Components

Component	Product
pol	Produces DNA polymerase / Produces endonuclease
gag	Codes for p24 and for proteins, including p17, p9, and p7
env	Codes for two glycoproteins: gp41, gp120

Viral Replication

The replication of HIV is complicated and involves several steps (Box 22-1). The HIV life cycle is that of a retrovirus. Retroviruses are so named because they reverse the normal flow of genetic information. In body cells the genetic material is DNA. When genes are expressed, DNA is first transcribed into messenger RNA (mRNA), which then serves as the template for the production of proteins. The genes of a retrovirus are encoded in RNA; before they can be expressed, the RNA must be converted into DNA. Only then are the viral genes transcribed and translated into proteins in the usual sequence.

Target Cells. The infectious process begins (Figure 22-1) when the gp120 protein on the viral envelope binds to the protein receptor, called CD4, located on the surface of a target cell. HIV-1 has a marked preference for the CD4+ subset of T lymphocytes. In addition to T lymphocytes, macrophages, peripheral blood monocytes, and cells in the lymph nodes, skin, and other organs also express measurable amounts of CD4 and can be infected by HIV-1. About 5% of the B lymphocytes may express CD4 and be susceptible to HIV-1 infection. Macrophages may play an important role in spreading HIV infection in the body, both to other cells and the target organs of HIV. Monocytes-macrophages enable HIV-1 to enter the immune-protected domain of the central nervous system—the brain, the spinal cord, and the remainder of the nervous system.

Fusion of the virus to the membrane of a host cell enables the viral RNA and reverse transcriptase to invade the cytoplasm of the cell. But CD4 receptors are not sufficient for HIV envelope fusion with the T4 cell membrane or for HIV penetration or entry into the interior of the cell. Chemokine coreceptors to CD4, which HIV uses to enter a host cell after binding to it, have been identified. β-Chemokines receptors are cell-surface proteins that bind small peptides. They are clsssified into three groups, depending on the location of the amino acid cysteine (C) in the peptide. These chemokine receptors are identified by the individual chemokine(s) that binds to them. In essence, the reference to a specific chemokine(s) also identifies its receptor. The first example of a coreceptor was CXCKR-4 (FUSIN R-4). Other coreceptors include CCKR-2 (R-2), CCKR-3 (R-3) and CC-CKR-5 (R-5). Current research involves exploring ways to block or fill the chemokine receptors with a harmless molecule, thus blocking the binding site of the HIV on the host cell.

Although some cells do not produce detectable amounts of CD4, they do contain low levels of messenger RNA encoding the CD4 protein, which indicates that they do produce

---

Box 22-1   Summary of HIV-1 Life Cycle

1. The virus attaches to the CD4 membrane receptor and sheds its protein coat, exposing its RNA core.
2. Reverse transcriptase converts viral RNA into proviral DNA.
3. The proviral DNA is integrated into the genome (genetic complement of the host cell).
4. New virus particles are produced as the result of normal cellular activities of transcription and translation. Once the viral genome is integrated into host cell DNA, the potential for viral production always exists, and the viral infection of new cells can continue.
5. New particles bud from the cell membrane.

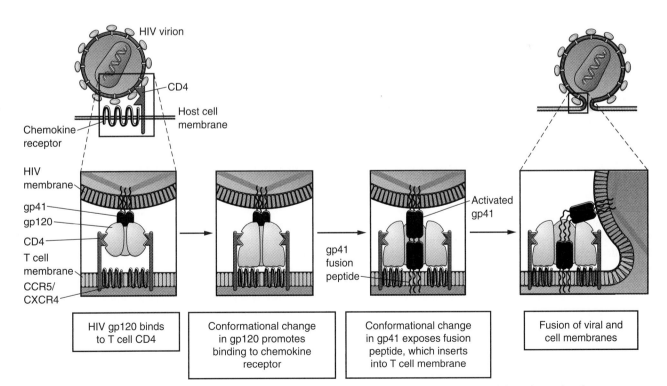

Figure 22-1   Mechanisms of HIV entry into a cell. In the model, depicted sequential conformational changes in gp120 and gp41 promote fusion of the HIV-1 and host cell membranes. The fusion peptide of activated gp41 contains hydrophobic amino acid residues that promote insertion into the host cell plasma membrane lipid bilayer. (Redrawn from Abbas AK, Lichtman AH, Pober JS: *Cellular and molecular immunology,* ed 4, Philadelphia, 2000, WB Saunders.)

some CD4. Because these cells can be infected by HIV in culture, the expression of only a very small amount of CD4 or an alternate receptor molecule may be necessary for HIV infection to take place. These cell types include certain cells of the brain, glial cells, a variety of malignant brain tumor cells, and some cells derived from cancers of the bowel. In addition, cells of the gastrointestinal system do not produce appreciable amounts of CD4, but gut cells called chromaffin cells do sometimes appear to be infected by HIV in vivo.

Replication. Retroviruses carry a single, positive-stranded RNA and use a special enzyme, called reverse transcriptase, to convert viral RNA into DNA. This reverses the normal process of transcription where DNA is converted to RNA—hence, the term *retrovirus.*

The life-cycle of the HIV-1 virus consists of five phases:
- The virus attaches and penetrates target cells such as lymphocytes that express the CD4+ receptor. After penetration, the virus loses its protein coat, exposing the RNA core.
- Reverse transcriptase converts viral RNA into proviral DNA.
- The proviral DNA is integrated into the genome (genetic complement of the host cell).
- New virus particles are produced as the result of normal cellular activities of transcription and translation.
- These new particles bud from the cell membrane. Once the viral genome is integrated into host cell DNA, the potential for viral production always exists and the viral infection of new cells can continue.

Immunologic activation of T-helper cells latently infected with HIV induces the production of multiple viral particles leading to cell death. The extensive destruction of T cells leads to the gradual depletion of CD4 lymphocytes. Progressive defects in the immune system include a severe B-cell failure, defects in monocyte function, and defects in granulocyte function.

EPIDEMIOLOGY

Incidence

Twenty years after the first clinical evidence of AIDS was reported, it has become the most devastating disease humankind has ever faced. HIV/AIDS is now the leading cause of death in sub-Saharan Africa. Worldwide, it is the fourth leading cause of death.

According to the Joint United Nations Program on HIV/AIDS, as of the end of 2002, the following trends of the worldwide epidemic (or pandemic) of HIV are evident:
- Today, 42 million people are estimated to be living with HIV/AIDS. Of these, 38.6 million are adults, 19.2 million are women, and 3.2 million are children less than 15 years old.
- During 2002 AIDS caused the deaths of an estimated 3.1 million people, including 1.2 million women and 610,000 children less than 15 years old.
- Women are becoming increasingly affected by HIV. Approximately 50%, or 19.2 million, of the 38.6 million adults living with HIV or AIDS worldwide are women.
- The overwhelming majority of people with HIV—approximately 95% of the global total—now live in the developing world.

The cumulative total of cases of AIDS reported to the Centers for Disease Control and Prevention (CDC) in 2001 is 24,855; for 2000 the cumulative total was 36,087. The total number of AIDS cases in the United States reported to CDC from 1982 to December 2001 was 816,149. Adult and adolescent AIDS cases total 807,075, with five times as many cases in males than in females. The percentage of AIDS cases in women has risen in recent years and is expected to continue to increase over the next several years. The majority of HIV-infected women are between 18 and 40 years old. In recent years throughout the United States, women of color (e.g., African-American women and women of Hispanic background) are disproportionately affected (>85%) by HIV. Through the same time period, 9,074 AIDS cases were reported in children under age 13 years. Total deaths of persons reported in the United States with AIDS are 467,910, including 5,257 children less than 15 years old, and 388 persons whose age at death is unknown.

Classification System

The new (Box 22-2) revised definition of HIV infection, which applies to any HIV (i.e., HIV-1 or HIV-2), incorporates the reporting criteria for HIV infection and AIDS into a single case definition. The revised criteria for HIV infection update the definition of HIV infection implemented in 1993; the revised HIV criteria apply to AIDS-defining conditions for adults and children, which require laboratory evidence of HIV.

Infectious Patterns

AIDS is present worldwide. In some countries (e.g., sub-Sahara Africa, Thailand, and India) >90% of HIV-1 infections are acquired through heterosexual transmission in contrast with 10% or less in the United States and Western Europe. Subtypes A, C, and D predominate in Africa; subtypes E and B are common in Thailand; and subtype B predominates in the United States and Western Europe. HIV-1 and HIV-2 are distinct but related viruses. The two viruses both can cause AIDS. HIV-1 is responsible for the main AIDS epidemic. The discovery of HIV-2 suggests that other HIVs may also exist.

Three infection patterns of HIV virus have been traced worldwide. Pattern 1 is found in North and South America, Western Europe, Scandinavia, Australia, and New Zealand. In these countries it is primarily a disease of homosexuals and intravenous (IV) drug abusers. The male to female ratio of reported AIDS cases in pattern 1 areas ranges from 10:1 to 15:1. Pattern 2 is found in Africa, the Caribbean, and some areas of South America. In the pattern 2 areas AIDS is primarily a heterosexual disease; the number of infected females and males is approximately equal. Pattern 3 is typically demonstrated in Eastern Europe, North Africa, the Middle East, Asia, and the Pacific, excluding Australia and New Zealand. In the pattern 3 areas relatively few cases of AIDS have been identified; most of the affected individuals have had contact with pattern 1 or pattern 2 countries.

HIV-2

In 1986 a second virus causing the AIDS, HIV-2, was discovered and is endemic in parts of West Africa. Epidemiologic data indicate that the prevalence of HIV-2 infections in

The revised definition of HIV infection, which applies to any HIV (e.g., HIV-1 or HIV-2), incorporates the reporting criteria for HIV infection and AIDS into a single case definition.

I. In adults, adolescents, or children ≥18 months,* a reportable case of HIV infection must meet at least one of the following criteria:

LABORATORY CRITERIA

Positive result on a screening test for HIV antibody (e.g., repeatedly reactive enzyme immunoassay), followed by a positive result on a confirmatory (sensitive and more specific) test for HIV antibody (e.g., Western blot or immunofluorescence antibody test)

OR

Positive result or report of a detectable quantity on any of the following HIV virologic (nonantibody) tests:

HIV nucleic acid (DNA or RNA) detection (e.g., DNA PCR or plasma HIV-1 RNA)†

HIV p24 antigen test, including neutralization assay

HIV isolation (viral culture)

OR

Clinical or other criteria (if the above laboratory criteria are not met)

Diagnosis of HIV infection, based on the laboratory criteria above, that is documented in a medical record by a physician

OR

Conditions that meet criteria included in the case definition for AIDS (17-19)

II. In a child less than 18 months old, a reportable case of HIV infection must meet at least one of the following criteria:

LABORATORY CRITERIA

Definitive

Positive results on two separate specimens (excluding cord blood) using one or more of the following HIV virologic (nonantibody) tests:

HIV nucleic acid (DNA or RNA) detection

HIV p24 antigen test, including neutralization assay, in a child greater than or equal to 1 month of age

HIV isolation (viral culture)

OR

Presumptive

A child who does not meet the criteria for definitive HIV infection but who has:

Positive results on only one specimen (excluding cord blood) using the above HIV virologic tests and no subsequent negative HIV virologic or negative HIV antibody tests

OR

Clinical or other criteria (if the above definitive or presumptive laboratory criteria are not met)

Diagnosis of HIV infection, based on the laboratory criteria above, that is documented in a medical record by a physician

OR

Conditions that meet criteria included in the 1987 pediatric surveillance case definition for AIDS

III. A child less than 18 months old born to an HIV-infected mother will be categorized for surveillance purposes as "not infected with HIV" if the child does not meet the criteria for HIV infection but meets the following criteria:

LABORATORY CRITERIA

Definitive

At least two negative HIV antibody tests from separate specimens obtained at ≥6 months old

OR

At least two negative HIV virologic tests‡ from separate specimens, both of which were performed at ≥1 month old and one of which was performed at ≥4 months old

AND

No other laboratory or clinical evidence of HIV infection (i.e., has not had any positive virologic tests, if performed, and has not had an AIDS-defining condition)

OR

Presumptive

A child who does not meet the above criteria for definitive "not infected" status but who has:

One negative EIA HIV antibody test performed at ≥6 months old and NO positive HIV virologic tests, if performed

OR

One negative HIV virologic test‡ performed at ≥4 months old and NO positive HIV virologic tests, if performed

OR

One positive HIV virologic test with at least two subsequent negative virologic tests,§ at least one of which is ≥4 months old; or negative HIV antibody test results, at least one of which is ≥6 months old

AND

No other laboratory or clinical evidence of HIV infection (i.e., has not had any positive virologic tests, if performed, and has not had an AIDS-defining condition).

OR

Clinical or other criteria (if the above definitive or presumptive laboratory criteria are not met)

Determined by a physician to be "not infected," and a physician has noted the results of the preceding HIV diagnostic tests in the medical record

AND

NO other laboratory or clinical evidence of HIV infection (i.e., has not had any positive virologic tests, if performed, and has not had an AIDS-defining condition)

IV. A child less than 18 months old born to an HIV-infected mother will be categorized as having perinatal exposure to HIV infection if the child does not meet the criteria for HIV infection (II) or the criteria for "not infected with HIV" (III).

From Centers for Disease Control and Prevention: MMWR recommendations and reports, 48 (RR13):29-31, Dec. 10, 1999.

* Children ≥18 months old but <13 years old are categorized as "not infected with HIV" if they meet the criteria in III.

†In adults, adolescents, and children infected by other than perinatal exposure, plasma viral RNA nucleic acid tests should NOT be used in lieu of licensed HIV screening tests (e.g., repeatedly reactive enzyme immunoassay). In addition, a negative (i.e., undetectable) plasma HIV-1 RNA test result does not rule out the diagnosis of HIV infection.

‡Draft revised surveillance criteria for HIV infection were approved and recommended by the membership of the Council of State and Territorial Epidemiologists at the 1998 annual meeting.

§HIV nucleic acid (DNA or RNA) detection tests are the virologic methods of choice to exclude infection in children less than 18 months old. Although HIV culture can be used for this purpose, it is more complex and expensive to perform and is less well standardized than nucleic acid detection tests. The use of p24 antigen testing to exclude infection in children less than 18 months old is not recommended because of its lack of sensitivity.

persons in the United States is extremely low (in the beginning of the year 2003, a total of 94 HIV-2 infected persons had been reported to the CDC).

The primary mode of transmission of HIV-2 is heterosexual contact, although HIV-2 infection has been reported in Europe in homosexual men, injecting drug users, transfusion recipients, and men with hemophilia.

Infection with HIV-2 can cause immunosuppression and the development of AIDS. The period between infection and disease may be longer and milder for persons with HIV-2 than for those with HIV-1. HIV-2 appears to be less harmful (cytopathic) to the cells of the immune system, and it reproduces more slowly than HIV-1. Compared with persons infected with HIV-1, those with HIV-2 are less infectious early in the course of infection. As the disease advances, HIV-2 infectivity seems to increase compared to HIV-1, but the duration of this increased infectivity is shorter.

In 1990 the U.S. Food and Drug Administration (FDA) licensed an enzyme immunoassay (EIA) test kit for detection of antibodies to HIV-2 in human serum or plasma. An additional combination procedure for screening for HIV-1/-2 was licensed in September 1991. However, the CDC does not recommend routine HIV-2 testing at HIV counseling and test sites or in settings other than blood centers. If HIV testing is to be performed, tests for antibodies to both HIV-1 and HIV-2 should be obtained if demographic or behavioral information suggests that HIV-2 infection might be present. Diagnosis of HIV-2 requires more specific supplementary tests, such as an HIV-2 Western blot assay.

Modes of Transmission

HIV enters the body in one of two ways. It can be transmitted as the virus itself or as a cell associated with HIV. The virus is held within leukocytes and carried in fluid (e.g., blood or semen) to the body of another person. In some cases the mode of viral transmission is associated with the viral subtype. HIV-1, subtype E, easily infects the Langerhans' cells, which are abundant in the cervical mucosa. In contrast, HIV-1 subtypes E and C are associated with heterosexual sex. Transmission of HIV is believed to be restricted to intimate contact with body fluids from an infected person; casual contact with infected persons has not been documented as a mode of transmission. Although the mode of transmission is considered to be predominantly sexual, the virus can be transmitted through contact with infected blood through blood transfusion (if the blood has not been screened for HIV) or by HIV-contaminated needles. Posttransfusion AIDS is now well documented from both cellular blood components and cell-free preparations such as unheated factor VIII concentrate and plasma. Although injuries occur in professional football competitions, bleeding injuries, especially lacerations, occur infrequently. The estimated risk for HIV transmission during such competition is considered to be extremely remote.

Babies born to HIV-infected women may become infected before or during birth or through breastfeeding after birth. The risk of HIV infection to children born to women with HIV is 20% to 30%. HIV-2 seems to be less transmissible from an infected woman to her fetus or newborn.

In the health care setting workers have been infected with HIV after being stuck with needles containing HIV-infected blood or, less frequently, after infected blood gets into a worker's open cut or a mucous membrane (for example, the eyes or inside of the nose). There has been only one instance of patients being infected by a health care worker in the United States; this involved HIV transmission from one infected dentist to six patients. Investigations have been completed involving more than 22,000 patients of 63 HIV-infected physicians, surgeons, and dentists, and no other cases of this type of transmission have been identified in the United States.

HIV has been isolated from blood, semen, vaginal secretions, saliva, tears, breast milk, cerebrospinal fluid (CSF), amniotic fluid, and urine. Only blood, semen, vaginal secretions, and breast milk have been implicated in the transmission of HIV to date. HIV has been found in saliva and tears in very low quantities from some AIDS patients. It is important to understand that finding a small amount of HIV in a body fluid does not necessarily mean that HIV can be transmitted by that body fluid. HIV has not been recovered from the sweat of HIV-infected persons. Contact with saliva, tears, or sweat has never been shown to result in transmission of HIV.

Sexual transmission, either heterosexual or male-male, is also a well-documented route of transmission. HIV is transmitted by infected cells and not free fluid. Relatively low levels of infective HIV particles are present in body fluids. However, genital secretion can contain substantial numbers of virus-infected cells. Up to 5% of white cells in seminal fluid can be HIV infected; approximately 10^6 mononuclear cells are found in seminal fluid. Seropositive individuals do not necessarily transmit the disease if their genital fluids do not contain a large number of infected cells.

Most transmission of HIV to organ/tissue recipients occurred before 1985, before the implementation of donor screening recommendations. Reports of transmission from screened, HIV-antibody negative organ or tissue donors have been rare. By early 2003 15 women were reported to have been infected through the use of anonymous donor sperm for artificial insemination. There are no U.S. federal regulations regarding HIV testing, and only a handful of states (California, Illinois, Ohio, Michigan, and New York) require HIV testing of semen donors.

Viral transmission can result from contact with inanimate objects, such as work surfaces or equipment recently contaminated with infected blood or certain body fluids, if the virus is transferred to broken skin or mucous membranes by hand contact.

SIGNS AND SYMPTOMS

It is not known when an exposed individual becomes infectious or how soon infected individuals develop serologic markers of infection. Infection with HIV produces a chronic infection with symptoms that range from asymptomatic to the end-stage complications of AIDS.

Typically patients in the early stages of HIV infection are either completely asymptomatic or may show mild, chronic lymphadenopathy. The early phase may last from many months to many years after viral exposure. Although the course of HIV-1 infection may vary somewhat among individual patients, a common pattern of development has been recognized. The newly revised HIV classification system provides uniform and simple criteria for categorizing conditions.

During the early period after primary infection, widespread dissemination of virus occurs and a sharp decrease in the number of CD4+ T cells in peripheral blood is manifested. The early burst of virus in the blood, viremia, is often accompanied by flulike symptoms that can be so severe that those suffering from them may seek help in hospital emergency rooms. An immune response to HIV develops with a concurrent decrease in detectable viremia. It was previously believed that the human immune system could drive the AIDS virus into a latent period that kept it inactive for years. Recently this view has been replaced with a new vision of a virus that is furiously creating copies of itself throughout the course of the disease, even when the patient appears healthy. Even when HIV cannot be detected in the blood (viremia), it infects (in large quantities) lymphatic tissues including the tonsils and lymph nodes throughout the body. The absence of viremia generally lasts until the end stage of the disease.

This phase is followed by a prolonged period of clinical latency (range, 7 to 11 years; median, 10 years). During the period of clinical latency, the patient is usually asymptomatic. Differences in the infecting virus, the genetic makeup of the host, and environmental factors (including concomitant infection) have been suggested as causes of the variation in the duration of clinical latency in persons not receiving antiretroviral therapy. Treatment with inhibitors of viral reverse transcriptase (e.g., zidovudine [Retrovir] and administration of prophylaxis for pneumonia caused by *Pneumocystis carinii*) has increased AIDS-free time in HIV-1 infected persons.

Opportunistic Infections

Since AIDS was first recognized 20 years ago, remarkable progress has been made in improving the quality and duration of life for HIV-infected persons in the industrialized world. During the first decade of the epidemic, this progress occurred because of improved recognition of opportunistic disease processes, improved therapy for acute and chronic complications, and introduction of chemoprophylaxis against key opportunistic pathogens. The second decade of the epidemic has witnessed extraordinary progress in developing highly active antiretroviral therapies (HAART) as well as continuing progress in preventing and treating opportunistic infections. HAART has reduced the incidence of opportunistic infections and extended life. In addition, prophylaxis against specific opportunistic infections continues to provide survival benefits even among persons who are receiving HAART.

The absolute number of CD4 T lymphocytes continues to diminish as the disease progresses. When the number of cells reaches a critically low level (<50 to 100×10^9/L), the risk of opportunistic infection increases. The period of susceptibility to opportunistic processes continues to be accurately indicated by CD4+ T lymphocyte counts for patients who are receiving HAART.

The end stage of AIDS is characterized by the occurrence of neoplasms and/or opportunistic infections (Box 22-3). Opportunistic infections noted with the greatest frequency are: *P. carinii* (Figure 22-2), cytomegalovirus, *Mycobacterium*

Box 22-3	Opportunistic Infections in Immunosuppressed and Immunodeficient Patients

Oral/esophageal candidiasis
Cytomegalovirus
Pneumocystis carinii
Herpes simplex
Entamoeba histolytica
Giardia lamblia
Herpes zoster
Atypical acid-fast bacilli
Shigella
Campylobacter
Cryptococcosis
Adenovirus
Hepatitis
Chlamydia
Salmonella
Syphilis
Anal candidiasis
Dientamoeba fragilis
Blastocystis hominis
Toxoplasmosis

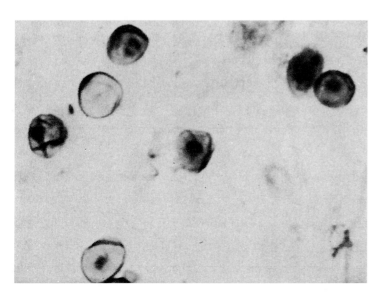

Figure 22-2   *Pneumocystis carinii* from tracheobronchial aspirate; stained with methenamine silver. (From Markell EK, Voge M: *Medical parasitology,* ed 5, Philadelphia, 1981, WB Saunders.)

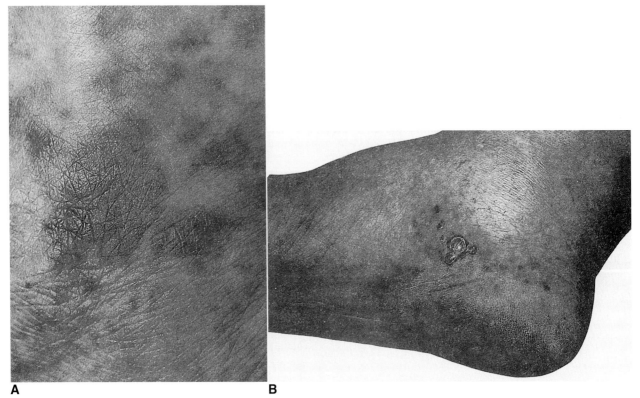

Figure 22-3 Kaposi's sarcoma. **A,** Early lesion consisting of violaceous macules and plaques. **B,** Purple nodules are most commonly seen on the lower legs. (From Habif TP: *Clinical dermatology,* ed 8, St Louis, 1985, Mosby.)

avium-intracellulare, Cryptococcus, Toxoplasma, Mycobacterium tuberculosis, herpes simplex, and *Legionella. Histoplasmosis capsulatum* is being recognized with increasing frequency. The most frequent malignancy observed is an aggressive, invasive variant of Kaposi's sarcoma (KS) (Figure 22-3), discovered in many cases on autopsy. Malignant B-cell lymphomas are being recognized with increasing frequency in patients with AIDS or at high risk for AIDS.

Kaposi's Sarcoma

KS was first described in 1872 by the dermatologist Moritz Kaposi. From the time of its identification until the current prevalence of AIDS, KS remained a rare tumor. Classic KS usually occurs in males. The tumor is usually present with one or more asymptomatic red, purple, or brown patches, plaque, or nodule skin lesions. The disease is often limited to single or multiple lesions usually localized to one or both lower extremities, especially involving the ankle and soles. Classic KS most commonly runs a relatively benign, indolent course for 10 to 15 years or more with slow enlargement of the original tumors and the gradual development of additional lesions. Up to one third of the patients with classic KS develop a second primary malignancy, most often non-Hodgkin's lymphoma. An excess incidence of Hodgkin's disease has been found in HIV-infected homosexual men.

Cryptosporidiosis

Cryptosporidiosis is a disease caused by the parasite *Cryptosporidium parvum.* As late as 1976 this parasite was not thought to cause disease in humans. In 1993 more than 400,000 people in Milwaukee, Wisconsin, became ill after drinking water contaminated with the parasite. In persons who are immunocompromised, cryptosporidiosis can be chronic and severe. The watery diarrhea can be prolonged and debilitating and may be fatal.

Persons at risk of severe cryptosporidiosis include persons with AIDS, persons who have cancer or organ or bone marrow transplants and who are taking drugs that weaken the immune system, and persons who are born with genetically weakened immune systems.

Disease Progression

Although a large enough dose of the right strain of HIV-1 can cause AIDS on its own, cofactors can influence the progression of disease development. Debilitated patients, weakened by a preexisting medical condition before HIV-1 infection, may progress toward AIDS more quickly than others (Figure 22-4). Stimulation of the immune system in response to later infections can also hasten disease progression. Other pathogenic microorganisms such as a herpes virus called human B-cell lymphotropic virus or human herpes virus 6 (HHV-6) can interact with HIV in a way that may increase the severity of HIV infection. HHV-6 is usually easily controlled by the immune system. If HIV compromises the immune system, however, HHV-6 may replicate more freely and become a health threat. The main host of HHV-6 is the B cell, but this virus can also infect T4 cells. If T cells are simultaneously infected by HIV, HHV-6 can stimulate the virus, which further impairs the immune system and promotes disease progression.

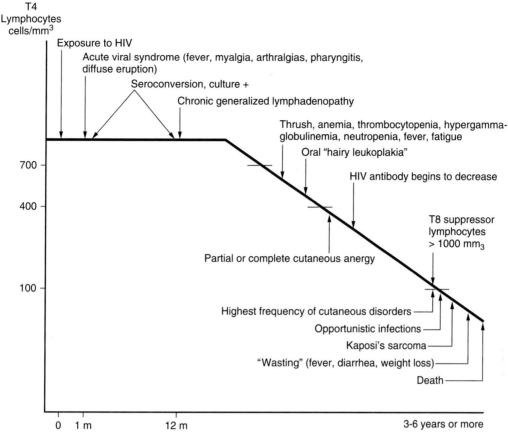

T4
Lymphocytes
cells/mm³

Exposure to HIV

Acute viral syndrome (fever, myalgia, arthralgias, pharyngitis, diffuse eruption)

Seroconversion, culture +

Chronic generalized lymphadenopathy

Thrush, anemia, thrombocytopenia, hypergamma-globulinemia, neutropenia, fever, fatigue

Oral "hairy leukoplakia"

HIV antibody begins to decrease

700

400

T8 suppressor
lymphocytes
> 1000 mm₃

Partial or complete cutaneous anergy

100

Highest frequency of cutaneous disorders

Opportunistic infections

Kaposi's sarcoma

"Wasting" (fever, diarrhea, weight loss)

Death

0   1 m   12 m   3-6 years or more

Figure 22-4   AIDS. Evolution of the disease. (Redrawn from Habif TP: *Clinical dermatology,* ed 2, St Louis, 1990, Mosby.)

The progressive decline of CD4 cells leads to a general decline in immune function and is the primary factor in determining the clinical progression of AIDS. Plasma HIV-1 RNA is a strong, CD4+ T-cell-independent predictor of a rapid progression to AIDS after HIV-1 seroconversion.

Infection with HIV is presently considered to lead to death. When the clinically apparent disease develops, patients usually die within 2 years with current treatment, but some exposed or HIV-1 infected patients never develop AIDS. Although scientists have known since 1986 that CD8 T cells, when stimulated, could release molecules capable of suppressing HIV, the identity of these substances eluded researchers for more than a decade. New research suggests that three large proteins, identified as alpha-defensins-1, -2, -3, could be major contributors to the CD8 antiviral factor that protects some patients against AIDS. In another new study, scientists at the National Institutes of Health have linked HIV-resistance to a different molecule secreted by CD8 T cells, called perforin. More studies related to each category of molecules are needed before either of these theories is confirmed.

Another recent study conducted at the National Institute of Allergy and Infectious Diseases examined variations in a gene called RANTES (*r*egulated-upon-*a*ctivation *n*ormal *T* *e*xpressed and *s*ecreted) in HIV-infected and HIV-resistant individuals. This study searched for changes in a single nucleotide polymorphism (SNP). The results were that one such SNP appears more often in HIV-positive compared to HIV-negative persons. In addition, this particular alteration in-creases the activity of the RANTES gene and is associated with up to twice the risk of HIV infection, but individuals with this SNP who are infected with HIV take about 40% longer to actually develop AIDS.

IMMUNOLOGIC MANIFESTATIONS

Cellular Abnormalities

HIV-1 has a marked preference for CD4+ subset of lymphocytes because the CD4 surface marker protein on these cells serves as a receptor site for the virus. Recent studies have demonstrated that immunologic activation, such as participation in an immune response to HIV-1 or to viruses in other cells, of T helper cells latently infected with HIV-1 induces the production of multiple viral particles leading to cell death. The extensive destruction of T cells leads to the gradual depletion of the CD4 type of lymphocytes. The major phenotypic cell populations affected by AIDS are CD4+ and CD8+ subsets of T lymphocytes. Normally this ratio is 2:1 in heterosexuals and 1.5:1 in homosexuals. A reversal of these subsets is evident in, but not diagnostic of, AIDS. In patients with AIDS it is less than 0.5:1. It is important to note that this results from a marked decrease in the absolute number of circulating helper or CD4 cells, rather than from an absolute increase in suppressor or CD8 cells. This abnormality exists in the lymph nodes and circulating T cells. A diminished CD4 or CD8 ratio (altered lymphocyte subpopulation) can also be seen in individuals with other disorders such as cutaneous T-cell lymphoma, systemic lupus erythematosus, and acute viral infections. The ratio, however, reverts back to normal after recovery from a viral infection in non-AIDS patients.

A decreased lymphocyte proliferative response to soluble antigens and mitogens exists in AIDS. Functional testing reveals a diminished response to pokeweed mitogen. This disease also demonstrates defective natural killer cell activity.

Alterations in Immune System

HIV is fragile, and as the virus particle leaves its host cell, a molecule called gp120 frequently breaks off the outer coat of the virus. gp120 can bind to the CD4 molecules of uninfected cells, and when that complex is recognized by the immune system, these cells can be destroyed. The lysis of infected cells and gp120-bound uninfected cells leads to the gradual depletion of the helper-n-inducer types of lymphocytes. Defects in immunity are related to this T-cell depletion. Progressive defects in the immune system also include a severe B-cell failure and defects in monocyte and granulocyte function.

Although HIV-1 destroys CD4 cells directly and hampers the immune system, this process does not cause the severe immune deficiency seen in AIDS. The severe deficiency can be explained only if the cells are also destroyed by other means. Several indirect mechanisms have been suggested. Infection by HIV can cause infected and uninfected cells to fuse into giant cells called syncytia, which are not functional. Autoimmune responses, in which the immune system attacks the body's own tissues, may also be at work. In addition, HIV-infected cells may send out protein signals that weaken or destroy other cells of the immune system. It is possible that the binding of HIV to a target cell triggers the release of the enzyme protease. Proteases digest proteins; if released in abnormal quantities, they might weaken lymphocytes and other cells and decrease cell survival. The decline in T cells and subsequent alteration of the immune mechanism are the underlying factors in progression of HIV infection.

Serologic Markers

Detection of Core Antigen

After initial infection the body mounts a vigorous immune response against the viremia. Immunologic activities include the production of different types of antibodies against HIV. Some antibodies neutralize it, others prevent it from binding to cells, and others stimulate cytotoxic cells to attack HIV-infected cells.

The time and sequence vary for the appearance and disappearance of antibodies specific for the serologically important antigens of HIV-1 during the course of infection. A "window" period of seronegativity exists from the time of initial infection to 6 or 12 weeks or longer thereafter. Through enzyme immunoassay methods based on defined HIV-1 proteins produced by recombinant DNA methods, antibodies specific for gp41 are detectable for weeks or months before assays specific for p24. The appearance of antibodies specific for p24, however, has been shown in several studies to precede that of anti-gp41 when serum specimens have been tested by Western blot analysis. This discrepancy in the sequence of antibody appearance is believed to be due to the greater sensitivity of the Western blot technique compared to viral lysate-based EIAs used for the detection of anti-p24. gp41 antibodies persist throughout the course of infection. Antibody specific for p24 not only rise to detectable levels after gp41 but can also disappear unpredictably and abruptly.

Increased production of core antigen is believed to be associated with a burst of viral replication and host cell lysis. The disappearance of antibody directed against p24 has been demonstrated to occur concomitantly with an increase in the concentration of core antigen in the serum. This parallel activity may be due to the sequestration of antibody in immune complexes, and the sudden decrease in anti-p24 is considered to be a grave prognostic sign in HIV-1-infected patients.

Antibodies to HIV-1

Antibodies to HIV-1 appear after a lag period of about 6 weeks between the time of infection and a detectable antibody response. Because of this, some virus-positive, antibody-negative individuals would escape initial screening assays.

In addition to a positive HIV antibody test in 85% to 90% of patients, increased antibody titers to viruses—such as cytomegalovirus, Epstein-Barr virus, hepatitis A and B, *Toxoplasma gondii*—and circulating immune (antigen-antibody) complexes can be found. Various other ancillary findings including polyclonal hypergammaglobulinemia, elevated levels of alpha interferon, alpha $(\alpha)_1$ thymosin, and beta microglobulin, as well as reduced levels of interleukin-1 or interleukin-2, have been noted.

Specific intrathecal synthesis of HIV antibody should be assessed simultaneously with an assay for total CSF IgM and for intrathecal synthesis of total IgG, as well as for intrathecal synthesis of IgG specific for an appropriate control organism such as adenovirus. In progressive encephalopathy related to AIDS, an increase in HIV antibody may suggest intrathecal synthesis compared to extrathecal synthesis.

DIAGNOSTIC EVALUATION

HIV infection is established by detecting antibodies to the virus, viral antigens, viral RNA/DNA, or by the "gold standard" viral culture. The standard test is for antibody detection. Laboratory evaluation of asymptomatic HIV-infected patients consists of assessment of cellular and humoral components (Table 22-4).

Screening of blood donors and patients at risk is usually done by serologic methods. In patients who have developed the signs and symptoms of AIDS, assessment of T lymphocytes and viral load concentrations are important, along with the diagnosis and treatment of opportunistic infections.

Both leukopenia and lymphocytopenia exist in the AIDS patient. Total leukocyte and absolute lymphocyte concentrations need to be periodically assessed. Additional testing includes viral load assay and resistance testing. Resistance testing is an in vitro method to measure resistance of HIV to antiretroviral agents. Resistance testing can aid in antiretroviral drug selection but it has limitations.

The common denominator of the disease is a deficiency of a specific subset of thymus-derived (T4) lymphocytes. Enumeration of lymphocyte subsets is usually performed by

TABLE 22-4   **Laboratory Assessment of Asymptomatic HIV-Positive Patients**

Test	Comments
HIV serology	Repeat test at 3 to 6 month intervals for patients with positive test results when no confirmatory assay is available, patient denies commonly accepted risk factors, assay performed with other than standard serology protocol, other reasons (e.g., undetectable viral load and normal CD4+ lymphocyte cell count).
Complete blood count	Repeat test at 3 to 6 month intervals or more frequently when a patient has low values and is receiving bone marrow toxic drugs.
CD4+ cell count and percentage	Repeat every 3 to 6 months or more often if needed. The CD4+ lymphocyte count is a standard test to stage the disease, formulate a differential patient diagnosis, and to make therapeutic decisions regarding antiviral treatment and prophylaxis for opportunistic pathogens. It is also a relatively reliable indicator of prognosis that complements the viral load assay. These two assays independently predict clinical progression and survival.
VDRL or RPR syphilis serology	Repeat annually
Hepatitis serology	Anti-HBs or anti-HBc, if a HBV vaccine candidate; screen for anti HAV (IgG), if an HAV vaccine candidate.
Cytomegalovirus (CMV) IgG	Optional
Toxoplasmosis (IgG)	Screen all patients, repeat if seronegative-negative, CD4+ cell count is low, and patient does not take *P. carinii* prophylaxis, and symptoms suggest toxoplasmosis encephalitis.
Serum chemistry	Repeat annually or more frequently in patients with abnormal results and who are receiving hepatotoxic or nephrotoxic drugs.
g6PD assay	Optional, except in susceptible hosts, patients receiving oxidant drugs, and patients with typical symptoms of g6PD deficiency.
Lipid profile	Therapeutic monitoring recommended for patients receiving certain antiviral regimens.
PPD skin test	Repeat annually in previously negative patients
PAP smear	Repeat at 6 months and then annually if results are normal.
Chest x-ray study	Suggested for patients with signs and symptoms of pulmonary disease or newly detected positive PPD.

From Bartlett JG, Gallant JE: *Medical management of HIV infection*, Baltimore, Md, 2002, Johns Hopkins Press.
CMV, Cytomegalovirus; *HIV,* human immunodeficiency virus; *Ig,* immunoglobulin; *PPD,* purified protein derivative; *VDRL* Venereal Disease Research Laboratories.

flow-cell cytometry. Various other ancillary findings including polyclonal hypergammaglobulinemia, elevated levels of alpha interferon, alpha (α)$_1$ thymosin, and beta microglobulin, as well as reduced levels of T-cell growth factor or interleukin-2, have been noted.

TESTING METHODS

HIV-1 Antibodies

Antibodies to HIV can be detected by EIA (specificity >99%, sensitivity >98%; see Table 22-5) or a newly FDA-approved assay, Ora Quick Rapid HIV-1 antibody test (Ora Sure Technologies, Bethlehem, PA) and confirmed by the immuno-Blot technique. The vast majority of, and probably all, seropositive patients are also infectious, as manifested by isolation of HIV from peripheral blood. The CDC estimates that one fourth of the approximately 900,000 infected people in the United States are not aware of being infected. Antibody testing by EIA remains the standard method for screening potential blood donors simultaneous testing for p24 antigenemia is considered unnecessary. Third-generation serologic assays demonstrate that seroconversion typically occurs 3 to 12 weeks after infection, but significant delays can occur in some individuals.

TABLE 22-5   **Causes of False-Positive and False-Negative HIV Enzyme Immunoassays**

False Positive	False Negative
Positive RPR (syphilis serology) test	Laboratory glove starch
Hematologic malignant disorder	Window period before seroconversion
DNA viral infections	Immunosuppressive therapy
Autoimmune disorders	Malignancies
Alcoholic hepatitis	Bone marrow transplantation
Vaccinations (e.g., hepatitis B, influenza)	Kits that mainly detect antibodies to p24
Chronic renal failure	
Renal transplantation	

Modified from Specialty Laboratories, Santa Monica, CA.
RPR, Rapid plasma reagent; *DNA,* deoxyribonucleic acid.

Western Blot Test

Before an HIV result is considered positive, the results should be both reproducible and confirmable by at least one additional test. The Western blot analysis is currently the standard method for confirming HIV-1 seropositivity. If the test is positive for bands gp41 and/or p24 in conjunction with a positive EIA test, it is regarded as a confirmatory test. The Western blot test appears to work best with samples that contain high levels of antibody.

In the Western blot procedure, purified HIV-1 viral antigens are electrophoresed on SDS gels, and the separated polypeptides are then transferred onto sheets of nitrocellulose paper incubated with the serum specimen. Any antibody that binds to the separated peptides present on the nitrocellulose paper is detected by a secondary antihuman antibody, conjugated to a suitable enzyme marker, and incubated with the appropriate enzyme substrate. Antibody specificities against known viral components (generally the core component p24 and envelope component gp41) are considered true-positive results, whereas antibodies specific against nonviral cellular contaminants are nonspecific, false-positive results. The Western blot technique, however, is time consuming and expensive. It is also open to considerable interpretation and has many sources of error. Variables in the test include:

- The technical skill and experience of the technologist performing the procedure
- Characteristics of the technical methodology
- General sensitivity of the Western blot technique in detecting antibodies specific for various HIV-1 antigens (especially during the window period of seronegativity)
- Frequent lack of specificity because of contamination of the viral reference preparation by histocompatibility and other antigens that electrophoretically migrate with p24 and gp41
- Variation in band reactivity patterns in sera from an individual over the course of HIV-1 infection

Indeterminate test results account for 4% to 20% of Western blot assays with positive bands for HIV-1 proteins. An indeterminate Western blot can be caused by a variety of factors. Causes of indeterminate results include:

- Serologic tests in the process of seroconversion; anti-p24 is usually the first antibody to appear
- End-stage HIV infection, usually with loss of core antibody
- Cross-reacting nonspecific antibodies, as seen with collagen-vascular disease, autoimmune diseases, lymphoma, liver disease, injection drug use, multiple sclerosis, parity, or recent immunization
- Infection with O strain or HIV-2
- HIV vaccine recipients
- Perinatally exposed infants who are seroconverting (losing maternal antibody)
- Technical or clerical error

In addition, nonspecific reactions producing indeterminate results in uninfected persons have occurred more frequently among pregnant women or mothers than among persons in other groups characterized by low HIV seroprevalence. The incidence of indeterminate Western blot results is relatively low. IFA can be used to resolve an EIA positive, Western blot-indeterminate sample.

The most important factor in evaluating indeterminate results is risk assessment. Patients in low-risk categories with indeterminate tests are almost never infected with either HIV-1 or HIV-2; repeat testing usually continues to show indeterminate results, and the cause of this pattern is infrequently established. Follow-up serology testing at 3 months is recommended to verify the previous results. Patients with indeterminate tests who are in the process of seroconversion usually have positive Western blot tests within 1 month; repeat tests at 1, 2, and 6 months are generally advocated with appropriate precautions to prevent viral transmission in the interim.

False-positive Western blot results, especially those with a majority of bands, are extremely uncommon. The frequency of false-positive Western blot results is extremely low.

HIV Antigen and Genome Testing

p24 Antigen

Enzyme immunoassay for HIV-1 antigen detects primarily uncomplexed p24 antigen. This procedure is applicable to blood or CSF testing as evidence of an active infection and can be diagnostic before seroconversion, can predict a patient's prognosis, and is useful for monitoring response to therapy. Disadvantages of the procedure include poor sensitivity, the inability to detect in patients with a high titer of p24 antibody, and the failure of the method to detect HIV-2 antigen. Antibodies to p24 antigen are a better predictive marker progression than p24 antigen.

PCR/DNA Amplification

This technique allows for the direct detection of HIV-1 by DNA amplification. This ultrasensitive PCR technique has revolutionized HIV-1 detection. In addition to confirmatory testing, DNA amplification can be used for the diagnosis of very early, postexposure HIV infection in the window period before production of antibodies.

The goal of direct detection of active virus in patient specimens by an ultrasensitive method is to detect less than 100 molecules of viral nucleic acid in the peripheral blood cells isolated from 1 mL of blood. This number is the assay target because as few as 1 in 10,000 lymphocytes express viral RNA in HIV-1 infected individuals. Therefore out of approximately 10^6 lymphocytes per mL of blood, about 100 contain viral nuclei acid, corresponding to 100 to 150 copies of HIV-1 DNA. The presence of HIV-1 DNA in lymphocytes of antibody-positive, asymptomatic persons can be used to confirm exposure to the virus; the presence of viral RNA might be a sensitive indication of viral replication and possibly an indication of further disease progression.

The basis of this technology lies in amplification of minute amounts of viral nucleic acid in lymphocyte DNA. In HIV-1-infected cells, the DNA template is a provirus that exists either as integrated or episomal DNA. After amplification, isotope or nonisotope methods can detect the amplified product. The most effective means of target amplification is the PCR. A pair of specific oligomer primers initiates DNA synthesis in combination with heat-stable Taq I DNA polymerase. After this first round of primer extension, the material is heated to denature the product from its template and cooled to 37° C to permit annealing of the primer molecules to the original template DNA, as well as to the newly synthesized DNA fragments. Primer extension is then resumed. By repetition of these cycles of denaturation, annealing, and extension, the original DNA can be increased exponentially.

Viral RNA can also be specifically amplified with some additional steps. The gag region is probably the best choice of a sequence for amplification. Detection of viral RNA and DNA in clinical specimens might prove to be a better indicator of biologically active virus than DNA detection alone. The presence of both provirus and viral RNA transcriptase would be a strong indication of viral replication.

Quantitation of HIV RNA in plasma is useful for determining free viral load, assessing the efficacy of antiviral therapy, and predicting progression and clinical outcome in AIDS patients.

Immunofluorescence Assay

IFA is commonly used to locate HIV-1 antigen in infected cells. Infected cells are treated with polyclonal or monoclonal antibody against p17 or p24. After being washed, the cells are incubated with fluorescein isothiocyanate or rhodamine conjugate as a secondary antibody, then are washed, mounted, and examined using a fluorescent microscope. The limitations of this technique include the need for expensive equipment and the fact that fluorescence fades quickly.

Immunohistochemical Staining

In this technique infected cells are incubated with HIV-1 antibody. After incubation the cells are treated with an enzyme-labeled secondary antibody (usually alkaline phosphatase or horseradish peroxidase), and an appropriate substrate is added. The cells are washed and examined using simple light microscopy. This method has the advantages of IFA but is simple and inexpensive and does not require extensive expertise. Morphologic changes can also be observed.

PREVENTION AND TREATMENT

Prevention

Health care personnel (HCP) should assume that the blood and other body fluids from all patients are potentially infectious. Therefore they should follow infection control precautions at all times. As of June 2001, occupational exposure to HIV has resulted in 57 documented cases of HIV seroconversion among HCP in the United States. To prevent transmission of HIV to HCP in the workplace, the CDC offers the following recommendations:

- Routine use of barriers (such as gloves and/or goggles) when anticipating contact with blood or body fluids
- Washing hands and other skin surfaces immediately after contact with blood or body fluids
- Careful handling and disposing of sharp instruments during and after use

Safety devices have been developed to help prevent needlestick injuries. If used properly, these types of devices may reduce the risk of exposure to HIV.

Although the most important strategy for reducing the risk of occupational HIV transmission is to prevent occupational exposures, plans for postexposure management of HCP should be in place. CDC has issued guidelines for the management of HCP exposures to HIV and recommendations for postexposure prophylaxis (PEP). Considerations that influence the rationale and recommendations for PEP include:

- The pathogenesis of HIV infection, particularly the time course of early infection
- The biologic plausibility that infection can be prevented or ameliorated by using antiretroviral drugs
- Direct or indirect evidence of the efficacy of specific agents used for prophylaxis
- The risk and benefit of PEP to exposed HCP

Continued work in the following areas is needed to reduce the risk of occupational HIV transmission to HCP. All health care organizations should train HCP in infection control procedures and on the importance of reporting occupational exposures. They should develop a system to monitor reporting and management of occupational exposures.

Transfusion-related AIDS can be virtually eliminated by careful screening of blood donors and blood products. Blood donor medical history standards have recently undergone extensive revision. The U.S. Public Health Service has recommended that all donated blood and plasma be tested for HIV antibody and, in addition, recommends that the blood or serum from donors of organs, tissues, or semen intended for human use be similarly tested and that the test result be used to evaluate the appropriate use of such materials from these donors. Abstinence from injection drug use and consistent use of clean equipment for those who are unable to cease injection drug use are further methods for reducing or eliminating the risk of contracting HIV.

Adopting and maintaining safe sex behaviors that prevent HIV exposure can significantly reduce the risk of contracting HIV. Safe sex behaviors include sexual abstinence, having sex only with an uninfected partner, and consistent condom use.

Treatment

At the present time there are 64 HIV and HIV-related FDA-approved medicines on the market in the United States. Antiretroviral agents from three traditional classes of drugs are available for the treatment of HIV infection:

1. *Nucleoside analog reverse transcriptase inhibitors (NRTIs).* The original NRTI was Zidovudine, AZT, which was approved in March 1987. Since then five additional nucleoside analog drugs have been approved. In 2001 the first nucleotide analog, Tenofovir, was approved for HIV treatment. It blocks HIV replication in a manner similar to the nucleoside analogs. NRTIs are potent in combination with other drugs. If used alone, resistance to HIV will develop. Some of the drugs in this class, (e.g., AZT) penetrate the blood-brain barrier.
2. *Non-nucleoside analog reverse transcriptase inhibitors (NNRTIs).* The first drug in this class, Nevirapine, was approved in June 1996. NNRTIs may interact with other cytochrome *p-450*-processed drugs (e.g. protease inhibitors). NNRTIs have a mixed ability to penetrate the blood-brain barrier.
3. *Protease inhibitors (PIs).* The first approved drugs in this class for the treatment of HIV were Ritonavir and Indinavir. Both drugs were approved in March 1996. PIs are very potent and may interact with other drugs using *cytochrome p450 metabolic pathways.* But poor absorption may affect potency.

Drugs in three new additional classes are now available:

1. *Fusion inhibitors.* The first drug in this class, Pentafuside (T20), went into Phase III clinical trials in early 2001. The mode of action of the drug is the prevention of HIV entry into the host cell.
2. *Integrase inhibitors.* The drug in this class, Zintevir, (AR-177) prevents HIV DNA from entering human DNA.
3. *Zinc Finger Inhibitors.* The drug in this class, Benzamide-disulfice, disrupts polyprotein formation essential for HIV replication.

New drugs are needed because resistant mutations that protect the virus against existing classes of antiretroviral drugs would be unlikely to also confer resistance to novel agents. In the beginning of 2003, 84 companies had 126 drugs and vaccines for AIDS and AIDS-related conditions in testing. Drug discovery and FDA approval currently take an average of 12 to 15 years and cost about $400 million for a drug to go from the laboratory to the drug store in the United States. For a new drug to be approved, it must be tested in three phases of a clinical trial for safety and efficacy before approval. Phase I, which takes about 1 year, includes from 20 to 80 healthy volunteers who are tested for the safety of a new drug. Phase II, which lasts about 2 years, expands the number of volunteers to 100 to 300 persons with the disease to assess the effectiveness of a drug and to observe for adverse side reactions. Phase III of a clinical trial, which lasts about 3 years, expands the number of patients with a specific disease to 1000 to 3000 patients to further verify effectiveness and to identify any specific negative side effects of the drug. Since the FDA Regulatory Modernization Act of 1997, the FDA review process has been streamlined to hasten approval of new therapies to treat severe diseases. Phase I and Phase II are now allowed to be combined to shorten the approval process. It now takes about 18 months for a drug to go through the review process for approval by the FDA. Only about one in five medicines that enters a clinical trial is approved.

New drugs are needed because resistant mutations that protect the virus against existing classes of antiretroviral drugs would be unlikely to also confer resistance to novel agents. Anti-HIV drugs under development include agents that interfere with other steps in the HIV life cycle (fusion inhibitors, and integrase inhibitors) and a second-generation NNRTI.

One new approach involves preventing HIV from invading the human cells in which it replicates, a concept known as entry inhibition. To gain entry to host cells, HIV binds to the cell's CD4 receptor in tandem with a coreceptor, usually CXCR5 or CXCR4. This process allows HIV to fuse with the cell membrane and inject its genes inside the cell. Patients with certain mutations in CCR5 are resistant to HIV infection. This finding has suggested to researchers that drugs that block this receptor could prevent the virus from invading cells. In addition to the new studies of drugs that prevent the virus from binding to host cell receptors, phase III clinical trials are under way for an agent called T-20 (a fusion inhibitor) which blocks a different event in viral invasion: the fusion of HIV with the host cell membrane. Another experimental viral entry inhibitor that appears to inhibit activity of gp120, the viral envelope protein that must interact with the host cell's CD4 receptor for HIV invasion to occur, is under development. Also in early phases of development is an experimental agent that is intended to block HIV at a later stage, after it has invaded cells. The compound, called S-1360, targets integrase, a viral enzyme that enables HIV to splice its DNA into the host cell's DNA. Human trials of the integrase inhibitor (AR-177) are now under way.

Also on the horizon are improved versions of NNRTIs. NNRTIs (e.g., EFV, nevirapine) target a key viral enzyme, reverse transcriptase, inhibiting its function by binding to a pocket near the enzyme's catalytic site. But NNRTI resistance can develop when HIV acquires one or more mutations that alter the binding pocket. The drug TMC-125, given as a single agent, performed as well as the 5-drug regimen containing drugs from all three currently licensed classes of anti-HIV medications.

Postexposure Prophylaxis

NRTI combinations that can be considered for PEP include zidovudine (ZDV) and lamivudine (3TC), 3TC and stavudine (d4T), and didanosine (ddI) and d4T. The addition of a third drug for PEP after high-risk exposures is based on demonstrated effectiveness in reducing viral burden in HIV-infected persons. Previously, indinavir or nelfinavir were recommended as first-choice agents for inclusion in an expanded PEP regimen. In 1998 the FDA approved efavirenz (EFV), an NNRTI; abacavir (ABC), a potent NRTI; and lopinavir/ritonavir (Kaletra), a PI, for PEP. Although side effects might be common with the NNRTIs, EFV might be considered for expanded PEP regimens, especially when resistance to PIs in the source person's virus is known or suspected. ABC has been associated with dangerous hypersensitivity reactions but, with careful monitoring, may be considered as a third drug for PEP. Kaletra is a potent HIV inhibitor that, with expert consultation, may be considered in an expanded PEP regimen. Lopinavir is a newly developed inhibitor that, when formulated with ritonavir, has antiviral activity superior to that of a nelfinavir-containing regimen by itself in the initial treatment of HIV-infected adults.

Recommendations for HIV PEP include a basic 4-week regimen of two drugs (ZDV and 3TC, d4T, or ddI and d4T) for most HIV exposures and an expanded regimen that includes the addition of a third drug for HIV exposures that pose an increased risk for transmission. When the source person's virus is known or suspected to be resistant to one or more of the drugs considered for the PEP regimen, the selection of drugs to which the source person's virus is unlikely to be resistant is recommended. In addition, consultation with local experts and/or the National Clinicians' Postexposure Prophylaxis Hotline ([PEPline] 1-888-448-4911) is advised under several special circumstances (e.g., delayed exposure report, unknown source person, pregnancy in the exposed person, resistance of the source virus to antiretroviral agents, or toxicity of the PEP regimen). Occupational exposures should be considered urgent medical concerns to ensure timely postexposure management.

Failure of PEP to prevent HIV infection in HCP has been reported in at least 21 instances. In 16 of the cases, ZDV was used alone as a single agent; in two cases, ZDV and ddI were used in combination; and in three cases more than three drugs were used for PEP. Guidelines for the treatment of HIV infection, a condition usually involving a high total body burden of HIV, include recommendations for the use of three drugs; however, the applicability of these recommendations to PEP remains unknown. In HIV-infected patients combination regimens have proved superior to monotherapy regimens in reducing HIV viral load, reducing the incidence of opportunistic infections and death, and delaying onset of drug resistance. A combination of drugs with activity at different stages in the viral replication cycle theoretically could offer an additional preventive effect in PEP, particularly for occupational exposures that pose an increased risk of transmission. Although the use of a three-drug regimen might be justified for exposures that pose an increased risk of transmission, whether the potential added toxicity of a third drug is justified for lower-risk exposures is uncertain.

Information from the National Surveillance System for Health Care Workers and the HIV Postexposure Registry indicates that nearly 50% of HCP experience adverse symptoms (e.g, nausea, malaise, anorexia, and headache) while taking PEP and that approximately 33% stop taking PEP because of adverse signs and symptoms. Some studies have shown that side effects and discontinuation of PEP are more common among HCP taking three-drug combination regimens for PEP compared with HCP taking two-drug combination regimens. Serious side effects, including nephrolithiasis, hepatitis, and pancytopenia have been reported with the use of combination drugs for PEP. Known or suspected resistance of the source virus to antiretroviral agents, particularly to agents that might be included in a PEP regimen, is a concern for persons making decisions about PEP. Resistance to HIV infection occurs with all of the available antiretroviral agents, and cross-resistance within drug classes is frequent. Recent studies have demonstrated an emergence of drug-resistant HIV among source persons for occupational exposures. Despite recent studies and case reports, the relevance of exposure to a resistant virus is still not well understood.

Vaccines

Following poor results from a phase II study, the HIV Vaccine Trials Network announced that it will not pursue a widely anticipated phase III study of two AIDS vaccines. The trial was to have been a three-armed study to test Aventis Pasteur's ALVAC-HIV and VaxGen's AIDSVAX B/B alone and in combination. Continued testing of vaccines is needed to determine whether they are more immunogenic in different doses, in different populations, and in combination with other candidate HIV vaccines (see Appendix D).

Case Study

History and Physical Examination

A 40-year-old man with a history of IV drug use comes to the emergency room because of a rash and fever. In addition, the patient is complaining of a several-day history of malaise, fatigue, fever, headache, and a sore throat.

Physical examination reveals a moderately ill-appearing male with a temperature of 38.8° C. He has a blanching erythematous, macular-papular rash evident over the trunk, back, and upper and lower extremities. In addition, his throat shows enlarged tonsils and broad-based ulcerations on the buccal mucosa.

He has a history of an episode of endocarditis 2 years ago. At that time, an HIV serology was performed. It was negative.

Laboratory Data

A complete blood count and liver function tests are ordered. The results of these tests show that the patient is anemic (hematocrit 38%). He also has a severely decreased total leukocyte count and a severely decreased absolute lymphocyte count. Some of his liver function tests are abnormal.

Questions and Discussion

1. What is a likely diagnosis of this patient's condition?
   The patient's history, physical examination, and laboratory data strongly suggest a diagnosis of acute HIV infection. Approximately 50% of those infected with HIV will have asymptomatic illness at the time of primary HIV infection. Acute Epstein-Barr virus (EBV) may produce an illness that is nearly indistinguishable from acute HIV, but some of the features that suggest HIV over EBV are mucosal ulcerations, rash, and the absence of atypical (variant) lymphocytes on the peripheral blood smear.

2. What is the natural history of this disease?
   The early phase of HIV infection may last from many months to many years after the initiation of infection. Typically, patients in the early stages of HIV infection are either completely asymptomatic or may show mild, chronic lymphadenopathy. When HIV first enters the body, the virus often replicates abundantly and free virus appears in CSF surrounding the brain and spinal cord and in circulating blood. Within a few weeks, the viral concentration in the bloodstream and CSF drops precipitously and the initial symptoms disappear.

   An unknown number of infected patients experience a brief, infectious, mononucleosis-like or flu-like illness with fever, malaise, and possibly a skin rash. Neurologic complaints may also be reported. These symptoms parallel the first wave of HIV replications and develop at about the time antibodies produced by the body against HIV can first be detected. This is usually between 2 weeks and 3 months after infection, rarely later. After HIV infection and any clinically manifested signs and symptoms, a person may remain symptom-free for years.

   From 2 to 10 years after HIV infection, replication of the virus flares again, and the infection enters its final stage. An average of 8 or 9 years may pass before AIDS is fully developed. The virus behaves differently, depending on the kind of host cell and the cell's own level of mitotic activity. In T cells, however, the virus can lie dormant indefinitely, but it can destroy the host cell in a burst of replication. HIV grows continuously, but slowly, in macrophages-monocytes. This slow growth of the virus saves the cell from destruction but probably alters its function.

   Clinical symptoms of the later phase of HIV infection include extreme weight loss, fever, and multiple secondary infections. The end stage of AIDS is characterized by the occurrence of neoplasms and/or opportunistic infections. Lethal *P. carinii* pneumonia has been a hallmark of AIDS. Other opportunistic infections, however, are frequent and may exist concurrently. Cryptosporidiosis and *H. capsulatum* are being recognized with increasing frequency.

   The most frequent malignancy observed is an aggressive, invasive variant of Kaposi's sarcoma, discovered in many cases through autopsy. Kaposi's sarcoma produces tumors in the skin and linings of internal organs, lymphomas, and cancers of the rectum and tongue. Malignant B-cell lymphomas are also being more commonly recognized in patients with AIDS or those at high risk for AIDS. Because certain lymphomas can develop quite early, it is hypothesized that B-cell hyperactivity plays a role in their development. Lymphomas and other cancers that appear late in HIV disease could also stem from the failure of the compromised immune system to recognize and destroy cancer cells.

3. What immunologic laboratory tests might be of value in establishing a diagnosis for this patient?

A screening test for infectious mononucleosis might be helpful to collaborate the absence of atypical lymphocytes on the patient's peripheral blood smear.

Approximately 7 to 14 days after exposure to HIV, there is a burst of viral replication that leads to detectable levels of p24 antigen in the blood. Antibody is not detectable initially; therefore an HIV antibody test would be negative. Patients with acute HIV infection will develop a positive antibody test within 6 months of their illness.

Follow-up serologic testing is important if p24 antigen testing is not done. Other tests that may be positive in this period before seroconversion are the PCR and viral culture.

Diagnosis

Acquired immunodeficiency syndrome

CHAPTER HIGHLIGHTS

HIV-1 is the predominant virus responsible for AIDS. In addition to the original HIV-1, a second AIDS-causing virus, HIV-2, was identified in 1985. In evolutionary terms, the two viruses are related and have a similar overall structure.

The HIV virus is a type D retrovirus. It is composed of structural proteins and glycoproteins that occupy the core and envelope regions of the particle. Retroviruses contain a single positive-stranded RNA with the genetic information of the virus and a special enzyme, called reverse transcriptase, in their core. Reverse transcriptase enables the virus to convert viral RNA into DNA. This reverses the normal process of transcription in which DNA is converted to RNA—hence the term *retrovirus*. The genomes of all known retroviruses are organized in a similar way. In the provirus, which is formed when complementary DNA synthesis is completed from the retroviral RNA template, viral core and envelope proteins and the enzyme reverse transcriptase are encoded by the gag, env, and pol genes, respectively, whereas viral gene expression is regulated by tat, trs, sor, and 3'orf gene products. The HIV life cycle is that of a retrovirus. The genes of a retrovirus are encoded in RNA; before they can be expressed, the RNA must be converted into DNA. Only then are the viral genes transcribed and translated into proteins in the usual sequence.

The infectious process with HIV begins when the gp120 protein on the viral envelope binds to the protein receptor, called CD4, located on the surface of a target cell. Fusion of the virus to the membrane of this host cell enables the viral RNA and reverse transcriptase to invade the cell's cytoplasm. HIV has a marked preference for the helper/inducer subset of T lymphocytes. These cells, however, are not the only cells

that have CD4 antigen embedded in their membrane. Macrophages, as many as 40% of the peripheral blood monocytes, and cells in the lymph nodes, skin, and other organs also express measurable amounts of CD4 and can be infected by HIV. In addition, about 5% of the B lymphocytes may express CD4 and be susceptible to HIV infection. Although some cells do not produce detectable amounts of CD4, they do contain low levels of messenger RNA encoding the CD4 protein, which indicates that they do produce some CD4. Because these cells can be infected by HIV in culture, the expression of only a very small amount of CD4 or an alternate receptor molecule may be necessary for HIV infection to take place. These cell types include certain cells of the brain, glial cells, a variety of malignant brain tumor cells, and some cells derived from cancers of the bowel. In addition, cells of the gastrointestinal system do not produce appreciable amounts of CD4, but gut cells called chromaffin cells do sometimes appear to be infected by HIV in vivo. This suggests that gastrointestinal infection may be what leads to the AIDS-associated weight loss and emaciation known in Africa as slim disease.

The viral replication cycle begins after HIV binds to the CD4 receptor and injects its core into the target cell. The core includes two identical strands of RNA. The enzyme DNA polymerase is responsible for converting the viral genetic information into DNA. Initially this enzyme makes a single-stranded DNA copy of the viral RNA. An associated enzyme, ribonuclease, destroys the original RNA, and the polymerase makes a second complementary copy of DNA using the first DNA strand as a template. The DNA polymerase and ribonuclease together are often called reverse transcriptase. After the viral genetic information is in the form of double-stranded DNA (the same form in which the cell carries its own genetic makeup), it migrates to the cell nucleus. A third viral enzyme, called an integrase, may then splice the HIV genome into the host cell's DNA. After the viral genome is integrated into the host DNA, the provirus will be duplicated together with the cell's own genes every time the cell divides. At this stage the HIV is permanent. The second half of the HIV life cycle (the production of new virus particles) takes place only sporadically and only in some infected cells.

AIDS has become a major cause of morbidity and mortality in the United States. The number of reported cases of AIDS has increased each year since the disease was first recognized. Transmission of HIV is believed to be restricted to intimate contact with body fluids from an infected person; casual contact with infected persons has not been documented as a mode of transmission. Although the mode of transmission is considered to be predominantly sexual, the virus can be transmitted through contact with infected blood. Although HIV has been isolated from blood, semen, vaginal secretions, saliva, tears, breast milk, CSF, amniotic fluid, and urine, only blood, semen, vaginal secretions, and possibly breast milk have been implicated in transmission of HIV to date. Various practices have been advocated for the prevention of HIV transmission. Sexual abstinence or the practice of safe sex is essential to curtailing HIV transmission. The screening of blood donors and donors of organs, tissues, and semen, as well as of blood products for HIV, has reduced the risk of HIV transmission to minimal levels.

The early phase of HIV-1 infection may last from many months to many years after initial infection. Typically patients in the early stages of HIV-1 infection are either completely asymptomatic or may show mild, chronic lymphadenopathy. HIV-1 causes a predictable, progressive derangement of immune function, and AIDS is just one late manifestation of that process. From 2 to 10 years after HIV infection, replication of the virus flares again and the infection enters its final stage. An average of 8 or 9 years may pass before AIDS is fully developed. The virus behaves differently depending on the kind of host cell and the cell's own level of mitotic activity. In T cells, however, the virus can lie dormant indefinitely, but it can destroy the host cell in a burst of replication. HIV grows continuously but slowly in macrophages-monocytes. This saves the cell from destruction but probably alters its function. The end stage of AIDS is characterized by the occurrence of neoplasms and/or opportunistic infections.

Lethal *P. carinii* pneumonia has been a hallmark of AIDS. Other opportunistic infections, however, are frequent and may exist concurrently. Infection with HIV is presently considered to lead to death. Several experimental treatments, however, are being tested. At present the interval from diagnosis of AIDS to death varies greatly. In developed countries 50% of patients die within 18 months of diagnosis and 80% die within 36 months.

Immunologic activities associated with HIV-1 infection include the production of different types of antibodies against HIV-1. Some antibodies neutralize it, others prevent it from binding to cells, and others stimulate cytotoxic cells to attack HIV-infected cells. A "window" period of seronegativity exists from the time of initial infection to 6 or 12 weeks or longer. With the use of enzyme immunoassay methods based on defined HIV-1 proteins produced by recombinant DNA methods, antibodies specific for gp41 are detectable for weeks or months before assays specific for p24. The appearance of antibodies specific for p24, however, has been shown in several studies to precede that of anti-gp41 when serum specimens have been tested by Western blot analysis. This discrepancy in the sequence of antibody appearance is believed to be due to the greater sensitivity of the Western blot technique compared to viral lysate-based EIAs used for the detection of anti-p24. gp41 antibodies persist throughout the course of infection. Antibody specific for p24 not only rises to detectable levels after gp41 but can also disappear unpredictably and abruptly in a short period of time. Increased production of core antigen is believed to be associated with a burst of viral replication and host cell lysis. The disappearance of antibody directed against p24 has been demonstrated to occur concomitantly with an increase in the concentration of core antigen in the serum. This parallel activity may be due to the sequestration of antibody in immune complexes; the sudden decrease in anti-p24 is considered to be a grave prognostic sign in HIV-1-infected patients.

Laboratory evaluation of HIV-infected patients consists of assessment of cellular and humoral components. Screening of blood donors and patients at risk is usually by serologic methods. In patients who have developed the signs and symptoms of AIDS, both the assessment of cellular concentrations and function and the diagnosis and treatment of opportunistic infections become important. Both leuko-penia and lymphocytopenia exist in the patient with AIDS. Total leukocyte and absolute lymphocyte concentrations need to be periodically assessed. The common denominator of the disease is a deficiency of a specific subset of thymus-derived (CD4) lymphocytes. Enumeration of lymphocyte subsets is usually performed by flow-cell cytometry. Decreased lymphocyte proliferative response to soluble antigens and mitogens, such as a diminished response to pokeweed mitogen, exists in this disorder.

Antibodies to HIV-1 are usually detected by EIA and confirmed by the Western blot technique. The Western blot analysis is currently the standard method for confirming HIV-1 seropositivity. If the test is positive for bands p41 and/or p24 in conjunction with a positive EIA, it is regarded as a confirmatory test.

REVIEW QUESTIONS

1. The major structural protein (core) of the HIV-1 virus is:
   A. gp41
   B. p24
   C. gp34
   D. gp140

2. The infectious process of AIDS begins when the gp120 protein on the viral envelope bends to the protein receptor, _____, on the surface of a target cell.
   A. CD 8
   B. CD 4
   C. p24
   D. p26

3. HIV can infect all of the following cells except:
   A. helper-inducer subset of T lymphocytes
   B. macrophages
   C. monocytes
   D. polymorphonuclear leukocytes

4. The most rapidly growing segment of the HIV-infected population is:
   A. homosexual males
   B. lesbians
   C. health care workers
   D. IV drug users and their sexual partners

5. In HIV infections, a window period of seronegativity exists from the time of initial infection to _____.
   A. 2 weeks
   B. 2 to 6 weeks or longer
   C. 6 to 12 weeks or longer
   D. 4 to 8 months or longer

6. HIV antibodies are usually detected by _____ (6) and confirmed by _____ (7).
   A. latex agglutination
   B. enzyme immunoassay
   C. enzyme inhibition
   D. radioimmunoassay

7.
   A. Southern blot
   B. Northern blot
   C. Western blot
   D. DNA hybridization

8. The AIDS-causing virus HIV has also been referred to as:
   A. human T-lymphotropic virus type III
   B. HTLV-III
   C. lymphadenopathy-associated virus (LAV)
   D. all of the above

9. HTLV-I was unique when it was isolated because it was the first:
   A. bovine infectious retrovirus
   B. canine infectious retrovirus
   C. human infectious retrovirus
   D. isolated AIDS virus

Questions 10-12. Fill in the blanks with the correct letter, choosing from the following answers:
   A. codes for p24 and for proteins including p17, p9, and p7
   B. codes for two glycoproteins: gp41, gp120
   C. produces DNA polymerase; produces endonuclease

Viral Genome Structural Components

Component	Product
pol	10. _____
gag	11. _____
env	12. _____

Questions 13-17. Arrange the HIV-1 life cycle events in proper order.

13. _____   A. Reverse transcriptase converts viral RNA into proviral DNA.

14. _____   B. New virus particles are produced as the result of normal cellular activities of transcription and translation. Once the viral genome is integrated into host cell DNA, the potential for viral production always exists and the viral infection of new cells can continue.

15. _____   C. New particles bud from the cell membrane.

16. _____   D. The virus attaches to the CD4 membrane receptor and sheds its protein coat, exposing its RNA core.

17. _____   E. The proviral DNA is integrated into the genome (genetic complement of the cell).

Questions 18-20. Match the characteristics to the three infectious patterns of HIV virus.

18. _____ Pattern 1: North and South America, Western Europe, Scandinavia, Australia, New Zealand

    A. primarily a disease of heterosexuals

19. _____ Pattern 2: Africa, Caribbean, some areas of South America

    B. few cases of AIDS

20. _____ Pattern 3: Eastern Europe, North Africa, the Middle East, Asia, the Pacific (excluding Australia and New Zealand)

    C. primarily a disease of homosexuals and IV drug abusers

21. The criteria for HIV infection for persons 13 years old and older include:
   A. repeatedly reactive screening test for HIV antibody
   B. specific HIV antibody identified by use of supplemental tests
   C. direct identification of the virus
   D. all of the above

22. After the early period of primary HIV infection, the patient enters a period of clinical latency that lasts a median of _____ years.
   A. 5
   B. 10
   C. 15
   D. 20

23. As AIDS progresses, the quantity of _____ diminishes, and the risk of opportunistic infection increases.
   A. HIV antigen
   B. HIV antibody
   C. CD4+T lymphocytes
   D. CD8+T lymphocytes

24. The clinical symptoms of the later phase of AIDS are:
   A. weight loss and decreased PMN cells
   B. extreme weight loss and fever
   C. multiple secondary (opportunistic) infections
   D. both B and C

25. The most frequent malignancy observed in AIDS patients is:
   A. *Pneumocystis carinii*
   B. Kaposi's sarcoma.
   C. toxoplasmosis.
   D. non-Hodgkin's lymphoma.

26. Sources of error in the Western blot test include:
    A. concentration of HIV antigen
    B. presence of other infectious agents
    C. the technical skill and experience of the technologist performing the test
    D. age of the blood specimen

27. All of the following methods have been developed to detect HIV-1 antigen except:
    A. transcriptase method
    B. synthetic peptide approach
    C. immunofluorescence assay
    D. immunohistochemical staining

28. All of the following methods have been developed to detect the presence of HIV-1 viral gene except:
    A. radioimmunoassay
    B. in situ hybridization
    C. Southern blot analysis
    D. DNA amplification

BIBLIOGRAPHY

Bartlett JG, Gallant JE: *Medical management of HIV 2001-2002* edition, Baltimore, 2001, Johns Hopkins Press.

Branca M: Chipping away at AIDS mystery, Bio-IT World, 1:20, 2002.

Gallo RC, Montagnier L: AIDS in 1988, *Sci Am* 259(4):40-51, 1988.

Goudsmit J et al: Expression of human immunodeficiency virus antigen (HIV-Ag) in serum and cerebrospinal fluid during acute and chronic infection, *Lancet* 2:177-180, 1986.

Goudsmit J et al: Intrathecal synthesis of antibodies to LAV/TLV-III specific IgG in individuals without AIDS or AIDS related complex, *N Engl J Med* 292:1231-1234, 1986.

Goudsmit J et al: Intrathecal synthesis of antibodies to HTLV-III in patients without AIDS or AIDS related complex, *Br Med J* 192:1231-1234, 1986.

Guidelines for the use of antiretroviral agents in HIV-infected adults and adolescents. Dept of Health and Human Services (DHHS) and the Henry J. Kaiser Family Foundation, February 4, 2002, website: www.hivatis.org.

Haseltine WA, Wong-Stall F: The molecular biology of the AIDS virus, *Sci Am* 259(4):52-63, 1988.

James E: Clinical clips—FDA approves rapid HIV test, *Advance Med Lab Prof* 14(25):12, 2002.

Miller LE: Effects of HIV on the immune system, *ADVANCE Medical Lab Professionals,* May 17, 1999, pp 12-17.

McCutchan FE: *Understanding the genetic diversity of HIV-1, AIDS 2000,* Philadelphia, 2000, Lippincott-Williams & Wilkins.

McDermott D et al: Chemokine promoter polymorphism affects risk of both HIV infection and disease progression in multicenter AIDS cohort study, *AIDS* 14:2671-2678, 2000.

Morbidity and Mortality Guidelines for national human immunodeficiency virus case surveillance, including monitoring for human immunodeficiency virus infection and acquired immunodeficiency syndrome, *MMWR.* 48(No. RR-13):1-11, 1999.

Morbidity and Mortality Weekly Report (MMWR): *Summary of notifiable diseases—United States,* 49(53):1-102, 2002.

Morbidity and Mortality Weekly Report (MMWR): *HIV and AIDS—United States, 1981-2000,* 50:430-434, 2001.

Morbidity and Mortality Weekly Report (MMWR): Public Health Service guidelines for the management and health-care worker exposures to HIV and recommendations for postexposure prophylaxis, *MMWR* 47(No. RR-7):1-28, 1998.

National Center for HIV, STD, and TB Prevention, Division of HIV/AIDS Prevention: US HIV and AIDS cases reported through December 2001, Year-end Edition, vol 13, no 2, Sept 25, 2002.

Redfield RR, Burke DS: HIV infection: the clinical picture, *Sci Am* 259(4):90-98, 1988.

Resnick L: Intra-blood-brain barrier synthesis of HIV specific IgG in patients with neurologic symptoms associated with AIDS or AIDS-related complex, *N Engl J Med* 313:1498-1502, 1985.

Salahuddin SZ: HTLV-III in symptom-free seronegative persons, *Lancet* 2:1418-1420, 1984.

Schim van der Loeff, MF, Aaby P: *Towards a better understanding of the epidemiology of HIV-2, AIDS,* Philadelphia, 1999, Lippincott Williams & Wilkins.

Sepkowitz, KA: AIDS—the first 20 years, *N Engl J Med* 344:1764-1772, 2001.

Shaw GM et al: HTLV-III infections in brains of children and adults with AIDS encephalopathy, *Science* 227:177-182, 1985.

Specialty Laboratories. Test Information, 2002, Website: www.specialtylabs.com.

Stephenson J: Scientists find some genes a bad omen for anti-HIV drug, *JAMA* 287(13):1637, 2002.

Stine G: *AIDS Update 2003,* Upper Saddle River, NJ, 2003, Prentice Hall.

Turgeon ML: *Clinical hematology,* ed 3, Philadelphia, 1999, Lippincott-Williams & Wilkins.

Turgeon ML: *Fundamentals of immunohematology,* ed 2, Baltimore, 1995, Williams & Wilkins.

US Department of Health and Human Services, Centers for Disease Control and Prevention: Human immunodeficiency fact sheet, retrieved 1-6-03, website: www.CDC.GOV/hiv/pubs/facts/hiv2.htm, updated 12-31-02.

US Department of Health and Human Services: Universal Precautions for prevention of transmission of HIV, hepatitis B virus, and other blood borne pathogens in health care settings, *MMWR* 37:377, 1988.

US Department of Health and Human Services: Update: acquired immunodeficiency syndrome and HIV infection among health care workers, *MMWR* 37:229, 1988.

US Department of Health and Human Services: Human immunodeficiency virus infection in the United States: a review of current knowledge, *MMWR* 36(Suppl 6):1-48, 1987.

Walmsley S et al: Lopinavir-ritonavir versus nelfinavir for the initial treatment of HIV infection, *N Engl J Med* 346:2039-2046, 2002.

Weber JN, Weiss RA: HIV infection: the cellular picture, *Sci Am* 259(4):100-109, 1988.

Weiss SH et al: Screening test for HTLV-III (AIDS agent) antibodies: specificity, sensitivity, and applications, *JAMA* 253:221-225, 1985.

Wong-Stall F, Gallo RC: Human T-lymphotropic retroviruses, *Nature* 317:395-403, 1985.

Part Four

Immunologically and Serologically Related Disorders

Chapter 23

Hypersensitivity Reactions

LEARNING OBJECTIVES

At the conclusion of this chapter, the reader should be able to:
• Define hypersensitivity reactions, including anaphylactic reactions.

• Compare Types I, II, III, and IV hypersensitivity reactions.
• Analyze related case studies.

The term *immunization,* or *sensitization,* describes an immunologic reaction dependent on the host's response to a subsequent exposure of antigen and not to any significant difference in the cellular and chemical events that follow the injection of the antigen. Small quantities of antigen, however, may favor sensitization by restricting the quantity of antibody formed. An unusual reaction (i.e., an allergic or hypersensitive reaction) that follows a second exposure to antigen reveals the existence of the sensitization. Hypersensitivity has traditionally been separated on the basis of time after exposure to an offending antigen. When this criterion is used, the terms *immediate* and *delayed* are appropriate. As described in Chapter 1, immediate hypersensitivity is antibody mediated, and delayed hypersensitivity is cell mediated.

ANAPHYLACTIC AND TYPE I REACTIONS

Type I hypersensitivity reactions can range from life-threatening anaphylactic reactions to milder manifestations associated with food allergies. Atopic allergies include hay fever, asthma, and food allergies.

Etiology

Atopic allergies are mostly naturally occurring, and the source of antigenic exposure is not always known. Atopic illnesses were among the first antibody-associated diseases demonstrating a strong familial or genetic tendency.

Several groups of agents cause anaphylactic reactions. The two most common agents are drugs (e.g., systemic penicillin) and insect stings. Insects of the order Hymenoptera (e.g., common hornet, yellow jacket, yellow hornet, and paper wasp) are representative examples of insects causing the most serious reactions.

Immunologic Activity

Mast cells (tissue basophils) are the cellular receptors for immunoglobulin E (IgE), which attaches to their outer surface. These cells are common in connective tissues, the lungs and uterus, and around blood vessels. They are also abundant in the liver, kidney, spleen, heart, and other organs. The granules contain a complex of heparin, histamine, and zinc ions, with the heparin existing in an approximate ratio of 6:1 with histamine. The actual heparin content is about 70 to 90 μg/10^6 cells; the histamine content is about 10 to 15 μg/10^6 cells. The release of histamine and heparin from mast cell granules occurs when the cells are exposed to specific immunologic or chemical agents. The cellular events during mast cell degranulation and the molecular events that follow degranulation occur within a few seconds.

Anaphylaxis is the clinical response to immunologic formation and fixation between a specific antigen and a tissue-fixing antibody. This reaction is usually mediated by IgE antibody and occurs in three stages:

- The offending antigen attaches to the IgE antibody fixed to the surface membrane of mast cells and basophils. Cross-linking of two IgE molecules is necessary to initiate mediator release from mast cells.
- Activated mast cells and basophils release various mediators.
- The effects of mediator release produce vascular changes, activation of platelets, eosinophils, and neutrophils, and activation of the coagulation cascade.

It is believed that physical allergies such as heat, cold, and ultraviolet light cause a physiochemical derangement of protein or polysaccharides of the skin and transform them into autoantigens responsible for the allergic reaction. Most, if not all, of these reactions are caused by the action of a self-directed IgE.

Anaphylactoid (anaphylaxis-like) reactions are clinically similar to anaphylaxis. They can be caused by immunologically inert materials that activate serum and tissue proteases and the alternate pathway of the complement system. They are not mediated by antigen-antibody interaction; instead offending substances act directly either on the mast cells, causing the release of mediators, or on the tissues (e.g., anaphylotoxins of the complement cascade—C3a, C5a). Direct chemical degranulation of mast cells may be the cause of anaphylactoid reactions resulting from the infusion of macromolecules such as proteins.

Signs and Symptoms

Local reactions consist of urticaria and angioedema at the site of antigen exposure of angioedema of the bowel after ingestion of certain foods. These reactions are severe but rarely fatal. Physical allergies to heat, cold, sunlight, and pressure are not as life threatening as those related to injectables.

Anaphylactic reactions are dramatic and rapid in their onset. The signs and symptoms of anaphylaxis are defined by the physiologic effects of the primary and secondary mediator on the target organs such as the cardiovascular or respiratory system, gastrointestinal tract, or the skin. Several important pharmacologically active compounds are discharged from mast cells and basophils during anaphylaxis (Table 23-1).

Histamine release leads to constriction of bronchial smooth muscle, edema of the trachea and larynx, and stimulation of smooth muscle in the gastrointestinal tract, which causes vomiting and diarrhea. The resulting breakdown of cutaneous vascular integrity results in urticaria and angioedema; vasodilation causes a reduction of circulating blood volume and a progressive fall in blood pressure leading to shock. Kinins also alter vascular permeability and blood pressure.

The body's natural moderators of anaphylaxis are the enzymes that decompose the mediators of anaphylaxis. Antihistamines have no effect on histamine release from mast cells or basophils. In humans antihistamines are effective antagonists of edema and pruritus, which is probably related to their blockage of a histamine-induced increase in capillary permeability. However, antihistamines are relatively less effective in humans in preventing bronchoconstriction.

Laboratory Evaluation

In vitro evaluation of type I hypersensitivity reactions can be by the older radioimmunosorbent test (RIST), radioallergosorbent test (RAST), and enzyme immunoassays. A nephelometric cryoprecipitation testing may also be used. The RIST procedure depends on the availability of an ^{125}I-labeled IgE myeloma protein and its specific antibody; the latter is used in the solid phase of this radioimmunoassay (RIA) procedure. Competition of IgE in any unknown serum sample with the radiolabeled myeloma protein is measured. It is a direct measure of total serum IgE and a typical competitive inhibition RIA test. RAST uses a specific allergen bound to a solid-phase carrier, which is then incubated with a serum sample containing an unknown amount of IgE specific for the allergen. The amount of label bound is only a measure of the allergen-specific IgE in the serum. Both the RIST and RAST tests have been adapted to the enzyme immunoassay method.

Advantages of in vitro testing include the lack of risk of a systemic hypersensitivity reaction and the lack of dependence on skin reactivity that can be influenced by drugs, disease, or the patient's age. Disadvantages of the RAST include limited allergen selection, reduced sensitivity compared with intradermal skin testing, and increased expense.

TABLE 23-1 Mediators of Anaphylaxis

Mediator	Primary Action
Histamine	Increases vascular permeability
	Promotes contraction of smooth muscle
Leukotrienes	Alters bronchial smooth muscle and enhances the effects of histamine on target organs
Basophil kallikrein	Generates kinins
Serotonin	Contracts smooth muscle
Platelet-activating factor	Enhances the release of histamine and serotonin from platelets that affect smooth muscle tone and vascular permeability
Eosinophil chemotactic factor of anaphylaxis	Attracts eosinophils to area of activity; these cells release secondary mediators that may limit the effects of primary mediators
Prostaglandins	Affect smooth muscle tone and vascular permeability

Healthy adults usually have 61 to 100 ng of IgE per milliliter of serum. IgE in cord serum is about 35% of the adult average. There is no correlation between maternal and newborn serum IgE levels, which indicates that fetal IgE synthesis can occur. In various atopic allergic diseases, especially hay fever and asthma, IgE levels may rise to nearly 6000 ng/mL. Values greater than 1000 ng/mL are considered pathologic.

CYTOTOXIC REACTIONS (TYPE II HYPERSENSITIVITY REACTIONS)

Cytotoxic reactions are characterized by the interaction of IgG or IgM antibody to cell-bound antigen. This binding of an antigen and antibody can result in the activation of complement and destruction of the cell (cytolysis) to which the antigen is bound. Erythrocytes, leukocytes, and platelets can be lysed by this process. Examples of cytotoxic reactions include immediate (acute) transfusion reactions and immune hemolytic anemias such as hemolytic disease of the newborn.

Transfusion Reactions

The term *transfusion reaction* generally refers to the adverse consequences of incompatibility between patient and donor erythrocytes. Transfusion reactions can include hemolytic (red cell lysing) reactions occurring during or shortly after a transfusion, shortened posttransfusion survival of red blood cells, an allergic response, or disease transmission.

Transfusion reactions can be divided into hemolytic and nonhemolytic types. Hemolytic reactions are associated with the infusion of incompatible erythrocytes. These reactions can be further classified into acute (immediate) or delayed in their manifestations (Box 23-1). Several factors influence

---

Box 23-1	**Types of Transfusion Reactions**

IMMEDIATE HEMOLYTIC

Intravascular hemolysis of erythrocytes

DELAYED HEMOLYTIC

Extravascular hemolysis of erythrocytes

IMMEDIATE NONHEMOLYTIC

Febrile reactions
Anaphylaxis
Urticaria
Noncardiac pulmonary edema
Fever and shock
Congestive heart failure
Myocardial failure

DELAYED NONHEMOLYTIC

Graft-vs-host disease
Posttransfusion purpura
Iron overload
Alloimmunization to erythrocytes, leukocytes, and/or platelet antigens or plasma proteins
Infectious disease

---

whether a transfusion reaction will be acute or delayed. These factors include:
- The number of incompatible erythrocytes infused
- The antibody class or subclass
- The achievement of the optimal temperature for antibody binding

Immediate Hemolytic Reactions

The most common cause of an acute hemolytic transfusion reaction is the transfusion of ABO-group incompatible blood. In patients with preexisting antibodies caused by prior transfusion or pregnancy, other blood groups may be responsible.

Epidemiology. Acute hemolytic reactions are the most serious and potentially lethal. Most fatalities resulting from acute hemolytic transfusion reactions occur in anesthetized or unconscious patients, with the immediate cause of death being uncontrollable hypotension.

Signs and Symptoms. Reactions can occur with the infusion of as little as 10 to 15 mL of incompatible blood. The most common initial symptoms are fever and chills, which mimic a febrile, nonhemolytic reaction caused by leukocyte incompatibility. Back pain, shortness of breath, pain at the infusion site, and hypotension are additional symptoms. In addition to shock, the release of thromboplastic substances into the circulation can induce disseminated intravascular coagulation and acute renal failure.

Immunologic Manifestations. Acute hemolytic reactions occur during or immediately after blood has been infused. Infusion of incompatible erythrocytes in the presence of preexisting antibodies initiates an antigen-antibody reaction with the activation of the complement, plasminogen, kinin, and coagulation systems. Other initiators of acute hemolytic reactions include bacterial contamination of blood or the infusion of hemolyzed erythrocytes. Many reactions demonstrate both extravascular and intravascular hemolysis. If an antibody is capable of activating complement and is sufficiently active in vivo, intravascular hemolysis occurs, producing a rapid increase of free hemoglobin in the circulation. The cause of the immediate clinical symptoms is uncertain, but it may be due to products released by the action of complement on the erythrocytes, which triggers multiple shock mechanisms.

Delayed Hemolytic Reaction

A delayed reaction may not express itself until 7 to 10 days posttransfusion. In contrast to an immediate reaction, a delayed reaction occurs in the extravascular spaces. These reactions are associated with decreased red cell survival because of the coating of the red cells (a positive direct antiglobulin test), which promotes phagocytosis and premature removal of the red cells by the mononuclear phagocytic system. If an antibody does not activate complement or does so very slowly, extravascular hemolysis occurs. Most IgG antibody-coated erythrocytes are destroyed extravascularly, mainly in the spleen.

A delayed hemolytic transfusion reaction may be of two types. It may represent an anamnestic antibody response in a previously immunized recipient on secondary exposure to transfused erythrocyte antigens, or it may result from primary alloimmunization. In an anamnestic response, the antibodies are directed against antigens to which the recipient has been previously immunized by transfusion or pregnancy.

Hemolytic Disease of the Newborn

Hemolytic disease of the newborn (HDN), previously called erythroblastosis fetalis, results from excessive destruction of fetal red cells by maternal antibodies. This condition in the fetus or newborn infant is clinically characterized by anemia and jaundice. If the hemoglobin breakdown product that visibly produces jaundice (bilirubin) reaches excessive levels in the newborn infant's circulation, it will accumulate in lipid-rich nervous tissue and can result in mental retardation or death.

Etiology

Antigens possessed by the fetus that are foreign to the mother can provoke an antibody response in the mother. Any blood group antigen that occurs as an IgG antibody is capable of causing HDN.

Although anti-A and anti-B are present in the absence of their corresponding antigens as environmentally stimulated (IgM) antibodies, infrequent IgG forms may be responsible for HDN because of ABO incompatibility. High titers of anti-A,B of the IgG type in group O mothers commonly cause mild HDN. Anti-A and anti-B antibodies are usually 19S (IgM) in character and as such are unable to pass through the placental barrier. In addition, the A and B antigens are not fully expressed on the erythrocytes of the fetus and newborn. In a survey of antibodies that have caused HDN, more than 70 different antibodies were identified.

Epidemiology

The incidence of HDN resulting from ABO incompatibility ranges from 1 in 70 to 1 in 180, with an estimated average of 1 in 150 births. The most frequent form of ABO incompatibility occurs when the mother is type O and the baby is type A or type B, usually type A.

Until the early 1970s the Rh antibody anti-D was the most frequent cause of moderate or severe forms of HDN and anti-D either alone or in combination with another Rh antibody; anti-C accounted for approximately 93% of the cases of non-ABO HDN. Since the development of modern treatment to prevent primary immunization to the D antigen, however, the frequency of HDN because of anti-D has significantly decreased.

Signs and Symptoms

HDN resulting from ABO incompatibility is usually mild in manifestations because of several factors: fewer A and B antigen sites on the fetal/newborn erythrocytes, weaker antigen strength of fetal/newborn A and B antigens, and competition for anti-A and anti-B between tissues and erythrocytes. The number and strength of A and B antigen sites on fetal erythrocytes are less than on adult red blood cell membranes. In addition, A and B substances are not confined to the red cells, so only a small fraction of IgG anti-A and anti-B that crosses the placenta combines with the infant's erythrocytes.

Manifestations of HDN caused by other antibodies can range from mild to severe. In addition to possible death in utero, newborn infants may demonstrate severe anemia and an increase in red blood cell breakdown products such as bilirubin. Accumulation of bilirubin causes jaundice and may result in mental retardation if methods are not applied to clear bilirubin from the infant's body.

Immunologic Mechanism

For antibody formation to take place, the mother must lack the antigen, and the fetus must express the antigen (gene product). The fetus would inherit the gene for antigen expression from the father. HDN results from the production of antibodies in the mother that have been stimulated by the presence of these foreign fetal antigens. The actual production of antibodies depends on a variety of factors: the genetic makeup of the mother, the antigenicity of a specific antigen, and the actual amount of antigen introduced into the maternal circulation.

Transplacental hemorrhage (TPH) can occur at any stage of pregnancy. Immunization resulting from TPH can result from negligible doses during the first 6 months in utero; however, significant immunizing hemorrhage usually occurs during the third trimester or at delivery. Fetal erythrocytes can also enter the maternal circulation as the result of physical trauma from an injury, abortion, ectopic pregnancy, amniocentesis, or normal delivery. Abruptio placentae, cesarean section, and manual removal of the placenta are often associated with a considerable increase in TPH.

An example of the normal pattern of immunization is demonstrated by the case of an Rh (D) negative mother whose primary immunization (sensitization) was due to either a previously incompatible Rh (D) positive pregnancy or a blood transfusion, which stimulates the production of low-titered anti-D, predominantly of the IgM class. Subsequent antigenic stimulation, such as fetal-maternal hemorrhage during pregnancy with an Rh (D) positive fetus, can elicit a secondary (anamnestic) response, which is characterized by the predominance of increasing titers of anti-D of the IgG class.

Immune antibodies subsequently react with fetal antigens. Erythrocytic antigens, as well as leukocyte and platelet antigens, can induce maternal immunization by the formation of IgG antibodies. In HDN the erythrocytes of the fetus become coated with maternal antibodies that correspond to specific fetal antigens. IgG antibodies, the only Ig is selectively transported to the fetus, are transferred from the maternal circulation to the fetal circulation through the placenta. The mechanism by which IgG passes through the placenta has not been definitely established. Most research on the subject of transplacental passage, however, supports the hypothesis that all IgG subclasses are capable of crossing the placental barrier between mother and fetus.

When the antigen and its corresponding antibody combine in vivo, increased lysis of red cells results. Because of this hemolytic process, the normal 45- to 70-day life span of the fetal erythrocytes is reduced. To compensate for red cell loss, the fetal liver, spleen, and bone marrow respond by increasing production of erythrocytes. Increased erythrocyte production outside of the bone marrow, extramedullary hematopoiesis, can result in enlargement of the liver and spleen and premature release of nucleated erythrocytes from the bone marrow into the fetal circulation. If increased production of erythrocytes cannot compensate for the cell being destroyed, a progressively severe anemia develops that can cause the fetus to develop cardiac failure with generalized edema and death in utero. Less severely affected infants continue to experience erythrocyte destruction after birth, which generates large quantities of unconjugated bilirubin. Bilirubin resulting from excessive hemolysis can produce the threat of accumulation of free bilirubin in lipid-rich tissue of the central nervous system.

Diagnostic Evaluation

The following procedures are generally used in either the prenatal or postnatal diagnostic evaluation of HDN:

- ABO blood grouping
- Rh testing
- Screening for irregular antibodies; identification and titering of any antibodies
- Amniocentesis (prenatal)
- Serum bilirubin of cord or infant blood
- Direct antiglobulin test of cord or infant blood
- Peripheral blood smear
- The Du Rosette or Kleihauer-Betke test

Prevention

Three independent research teams showed that a passive antibody, Rh IgG, could protect most Rh-negative mothers from becoming immunized after the delivery of Rh (D)-positive infants or similar obstetric conditions. In 1968, Rh IgG was licensed for administration in the United States. Since that time a dramatic decrease in the incidence of HDN caused by anti-D has taken place, although complete elimination may never occur because of the cases in which anti-D is formed before delivery. All pregnant Rh-negative women should receive Rh IgG, even if the Rh status of the fetus is unknown because fetal D antigen is present on fetal erythrocytes as early as 38 days from conception.

IMMUNE COMPLEX (TYPE III) REACTIONS

The formation of immune complexes under normal conditions protects the host because these complexes facilitate the clearance of various antigens and invading microorganisms by the phagocytic system. In immune complex reactions, however, antigen-antibody complexes form in the soluble or fluid phase of tissues or in the blood and assume unique biologic functions such as interaction with complement and with cellular receptors. Examples of type III reactions include the Arthus reaction (Figure 23-1), serum sickness, and certain aspects of autoimmune disease such as glomerulonephritis in systemic lupus erythematosus. Circulating soluble immune complexes are responsible for or associated with a variety of human diseases in which both exogenous and endogenous antigens can trigger a pathogenic immune response and result in immune complex disease (Table 23-2).

These reactions are caused by IgG, IgM, or possibly other antibody types. Immune complexes can exhibit a spectrum of biologic activities, including suppression or augmentation of the immune response by interacting with B and T cells; inhibition of tumor cell destruction; and deposition in blood vessel walls, glomerular membranes, and other sites. These deposits interrupt normal physiologic processes because of tissue damage secondary to the activation of complement and resulting activities such as mediating immune adherence and attracting leukocytes and macrophages to the sites of immune complex deposition. The release of enzymes and possibly

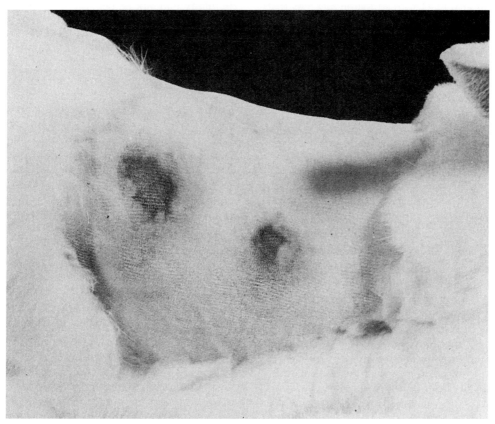

Figure 23-1   The Arthus reaction. In these two reactions of the skin of a rabbit, the larger reaction has an extensive zone of erythema and edema surrounding its necrotic center. (From Markell EK, Voge M: *Medical parasitology,* ed 5, Philadelphia, 1981, WB Saunders.)

TABLE 23-2	Diseases Associated With Immune Complexes
Type	**Examples**
Autoimmune diseases	Rheumatoid arthritis, systemic lupus erythematosus, Sjögren's syndrome, mixed connective tissue disease, systemic sclerosis, glomerulonephritis
Neoplastic disease	Solid and lymphoid tumors
Infectious disease	Bacterial infective endocarditis, streptococcal infection, viral hepatitis, infectious mononucleosis

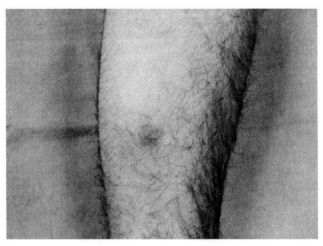

Figure 23-2   A delayed skin reaction exhibiting an erythematous but nonedematous zone 15 mm in diameter at 48 hours. A control site, inoculated higher on the forearm, shows no reaction at this time. (From Barrett JT: *Textbook of immunology,* ed 5, St Louis, 1988, Mosby.)

other agents damages the tissues. The three general anatomic sites of antigen-antibody interactions are:

- Antibody can react with soluble antigens in the circulation and form immune complexes that may disseminate and lodge in any tissue with a large filtration area and cause lesions of immune complex disease.
- Antibody can react with antigen secreted or injected locally into the interstitial fluids. The classic example of this is the experimental Arthus reaction, which is the basic model of local immune complex disease.
- Antibody can also react with structural antigens that form part of the cell surface membranes or with fixed intercellular structures such as the basement membranes. The systemic immune complex disease, serum sickness, is an example of soluble and tissue-fixed antigen involvement.

Acute serum sickness develops within 1 to 2 weeks after initial exposure or repeated exposure by injection of heterologous serum protein. There is no preexisting antibody, and the disease appears as antibody formation begins. The hallmark of serum sickness is the protracted interaction between antigen and antibody in the circulation with the formation of antigen-antibody complexes in an environment of antigen excess. Chronic serum sickness can be experimentally induced if small amounts of antigen are given daily and represent just enough antigen to balance antibody production.

TYPE IV CELL-MEDIATED REACTIONS

Cell-mediated immunity consists of immune activities that differ from antibody-mediated immunity. Cell-mediated immunity is moderated by the link between T lymphocytes and phagocytic cells (i.e., monocytes-macrophages). Lymphocytes (T cells) do not recognize the antigens of microorganisms or other living cells but are immunologically active through various types of direct cell-to-cell contact and by the production of soluble factors. The delayed type reaction is cell mediated and involves antigen-sensitized T cells, which respond directly or by the release of lymphokines to exhibit contact dermatitis and allergies of infection (Figure 23-2).

Cell-mediated immunity is responsible for the following immunologic events:

- Contact sensitivity
- Delayed hypersensitivity
- Immunity to viral and fungal antigens
- Immunity to intracellular organisms
- Rejection of foreign tissue grafts
- Elimination of tumor cells bearing neoantigens
- Formation of chronic granulomas

Under some conditions the activities of cell-mediated immunity may not be beneficial. Suppression of the normal adaptive immune response (immunosuppression) by drugs or other means is necessary in conditions such as organ transplantation, hypersensitivity, and autoimmune disorders.

Case Study

Mr. R.M., a 60-year-old Caucasian man, was stung by a bee while gardening. He had been stung once before earlier in the summer. Within a few seconds, his hand began to itch and he began to experience abdominal cramping. He subsequently began experiencing difficulty breathing. Fortunately, he was able to reach a first aid kit in his garage. Inside of the kit was an EpiPen (injectable epinephrine) that his wife kept for herself because she was allergic to bee venom. He used the pen and began to feel somewhat better. He immediately had his wife drive him to the hospital.

He was asymptomatic on arrival at the hospital. R.M. had no history of adverse reactions to bee venom or antibiotics. Because of the nature of the incident, a diagnosis of anaphylactic shock due to bee venom sensitivity was made. An IgE level was ordered. The results indicated a level more than twice the (normal) reference range value. In addition, a follow-up skin test was performed. The patient was extremely positive for bee venom.

Box 23-2	**Case Study Laboratory Results**

| Mrs. C.C. | Group A; Rh D-negative | Irregular antibody screen = positive anti-D (1:8) |
| Mr. C.C. | Group A; Rh D-positive | (CDe/CDe) |

Questions and Discussion

1. What is the mechanism involved in anaphylaxis?

    The term anaphylaxis is used to describe a systemic clinical syndrome caused by IgE mediated degranulation of tissue basophils (mast cells) and peripheral blood basophils. Susceptible individuals exposed to a sensitizing antigen produce specific IgE antibodies that bind to high affinity IgE receptors found on mast cells and basophils. The receptor binds the Fe portion of the antibody leaving the Fab binding sites available to interact with antigen. The avidity of this Fe binding reaction is high; the dissociation of IgE from the receptors is slow. If a repeat exposure occurs, the antigen is bound by the IgE receptor complexes, which causes receptor-mediated activation of the cells with release of mediators. The rapid release of massive amounts of mediators is responsible for the clinical manifestations of anaphylaxis.

2. What types of agents can induce anaphylactic shock?

    The IgE-mediated mast cell degranulation can be triggered by a variety of agents: antibiotics (e.g., penicillins, cephalosporins), pharmacologic agents (e.g., streptokinase, vaccines), foods (e.g., peanuts, shellfish), and foreign proteins (e.g., latex, bee venom).

    Mast cell degranulation can also occur by IgE independent pathways. In this situation, prior exposure is not a prerequisite because specific IgE antibodies are not involved. Three putative mechanisms of anaphylactoid reactions are blood, blood products, and Igs; certain therapeutic and diagnostic agents; and reaction to nonsteroidal antiinflammatory drugs (NSAIDs).

    Blood, blood products, and Igs can cause an anaphylactoid reaction because of the formation of immune complexes with subsequent complement activation and production of C3a and C5a. C3a and C5a are capable of degranulating mast cells directly and increase vasopermeability, which can induce hypotension and shock.

    Certain therapeutic and diagnostic agents (e.g., opiates, muscle relaxants, and radiographic contrast media) are also capable of directly causing mast cell degranulation and anaphylaxis.

    Reaction to NSAIDs (e.g., aspirin) can be observed in a minority (5% to 10%) of patients with asthma. The ability of these agents to cause anaphylaxis appears to correlate with their unknown mode of action in inhibiting prostaglandin synthesis.

Diagnosis

Type I Hypersensitivity Reaction

Case Study

Mrs. C.C., a 35-year-old gravida 4 para 1+2, was seen by her gynecologist when she was 8 weeks pregnant. Her first pregnancy 4 years ago was unremarkable. The patient reported that her second and third pregnancies had resulted in a stillbirth at 36 weeks and a spontaneous abortion at 10 weeks of gestation. Her medical history revealed no history of blood transfusions. She remembered being vaccinated for rubella. Her medical records had been destroyed in a fire at the clinic. Repeat blood grouping and Rh testing, and an irregular antibody screen were ordered (Box 23-2).

Mrs. C.C. returned in 2 weeks for a repeat anti-D titer. The titer had risen to 1:16. At 17 weeks of gestation, an amniocentesis was performed. Severe hemolysis was demonstrated and an intrauterine transfusion of the fetus was carried out using fresh, washed, cytomegalovirus screening test–negative, group O, Rh D negative blood. Because of the continuing risk to the fetus, a caesarean section was performed at 36 weeks of gestation. On the delivery, the baby was noted to be jaundiced and pale. The first of three exchange transfusions were performed. Phototherapy was also used to degrade the bilirubin deposited in the skin. The baby made an uneventful recovery with no signs of kernicterus and was discharged from the hospital 5 days after birth.

Questions and Discussion

1. What is the mechanism of HDN?

    Destruction of fetal red blood cells can occur when maternal IgG specific for antigens on the baby's red blood cells cross the placental barrier. The cells become coated by the antibody in vivo and are destroyed by the fetal phagocytic system. Unborn babies can die in utero or live born babies can present with symptoms of anemia, jaundice, or cardiac failure at birth.

    Before the availability of prophylactic therapy for Rh disease caused by the D antigen, most severe cases of HDN were attributable to the D antigen of the Rh blood group system. The mother lacks the D antigen; the baby possesses the D antigen. Initial maternal exposure to fetal red cells causes a primary IgM antibody response, which often occurs as a result of transplacental hemorrhage at birth. The first child is not usually affected. Subsequent Rh D positive children are at risk from the antibodies because they are of the IgG class and so cross the placenta freely.

Many D negative mothers do not become sensitized to the D antigen of the fetus because of maternal-fetal ABO blood group incompatibility. The most common examples occur if the mother is group O and the baby is group A. If such an incompatibility exists, fetal red cells entering the maternal circulation will be coated with the mother's isoantibody and destroyed before they have a chance to provoke a D-antigen-specific antibody response. Many cases of ABO incompatibility occur with group O mothers who have an increased incidence of IgG anti-B and anti-A antibodies. Most infants with ABO HDN are mildly affected. Phototherapy normally resolves the jaundice, with less than 0.05% of babies requiring exchange transfusions.
2. What prophylactic measures are used to prevent HDN due to the D antigen?

Anti-D antibodies are administered to eligible Rh D negative women immediately after birth of an Rh D positive child. The prevention mechanism is believed to be that the injected antibody coats the baby's D positive cells circulating in the mother's blood. The coated cells are removed by the mononuclear phagocytic system and no immunologic exposure to the D antigen occurs.

Diagnosis

Type II hypersensitivity reaction

Case Study

Z.Z.'s medical history included frequent sore throats as a child. He had been treated with antibiotics, particularly penicillin. Eventually he developed a rash. He was told that he had developed an allergy to penicillin and that he should not have it again.

A decade later he developed a urinary tract infection for which he was treated with an antibiotic, trimethoprim. The therapy was for 8 days. A few days after completing the regimen, he developed a headache and some itchy bumps on his skin. The next day he had sore and swollen joints. His physician confirmed that the rash was urticaria. He also had an elevated temperature and swollen glands in his neck. The diagnosis of a drug allergy was made. The patient was given antihistamines. If this medication failed to alleviate the symptoms, more aggressive steroid therapy would be pursued.

His symptoms did not improve and he was started on an oral corticosteroid, prednisone. Three weeks later, the patient returned to his physician. He was asymptomatic.

Questions and Discussion

1. What is the likely mechanism of the reaction?

The symptoms of rash, headache, and joint pain are the hallmarks of an allergic drug response. A delayed onset reflects the need for antigen to remain in the circulation for a prolonged period in order for a sufficient amount of antibody to be synthesized. Once an adequate titer of antibody has been pro-

duced, circulating antigen-antibody complexes are formed which "precipitate" out in various target tissues. Wherever the complexes are sited, complement can be fixed, and local damage occurs. Local damage can be manifested as inflammation of the joints and skin. Anaphylatoxins, C3a and C5a, can directly release histamine from mast cells. This activity can lead to a confusing picture of a type III hypersensitivity reaction presenting clinically as anaphylactic shock.
2. What kinds of agents can lead to drug reactions?

A variety of drugs can cause reactions by activating effector pathways by nonimmunologic means. Opiates, for example, can cause the release of mediators from mast cells by direct action on the cell without the involvement of IgE. Other agents leading to drug reactions include x-ray contrast media, which activates the alternative pathway of complement and can produce anaphylatoxins (C3a and C5a) and can lead to anaphylactic shock.

Drugs (e.g., aspirin and NSAIDs) alter arachidonic acid pathways and can produce anaphylactic shock.

Diagnosis

Type III hypersensitivity reaction

Case Study

This 19-year-old college student went to the Student Health Services because she had slowly developed a rash on both ear lobes, the hands and wrist, and around her neck.

Her past medical history revealed that as a child she had suffered from eczema. Later on during her early teens she had facial acne for which she was given tetracycline. Physical examination revealed a rash consisting of erythema and small blisters. There was marked excoriation because of the itching. Her hands were red, scaly, and dry. The rash on her hands looked very different to the eruptions on her neck and ears. A contact hypersensitivity was suspected.

Follow-up patch tests included a standard battery of agents: rubber, cosmetics, plant extracts, perfumes, nickel, and makeup. Strongly positive reactions for rubber and nickel were observed.

The student was advised to eliminate contact with rubber (e.g., rubber gloves) used at home or on the job. Her jewelry probably contained nickel and was believed to be the source of the irritation to her earlobes, neck, and wrists. She was advised to wear only nickel-free jewelry. A mild corticosteroid cream was prescribed to be used until her symptoms disappeared.

Questions and Discussion

1. Why did the jewelry cause a rash?

A contact allergy is a classic example of a type IV hypersensitivity. The reaction itself is one of eczema where the external agent comes into contact with the skin. The most common causative agents are haptens (e.g., metals such as nickel, chemicals, poison ivy, and poison oak). Drugs that are topically applied can also be a source of contact dermatitis.

Haptens are small molecules that are too small themselves to elicit an immunologic response. When these small molecules penetrate the epidermis, however, they form covalent bonds with body proteins and produce the immunogenic hapten-carrier complex.

2. What is the mechanism of type IV hypersensitivity involvement in contact eczema?

There are two main phases of a contact hypersensitivity reaction:

a. Sensitization is the first phase and can take up to 2 weeks. During this stage the hapten has combined with the carrier protein and been processed by the Langerhans' cells in the epidermis. These cells migrate to the paracortical area of the draining lymph node where major histocompatibility complex class II molecules present the antigen to CD4+ lymphocytes leading to clonal expansion.

b. Elicitation is the phase that involves the Langerhans' cells. After the application of the contact agent to the skin, there is a decrease in the resident population of Langerhans' cells in the epidermis. Presentation of the antigen occurs in the skin and local lymph node with the release of cytokines from many types of cells. There is also evidence of mast cell degranulation after contact with the allergen. This leads not only to mediator release but to further production of cytokines as well. Tumor necrosis factor-alpha and interleukin-1 induce adhesion molecules on endothelial cells, which produce the signal for mononuclear cell migration into the skin, peaking at 48 to 72 hours.

Diagnosis

Type IV hypersensitivity reaction

CHAPTER HIGHLIGHTS

The term *immunization,* or *sensitization,* is used to describe an immunologic reaction dependent on the response of the host to a subsequent exposure of antigen. Hypersensitivity has traditionally been separated on the basis of time after exposure to an offending antigen. When this criterion is used, the terms *immediate* and *delayed* are appropriate.

Type I hypersensitivity reactions can range from life-threatening anaphylactic reactions to milder manifestations associated with food allergies. Anaphylaxis is the clinical response to immunologic formation and fixation between a specific antigen and a tissue-fixing antibody. This reaction is usually mediated by IgE antibody and occurs in three stages. Anaphylactoid (anaphylaxis-like) reactions are clinically similar to anaphylaxis. They can be caused by immunologically inert materials that activate serum and tissue proteases and the alternate pathway of the complement system.

In vitro evaluation of Type I hypersensitivity reactions can be by RIST, RAST, and enzyme immunoassays. The advantages of in vitro testing include the lack of risk of a systemic hypersensitivity reaction, and the lack of dependence on skin reactivity that can be influenced by drugs, disease, or the age of the patient. Disadvantages of the RAST include limited allergen selection, reduced sensitivity compared with intradermal skin testing, and increased expense.

Cytotoxic reactions are characterized by the interaction of IgG or IgM antibody to cell-bound antigen. This binding of an antigen and antibody can result in the activation of complement and cytolysis to which the antigen is bound. Erythrocytes, leukocytes, and platelets can be lysed by this process. Examples of cytotoxic reactions include immediate (acute) transfusion reactions and immune hemolytic anemias such as hemolytic disease of the newborn.

Transfusion reactions can be divided into hemolytic and nonhemolytic types. Hemolytic reactions are associated with the infusion of incompatible erythrocytes. These reactions can be further classified into acute or delayed in their manifestations.

The most common cause of an acute hemolytic transfusion reaction is the transfusion of ABO-incompatible blood. Other initiators of acute hemolytic reactions include bacterial contamination of blood or the infusion of hemolyzed erythrocytes. A delayed reaction may not express itself until 7 to 10 days after transfusion.

HDN is another example of a cytotoxic (type II) reaction. This condition in the fetus or newborn infant is clinically characterized by anemia and jaundice and is caused by antibodies in the mother that are stimulated by fetal antigens. The most frequent form of ABO incompatibility occurs when the mother is type O and the baby is type A or type B, usually type A.

However, in immune complex reactions antigen-antibody complexes form in the soluble or fluid phase of tissues or in the blood and assume unique biologic functions such as interaction with complement and with cellular receptors. Examples of type III reactions include the Arthus reaction, serum sickness, and certain aspects of autoimmune disease.

Cell-mediated immunity consists of immune activities that differ from antibody-mediated immunity. Cell-mediated immunity is moderated by the link between T lymphocytes and phagocytic cells. Cell-mediated immunity is responsible for contact sensitivity, delayed hypersensitivity, immunity to viral and fungal antigens, immunity to intracellular organisms, rejection of foreign tissue grafts, elimination of tumor cells bearing neoantigens, and formation of chronic granulomas.

REVIEW QUESTIONS

Questions 1-4. Match the following types of hypersensitivity reactions with their respective type of reaction.

1. Type I
2. Type II
3. Type III
4. Type IV
   A. cytotoxic
   B. cell-mediated
   C. immune complex
   D. anaphylactic

5. With which cell type are anaphylactic reactions associated?
   A. T lymphocyte
   B. B lymphocyte
   C. monocyte
   D. mast

6. Type III reactions are exemplified by all of the following except:
   A. Arthus reaction
   B. serum sickness
   C. glomerulonephritis
   D. shingles

7. Type IV reactions are responsible for all of the following except:
   A. contact sensitivity
   B. delayed hypersensitivity
   C. immunity to viral and fungal antigens
   D. immunity to bacteria

8. Type I hypersensitivity reactions can be associated with:
   A. food allergies
   B. hay fever
   C. asthma
   D. all of the above

9. The most common agents that cause anaphylactic reactions are:
   A. drugs and food
   B. drugs and insect stings
   C. poison ivy and insect stings
   D. food and insect stings

Questions 10-12. Arrange the sequence of events in anaphylaxis in the proper sequence.

10. _____   A. The effects of mediator release produce vascular changes, activation of platelets, eosinophils, and neutrophils, as well as activation of the coagulation cascade.
11. _____   B. The offending antigen attaches to the IgE antibody fixed to the surface membrane of mast cells and basophils.
12. _____   C. Activated mast cells and basophils release various mediators.

Questions 13-18. Complete the table, choosing from the possible answers provided.

Possible answers to questions 13-15
   A. enhances the effects of histamine on target organs
   B. increases vascular permeability and promotes contraction of smooth muscle
   C. generates kinins
   D. contracts smooth muscle

Possible answers to questions 16-18
   A. affects smooth muscle tone and vascular permeability
   B. enhances the release of histamine and serotonin
   C. attracts cells to area of activity; these cells release secondary mediators that may limit the effects of primary mediators
   D. alters bronchial smooth muscle

Mediators of Anaphylaxis

Mediator	Primary action
Histamine	13. _____
Leukotrienes	14. _____
Serotonin	15. _____
Platelet-activating factor	16. _____
Eosinophil chemotactic factors of anaphylaxis	17. _____
Prostaglandins	18. _____

19. In vitro evaluation of type I hypersensitivity reactions can include:
    A. RIST
    B. RAST
    C. neither A nor B
    D. both A and B

20. Cytotoxic reactions are characterized by:
    A. interaction of IgG to soluble antigen
    B. interaction of IgG to cell-bound antigen
    C. interaction of IgM to soluble antigen
    D. interaction of IgM or IgG to cell-bound antigen

21. An example of a delayed nonhemolytic (type II hypersensitivity reaction) is:
    A. febrile reaction
    B. graft-vs-host disease
    C. urticaria
    D. congestive heart failure

22. Under normal conditions immune complexes protect the host because:
    A. complexes facilitate the clearance of various antigens
    B. complexes facilitate the clearance of invading microorganisms
    C. they interact with complement
    D. both A and B

23. Immune complexes can:
    A. suppress or augment the immune response by interacting with T and B cells
    B. inhibit tumor cell destruction
    C. deposit in blood vessel walls
    D. all of the above

24. The general anatomic site(s) of antigen-antibody interaction is (are):
    A. any tissue with a large filtration area
    B. interstitial fluids
    C. cell surface membranes or fixed intercellular structures
    D. all of the above

25. Type IV hypersensitivity reactions are responsible for all of the following except:
    A. contact sensitivity
    B. elimination of tumor cells
    C. rejection of foreign tissue grafts
    D. serum sickness

BIBLIOGRAPHY

Altman LC, editor: *Clinical allergy and immunology,* Boston, 1984, GK Hall.

Anderson DC, Stiehm R: Immunization, *JAMA* 268(20):2959-2963, 1992.

Bochner BS, Lichtenstein LM: Anaphylaxis, *N Engl J Med* 324(25):1785-1790, 1991.

Gardner P, Schaffner W: Immunization of adults, *N Engl J Med* 328(17):1252-1258, 1993.

Homburger HA: The laboratory evaluation of allergic diseases: Part I, *Lab Med* 22(11):780-782, 1991.

Homburger HA: The laboratory evaluation of allergic diseases: Part II, *Lab Med* 22(12):845-848, 1991.

Ishizaka K: Regulation of IgE biosynthesis, *Hosp Pract* 20:53-41, 1989.

Kaitin KI: Graft-versus-host disease, *N Engl J Med* 325(5):357-358, 1991.

Kaplan AP, editor: *Allergy,* New York, 1985, Churchill Livingstone.

Lawlor GJ, Rosenblatt HM: Anaphylaxis. In Lawlor GJ, Rosenblatt HM, editors: *Manual of allergy and immunology,* ed 2, Boston, 1988, Little, Brown.

Lockey RF, Bukantz SC, editors: *Principles of immunology and allergy,* Philadelphia, 1987, WB Saunders.

Lockey RF: Future trends in allergy and immunology, *JAMA* 268(20):2991-2992, 1992.

Luban NLC: The new and the old-molecular diagnostics and hemolytic disease of the newborn, *N Engl J Med* 329(9):658-660, 1993.

Mann R, Neilson EG: Pathogenesis and treatment of immune-mediated renal disease, *Med Clin N Am* 69(4):715-719, 1985.

McDougal JS, McDuffie FC: Immune complexes in man: detection and clinical significance, *Adv Clin Chem* 24:1-59, 1985.

Peter G: Childhood immunizations, *N Engl J Med* 327(25):1794-1800, 1992.

Sly MR: *Textbook of pediatric allergy,* New Hyde Park, NY, 1985, Medical Examination Publishing Co.

Sussman GL, Tarlo S, Dolovich J: The spectrum of IgE-mediated responses to latex, *JAMA* 265(21): 2844-2847, 1991.

Turgeon ML: *Fundamentals of immunohematology,* ed 2, Baltimore, 1995, Williams & Wilkins.

U.S. Dept of Health and Human Services: Update on adult immunization, *MMWR* 40(RR-12):1-52, 1991.

Valentine MD: Anaphylaxis and stinging insect hypersensitivity, *JAMA* 268(20):2830-2833, 1992.

Walker RH: *AABB technical manual,* ed 11, Bethesda, Md, 1993, American Association of Blood Banks.

Chapter 24

Immunoproliferative Disorders

LEARNING OBJECTIVES

At the conclusion of this chapter, the reader should be able to:

• Compare the general characteristics of monoclonal and polyclonal gammopathies.

• Describe and compare the etiology, epidemiology, signs and symptoms, immunologic manifestations, and diagnostic

evaluation of multiple myeloma and Waldenström's primary macroglobulinemia.

• Explain and contrast the characteristics of other monoclonal disorders.

• Analyze a representative case study.

Hypergammaglobulinemias are either monoclonal or polyclonal in nature. A monoclonal gammopathy, which can be either a benign or malignant condition, results from a single clone of lymphoid-plasma cells producing elevated levels of a single class and type of immunoglobulin (Ig). The elevated Ig is referred to as a monoclonal protein, M protein, or paraprotein. Disorders in this category of plasma cell dyscrasias include multiple myeloma, Waldenström's macroglobulinemia (WM), light-chain deposition disease, and heavy-chain diseases. In comparison, a polyclonal gammopathy is classified as a secondary disease and characterized by the elevation of two or more Igs by several clones of plasma cells.

GENERAL CHARACTERISTICS OF MONOCLONAL GAMMOPATHIES

Monoclonal gammopathies are characterized by an uncontrolled proliferation of a single clone of plasma cells at the expense of other clones. Monoclonal gammopathy of undetermined significance is an asymptomatic laboratory deviation that may evolve into a disorder such as multiple myeloma in about one fourth of cases.

The stimulus for proliferation is unknown, but it is not believed to be antigenic. This dysfunction, however, leads to the synthesis of elevated quantities of one homogeneous Ig or of Ig subunits and an associated immunodeficiency because of decreased levels of normal Igs.

Serum and urine electrophoresis patterns and other Ig assays can demonstrate strikingly abnormal results in disorders such as multiple myeloma and WM. The gamma region of the electrophoresis pattern can show a dense, highly restricted band from uncontrolled proliferation of one cell clone, whereas the other normal Igs are deficient. Clinical interpretation of some patterns, however, can be difficult. In contrast, some symptomatic patients do not exhibit the characteristic monoclonal band or spike in their serum protein patterns. This is often the case with light-chain disease (LCD), where only kappa or lambda monoclonal light chains are synthesized by the clone. These low-molecular-weight Ig fragments are filtered through the glomerulus and into the urine, which produces a serum electrophoresis pattern that suggests hypogammaglobulinemia with either a very faint monoclonal band or no band at all. These also suggest the possibility of the presence of a nonsecretory clone, which produces no monoclonal Igs and frequently demonstrates hypogammaglobulinemia because of the inhibition of normal clones.

GENERAL CHARACTERISTICS OF POLYCLONAL GAMMOPATHIES

A polyclonal gammopathy is a common protein abnormality. It is defined as an increase in more than one Ig and involves several clones of plasma cells. In contrast to a monoclonal protein, a polyclonal protein consists of one or more heavy-chain classes and both light-chain types. Polyclonal increases are exhibited as secondary manifestations of infection or inflammation. They are commonly seen in chronic infections; chronic liver disease, especially chronic active hepatitis; rheumatoid connective tissue (autoimmune) diseases; and lymphoproliferative diseases.

A polyclonal protein is characterized by a broad peak or band, usually of gamma mobility, on electrophoresis; by a thickening and elongation of all heavy- and light-chain arcs on immunoelectrophoresis; and by the absence of a localized band on immunofixation. A polyclonal gammopathy, therefore, resembles a normal pattern with the serum staining more intensely. A selective polyclonal increase is of special interest because only one class of Ig is significantly elevated; however, the increase is polyclonal because Ig is produced by several clones of plasma cells, and both kappa and lambda types are produced. Quantitation by specific assay procedures of the Igs demonstrates which Ig is increased. Immunofixation is not recommended in cases of polyclonal gammopathy because it presents no additional information.

MULTIPLE MYELOMA

Multiple myeloma (also referred to as plasma cell myeloma, myelomatosis, or Kahler's disease) is characterized by a neoplastic or potentially neoplastic proliferation of a single clone of plasma cells that produce a specific type of Ig. The synthesized Ig, often referred to as M protein, myeloma protein, or paraprotein, is monoclonal. It consists of one heavy-chain and one light-chain class.

Etiology

The cause of multiple myeloma is unknown. Radiation may be a factor in some cases; the possibility of a viral cause has been suggested. Other possible factors may be environmental stimulants such as exposure to asbestos, benzene, or industrial toxins. The likelihood of a genetic factor in some cases is supported by well-documented reports of familial clusters with multiple myeloma.

Epidemiology

Multiple myeloma is the most common form of dysproteinemia. It accounts for 1% of all types of malignant diseases and 10% of hematologic malignancies. The general incidence is estimated to be 4 cases per 100,000 per year in the United States. About 10,000 Americans die each year from multiple myeloma.

Onset of this disorder is between the ages of 40 and 70 years, with a peak incidence in the seventh decade. It is uncommon (<2% of cases) in patients less than 40 years old. In general, patients with LCD and with IgD myeloma are younger than those with IgG or IgA myeloma and have a poorer prognosis because of their high incidence of nephropathy. Males are afflicted with the disease in approximately 62% of cases. The male-to-female ratio is 1.6:1. In addition, African-Americans are afflicted twice as often as Caucasians.

IgG myeloma is the most common form of multiple myeloma (Table 24-1). Four subtypes of IgG heavy chains are known to exist among patients with IgG myeloma. Cases of IgG myeloma are distributed as follows: 65% are gamma G1, 23% are gamma G2, 8% are gamma G3, and 4% fall into the gamma G4 subclass. The only subclass-dependent difference is the greater propensity for patients with IgG3 myeloma to experience hyperviscosity syndrome similar to the manifestation in WM.

Multiple myeloma runs a progressive course, with most patients dying within 1 to 3 years. The beta-2 microglobulin level at the time of initial evaluation has been adopted as a predictor of outcome. If the serum beta-2 microglobulin level is elevated at the start of therapy, the prognosis is less favorable. The major causes of death are overwhelming infection (sepsis) and renal insufficiency. In cases of sepsis, the death rate exceeds 50% despite antibiotic therapy.

Signs and Symptoms

The signs and symptoms of multiple myeloma include bone pain, typically in the back or chest, and weakness, fatigue, and pallor associated with anemia or abnormal bleeding. In all, 20% of patients exhibit hepatomegaly and 5% demonstrate splenomegaly. In some cases the major manifestations of disease result from acute infection, renal insufficiency, hy-

TABLE 24-1 Distribution of Immunoglobulin Types Produced in Patients Having Multiple Myeloma

Type of Protein	Multiple Myeloma (%)
IgM	12
IgG	52
IgA	22
IgD	2
IgE	Rare
Light chains (kappa or lambda)	11
Heavy chains	Rare
Monoclonal proteins	<1
Nonsecretory myeloma	1

percalcemia, or amyloidosis. Weight loss and night sweats are not prominent until the disease is advanced. Bone pain, anemia, and renal insufficiency constitute a triad of signs and symptoms strongly suggestive of multiple myeloma.

In 1975 a staging system for myeloma was developed. This system defines indolent versus severe disease and determines a basis for therapy. Patients are divided into three groups. Establishment of the classifications is based on production of IgG by plasma cells and the total quantity of IgG in the body. The number of abnormal plasma cells is correlated with hemoglobin, serum calcium, serum IgG peak, and the presence or absence of lytic bone lesions. Renal function is also considered important because kidney function is important to survival and because IgG light chains can damage the kidneys. Some physicians use a simpler system of staging based on serum albumin, hemoglobin, and beta-2 microglobulin.

Skeletal Abnormalities

About 90% of patients who have multiple myeloma suffer from broadly disseminated destruction of the skeleton, which is responsible for the predominance of bone pain. These abnormalities consist of punched-out lytic areas (Figures 24-1), osteo-

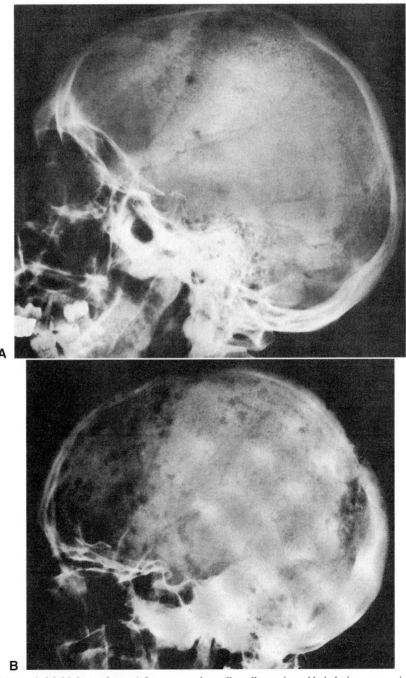

A

B

Figure 24-1　A, Multiple myeloma. A few scattered, small, well-marginated lytic lesions appear in calvarium. These are located in normally mineralized bone. Multiple lytic lesions can also be seen in the mandible. **B,** Multiple myeloma. Multiple circumscribed lytic lesions crowd bones throughout. Lesions are still discrete, and margins of most are fairly sharp. (From Newton TH, Potts DG: *Radiology of the skull and brain,* vol 1, book 2, St Louis, 1971, Mosby.)

porosis, and fractures in about 80% of patients. The vertebrae, skull, thoracic cage, pelvis, and proximal humeri and femurs are the most frequent sites of involvement.

Hematologic Features

Diagnosis of multiple myeloma depends on the demonstration of an increased number of plasma cells in a bone marrow aspirate and/or biopsy and supporting laboratory results (discussed later under Diagnostic Evaluation). Although the bone marrow is typically involved, the disorder may involve other tissues. For example, a positive correlation exists between the production of osteoclast-activating factor by bone marrow cells and the extent of skeletal destruction. Other hematologic factors contributing to the signs and symptoms of pallor and anemia include bleeding, qualitative platelet abnormalities, inhibition of coagulation factors by M protein, and thrombocytopenia. Intravascular coagulation may be manifested.

Renal Disorders

Acute renal failure occurs in about 5% to 10% of patients. Although acute renal failure may occur at any time in the course of myeloma, it is not uncommon for it to be the initial manifestation of disease. Acute renal failure has been observed after infection, hypercalcemia, dehydration, and intravenous urography. Serum creatinine levels are elevated in about half of these patients, and approximately one third suffer from hypercalcemia.

Chronic renal failure is a common development in patients with multiple myeloma. As many as two thirds of patients display serum creatinine levels of greater than 1.5 mg/dL, and 10% to 20% may develop end-stage renal disease. Patients with IgD or light-chain myeloma are much more likely to develop renal failure than those with IgG or IgA myeloma. Proteinuria is a common finding, with over half of all multiple myeloma patients excreting abnormal amounts of Bence-Jones (BJ) protein (light chains). Patients with BJ proteinuria are much more likely to have renal tubular defects than those without BJ protcinuria. It has been suggested that BJ proteins may have a deleterious effect on renal function via at least two mechanisms. In one mechanism, renal failure may occur as a result of intratubular precipitation of BJ protein and subsequent intrarenal obstruction. When the distal end collecting tubules become obstructed by large casts consisting mainly of BJ protein, it may be referred to as myeloma kidney. The second mechanism of renal failure may be a function of direct tubular cell injury. As a result of these tubular defects, abnormalities in urinary concentrating ability and renal acidification are observed. Although the presence of a large concentration of BJ proteinuria is usually associated with some degree of renal dysfunction, some patients excrete large amounts of BJ protein for years and maintain renal function. Lambda light chains have been implicated in nephrotoxicity, but their role has not been firmly established.

Neurologic Features

Pain is a common characteristic of multiple myeloma, often caused by compression of the spinal cord or nerves. Compression produces back pain, with weakness or paralysis of the lower extremities and bowel or bladder incontinence.

Infectious Diseases

The most frequent cause of death is infection. Patients with multiple myeloma have increased susceptibility to infectious microorganisms because of an inability to cope with bacterial infections and certain viral diseases. Increased susceptibility principally results from defective antibody synthesis caused by the crowding out and suppression of normal plasma cell precursors.

Repeated bouts of sepsis, often resulting from recurrent infection by microorganisms such as pneumococci or gram-negative bacteria, are common. Pneumonia, pyelonephritis, meningitis, and arthritis are the leading forms of sepsis; when bacteremia ensues, the death rate is high.

Immunologic Manifestations

In approximately 20% of patients, multiple myeloma is diagnosed by chance in the absence of symptoms, usually after screening laboratory studies have revealed an increased serum protein concentration. Multiple myeloma cells express not only cytoplasmic Igs, the hallmark of plasma cells, but early B, T, natural killer, myeloid, erythroid, and megakaryocytic cell markers as well. These phenotype features are consistent with the hypothesis that multiple myeloma may originate from a transformed early hematopoietic progenitor cell, which explains the occasional coincidence of multiple myeloma and acute myelogenous leukemia.

Interleukin-6 (IL-6) is considered the major growth factor for multiple myeloma. Activated bone marrow stromal cells are thought to trap circulating multiple myeloma progenitor cells as the primary target of IL-6 and other cytokines, resulting in an avalanche effect of tumor cell replication with expansion and differentiation of monoclonal plasma cells. These effects are mediated by the same cytokines involved in normal hematopoiesis. In addition, IL-6 and other cytokines also function as osteoclast-activating factors. IL-6 may account for multiple myeloma-associated anemia and for the lack of thrombocytopenia because of its stimulation of megakaryopoiesis.

Patients with multiple myeloma have defects in humoral but not in cellular immunity. Humoral immunity is disrupted because plasma cell tumors induce suppression of antibody synthesis by normal Ig-secreting cells, and the production of antiidiotype antibodies suffers proportionately. In addition, selective impairment occurs in the formation of normal antibodies because of increased Ig catabolism and the release of a protein that incites macrophages to suppress synthesis of normal Igs by myeloma cells. Depression of normal humoral immunity accounts for the high susceptibility of patients with multiple myeloma to bacterial infection. The normal functioning of cellular immunity, however, is demonstrated by normal resistance to fungal and most viral infections and by normal delayed-type hypersensitivity to skin-testing antigens.

Initially in vivo myeloma clones are subject to control by the immune network through specific idiotype-antiidiotype mechanisms. Each of the million or more potential Ig variants in every individual carries singular determinants designated idiotypes. Antiidiotypic antibodies directed against autologous Ig are elicited during a normal immune response. The presumed mission of antiidiotypic antibodies is to help terminate the immune response by binding complementary idiotypes to form endogenous immune complexes that are removed from the circulation. The antiidiotype antibodies in turn stimulate production of antibodies to antiidiotype, and so on, to create a modulating network that includes T cells, which recognize idiotype antigens by means of their unique antigen receptors. Antiidiotype and idiotype-sensitized T cells collaborate most efficiently during highly restricted responses, during which both antibodies and lymphocytes that specifically recognize the dominant idiotype are activated. These can either inhibit or enhance the response of lymphocytes to receptors expressing the idiotype. The overall net direction of the response is determined by the functional influence of T cells linked by antiidiotype receptor interactions to their molecular targets on B cells. In multiple myeloma, idiotype expression is carried to an extreme. Monoclonal paraprotein secreted by plasma cell tumors induces a multitude of immunologic responses capable of acting in concert to contain or modulate tumor growth.

The earliest detectable monoclonal B cell, as identified by idiotypic structures of the myeloma protein, is the transitional form-bearing surface IgM, IgD, and IgG. This and the finding that precursor (early) B cells destined to become myeloma cells possess surface IgG (sIgG) indicate that the myeloma tumor clone includes memory B cells that can mature into plasma cells. Use of antiidiotypic antibodies in identifying IgA myeloma clones has revealed clonal expression at the pre-B state, a finding supported by the observation that B cells in the circulation of myeloma patients are clonally frozen at the pre-B stage. As maturing B cell members of the malignant clone differentiate in the marrow, they lose IgD and IgM in that order, accumulate sIgG, and finally shed sIg to become IgG-producing mature plasma cells as programmed by the mutant precursor cell. Thus the mature myeloma cell contains abundant cytoplasmic (secretory) IgG but no sIg. IgA myeloma cells proceed along the same normal differentiation scheme of B cell maturation. Although multiple myeloma-associated tumors disseminate widely, the disease is spread through release into the blood circulation of clonal precursors that show lymphoid rather than plasma cell morphology.

The most consistent immunologic feature of multiple myeloma is the incessant synthesis of a dysfunctional single monoclonal protein or of Ig chains of fragments, with concurrent suppression of the synthesis of normal functional antibody. In 99% of myeloma patients, an M component is usually found in serum, urine, or both. Different types of M components are associated with various clinical syndromes.

Diagnostic Evaluation

Hematologic Assessment

A normochromic normocytic anemia is present in about two thirds of patients at the time of diagnosis. In part, anemia is related to the hypervolemia caused by the increase in plasma volume because of monoclonal protein production. Rouleaux formation is a common finding on peripheral blood smears. The leukocyte count can be normal, although about one third of patients suffer from leukopenia. Relative lymphocytosis is usually present. If lymphocyte subsets are examined, a reduction in CD4+ (helper) and an increase in CD8+ (suppressor) blood lymphocytes can be noted. Defects in the proliferative responses of lymphocytes to mitogens or antigens are explained by the large portion of B cells in multiple myeloma that originate from the malignant stem cell clone. Few mature plasma cells are seen in the circulation except at the terminal phase of the disease, but the covert presence of the malignant B cell clone can be unmasked by the laboratory use of monoclonal antibodies or by transforming agents such as phorbol esters. In rare cases in the terminal stages, plasmablasts and proplasmacytes may amount to 50% of the leukocytes in the peripheral blood.

Bleeding is commonly seen. Platelet abnormalities, impaired aggregation of platelets, and interference with platelet function by the abnormal monoclonal protein contribute to bleeding. Inhibitors of coagulation factors and thrombocytopenia from marrow infiltration of plasma cells or chemotherapy may also contribute to bleeding. Some patients have a tendency toward thrombosis, which may be manifested by a shortened coagulation time, and increased fibrinogen and factor VIII.

Diagnosis of multiple myeloma, however, depends on the demonstration of an increased number (>10%) of plasma cells in a bone marrow aspirate (Figure 24-2) and/or biopsy and supporting laboratory results.

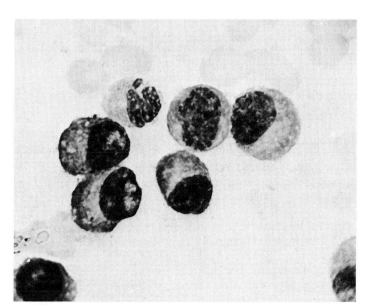

Figure 24-2 Myeloma cells in a bone marrow aspirate. (From Bauer JD: *Clinical laboratory methods,* ed 9, St Louis, 1982, Mosby.)

Another useful laboratory test is the plasma cell labeling index. One method uses thymidine labeled with tritium in cultures of suspected myeloma cells. The amount of thymidine taken up (thymidine labeling index) reflects the growth rate of the myeloma cells. Generally patients with myeloma will have a higher labeling index than those with benign gammopathy or smoldering myeloma. This index therefore distinguishes between benign and malignant entities. A newer method of cell labeling uses a simpler and more rapid immunofluorescent assay to determine the labeling index. This method appears to be useful in identifying active myeloma and is being assessed in clinical studies for correlation with response or lack of response to therapy.

Bence-Jones Proteins

BJ proteins may be demonstrated in the urine. In about 10% of multiple myeloma patients, only BJ proteins are produced, with no complete IgM, IgG, or IgA. BJ proteins are single-peptide chains with a molecular weight of 20,000 or 22,000, but dimerization occurs spontaneously to form molecules with a molecular weight of 40,000 or 44,000.

BJ proteins are monoclonal kappa or lambda Ig light chains not attached to the heavy-chain portion of the Ig molecule. BJ proteins are seen in two types of syndromes:

- In conjunction with a typical monoclonal gammopathy
- In free LCD

Very small amounts of BJ protein in serum can be associated with significant clinical problems, especially pathologic renal changes. Free light chains filter through the glomeruli almost without obstruction because of their small molecular size and accumulate in the tubules. Renal impairment can result from the toxicity of the light chains. Pathologic changes can range from relatively benign tubular proteinuria to acute renal failure or amyloidosis.

BJ protein can be detected in serum, urine, or both. The level of monoclonal light chains in serum or urine, however, is related to filtration, resorption, or catabolism of the protein by the kidneys. During the early stages of renal disease, when the kidneys are only mildly affected, excretion and reabsorption continue normally, but only partial catabolism occurs. At this point, BJ protein may be detected in the serum but not in the urine. Progressive renal involvement impairs reabsorption, so that diminished reabsorption with decreased catabolism results in free light chains in both serum and urine. Later, as resorption is totally blocked, light chains are present in urine only. In terminal stages of renal disease, uremia occurs, renal clearance is affected, and BJ protein again appears in the serum.

BJ proteins are unusual in their response to heating. They are soluble at room temperature, become insoluble near 60° or 70° C, then resolubilize at 80° C. This pattern reverses when the temperature is lowered, which is a characteristic unique to BJ protein.

Serologically all BJ proteins (L chains) are not identical. However, two types, kappa and lambda, exist. BJ proteins will react with antisera to the L chains of IgG, and L chains react with antisera to BJ protein.

Immunologic Testing

Each monoclonal protein (M protein or paraprotein) consists of two heavy-chain polypeptides of the same class and

---

Box 24-1   Monoclonal Gammopathies

I. Malignant monoclonal gammopathies
   A. Multiple myeloma (IgG, IgA, IgD, IgE, and free light chains)
   B. Plasmacytoma
   C. Malignant lymphoproliferative diseases
   D. Heavy-chain diseases
   E. Amyloidosis
II. Monoclonal gammopathies of undetermined significance
   A. Benign (IgG, IgA, IgD, IgM, and rarely, free light chains)
   B. Associated with neoplasms of cell types not known to produce monoclonal proteins
   C. Biclonal gammopathies

---

subclass and two light-chain polypeptides of the same type. The different monoclonal proteins are designated by capital letters corresponding to the class of their heavy chains, which are designated by Greek letters: gamma in IgG, alpha in IgA, mu in IgM, delta in IgD, and epsilon in IgE. The subclasses are IgG1, IgG2, IgG, and IgG4, or IgA1 and IgA2, and their light-chain types are kappa and lambda. A monoclonal protein is characterized by a narrow peak or a localized band on electrophoresis; by a thickened, bowed arc on immunoelectrophoresis; and by a localized band on immunofixation. Many different entities are associated with M proteins (monoclonal gammopathies) (Box 24-1).

Electrophoresis (Figure 24-3) of the serum or urine reveals a tall, sharp peak on the densitometer tracing or dense localized band in a majority of cases of multiple myeloma. A monoclonal protein is demonstrable in the serum and urine in 90% of patients. In all, 60% of patients exhibit IgG, 20% IgA, 10% light chain only (BJ proteinemia), and 1% IgD. Electrophoresis of urine shows a globulin peak in 75% of cases, mainly albumin in 10% of patients, and a normal pattern in 15%. When an M spike is observed on serum protein electrophoresis, the suggested sequence of testing (Table 24-2) includes testing by immunoelectrophoresis and immunofixation. Screening for cryoglobulins and viscosity may also be warranted.

Most patients demonstrate complex karyotype abnormalities with chromosomal gains, deletions, and translocations, some of which are identical to those observed in certain B cell lymphomas. The number of chromosomal aberrations is of sufficient extent to be detected on flow analysis of DNA content, which is aneuploid in about 80% of patients. Most patients exhibit a slight nuclear DNA excess of 5% to 10%; hypoploidy is observed in only 5% to 10% of patients and is strongly associated with resistance to standard chemotherapy. Deletions of chromosomes 13 and 17 have been observed.

DNA hybridization or blotting technology is the newest technology available and can be used to detect abnormal gene arrangements and mutations in cellular oncogenes. Although the gene product of monoclonal antibodies is the method of detection, DNA probes that can detect the abnormal gene are now available. Blotting techniques may someday replace the current approach to the laboratory evaluation of monoclonal gammopathies.

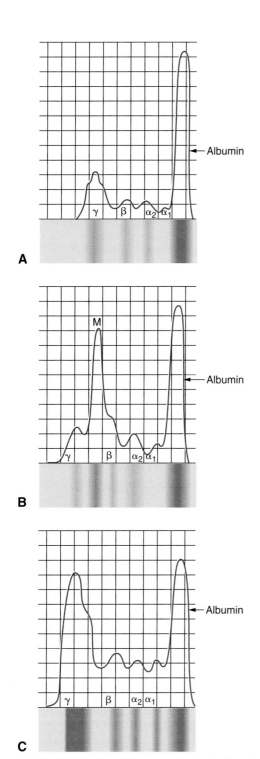

Figure 24-3 Serum electrophoretic patterns. **A,** Normal patient. **B,** A patient with multiple myeloma. **C,** A patient with Waldenström's macroglobulinemia.

TABLE 24-2	Suggested Sequence of Immunologic Testing for Monoclonal Proteins

M Spike on Serum Protein Electrophoresis

Serum	Urine
Immunoelectrophoresis	Screening of urine for increased protein, (e.g., sulfosalicylic acid)
Immunofixation	Total protein assay of a 24-hour urine specimen
Quantitation of immuno-globulins by radial immunodiffusion or nephelometry	Urinary protein electrophoresis
Screening for cryoglobulins	Urinary immunoelectro-phoresis
Determination of serum viscosity, if IgM, IgA, or IgG, or signs and symp-toms suggestive of hyperviscosity	Immunofixation

exist. A greater frequency of IgM monoclonal proteins, as well as quantitative abnormalities, has been observed in some relatives of patients with WM.

WM is a malignant offshoot of B-cell development before the myelomas; therefore the sole gene product is IgM. Patients with WM have chromosomal rearrangements characteristic of B-cell neoplasia, including t(8:14) and trisomy 12.

Epidemiology

WM is about one-tenth as frequent as multiple myeloma. This disorder has an age-specific incidence; it is most commonly found in older individuals, with a mean age of onset of 60 to 64 years. No significant differences in the incidence of WM occur between males and females. Disease onset is usually insidious, and the median survival is approximately 3 years after diagnosis.

Signs and Symptoms

The signs and symptoms of WM have an indolent progression over a period of many years. Initially the onset of the disease is slow and insidious, with the pace of manifestations determined by the rate of proliferation of the IgM-secreting clone. Most of the clinical signs and symptoms of disease stem from intravascular accumulation of high levels of IgM macroglobulin. When the IgM is precipitable at cold temperatures, as it is in 37% of cases, clinical manifestations of cold sensitivity such as Raynaud's phenomenon, arthralgias, purpura of the extremities, renal insufficiency, and peripheral vascular occlusions may develop. Cold hypersensitivity can occur when serum IgM levels exceed 2 to 3 g/dL and the protein precipitates at temperatures exceeding 20° C.

Although the patient experiences weakness and fatigue, it is usually the onset of bleeding from the gums or nose that arouses concern. Patients suffer from weight loss, and the incidence of infection is twice the normal rate. As the disease

WALDENSTRÖM'S PRIMARY MACROGLOBULINEMIA

Etiology

Waldenström's primary macroglobulinemia (WM), or simply macroglobulinemia, is a malignant lymphocyte-plasma cell proliferative disorder that exhibits abnormally large amounts of Ig of the 19S-IgM type. The cause of this disorder is unknown, but a possible genetic predisposition may progresses, about 40% of patients develop hepatomegaly, splenomegaly, and lymphadenopathy. Occasionally the clinical manifestations may simulate diffuse lymphoma. Specific dysfunctions and abnormalities occur in a variety of body systems.

Skeletal Features

In contrast to multiple myeloma, bone pain is virtually nonexistent in WM. Diffuse osteoporosis may be seen, but bone lesions are extremely rare.

Hematologic Abnormalities

Patients with WM usually suffer from chronic anemia and bleeding episodes. Bleeding problems in the form of bruising, purpura, and bleeding from the mouth, gums, nose, and gastrointestinal tract are common. The quantities of circulating platelets may be normal or decreased, but the most notable alteration is a disturbance in platelet function. Therefore thrombocytopenia or hyperviscosity may contribute to the bleeding disorder.

In addition to anemia caused by chronic or recurrent bleeding, the decrease in red blood cells becomes more severe as the disease progresses because of a dilutional effect caused by increased Ig production. In addition, the presence of macroglobulin also produces an increased erythrocyte sedimentation rate. Microscopic examination of a peripheral blood smear usually reveals normocytic and frequently hypochromic red cells with striking rouleaux formation. The total blood leukocyte count is either normal or slightly depressed because of moderate neutropenia. In a terminal patient, the blood may be inundated with malignant lymphoplasmacytic cells.

Renal Dysfunction

Renal function becomes mildly or moderately impaired in about 15% of WM patients. Nephrosis is uncommon. BJ proteinuria, however, is present in about 70% of WM patients, but the quantity of light chains excreted is much less than in multiple myeloma.

Glomerular lesions are the predominant form of renal injury. IgM collects on the endothelial side of the basement membrane of the kidney, and sometimes these macroglobulin accumulations obstruct glomerular capillaries.

Ocular Manifestations

Blurred vision is a frequent abnormality of WM. Rouleaux induced by elevations of IgM causes distention of veins and capillaries; retinal oxygenation diminishes as rouleaux-inducing IgM rises. As a result of increased IgM levels, retinal hemorrhage, exudate formation, and varicosities develop, which can lead to more permanent retinal damage unless IgM levels are lowered by therapy.

Neuropsychiatric Problems

The most common serious neurologic consequence of the slowed cerebral perfusion caused by macroglobulinemia is acute cerebral malfunction beginning with headache, fluctuating confusion, forgetfulness, and slowed mentation. This can progress to somnolence, stupor, and coma-diffuse brain syndrome, sometimes called coma paraproteinaemicum. Neurologic abnormalities can be improved by reduction of plasma viscosity.

Polyneuropathy affects 5% to 10% of patients with WM. This condition is associated with an increase in spinal fluid protein and deposits of monoclonal IgM on myelin sheaths. Monoclonal IgM found in the plasma and attached to damaged nerves has been shown in some instances to share idiotypic determinants. This suggests that polyneuropathy of WM may be an autoimmune process caused by monoclonal IgM possessing antibody activity for a component of nerve tissue.

Cardiopulmonary Abnormalities

Congestive heart failure becomes a serious problem in patients with chronic uncontrolled WM. About 90% of IgM remains trapped in the circulating plasma and exerts an unbalanced transendothelial osmotic effect sufficient to cause marked expansion of the plasma volume. This in turn creates a dilutional anemia and augments cardiac filling and cardiac output. As a result, increased cardiac output and blood viscosity overwork the myocardium.

About 10% of patients develop pulmonary lesions. Pulmonary tumors, diffuse infiltrates, and pleural involvement are all about equally represented. The signs and symptoms of pulmonary dysfunction include coughing and dyspnea.

Cutaneous Manifestations

Cold sensitivity is a frequent manifestation of WM; however, skin lesions are uncommon. A small number of patients develop flat, violaceous, macular skin lesions caused by dense infiltration by lymphoplasmacytoid cells. Pink, pearly looking papules caused by dense deposits of IgM may be exhibited.

Immunologic Manifestations

The basic abnormality in this macroglobulinemia is uncontrolled proliferation of B lymphocyte-plasma cells. As a result, there is a heavy accumulation of monoclonal IgM in the circulating plasma and of plasmacytoid lymphocytes in the bone marrow.

In many cases WM is associated with mixed cryoglobulinemia, which reflects the binding of IgG or IgA antiidiotypic antibody to the mutant IgM. In a small number of patients, dysplastic tumor cells secrete 7S IgM monomers, mu chains, or other monoclonal Igs or fragments. Therefore the major IgM production indicates that the Ig (gene) lesion sometimes degenerates and codes for more than one M component.

Diagnostic Evaluation

Hematologic Assessment

Microscopic examination of a bone marrow aspirate reveals that the lymphocyte-plasma cells vary morphologically from small lymphocytes to obvious plasma cells. Frequently the cellular cytoplasm is ragged and may contain Periodic Acid–Schiff's (PAS) stain–positive material probably identical to the circulating macroglobulin.

The total peripheral blood leukocyte count is usually normal with an absolute lymphocytosis. Moderate-to-severe degrees of anemia are frequently observed on peripheral blood smears as well as rouleaux formation. The patient's plasma volume may be greatly increased and the erythrocyte sedimentation rate (ESR) is increased.

Platelet counts are usually normal. Faulty platelet aggregation and release of platelet factor 3 are caused by nonspecific coating of platelets by IgM. The most common coagulation defect is a prolonged thrombin time as the result of the binding of M component to fibrin monomers and resultant gel clotting of IgM-coated fibrin. Bleeding abnormalities, however, can be demonstrated by a variety of procedures. These procedures include:

- Faulty platelet adhesiveness
- Defective platelet aggregation
- Abnormal release of platelet factor 3
- Impaired clot retraction
- Prolonged bleeding time
- Positive tourniquet test
- Prolonged thrombin/prothrombin time test
- Decreased levels of factor VIII

Immunologic Assessment

Electrophoresis of serum usually demonstrates the overproduction of IgM (19S) antibodies. Diagnosis is made by demonstration of a homogenous M component composed of monoclonal IgM. Quantitation of Igs reveals IgM levels ranging from 1 to 12 g/dL (usually more than 3 g/dL), and it accounts for 20% to 70% of the total proteins. Characteristically, blood samples are described as having hyperviscosity.

In addition, cryoglobulins can be detected in the patient's serum. Cryoglobulins are proteins that precipitate or gel when cooled to 0° C and dissolve when heated. In most cases monoclonal cryoglobulins are IgM or IgG. Occasionally the macroglobulin is both cryoprecipitable and capable of cold-induced, anti-i–mediated agglutination of red cells. IgM may also occasionally be a pyroglobulin, which precipitates on heating to 50° to 60° C but does not redissolve on cooling or intensified heating as do typical BJ pyroglobulins. Many cryoglobulins have the ability to fix complement and initiate an inflammatory reaction similar to antigen-antibody complexes.

Cryoglobulins have been classified into three types. Type I classification is composed of a single class. IgM and IgG classes are most common; IgA or light-chain single cryoglobulins are seen less frequently. Type I constitutes about 25% of cryoglobulins and is generally associated with multiple myeloma, macroglobulinemia, and other rarer neoplastic proliferations of plasma cells and lymphocytes.

Type II cryoglobulins consist of two forms. The monoclonal form always has rheumatoid factor activity and usually is an IgM with kappa light chains. The second form is polyclonal IgG, which reacts with the monoclonal IgM rheumatoid factor.

Type III is a mixed cryoglobulin in which both constituent Igs are polyclonal. More than 90% of type III cryoglobulins contain IgM rheumatoid factor and IgG. Type III cryoglobulins are seen in a variety of autoimmune, systemic rheumatic diseases, and persistent infections with immune complexes (e.g., bacterial endocarditis).

OTHER MONOCLONAL DISORDERS
Light-Chain Disease

Light-chain disease represents about 10% to 15% of monoclonal gammopathies, ranking behind IgG and IgA myelomas, which represent about 60% and 15%, respectively. The incidence of light-chain disease is about as frequent as WM. In light-chain disease only kappa or lambda monoclonal light chains or BJ proteins are produced.

Diagnostic evaluation of suspected light-chain disease is similar to the protocol for any lymphoproliferative disorder, but certain changes in approach are necessary because of the low levels of paraprotein that can be involved. Agarose high-resolution protein electrophoresis of serum and urine should be done to determine the total protein concentration. A 24-hour urine specimen should be examined electrophoretically because almost all of the protein may be BJ protein. Visual examination of the electrophoresis pattern is essential because a small light-chain band frequently does not exhibit a significant peak on densitometric scanning. Serum protein electrophoresis patterns from patients with monoclonal gammopathies may demonstrate:

- A typical well-defined monoclonal band
- A somewhat broad, diffuse band caused by polymerization of monoclonal protein
- A normal gamma region
- Hypogammaglobulinemia

Heavy-Chain Disease

As the name heavy-chain disease implies, this abnormality is characterized by the presence of monoclonal proteins composed of the heavy-chain portion of the Ig molecule. The name Franklin's disease is synonymous with gamma heavy-chain disease. Alpha heavy-chain disease is the most frequent of the heavy-chain gammopathies and is frequently seen in men of Mediterranean descent. Mu heavy-chain disease is rare.

Heavy chains may be detected in serum or urine or both (depending on the class of heavy chain involved). When heavy-chain disease is suspected, nonspecific anti-FAB antisera should be used for definitive testing. The serum sample should also be diluted and retested with kappa and lambda light-chain antisera to rule out prozoning caused by antigen excess.

Gammopathies With More Than One Band

In some cases more than one monoclonal band is produced. Although gammopathies with two bands may represent a true biclonal condition, routine laboratory techniques cannot distinguish between the various mechanisms that could produce two or more monoclonal bands. Therefore a serum specimen with an IgG kappa and an IgA lambda band should be appropriately reported as a gammopathy with IgG kappa and IgA lambda monoclonal bands. The appearance of more than one band on electrophoresis is often associated with advanced gammopathies, where the asynchronous production of the components of the Ig molecule occurs. In such cases synthesis of an intact monoclonal Ig and an excess of monoclonal light chains may be observed. An example of the demonstration of more than one band on electrophoresis can include cases where the pentameric IgM breaks down into 7S subunits, which show up on electrophoresis as one or more "extra" monoclonal bands. In addition, monoclonal IgA molecules have a tendency to dimerize, and the resulting dimer often has a different mobility than the monomer parent molecule.

Case Study

History and Physical Examination

A 58-year-old male nuclear power plant worker sees his family physician because of increasing fatigue and weakness. He also reports pain in his lower back and arms when he walks. Physical examination reveals that the man has pale mucous membranes and hepatosplenomegaly. The physician orders a complete blood count (CBC) and urinalysis. A follow-up appointment is scheduled for the following week.

Laboratory Data

The CBC reveals that the patient has anemia. His leukocyte count and differential count are normal, except for a rouleaux (rolled coin) appearance of the red blood cells. The result of urinalysis is normal. The patient is called and requested to return to the laboratory for additional tests. The physician orders the following tests: ESR, kidney screening profile, liver blood profile, and radiographic skeletal survey, with the following results:

ESR: 50 mm/hr
Kidney profile: normal
Liver profile: normal, except for increased globular protein
Skeletal survey: bone lesions in various sites

Questions and Discussions

1. What follow-up laboratory tests might be ordered to assist in establishing a definitive diagnosis?

    In this case, further investigation of the increased serum globular protein is ordered. A serum electrophoresis and immunoelectrophoresis reveal the presence of an abnormal protein, a 7S Ig. A monoclonal gammopathy, which can be either a benign or malignant condition, results from a single clone of lymphoid-plasma cells, producing elevated levels of a single class and type of Ig. The elevated Ig is referred to as a monoclonal protein, M protein, or paraprotein. Disorders in this category of plasma cell dyscrasias include multiple myeloma, WM, light-chain deposition disease, and heavy-chain diseases.

    Serum and urine electrophoresis patterns and other Ig assays can demonstrate strikingly abnormal results in disorders such as multiple myeloma and WM.

2. What is the nature of the protein found in the urine?

    BJ protein is identified in the urine. BJ protein precipitates when heated to 56° C and dissolves when heated to boiling, and reprecipitates with cooling. On electrophoresis, this protein will reflect its monoclonal nature and appear in the beta or gamma region.

3. What is the most significant laboratory finding in this disorder?

    The presence of increased plasma cells is significant in establishing the diagnosis. Laboratory tests, particularly serum and urine electrophoresis, are important adjuncts.

4. What type of immunologic defects exist in this disease process?

    Patients with multiple myeloma have defects in humoral, but not cellular, immunity. Humoral immunity is disrupted because plasma cell tumors induce suppression of antibody synthesis by normal Ig-secreting cells; the production of antiidiotype antibodies suffers proportionately. In addition, selective impairment occurs in the formation of normal antibodies because of increased Ig catabolism and the release of a protein that incites macrophages to suppress synthesis of normal Igs by myeloma cells. Depression of normal humoral immunity accounts for the high susceptibility of these patients to bacterial infection. The normal functioning of cellular immunity, however, is demonstrated by normal resistance to fungal and most viral infections and normal delayed-type hypersensitivity to skin testing antigens.

5. Does this patient have a risk of occupational exposure?

    Yes. Nuclear plant workers have an increased likelihood of developing multiple myeloma. Older workers, especially 45 years and older, with cumulative radiation doses of 5 rem (roentgen equivalent, man) or more were found to have nearly 3.5 times the chance of dying from multiple myeloma than workers at the same plants with cumulative doses of less than 1 rem. A rem represents a dosage of radiation that has the same biologic effect as 1 roentgen of x-ray or gamma-ray radiation.

Reference

Bureau of National Affairs: *BNA's Safety Net* 3(8):57, 2000.

Diagnosis

Multiple Myeloma

CHAPTER HIGHLIGHTS

Hypergammaglobulinemias are either monoclonal or polyclonal in nature. A monoclonal gammopathy can be either a benign or malignant condition that results from a single clone of lymphoid-plasma cells producing elevated levels of a single class and type of Ig. The elevated Ig is referred to as a monoclonal protein, M protein, or paraprotein. A polyclonal gammopathy, however, is classified as a secondary disease and is characterized by the elevation of two or more Igs by several clones of plasma cells. In monoclonal gammopathies such as multiple myeloma and WM, serum and urine electrophoresis patterns and other Ig assays can demonstrate strikingly abnormal results. In contrast to a monoclonal protein, a polyclonal protein consists of one or more heavy-chain classes and both light-chain types. Polyclonal increases are exhibited as secondary manifestations of infection or inflammation.

Multiple myeloma, a neoplastic or potentially neoplastic proliferation of a single clone of plasma cells, produces a specific type of Ig. The cause of this disorder is unknown. Radiation may be a factor; the possibility of a viral cause has also been suggested. Other possible factors in the etiology may be environmental stimuli; the likelihood of a genetic factor in some cases is supported by reports of familial clusters with multiple myeloma. Multiple myeloma is the most common form of dysproteinemia. IgG myeloma is the most common form of multiple myeloma, with four subtypes of IgG heavy chains known to exist among patients with IgG myeloma. The signs and symptoms of multiple myeloma include bone pain, typically in the back or chest; weakness; fatigue; and pallor associated with anemia or abnormal bleeding. Bone pain, anemia, and renal insufficiency constitute a triad of signs and symptoms strongly suggestive of multiple myeloma. Proteinuria is a common finding in more than half of all patients excreting abnormal amounts of BJ protein (light chains). Patients have defects in humoral but not cellular immunity. Humoral immunity is disrupted because plasma cell tumors induce suppression of antibody synthesis by normal Ig-secreting cells; the production of antiidiotype antibodies suffers proportionately. Selective impairment occurs in the formation of normal antibodies because of increased Ig catabolism and the release of a protein that incites macrophages to suppress synthesis of normal Igs by myeloma cells. Depression of normal humoral immunity accounts for the high susceptibility of multiple myeloma patients to bacterial infection. However, the normal functioning of cellular immunity is demonstrated by normal resistance to fungal and most viral infections and normal delayed-type hypersensitivity to skin-testing antigens. Laboratory diagnosis includes electrophoresis of the serum or urine, which can reveal a tall, sharp peak on the densitometer tracing or a dense localized band in a majority of cases. A monoclonal protein is demonstrable in the serum and urine in 90% of patients. DNA hybridization or blotting technology is the newest technology available and can be used to detect abnormal genes in B cells. Although the gene product of monoclonal antibodies is the method of detection, DNA probes, which can detect the abnormal gene, are now available. Blotting techniques may some day fully or partially replace the current approach to the laboratory evaluation of monoclonal gammopathies.

WM, or simply macroglobulinemia, is a malignant lymphocyte-plasma cell proliferative disorder that exhibits abnormally large amounts of Ig of the 19S-IgM type. The cause of this disorder is unknown, but a possible genetic predisposition may exist. The signs and symptoms of WM have an indolent progression over a period of many years. Initially the onset of the disease is slow and insidious, with the pace of manifestations determined by the rate of proliferation of the IgM-secreting clone. Most of the clinical signs and symptoms of disease stem from intravascular accumulation of |high levels of IgM macroglobulin. The basic abnormality in this macroglobulinemia is uncontrolled proliferation of B lymphocyte-plasma cells. As a result, there is a heavy accumulation of monoclonal IgM in the circulating plasma and of plasmacytoid lymphocytes in the bone marrow. In many cases WM is associated with mixed cryoglobulinemia, which reflects the binding of IgG or IgA antiidiotypic antibody to the mutant IgM. In a small number of patients, dysplastic tumor cells secrete 7S IgM monomers, mu chains, or other monoclonal Igs or fragments. Therefore, in addition to the major IgM production, the lesion sometimes degenerates and codes for more than one M component. Laboratory diagnosis includes electrophoresis of serum, which usually demonstrates the overproduction of IgM (19S) antibodies. Diagnosis is made by demonstration of a homogeneous M component composed of monoclonal IgM. Blood samples characteristically display hyperviscosity. In addition, cryoglobulins can be detected in the patient's serum.

Other monoclonal disorders include LCD and heavy-chain disease. LCD represents about 10% to 15% of monoclonal gammopathies. The incidence of LCD is about as frequent as WM. In LCD only kappa or lambda monoclonal light chains or BJ proteins are produced. Diagnostic evaluation of suspected LCD is similar to the protocol for any lymphoproliferative disorder, but there are certain changes in approach because of the low levels of paraprotein that can be involved. Agarose high-resolution protein electrophoresis of serum and urine should be done to determine the total protein concentration. A 24-hour urine specimen should be examined electrophoretically because almost all of the protein may be BJ. Visual examination of the electrophoresis pattern is an essential part of the interpretation because a small light-chain band frequently does not exhibit a significant peak on densitometric scanning.

As the name heavy-chain disease implies, this abnormality is characterized by the presence of monoclonal proteins composed of the heavy-chain portion of the Ig molecule. Alpha heavy-chain disease is the most frequent of the heavy-chain gammopathies; mu heavy chain-disease is rare. Heavy chains may be detected in serum or urine or both (depending on the class of heavy chain involved). When heavy-chain disease is suspected, nonspecific anti-FAB antisera should be used for definitive testing. The serum sample should also be diluted and retested with kappa and lambda light-chain antisera to rule out prozoning caused by antigen excess.

In some cases gammopathies with more than one monoclonal band exist. Although gammopathies with two bands may represent a true biclonal condition, routine laboratory techniques cannot distinguish between the various mechanisms able to produce two (or more) monoclonal bands. A serum specimen with an IgG kappa and an IgA lambda band should be appropriately reported as a gammopathy with IgG kappa and IgA lambda monoclonal bands. The appearance of more than one band on electrophoresis is often associated with advanced gammopathies, where the asynchronous production of the components of the Ig molecule occurs. In such cases synthesis of an intact monoclonal Ig and an excess of monoclonal light chains may be observed.

REVIEW QUESTIONS

1. Polyclonal gammopathies can be exhibited as a secondary manifestation of all of the following except:
   A. chronic infection
   B. chronic liver disease
   C. multiple myeloma
   D. rheumatoid connective disease

2. What is the most frequent cause of death in a patient with multiple myeloma?
   A. skeletal destruction
   B. chronic renal failure
   C. neurologic disorders
   D. infectious disease

3. Patients with multiple myeloma have defects in:
   A. cellular immunity
   B. humoral immunity
   C. synthesis of normal immunoglobulins
   D. both B and C

4. What is (are) the most consistent immunologic feature(s) of multiple myeloma?
   A. synthesis of dysfunctional single monoclonal proteins
   B. synthesis of Ig chains or fragments
   C. the presence of M protein in serum and/or urine
   D. all of the above

5. Bence-Jones proteins are soluble at room temperature, become insoluble near _____ (5), and then resolubilize at _____ (6).
   A. 37° C
   B. 50° C
   C. 65° C
   D. 80° C

6.
   A. 37° C
   B. 50° C
   C. 65° C
   D. 80° C

7. M proteins are associated with all of the following malignant conditions except:
   A. multiple myeloma
   B. plasma cytoma
   C. malignant lymphoproliferative diseases
   D. lymphoma

8. Cryoglobulins are proteins that precipitate at _____.
   A. −18° C
   B. 4° C
   C. 0° C
   D. 4° C

9. The elevated levels of a single class and type of immunoglobulin is referred to as:
   A. monoclonal protein
   B. M protein
   C. paraprotein
   D. all of the above

Questions 10 and 11. Fill in the blanks, choosing from the following answers:

Possible answers to question 10.	Possible answers to question 11.
A. beta	A. lambda
B. gamma	B. alpha
C. kappa	C. beta
D. alpha	D. gamma

In light-chain disease only (10) _____ or (11) _____ monoclonal light chains are synthesized by a one-cell clone.

12. Multiple myeloma is also referred to as:
    A. plasma cell myeloma
    B. Kahler's disease
    C. myelomatosis
    D. all of the above

13. Most patients with multiple myeloma manifest:
    A. bone pain
    B. acute renal failure
    C. no symptoms
    D. hepatomegaly and splenomegaly

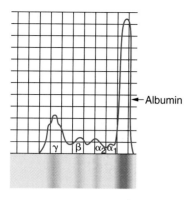

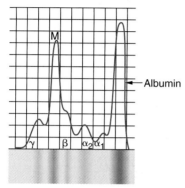

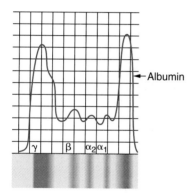

14. The figure above represents the serum electrophoresis of a patient with:
    A. Waldenström's macroglobulinemia
    B. multiple myeloma
    C. no protein abnormality
    D. polyclonal gammopathy

15. Patients with Waldenström's macroglobulinemia exhibit abnormally large amounts of:
    A. IgM
    B. IgG
    C. IgE
    D. IgA

16. Light chain disease represents about _____ % of monoclonal gammopathies.
    A. 5-10
    B. 10-15
    C. 15-25
    D. 25-50

BIBLIOGRAPHY

Alexanian R, Dimopoulos M: The treatment of multiple myeloma, *N Engl J Med* 330(7):484-489, 1994.

American Cancer Society: *How is multiple myeloma diagnosed?* website: www.cancer.org.

Aucouturier P et al: Heavy-chain deposition disease, *N Engl J Med* 329(19):1389-1393, 1993.

Barlogie B, Alexanian R, Jagannath S: Plasma cell dyscrasias, *JAMA* 268(20):2946-2951, 1992.

Caroscio JT: Quantitative CSF IgG measurements in multiple sclerosis and other neurologic diseases, *Arch Neurol* 40:409-413, 1983.

Hoffman EG: Laboratory evaluation of monoclonal gammopathies, *Can J Med Technol* 49(2):99-115, 1987.

Jandl JA: Multiple myeloma and other differentiated B cell malignancies. In Jandl JA: *Blood,* Boston, 1988, Little, Brown.

Keren DF, Morrison N, Gulbranson R: Evolution of a monoclonal gammopathy, *Lab Med* 25(5):313-317, 1994.

Keshgegian AA, editor: Oligoclonal immunoglobulins in cerebrospinal fluid in multiple sclerosis, *Clin Chem* 26(9):1340-1345, 1980.

Killingsworth LM: Clinical applications of protein determination in biological fluids other than blood, *Clin Chem* 28(5):1093-1258, 1982.

Killingsworth LM, Warren BM: *Immunofixation for the identification of monoclonal gammopathies,* Beaumont, Tex, 1986, Helena Laboratories.

Konrad RJ et al: Myeloma-associated paraprotein directed against the HIV-1 p24 antigen in an HIV-1-seropositive patient, *N Engl J Med* 328(25):1817-1819, 1993.

Kyle A: Evaluation of monoclonal proteins in serum and urine. In Stein J, editor: *Internal medicine,* ed 2, Boston, 1987, Little, Brown.

Kyle A: Multiple myeloma and the dysproteinemias. In Stein J, editor: *Internal medicine,* ed 2, Boston, 1987, Little, Brown.

Kyle RA: "Benign" monoclonal gammopathy—after 20 to 35 years of follow-up, *Mayo Clin Proc* 68:26-36, 1993.

Mayo Clinic Myeloma Amyloidosis Monoclonal Gammopathy Group, website: www.mayo.edu.

Papadopoulos NM et al: A unique protein in normal human cerebrospinal fluid, *Clin Chem* 29(10):1842-1844, 1983.

Ritzmann EE: Immunoglobulin abnormalities. In Ritzmann S, editor: *Serum protein abnormalities, diagnostic and clinical aspects,* Boston, 1976, Little, Brown.

Smolens P, Stein JH: Renal manifestations of dysproteinemias. In Stein J, editor: *Internal medicine,* ed 2, Boston, 1987, Little, Brown.

Turgeon ML: *Clinical hematology,* ed 3, Philadelphia, 1999, Lippincott Williams & Wilkins.

Chapter 25

Autoimmmune Disorders

LEARNING OBJECTIVES

At the conclusion of this chapter, the reader should be able to:
- Describe the nature of autoimmune disorders.
- Compare organ-specific and organ nonspecific characteristics.

- Explain the role of T and B cells in autoimmunity.
- Describe organ-specific and midspectrum disorders.
- Analyze representative case studies.

THE NATURE OF AUTOIMMUNITY

Autoimmunity represents a breakdown of the immune system's ability to discriminate between self and nonself. More than 40 autoimmune diseases occur in 5% to 10% of the general population. Various organs and tissues of cardiopulmonary, dermatologic, endocrine, gastrointestinal, hematopoietic, and neuromuscular systems can be affected in autoimmune disorders.

Autoimmune diseases are characterized by the persistent activation of immunologic effector mechanisms that alter the function and integrity of individual cells and organs. The sites of organ or tissue damage depend on the location of the immune reaction.

The term *autoimmune disease* is used when demonstrable immunoglobulins (Igs) (autoantibodies) or cytotoxic (T) cells display specificity for self-antigens or autoantigens (Table 25-1) and contribute to the pathogenesis of the disease. The variety of signs and symptoms seen in patients with autoimmune diseases reflects the various forms of the immune response.

It is also important to note that autoantibodies may be formed in patients secondary to tissue damage or when no evidence of clinical disease exists. Unlike autoimmune

TABLE 25-1	Examples of Autoimmune Diseases and Associated Abnormalities

Clinical Diagnosis	Autoantigen
Addison's disease	p450 enzymes
Crohn's disease	p-ANCA, pancreatic acinar cells
Ovarian failure/infertility	p450 enzymes
Pernicious anemia	Parietal cells
Ulcerative colitis	p-ANCA

disease, autoantibodies can occur as immune correlates of conditions such as blood transfusion reactions. In addition, autoantibodies can be demonstrated in hemolytic disease of the newborn and graft rejection, or result from disorders such as serum sickness, anaphylaxis, or hay fever, when the immune response is clearly the cause of the disease.

THE SPECTRUM OF AUTOIMMUNE DISEASE

Many disorders are believed to be related to immunologic abnormalities, and the identification of additional diseases grows continually. Autoimmune diseases exhibit a full spec-

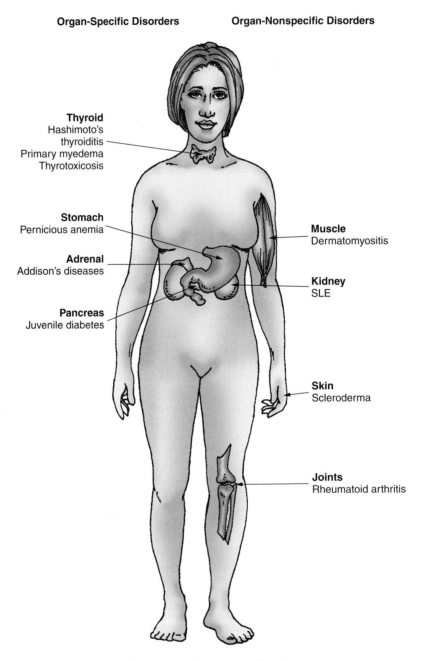

Organ-Specific Disorders

Organ-Nonspecific Disorders

Thyroid
Hashimoto's thyroiditis
Primary myedema
Thyrotoxicosis

Stomach
Pernicious anemia

Adrenal
Addison's diseases

Pancreas
Juvenile diabetes

Muscle
Dermatomyositis

Kidney
SLE

Skin
Scleroderma

Joints
Rheumatoid arthritis

Figure 25-1 Autoimmune disorders.

trum of tissue reactivity (Figure 25-1). At one extreme are organ-specific diseases such as Hashimoto's disease of the thyroid; at the other extreme are diseases that manifest themselves as nonorgan-specific diseases such as systemic lupus erythematosus (SLE) and rheumatoid arthritis (RA) (Box 25-1). In organ-specific diseases, both the lesions produced by tissue damage and the autoantibodies are directed at a single target organ (e.g., the thyroid). Midspectrum disorders are characterized by localized lesions in a single organ and by organ-nonspecific autoantibodies. An example of a midspectrum disorder is primary biliary cirrhosis. In this disorder the small bile duct is the main target of inflammatory cell infiltration, but the serum autoantibodies are mainly mitochondrial antibodies and are not liver specific. Organ-nonspecific disorders are characterized by the presence of both lesions and autoantibodies not confined to any one organ. A summary of the features of organ-specific and organ-nonspecific disorders is presented in Table 25-2. Characteristics of some of the organ-specific and midspectrum disorders are discussed later in this chapter. The organ-nonspecific disorders of SLE and RA are discussed in detail in Chapters 26 and 27.

Box 25-1 Examples of Autoimmune Diseases

Active chronic hepatitis
Addison's disease
Autoimmune atrophic gastritis
Autoimmune hemolytic anemia
Dermatomyositis
Discoid lupus erythematosus
Goodpasture's syndrome
Hashimoto's thyroiditis
Idiopathic thrombocytopenic purpura
Juvenile diabetes
Multiple sclerosis
Myasthenia gravis
Pemphigus vulgaris
Pernicious anemia
Primary biliary cirrhosis
Primary myxedema
Rheumatoid arthritis
Scleroderma
Sjögren's syndrome
Systemic lupus erythematosus
Thyrotoxicosis

FACTORS INFLUENCING THE DEVELOPMENT OF AUTOIMMUNITY

Autoimmunity begins with an abnormal interaction of T and B lymphocytes with autoantigens. No single theory or mechanism has been identified as a cause. The potential for autoimmunity, if given appropriate circumstances, is constantly present in every immunocompetent individual because lymphocytes that are potentially reactive with self-antigens exist in the body. Antibody expression appears to be regulated by a complex set of interacting factors. These influences include:
- Genetic factors
- Age
- Exogenous factors

TABLE 25-2 Summary of Organ-Specific and Organ-Nonspecific Disorders

Similarities

1. Circulating autoantibodies react with normal body constituents
2. Increased immunoglobulin concentration in serum often found
3. Antibodies may appear in each of the main immunoglobulin classes
4. Disease process not always progressive; exacerbations and remissions occur
5. Autoantibody tests of diagnostic value

Differences

Organ-Specific	Organ-Nonspecific
Antibodies and lesions are organ specific	Antibodies and lesions are nonorgan-specific
Clinical and serologic overlap (e.g., thyroid, stomach, adrenal glands, kidney)	Overlap of SLE, RA, and other connective tissue disorders
Antigens only available to lymphoid system in low concentrations	Antigens accessible at higher concentrations
Antigens evoke organ-specific antibodies in normal animals with complete Freund's adjuvant	No antibodies produced in animals with comparable stimulation
Familial tendency to develop organ-specific autoimmunity	Familial tendency to develop connective tissue disease
	Questionable abnormalities in immunoglobulin synthesis in relatives
Lymphoid invasion, parenchymal destruction by questionable cell-mediated hypersensitivity or antibodies	Lesions caused by deposition of antigen-antibody (immune) complexes
Tendency to develop cancer in the organ	Tendency to develop lymphoreticular neoplasia

SLE, Systemic lupus erythematosus; *RA,* rheumatoid arthritis.

Genetic Factors

Although a direct genetic etiology has not been established in autoimmune disease, there is a tendency for familial aggregates to occur. In addition, a tendency for more than one autoimmune disorder to occur exists in the same individual. For example, patients with Hashimoto's disease have a higher incidence of pernicious anemia than would be expected in a random population matched for age and sex.

Another factor related to genetic inheritance is that autoimmune disorders and autoantibodies are found more frequently in women than in men.

The presence of certain human leukocyte antigens (HLAs) is also associated with an increased risk of certain autoimmune states.

Age

Autoantibodies are manifested infrequently in the general population. The incidence of autoantibodies, however, increases steadily with age, reaching a peak at around 60 to 70 years.

Exogenous Factors

Ultraviolet radiation, drugs, viruses, and chronic infectious disease may all play a role in the development of autoimmune disorders. These factors may alter antigens, which the body then perceives as nonself.

IMMUNOPATHOGENIC MECHANISMS

An Overview of Immunopathogenicity

Autoimmune disease is usually prevented by the normal functioning of immunologic regulatory mechanisms. When these controls dysfunction, antibodies to self-antigens may be produced and bind to antigens in the circulation to form circulating immune complexes or to antigens deposited in specific tissue sites.

The mechanisms governing the deposition in one organ or another are unknown; however, several mechanisms may be operative in a single disease. Wherever antigen-antibody complexes accumulate, complement can be activated, with the subsequent release of mediators of inflammation. These mediators increase vascular permeability, attract phagocytic cells to the reaction site, and cause local tissue damage. Alternatively, cytotoxic T cells can directly attack body cells bearing the target antigen, which releases mediators that amplify the inflammatory reaction. Autoantibody and complement fragments coat cells bearing the target antigen, which leads to destruction by phagocytes or by antibody-seeking K-type lymphocytes.

An individual may develop an autoimmune response in a variety of immunogenic stimuli (Table 25-3).

These responses may be caused by:
- Antigens that do not normally circulate in the blood. The hidden, or sequestered, antigen theory is one of the earliest views with respect to organ-specific antibodies. According to this theory, antigens are sequestered within the organ, and because of the lack of contact with

TABLE 25-3	Examples of Antigens Implicated in Autoimmune Endocrine Diseases
Disorder	**Antigen**
Hashimoto's disease	Thyroglobulin
	Thyroid peroxidase
	Thyrotropin receptor
Graves' disease	Thyrotropin receptor
	Thyroid peroxidase
	Thyroglobulin
	64-kd antigen
	70-kd heat shock protein
Type 1 diabetes	Insulin/proinsulin
	Insulin receptor
	Glutamic acid decarboxylase
	B cell release granule
	Pancreatic cytokeratin
	64-kd antigen
	Glucagon
	65-kd heat shock protein
Addison's disease	Adrenal cortical cells
	55-kD microsomal antigen
Idiopathic hypoparathyroidism	200-kD and 130-kD
	Endothelial antigen
	Mitochondrial antigen

the mononuclear phagocytic system, they fail to establish immunologic tolerance. Any conditions producing a release of antigen would then provide an opportunity for autoantibody formation. This situation is true when sperm cells or lens and heart tissues are released directly into the circulation, and autoantibodies are formed. Unmodified extracts of tissues involved in organ-specific autoimmune disorders, however, do not readily elicit antibody formation.
- Altered antigens that arise because of chemical, physical, or biologic processes such as hapten complexing, physical denaturation, or mutation
- A foreign antigen that is shared or cross-reactive with self-antigens or tissue components
- Mutation of immunocompetent cells to acquire a responsive to self-antigens
- Loss of the immunoregulatory function by T-cell subsets

Comprehension of the mechanism of autoimmunity requires an understanding of the regulation of the immune response. The immune response involves interaction of cellular elements such as lymphocytes and macrophages, antigen, antibody, immune complexes, and complement.

T Cells

Helper and suppressor T cells act together to establish an immunoregulatory balance, which determines the level of immunologic response to a particular antigen. A disequilibrium resulting from either an expansion of helper T cells or a deficiency of suppressor T cells could trigger potentially autoreactive B-cell clones to produce autoantibodies.

Autoreactive T cells can also be demonstrated. Self-reactive effector T cells have been generated when lymphocytes have been cultured with a variety of autologous tissues in the presence of an agent such as mitogenicin lectin. It is believed that the body, under normal conditions, has a homeostatic mechanism to prevent them from being triggered. Presumably these cells are unresponsive because of clonal deletion, T-cell suppression, or failure of autoantigen presentation.

B Cells

Intrinsic abnormalities in the B cells themselves can contribute to autoimmunity. According to the theory of B-cell abnormality, inappropriate or outlaw B cells are triggered by unknown stimuli. They escape T-cell control and may even interact or destroy T cells by producing anti-T- cell antibodies.

Macrophages

Abnormalities of macrophages, particularly those expressing Ia antigens, also may contribute to autoimmunity. A major aspect of immunologic control resides with this important cell population.

SELF-RECOGNITION (TOLERANCE)

Self-recognition of membrane idiotypic receptors and the major histocompatibility complex (MHC) antigens appear fundamental to facilitating the regulatory interactions between cells. Many of these interactions are mediated through the production of highly specific soluble fraction that contains Ia and idiotypic determinants and transmits signs from one cell to another.

Whether the immunologic response to any given antigen will be expressed as immunity or tolerance is probably determined by a regulatory equilibrium, primarily established by the balance between helper and suppressor T cells. This equilibrium appears to be controlled by immune response (Ir) genes linked to the MHC and expressed on the surface of lymphocytes and macrophages as the Ia antigens. In addition, a new theory suggests that aberrant Ia expression on inflamed cells, such as thyroid cells in autoimmune thyroiditis, could lead to inappropriate antigen presentation by these cells, immune cell activation, and ultimately, to organ-specific autoimmune disease.

Self-tolerance is induced by at least two mechanisms involving contact between antigen and immunocompetent cells:

- Elimination of the small clone of immunocompetent cells programmed to react with the antigen (Burnet's clonal selection theory).
- Induction of unresponsiveness in the immunocompetent cells through excessive antigen binding to them and/or through triggering of a suppressor mechanism. The normal immune response is modulated by both antigen-specific and nonspecific suppressor cell activity.

The major mechanism in antigen-specific suppression of antibody response appears related to an antiidiotypic immune response induced by the antigen-binding site (idiotype) unique for a particular antibody. In the opposite situation, prolonged antigen stimulation, such as in certain chronic infections, leads to polyclonal activation of the B-cell response with a resultant polyclonal hypergammaglobulinemia (see

Chapter 24) for a complete discussion of polyclonal and monoclonal hypergammaglobulinemias).

Receptors for antigens on B cells have the same antigen-binding configurations as the antibody molecules secreted by these cells. In addition, components of the antibody molecule itself elicit the formation of antiidiotype antibody, which can react with antigen receptors on the cell surface and thus control the immune response. Antibody molecules with the same configuration are known as idiotypes and will be represented on the antigen receptor on B cells.

Both T and B cells appear to be targets of suppression by antiidiotypic reactivities represented by antibody and possibly also by specifically reactive T cells. In autoimmunity, T and B cells with antiidiotypic specificity could have the normal function of limiting the immune response to extrinsic antigens. Some types of suppressor T cells may also operate this way. The likelihood that antiidiotype antibodies occur naturally as molecules that are reactive with antigen receptor on T and B cells forms the basis of Jerne's network theory of self-regulation.

MAJOR AUTOANTIBODIES

Major autoantibodies can be detected in different diseases. Many diagnostic laboratory tests are based on detecting these autoimmune responses. Commonly encountered autoantibodies include thyroid, gastric, adrenocortical, striated muscle, acetylcholine receptor, smooth muscle, salivary gland, mitochondrial, reticulin, myelin, islet cell, and skin. Antibodies to antinuclear antibodies, which are discussed in detail in Chapter 26, include DNA, histone, and nonhistone protein antibodies. The action of specific autoantibodies and their use in medical diagnosis are:

- Acetylcholine receptor binding antibody: measures antibody to acetylcholine receptors at neuromuscular junctions of skeletal muscle. Useful in the diagnosis of myasthenia gravis.
- Acetylcholine receptor (AcHR) blocking antibody: measures antibodies to acetylcholine receptors. Found in about one third of patients with myasthenia gravis.
- Antiadrenal antibody: measures antibodies to adrenal cortex cells. High antibody titers are characteristic of autoimmune hypoadrenalism in about three fourths of cases, but they are not found in tuberculous Addison's disease.
- Anticardiolipin antibody: antibodies directed to cardiolipin are present in patients with SLE associated with arterial and venous thromboses and in those with placental infarcts in early pregnancy with or without SLE. Elevation may be predictive of risk of thrombosis or recurrent spontaneous abortions of early pregnancy. They are also called lupus anticoagulant or phospholipid antibodies.
- Anticentriole antibody: measures antibodies to the cellular ultrastructures, centrioles. The appearance of these antibodies is unusual but can be demonstrated in systemic sclerosis.
- Anticentromere antibody: measures anticentromere (antikinetochore) to chromosomal centromeres. Most patients with calcinosis, Raynaud's phenomenon, esophageal dysfunction, sclerodactyly, and telangiectasia (CREST) syndrome demonstrate these antibodies. They

can also be exhibited by about one third of patients with Raynaud's disease and approximately 10% of patients with systemic sclerosis.

- Anti-DNA antibody: measures antibody to DNA. Increased amounts (>25% by membrane assay) and decreased quantities of the C4 complement component confirm the diagnosis of SLE. These tests are also useful in monitoring the activity and exacerbations of SLE. The absence of anti-DNA is demonstrated in about one fourth of patients with SLE.

- Antiglomerular basement membrane antibody: measures the amount of antibody to glomerular basement membrane (anti-GBM). High titers are suggestive of Goodpasture's disease or anti-GBM nephritis. The test is also useful for monitoring anti-GBM nephritis. Negative results, however, do not rule out Goodpasture's disease.

- Antiintrinsic factor antibody: measures antibody to intrinsic factor (IF). The presence of IF-blocking antibodies is diagnostic of pernicious anemia and found in approximately 60% of cases.

- Antiislet cell antibody: measures antibody to the islet cells of the pancreas. This test is useful as an early marker of beta pancreatic cell destruction.

- Anti-liver and kidney microsomes (anti-LKM) antibody: measures antibody to components of renal and hepatic microsomes. The presence of a high titer is diagnostic of hepatic disease and suggests aggressive disease.

- Antimitochondrial antibody: measures antibody to the cellular ultrastructures, mitochondria. A high titer strongly suggests primary biliary cirrhosis (PBC); the absence of mitochondrial antibodies is strong evidence against PBC. Other forms of liver disease frequently exhibit low mitochondrial antibody titers.

- Antimyelin antibody: measures antibody to components of the myelin sheath of nerves or myelin basic protein. Antibodies to myelin are associated with multiple sclerosis or other neurologic diseases. Myelin antibodies are not detectable in the cerebrospinal fluid (CSF) of patients with multiple sclerosis.

- Antimyocardial antibody: measures antibody to components of the myocardium. The presence of myocardial antibodies is diagnostic of Dressler's (cardiac injury) syndrome or rheumatic fever.

- Antineutrophil antibody: autoantibody producing a characteristic granular cytoplasmic staining pattern (c-ANCA) to cytoplasmic constituents of neutrophilic granulocytes. Antineutrophil cytoplasmic antibody has been described as a sensitive and specific marker for active Wegener's granulomatosis, a systemic vasculitides. Antibody producing a perinuclear staining of neutrophils (p-ANCA) occurs in a wide range of diseases.

- Antinuclear antibody (ANA): measures antibody to nuclear antigens. Antinuclear antibodies are found in most (99%) patients with untreated SLE.

- Antiparietal cell antibody: measures antibody to parietal cells (large cells on the margin of the peptic glands of the stomach). Most (80%) patients with pernicious anemia have parietal cell antibodies. In the presence of parietal cell antibodies, gastric biopsy almost always demonstrates gastritis. Low antibody titers to parietal cells are often found with no clinical evidence of pernicious anemia or atrophic gastritis and are sometimes seen in elderly patients.

- Antiplatelet antibody: measures immunologically attached IgG on platelets. The presence of platelet antibodies, measured indirectly, is associated with immune thrombocytopenia SLE.

- Antireticulin antibody: measures antibody to reticulin, an albuminoid or scleroprotein substance present in the connective framework of reticular tissue. Most (80%) cases of childhood gluten-sensitive enteropathy demonstrate reticulin antibodies. These antibodies can also be found in dermatitis herpetiformis, adult gluten-sensitive enteropathy, and in about one fifth of patients with chronic heroin addiction.

- Antirheumatoid arthritis nuclear antigen (anti-RANA) (also called RA precipitin): measures an antibody to a component of the Epstein-Barr virus (EBV). The antibody is found in most patients with RA and in about 15% of patients with SLE. Anti-RANA is not useful in diagnosis or differential diagnosis of arthritis.

- Antiribosome antibody: measures the presence of antibody to the cellular organelles, ribosomes. Ribosomal antibodies are found in about 10% of patients with SLE.

- Antinuclear ribonucleoprotein (anti-nRNP) antibody: measures an ANA, nuclear ribonucleoprotein. A high titer of this antibody is characteristic of mixed connective tissue disease (MCTD) or undifferentiated connective tissue disease. In MCTD, anti-nRNP is found in the absence of various other ANAs. Low titers of anti-nRNP are seen in about one third of patients with SLE and are typically found in association with other ANAs such as anti-DNA or anti-Sm.

- Anti-Scl or Anti-Scl-70 antibody: measures an antibody to a basic nonhistone nuclear protein. The presence of anti-Scl is diagnostic of systemic sclerosis; however, it is demonstrable in only about one fifth of patients with systemic sclerosis.

- Antiskin antibody (dermal-epidermal): measures antibody to the basement membrane area of the skin. Antibodies are present in more than 80% of patients with bullous pemphigoid, but the absence of antibodies does not rule out the disorder.

- Antiskin (interepithelial) antibody: measures antibody to intercellular substance of the skin. Antibodies can be detected in most (90%) patients with pemphigus; the absence of demonstrable antibody usually excludes the diagnosis. The presence of antibodies is also useful in evaluating blistering disease. A rising antibody titer may indicate an impending relapse of pemphigus, and a falling titer is suggestive of effective control of the disease.

- Anti-Sm antibody: measures Sm (Smith) antibody to acidic nuclear protein. Sm antibody is demonstrated by about one third of patients with SLE. Presence of the antibody confirms the diagnosis of SLE, but the absence of antibody does not exclude the diagnosis.

- Antismooth muscle antibody: measures antibody to components of smooth muscle. A high and persistent titer is suggestive of the autoimmune form of chronic active hepatitis. Antismooth muscle antibodies are also seen in viral disorders such as infectious mononucleosis.

- Antisperm: evaluates the presence of sperm antibodies. Half of vasectomized men demonstrate the antibody, as well as 40% of men and women with fertility problems.
- Anti-SS-A (SS-A precipitin; anti-Ro) antibody: detects the presence of antibody to acidic nucleoprotein of human spleen extract. SS-A precipitins are demonstrable in more than 70% of patients with Sjögren's syndrome-sicca complex and are often found in a subset of these patients at risk for vasculitis. The antibody is also found in one third of patients with SLE and in those with Sjögren's syndrome-RA or the annular variety of subacute cutaneous lupus erythematosus. In neonatal lupus erythematosus autoantibodies to SS-A, discoid skin lesions and congenital heart blocks are common.
- Anti-SS-B (SS-B precipitin, anti-La) antibody: is demonstrated by most patients with Sjögren's syndrome-SLE. One half to three fourths of patients with Sjögren's syndrome have the antibody; it is frequently found in a subset of these patients at risk for vasculitis.
- Antistriational antibody: measures antibody to components of striated muscle. Antibodies to striated muscles may be detected in patients with myasthenia gravis or thymoma, or in those undergoing penicillamine treatment. Absence of the antibody in patients with myasthenia gravis generally rules out the presence of thymoma.
- Antithyroglobulin and antithyroid microsome antibody: evaluates the presence of antibodies to the thyroid components: thyroglobulin, an iodine-containing protein secreted by the thyroid gland and stored within its colloid substance; and thyroid microsomes, particles derived from the endoplasmic reticulum. The presence of microsome antibodies is considered predictive of an elevated thyroid-stimulating hormone (TSH) level. A positive thyroid antibody test and an elevated TSH titer are associated with a risk of hypothyroidism. Absence of both antibodies is strong evidence against autoimmune thyroiditis.
- Cardiolipin antibodies: also referred to as phospholipid antibodies and lupus anticoagulants.
- Histone reactive antinuclear antibody (HRANA): measures the presence of HRANA. A high titer of HRANA is highly suggestive of drug-induced (e.g., hydralazine) lupus erythematosus. HRANA may occasionally be demonstrated in patients with SLE.
- Jo-1 antibody: detects precipitins to an acidic nuclear protein from calf thymus. Approximately one third of patients with uncomplicated polymyositis and some patients with dermatomyositis demonstrate this antibody.
- Ku antibody: detects precipitins to an acidic nuclear protein from calf thymus. About half of patients with overlapping signs and symptoms of scleroderma and polymyositis demonstrate Ku precipitins.
- Mi-1-antibody: detects antibodies to an acidic nuclear protein from calf thymus. Some patients with dermatomyositis and polymyositis demonstrate Mi-1-antibodies.
- PM-1 antibody: detects antibodies to an acidic nuclear protein from calf thymus. These precipitins are found in most (87%) patients with polymyositis-scleroderma. More than half the patients suffering from polymyositis demonstrate the antibody, but it is detected in less than one fifth of patients with dermatomyositis.

ORGAN-SPECIFIC AND MIDSPECTRUM DISORDERS

Cardiovascular Disorders

The primary immunologic diseases of the blood vessels are termed vasculitis; those of the heart are called carditis.

Vasculitis

Deposition of circulating immune complexes is considered directly or indirectly responsible for many forms of vasculitis. The inflammatory lesions of blood vessels produce variable injury or necrosis of the blood vessel wall. This may result in narrowing, occlusion, or thrombosis of the lumen, or the formation of aneurysms or rupture. Vasculitis occurs as a primary disease process or as a secondary manifestation of another disease (e.g., RA).

Vasculitis is characterized by inflammation within blood vessels, which often results in a compromise of the vessel lumen with ischemia. Ischemia causes the major manifestations of the vasculitic syndromes and determines the prognosis. Any size and type of blood vessel may be involved. Therefore the vasculitic syndromes are a heterogeneous group of diseases (Table 25-4).

Antibody specific to endothelial cells also contributes to immune vasculopathy. Antiendothelial antibodies are autoantibodies directed against antigens in the cytoplasmic membrane of endothelial cells.

Carditis

The heart shares with other organs a susceptibility to immune-mediated injury. Numerous cardiac diseases are characterized by the presence of inflammatory cells within the myocardium resulting from immune sensitization to endogenous or exogenous cardiac antigens. The consequent reaction of cardiac myocytes to immune injury can range from reversible modulation of their electrical and mechanical

TABLE 25-4 **Examples of the Classification of Vasculitic Syndromes**

Systemic necrotizing arteritis
   Polyarteritis nodosa
   Allergic angiitis and granulomatosis
   Overlap syndrome
Hypersensitivity vasculitis
   Henoch-Schönlein purpura
   McDuffie's syndrome
Wegener's granulomatosis
Lymphomatoid granulomatosis
Giant cell arteritis
   Takayasu arteritis
Mucocutaneous lymph node syndrome (Kawasaki's disease)
Behçet's disease
Thromboangiitis obliterans
Central nervous system vasculitis
Miscellaneous
   Cogan's syndrome
   Eales disease
   Hypereosinophilic syndrome with vasculitis

capabilities to cell death. Carditis can be caused by a variety of conditions including acute rheumatic fever, Lyme disease, and cardiac transplantation rejection.

Myocardial contractility can be impaired by cell-mediated injury or local release of cytokines. The study of immune cardiac disease has entered a period of rapid expansion. Primary idiopathic myocarditis is an autoimmune disease characterized by infiltration of the heart by macrophages and lymphocytes. The mechanisms by which immune cells and factors localize in the myocardium, modulate myocyte function, and remodel myocardial architecture are underway.

A diagnosis of acute rheumatic fever requires differentiation from other immunologic and infectious diseases. The immunologic basis for rheumatic heart disease has been suspected for a long time. Patients with rheumatic heart disease exhibit antimyocardial antibodies that bind in vitro to foci in the myocardium and heart valves. These antibodies may be responsible for the deposition of Ig and complement components found in the same area of rheumatic heart disease tissues at autopsy.

Antimyocardial antibodies appear to be strongly cross-reactive with streptococcal antigens, but they are not toxic to heart tissue unless the latter is damaged previously by some other cause. Because antimyocardial antibodies are commonly found in patients who have recently suffered a myocardial infarction or have had a recent streptococcal infection (see Chapter 14) without cardiac sequela, detection of these antibodies has not been a particularly useful differential diagnostic test for cardiac injury. The presence of myocardial antibodies, however, is diagnostic of Dressler's syndrome (cardiac injury) or rheumatic fever.

Collagen-Vascular Disorders

Progressive Systemic Sclerosis (Scleroderma)
Scleroderma is a collagen-vascular disease of unknown etiology that assumes various forms. Eosinophilic fasciitis is considered by some to be a variant of scleroderma.

Development of scleroderma has been associated with a number of occupations and drugs. Occupational exposure to vinyl chloride, vibratory stimuli, and silicosis have been associated with subsequent development of scleroderma. Drug-induced cases include bleomycin sulfate, tryptophan, and carbidopa as causes.

Epidemiology. Scleroderma occurs in all races. It is three times more frequent in women than in men.

Signs and Symptoms. Scleroderma is characterized by fibrosis in skin and internal organs and by arterial occlusions with a distinct proliferative pattern. Initial symptoms usually appear in the third decade of life. Raynaud's phenomenon is the most frequent manifestation. The disease is slowly progressive and chronically disabling, but it can be rapidly progressive and fatal.

Immunologic Manifestations. Idiopathic scleroderma is considered an autoimmune disease because of the autoantibodies associated with it and the overlap syndromes of scleroderma-polymyositis and scleroderma-SLE.

Antinuclear antibodies are formed in 40% to 90% of patients to (1) extractable nuclear antigens, (2) the nucleolus, (3) the centromere, and (4) Scl-70. The anticentromere antibody is sensitive and is specific for patients with a subset of scleroderma with CREST syndrome.

In addition, T-cell hyperactivity correlates with disease activity. Activated T cells can result in both the vascular changes and the increased collagen production in scleroderma. It is now thought that both the vascular disorder and fibrosis result from this cellular immune activation. Vascular injury could be mediated by cytokines or direct cell-cell interaction by activated lymphocytes and endothelial cells.

Signs and Symptoms. Systemic sclerosis is a chronic multisystem disorder that causes thickening of the skin (scleroderma) and involves other organ systems.

In more than half the cases, Raynaud's phenomenon occurs before the onset of other manifestations. Skin manifestations can proceed through the stages of pitting edema, a sclerotic "hidebound" stage, and a final stage of atrophy or softening and a return toward normal. Articular complaints are common. Hypomotility of the gastrointestinal tract is the second most common clinical feature.

Eosinophilia-Myalgia Syndrome
Many people exposed to the agent causing eosinophilia-myalgia syndrome (EMS) may develop illness. Patients develop severe myalgia. More than half of patients with EMS develop scleroderma-like manifestations.

The single most important predictor of the disorder is ingestion of contaminated L-tryptophan. The association of ingestion of L-tryptophan with a systemic disease now called EMS was first observed in 1989. Some patients have died from the L-tryptophan.

L-Tryptophan was widely used after it was introduced in 1974 as an over-the-counter nostrum for various ailments such as insomnia, premenstrual syndrome, and anxiety. Medical professionals were also known to recommend its use for neuropsychiatric or fibromyalgia disorders.

Endocrine Gland Disorders

Numerous endocrine gland disorders are attributable to an autoimmune process. Several of the classic and more common disorders are discussed in this section.

Thyroid
The clinical spectrum of autoimmune thyroid disease is very broad. There are two major forms of autoimmune thyroid disease—chronic autoimmune thyroiditis and Graves' disease. Lymphoid (Hashimoto's) chronic thyroiditis is a classic example of an organ-specific autoimmune disorder. Other autoimmune disorders affecting the thyroid gland include transient thyroiditis syndrome and idiopathic hypothyroidism.

Lymphoid (Hashimoto's) Chronic Thyroiditis
Etiology. The exact mechanism of the disorder is unknown, but it is believed to be related to an autoimmune process in which the development of circulating cytotoxic antibodies eventually destroys the thyroid gland, producing hypothyroidism. This disorder is associated with the presence of HLA-DR4 and -DR5. However, these associations are not consistent in different races and ethnic groups.

Epidemiology. This disorder can occur at any age but it is most commonly first diagnosed in the third to fifth decade of life and is much more common in women than in men. The fibrous variant of the disease is more often present in middle-age and older patients.

The mode of inheritance is unknown. However, a strong possibility of a genetic tendency to inherit the trait for the development of antibodies against the thyroid gland exists. It is common to have multiple members of a family suffer from the same disease. (e.g., Graves' disease or lymphoid thyroiditis).

Signs and Symptoms. Lymphoid thyroiditis is believed to be the most common cause of sporadic goiter. Characteristically there is a firm, diffusely enlarged, nontender thyroid gland that may be lobulated. Hypothyroidism, however, is a common late sequela of lymphoid thyroiditis, and patients are usually euthyroid when first seen by a physician. Some individuals have clinical and pathologic evidence of the coexistence of both Graves' disease and lymphoid (Hashimoto's) thyroiditis. Histologically, Hashimoto's thyroiditis is characterized by diffuse lymphocytic infiltration (Figure 25-2).

Immunologic Manifestations

Patients with lymphoid thyroiditis, as well as other autoimmune thyroid disorders, can demonstrate histologic and immunologic manifestations of the disease. Antibodies to thyroid constituents may be observed in these patients. Antibodies to the following list of constituents may be demonstrated serologically:

- Thyroglobulin
- Thyroid microsome
- Second colloid antigen (CA2 antigen)
- Thyroid membrane receptors
- Thyronine (T_4) and triiodothyronine (T_3)

Thyroglobulin. Antithyroglobulin (TgAb) was the first antibody discovered against a thyroid protein, thyroglobulin. Immunofluorescent laboratory methods using fluorescein-labeled antihuman Ig can demonstrate the binding of antithyroglobulin antibody to thin sections of thyroid tissue in abnormal conditions or in approximately 4% of the normal population. It has also been noted that a gradual increase in the frequency of positive titers occurs in the female population with aging. The absence of antithyroglobulin antibodies, however, does not exclude the diagnosis of lymphoid (Hashimoto's) thyroiditis; conversely, the presence of antibodies does not establish the diagnosis because it can be positive in Graves' disease and is occasionally positive in thyroid cancer and subacute thyroiditis. Testing for antibody may also be used to monitor patients with thyroid cancers.

Thyroid Microsomes. Antibodies directed against thyroid microsomes, antithyroid microsomal antibodies or antithyroperoxidase antibodies (TPO Ab) can be detected in about 7% of the population, with titers ranging from 1:100 to 1:1600. Even a low titer of antithyroid antibodies correlates with a degree of thyroid involvement by an autoimmune process. The absence of antibodies has been documented in diagnosed cases of autoimmune thyroiditis, which may be explained by special characteristics of the antibody or by the fact that it forms complexes with thyroglobulins in the circulation and escapes detection. The presence of such circulating complexes has been documented in patients with thyroid autoimmune disorders.

Second Colloid Antigen. CA2 antigen is directed against a colloid protein and can be detected by immunofluorescent examination. Antibody to CA2 is present in about 50% of patients who have subacute thyroiditis, and it is detectable in some patients with Hashimoto's thyroiditis whose sera show no other evidence of abnormal antibodies.

Thyroid Membrane Receptors. The thyroid membrane receptors are a group of IgG antibodies that interact with receptors on thyroid membranes. They often produce hyperthyroidism that manifests itself clinically, chemically, and histologically. At present the classification of these IgG antibodies is operational, based on their method of detection.

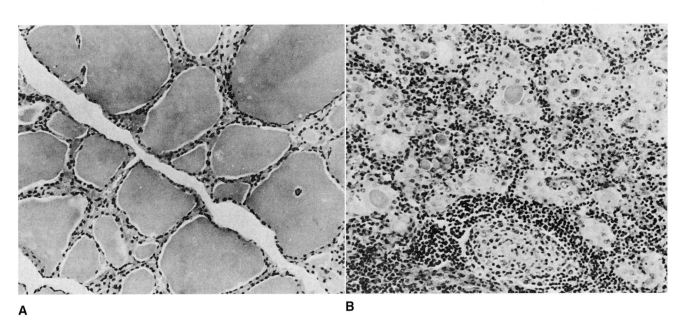

A   **B**

Figure 25-2   A comparison of the histologic architecture of the thyroid gland of a normal patient, **A,** and a patient with Hashimoto's disease, **B,** In the normal thyroid colloid fills the vesicles, but in a diseased gland only isolated deposits of colloid are seen. The cell infiltrate is lymphoid in nature. In the lower center is a germinal center. (From Anderson JR, Buchanan WW, Goudie RB: *Autoimmunity,* Springfield, Ill, 1967, Charles C Thomas.)

Long-acting thyroid stimulator (LATS) and long-acting thyroid stimulator protector (LATS-P) assays are of importance.

Thyronine and Triiodothyronine. Antibodies to T_4 and T_3 have been found in several patients, most of whom had evidence of a thyroid autoimmune process such as goiter and hypothyroidism. In these cases the underlying autoimmune process is most likely responsible for the hypothyroidism rather than hormone binding by the circulating antithyronine antibodies.

Diagnostic Evaluation

Fine-needle aspiration biopsy of the thyroid is useful in conjunction with clinical evaluation and serologic studies in the diagnosis of lymphocytic (Hashimoto's) thyroiditis.

Histologic examination of thyroid tissue demonstrates variable infiltration of the entire gland with lymphocytes. Germinal lymphoid centers are characteristic, and destruction and distortion of normal thyroid follicles are apparent. The thyroid cells remain intact but are hypertrophied, although the usual heterogeneity of small, enlarged thyroid follicles, some containing flat epithelium, also can be seen. In advanced cases, there is almost complete destruction of normal thyroid tissue, with replacement by lymphocytes or fibrous tissue.

When the disease produces hypothyroidism, a slight increase in the plasma TSH concentration can usually be demonstrated in the early phase, followed by a fall in serum thyroxine and eventually by a fall in serum triiodothyronine. Antithyroglobulin and/or antithyroid microsomal antibodies are found in moderate-to-high titers in more than 50% of patients, but the presence of antimicrosomal antibodies is considered to be more diagnostic.

Antibodies directed against thyroid microsomal antigen (thyroid peroxidase antibody [anti-TPO]) can be detected by various techniques (Table 25-5). Chemiluminescent immunoassay is commonly performed to detect anti-TPO autoantibodies. TPO plays a significant role in the biosynthesis of thyroid hormones by catalyzing both the iodination of tyrosyl residues in thyroglobulin and the coupling of the iodotyrosyl residues to form thyroxine (T_4) and triiodothyronine (T_3). Autoantibodies produced against TPO are capable of inhibiting the enzyme activity. They are also complement fixing antibodies that can induce cytotoxic changes in cells and consequently cause thyroid thyroid dysfunction. More than 90% of patients with autoimmune thyroiditis (Hashimoto's thyroiditis) have anti-TPO. Antibodies to TPO have also been found in most patients with idiopathic hypothyroidism (85%) and Graves' disease (50%).

Pancreas

Insulin-Dependent Diabetes Mellitus

Etiology. Insulin-dependent diabetes mellitus (IDDM) or type 1 diabetes mellitus is a disorder of deficient insulin production caused by immune destruction of the B cells of the pancreatic islets. The only definitively identified environmental factor causing IDDM is congenital rubella infection. Reports of association between diabetes and infections with coxsackievirus B and several other viruses suggest the possibility of other triggers for the disease.

Genetic susceptibility factors have been identified. IDDM

TABLE 25-5	Antithyroid Antibody Tests
Antigen	**Test To Identify Antibody**
Thyroglobulin	Indirect immunofluorescence on fixed thyroid tissues
	Tanned RBC hemagglutination
	Immunometric assays (IMA) or sandwich methods
	Radioimmunoassay (RIA)
Microsomal antigen	Enzyme–linked immunosorbent assay (ELISA)
Second colloid antigen (CA2)	Indirect immunofluorescence
Thyroid membrane receptors	Long-acting thyroid stimulator (LATS)
	Long-acting thyroid stimulator protector (LATS-P)
	In vitro assays for thyroid-stimulating immunoglobulin (TSI) or TSH-binding inhibition (TBI)
Triiodohyronine (total T_3)	Radioimmunoassay using different separation methods
	Electrophoresis with radioactive-labeled thyronines

is associated with HLA-DR3, -DR4, DQ2, and DQ8 antigens. A total of 90% of Caucasian patients with IDDM have either one or both of these antigens. The presence of both DR3 and DR4 antigens yields an even higher risk of disease development than the additive susceptibility from either antigen, suggesting that other MHC-related genes may be involved in pathogenesis. Another HLA antigen, DR2, is found less frequently in people with diabetes than in the general population, indicating that this antigen is associated with some type of protective effect. HLA-DQw8 is associated with a twofold to sixfold increased risk for diabetes. Several lines of investigation have implicated the CD4+ T lymphocyte as central in the immune process that leads to the development of diabetes.

Epidemiology. IDDM was previously called juvenile-onset disease because of the time of life in which it often presents; 10% of people with diabetes have IDDM, and approximately 10,000 new cases are diagnosed each year. Most patients develop IDDM in childhood or early adolescence, but it may occur any time. Approximately 95% of patients who develop clinical diabetes before the age of 30 years have IDDM.

Signs and Symptoms. The central clinical feature is the requirement for exogenous insulin to maintain euglycemia.

Immunologic Manifestations. T cells of the CD4+ type are responsible for initiating the immune response to the islets that results in islet cell autoantibodies and B cell destruction.

Patients with IDDM have several types of autoantibodies; the more tested are:

- Antiinsulin (IAA)
- Antiglutamic acid decarboxylase (GAD)

- Antiislet cell antigen 2 (IA-2)
- Antibodies reacting with the cells of the pancreatic islets have been found in patients with diabetes accompanying autoimmune endocrine disorders. Autoantibodies to islet-related antigens precede the development of clinical IDDM by a prolonged period, often several years. A higher incidence of these antiislet cell antibodies, however, has been demonstrated in patients with IDDM.

An Ig in the sera of patients with insulin-resistant diabetes appears to bind to a tissue receptor for insulin, which prevents some of the biologic effects of insulin. In addition, antibodies that bind to and possibly kill pancreatic islet cells have been found in most young patients with IDDM.

A small subgroup of patients with IDDM has demonstrated antireceptor antibody (InR), an IgG class of antibodies directed against the insulin receptor. Antibodies to InR may be directed to the binding site or to determinants away from the binding site for insulin. This condition is predominant in non-Caucasian females of all ages.

Antiislet cell antigen 2 (IA-2) is directed against a phosphatase-type transmembrane 37-kD islet beta-cell antigen (ICA512).

Adrenal Glands

Idiopathic adrenal atrophy is the primary cause of Addison's disease. It is believed that many of these cases are autoimmune in etiology. Women are afflicted twice as often as men. The disease usually presents in the third and fourth decade of life. Although a great potential exists for morbidity, it has a relatively low incidence. The adult form of Addison's disease is associated with HLA class II antigens DR3 and DR4.

Idiopathic Addison's disease is usually diagnosed in patients because of low serum cortisol levels in the presence of elevated levels of corticotropin. Most (approximately 80%) patients manifest serum antibodies against cortical elements, probably microsomal. Some cases demonstrate antibodies against adrenal cell surfaces. These antibodies generally bind to components in the adrenal cortex but affect only individual zones. Antibodies are generally low in titer and are not a direct reflection of adrenal cell damage. In women with premature ovarian failure, autoimmune destruction of the ovarian stroma has been observed.

Pituitary Gland

Sheehan's syndrome, lymphocytic adenohypophysitis, is a disorder that causes rapid decline in pituitary function. This disorder is most commonly seen in postpartum women. Antibodies against pituitary cells are observed in some patients. The disorder is distinguished by a mononuclear infiltrate of the pituitary gland and hypophysis.

Parathyroid Gland

Idiopathic hypoparathyroidism occurs both as a childhood disorder in type I polyglandular syndrome, and less commonly as an isolated disorder in adults. It is associated with complement-mediated cytotoxicity of parathyroid cells, indicating a specific immune response to the parathyroid. Several antigens have been associated with this disorder, including endothelial cell proteins and mitochondria.

Polyglandular Syndromes

Three syndromes of associated endocrinopathies have been defined as the polyglandular syndromes.

- Type I syndrome: involves mucocutaneous candidiasis and associated endocrinopathies that begin in early childhood. Patients initially develop candidiasis and hypoparathyroidism, but more than half the patients also develop Addison's disease. Gonadal failure, alopecia, and chronic hepatitis are also seen. Patients have organ-specific autoantibodies and poorly defined defects in cell-mediated immunity.
- Type II syndrome: involves the combined occurrence of either IDDM or autoimmune thyroid disease with Addison's disease. It is also called Schmidt's syndrome. This type of disorder is seen primarily in women in the second or third decades of life. Most cases are familial, but the mode of inheritance is unknown. There is a strong association with HLA-DR3.
- Type III syndrome: defined as the co-occurrence of autoimmune thyroid disease with two other autoimmune disorders, including IDDM, pernicious anemia, or a nonendocrine, organ-specific autoimmune disorder such as myasthenia gravis. These patients do not have Addison's disease. The HLA-DR3 allele is present in more than 50% of cases. Patients in this category are overwhelmingly female.

Reproductive Disorders

Antibodies against cytoplasmic components of different cells of the ovary have been demonstrated in Addison's disease and in premature ovarian failure. Premature ovarian failure may be an immune disorder causing reproductive failure and eventually early menopause. A prevalence of smooth-muscle antibody, antinuclear antibody, and antiphospholipid antibodies has been found in women with unexplained infertility. In addition, autoantibodies to the ovary and gonadotropin receptors are measured in many women with polyendocrinopathies.

In cases of endometriosis, a defect in natural killer cell activity exists. This results in decreased cytotoxicity for autologous endometrial cells. Reduced T-lymphocyte-mediated cytotoxicity to endometrial cells has also been found.

A sizable proportion of pregnancy losses may be due to immunologic factors. The fetus is an immunogenic allograft that evokes a protective immune response from the mother, which is necessary for implantation and growth. The mechanism of pregnancy loss is hypothesized to involve two antiphospholipid antibodies. Lupus anticoagulant and anticardiolipin antibodies are directed against platelets and vascular endothelium. This causes vascular destruction and thrombosis, which leads to fetal death and abortion. There is no evidence of a direct immunologic attack on the embryo. A human fetus is capable of survival in utero if it does not share a significant number of maternal MHC antigens, especially HLA-B and -DR, and DQ loci.

Antisperm antibodies have been detected in the serum of both men and women, in cervical mucus of women, in seminal fluid of men, and attached to sperm cells. In seminal fluid, the immobilizing antibodies to sperm are usually of

IgG class, and the agglutinating antibodies are IgA. Elevated levels of antibodies to sperm have been found in more than 40% of males after vasectomy but only occasionally in males with primary testicular agenesis. Allergy-like reactions to seminal fluid have also been observed. These reactions range from local reactions to systemic reactions, including life-threatening anaphylaxis. The allergen is usually one or more prostatic proteins, but it can include IgE to spermatozoa.

Exocrine Gland Disorder

Sjögren's Syndrome

Etiology. This disorder is a chronic inflammatory disease of unknown etiology that affects lacrimal, salivary, and other excretory glands. It results in keratoconjunctivitis sicca and xerostomia.

As with RA and SLE, etiologic factors considered are infection, abnormalities of immune regulation, and genetic factors. Development of Sjögren's syndrome is strongly associated with HLA-B8 and HLA-DR3. Infectious origin is suggested. Clear evidence for excessive B-cell activity has been demonstrated, but it is not known whether this is due to B- or T-cell abnormalities.

Epidemiology. A primary form is not associated with other diseases; a secondary form is associated with RA and other connective tissue diseases. A total of 90% of patients are women. A 44-fold increased incidence of lymphoma has been noted in patients with Sjögren's syndrome.

Signs and Symptoms. The main clinical manifestations (Table 25-6) of Sjögren's syndrome are dry eyes, dry mouth, and recurrent salivary gland pain and swelling. Hoarseness, chronic cough, and increased incidence of infection have been observed. Dryness of the vagina leads to dyspareunia and itching. Dysphagia and atrophic gastritis can also be present. Extraglandular involvement results in interstitial pneumonitis and fibrosis. Renal tubular acidosis and vasculitis involving peripheral nerves and the central nervous system (CNS) can also result from Sjögren's syndrome.

Immunologic Manifestations. The immunologic characteristics of Sjögren's syndrome include hypergammaglobulinemia, ANAs, rheumatoid factor, autoantibodies to salivary duct and other antigens, and lymphocyte and plasma cell infiltration of involved tissue. Antibodies are usually polyclonal and may result in the hyperviscosity syndrome and hypergammaglobulinemic purpura. ANA speckled or homogeneous patterns are present in 65% of patients and are present more frequently in primary Sjögren's syndrome. Antibodies to Sjögren's syndrome-A antigen have been associated with vasculitis in primary Sjögren's syndrome. Antibodies to Sjögren's syndrome-B antigen are nearly always found in association with Sjögren's syndrome-A and only occur in SLE and Sjögren's syndrome. Rheumatoid factor is found in 90% of cases. A novel autoantibody, anti-alpha-Fodrin, has been found in the sera of a majority of patients with primary Sjögren's syndrome. This antibody is possibly pathophysiologically associated with some extraglandular manifestations characteristically seen in patients with Sjögren's syndrome.

Autoantibodies to salivary duct antigens are frequently detected in patients with secondary Sjögren's syndrome. They are also common in one fourth of cases with RA without Sjögren's syndrome. Mitochondrial antibodies are detected in 10% of patients with primary Sjögren's syndrome

TABLE 25-6	Criteria for Diagnosis Sjögren's Syndrome
Four or More of the Following Criteria Must Be Present	
Ocular symptoms	Daily dry eyes for 3 months, sand or gravel feeling in eyes
Oral symptoms	Daily dry mouth for 3 months or recurrent or persistent swollen glands
Ocular signs	Post-Schirmer test or a rose bengal score >4
Histopathology	Aggregates of ≥50 mononuclear cells /4 mm² of glandular tissue
Autoantibodies	Presence of anti-Ro (SS-A), anti-La (SS-B), or antinuclear antibodies (ANA), or rheumatoid factor.

From Vitali C: Preliminary criteria for the classification of Sjögren's syndrome. Results of a prospective concerted action supported by the European community, *Arthritis Rheum* 36:36, 1993.

and rarely in patient's with secondary Sjögren's syndrome and RA. Patients with primary Sjögren's syndrome also have higher levels of antibodies to the thyroid gland, gastric parietal cells, pancreatic epithelial cells, and smooth muscle. Lymphocytyic infiltration of the exocrine glands of the eyes, mouth, nose, lower respiratory tract system, gastrointestinal system, and vagina occurs. The infiltrate is composed of B and T cells. In tissue culture these cells produce large amounts of IgM and IgG. T cells are predominantly helper cells.

Gastrointestinal Disorders

Atrophic Gastritis and Pernicious Anemia

Immunologic Findings. Antibodies against a lipoprotein cytoplasmic component of gastric parietal cells can be detected by immunofluorescence in up to 90% of patients with pernicious anemia (PA) and in about 60% of patients with atrophic gastritis without hematologic abnormalities. These antibodies may also be demonstrated in patients with other autoimmune diseases such as thyroiditis. In addition, antibodies can be found in asymptomatic patients and in persons more than 60 years old.

Histologic Findings. The histologic findings in atrophic gastritis, which almost always accompanies PA, is characterized by lymphocytic infiltration and the absence of parietal and chief cells. The lesions are associated with decreased synthesis of gastric acid and intrinsic factor. IF normally binds ingested vitamin B_{12} at one site and binds to receptors in the distal ileum at another site. In this manner vitamin B_{12} transport across the ileum is affected.

Vitamin B_{12} (Cobalamin) Transport. Cobalamin transport is mediated by three different binding proteins (Table 25-7) capable of binding the vitamin at its required physiologic concentrations: IF, transcobalamin II, and the R proteins.

IF, a glycoprotein, is synthesized and secreted by the parietal cells of the mucosa in the fundus region of the stomach in several mammalian species, including humans. In a healthy state, the amounts of IF secreted by the stomach

TABLE 25-7 Vitamin B$_{12}$ (Cobalamin)-Binding Proteins

	Intrinsic Factor	Transcobalamin II	R Proteins
Source	Stomach	Liver, other tissues	Leukocytes, ? other tissues
Function	Intestinal absorption	Delivery to cells	Excretion storage
Membrane receptors	Ileal enterocytes	Many cells	Liver cells

greatly exceed the quantities required to bind ingested cobalamin in its coenzyme forms. At a very acidic pH, cobalamin splits from dietary protein and combines with IF to form a vitamin-IF complex. Binding by IF is extraordinarily specific and is lost with even slight changes in the cobalamin molecule. This complex is stable and remains unabsorbed until it reaches the ileum. In the ileum the vitamin-IF complex attaches to specific receptor sites present only on the outer surface of microvillus membranes of ileal enterocytes.

The release of this complex from the mucosal cells, with subsequent transport to the tissues, depends on transcobalamin II (TC II). TC II is a plasma polypeptide synthesized by the liver and probably several other tissues. Like IF, TC II, which turns over very rapidly in the plasma, acts as the acceptor and principal carrier of the vitamin to the liver and other tissues. Receptors for TC II are observed on the plasma membranes of a wide variety of cells. TC II is also capable of binding a few unusual cobalamin analogs. TC II also stimulates cobalamin uptake by reticulocytes.

The R proteins compose an antigenically cross-reactive group of cobalamin-binding glycoproteins. The R proteins bind cobalamin and various cobalamin analogs. Their function is unknown, but they appear to serve as storage sites and as a means of eliminating excess cobalamin and unwanted analogs from the blood circulation through receptor sites on liver cells. R proteins are produced by leukocytes and perhaps other tissues. They are present in plasma as transcobalamin I and transcobalamin III, as well as in saliva, milk, and other body fluids. Transcobalamin I probably serves only as a backup transport system for endogenous cobalamin. Endogenous vitamin is synthesized in the human gastrointestinal tract by bacterial action, but none is adsorbed.

Autoimmune Liver Disease

Autoimmune processes are believed to be the possible cause of chronic liver disease. Hypergammaglobulinemia, prominent lymphocyte and plasma cell inflammation of the liver, and the presence of one or more circulating tissue antibodies are commonly manifested. These manifestations suggest an organ-localized autoimmune pathogenesis.

Chronic active hepatitis, for example, is an inflammatory condition most common in young women. It is characterized by prominent lymphocyte and plasma cell inflammatory changes, which start in the portal tracts. In some cases this condition results from a chronic viral infection or inflammation, but in other cases a number of immunologic abnormalities are present to varying degrees, in addition to hypergammaglobulinemia and an elevated erythrocyte sedimentation rate. A defect in immunoregulation is commonly demonstrated, which possibly leads to unrestrained Ig production. These patients display ANAs and antismooth muscle antibodies. A high and persistent titer of antismooth antibodies is suggestive of the autoimmune form of chronic active hepatitis or viral disorders such as infectious mononucleosis.

In some cases this disease is referred to as lupoid hepatitis. Patients with aggressive chronic active hepatitis have a poor prognosis, and a significant rate of mortality is reported 5 years after diagnosis.

Idiopathic Biliary Cirrhosis

Idiopathic biliary cirrhosis is a slowly progressive disease that starts as an apparently noninfectious inflammation in the bile ducts of young to middle-age women. An increased familial incidence has been noted.

Patients exhibit increased serum IgM; depression of cellular immunity, with prominent decreases in suppressor T cells common; and associated autoimmune disorders. It is believed that tissue damage results from an unmodulated attack against host tissue antigens. Antimitochondrial antibodies directed against the cellular ultrastructures, mitochondria, can be displayed. A high titer of these strongly suggests primary biliary cirrhosis (PBC); the absence of mitochondrial antibodies is strong evidence against PBC. Other forms of liver disease, however, frequently exhibit low mitochondrial antibody titers.

Inflammatory Bowel Disease

The mucosal immune system is composed of afferent lymphoid tissues and efferent lymphoid tissues, with several unique features that facilitate host defense at mucosal surfaces. One unique feature is the tendency of cells originating in the mucosal follicles to migrate to the diffuse lymphoid areas. Another unique feature of the mucosal immune system is that B cells in mucosal follicles tend to differentiate into cells that produce polymeric IgA. The ability of IgA to use the polymeric Ig transport receptor on the surface of mucosal epithelial cells (secretory component) allows the molecules to gain ready access to the mucosal surface. A final unique feature of the mucosal immune system is the capacity of the mucosal follicles to elaborate populations of T cells with functions adapted to the mucosal environment.

Idiopathic inflammatory bowel disease (IBD) is an immunologically mediated group of disorders characterized by a chronic, relapsing inflammatory response. One form of IBD, ulcerative colitis (UC), is limited to the large bowel (colon) and is characterized by superficial ulceration manifesting first in the rectum and then extending proximally as a continuous lesion. Longstanding UC is associated with epithelial cell dysplasia and carcinoma. Another form of IBD is Crohn's disease. The terminal ileum and ascending large bowel are typically involved in Crohn's disease. Environmental influences are suspected.

Antibodies directed against colon components are commonly found in the serum of patients with chronic UC, Crohn's disease, and in some cases of regional ileitis. There is evidence that lymphocytes from some patients with IBD are cytotoxic for human fetal colon tissue. However, it is not clear whether antibody-dependent cellular cytotoxicity plays a role in the disease. Other manifestations of uncertain significance are the presence of circulating immune complexes and the depressed capacity to express delayed hypersensitivity (anergy), which occurs commonly but not consistently in IBD.

Elevation of several cytokines with important immunoregulatory and proinflammatory activities has been demonstrated during active IBD. These cytokines, including interleukin-1 (IL-1), IL-6, and IL-8, may play an important role in the initiation and amplification of the immune responses leading to intestinal injury. There is also increasing evidence that IL-1 is activated early in the cascade of events leading to inflammation. Therefore IL-1 has been implicated as a primary target for therapeutic intervention in the treatment of several inflammatory diseases, including IBD.

Other Immunologic Disorders of the Gastrointestinal Tract

Examples of other immunologic disorders related to the gastrointestinal and hepatobiliary tracts include allergy of the gastrointestinal tract, Whipple's disease, immunoproliferative intestinal disease (alpha heavy-chain disease), and infectious hepatitis (discussed in Chapter 20). Allergy of the gastrointestinal tract is an IgE-mediated hypersensitivity to food substances that involves the gastrointestinal tract and, in some cases, the skin and lungs. Examples of systemic autoimmune disease caused by mucosal immune abnormalities are IgA nephropathy (Berger's disease), Henoch-Schönlein purpura, and diseases associated with the presence of circulating IgA complexes in the kidney and vasculature. Immunoproliferative intestinal disease is characterized by monoclonal B cells that produce an aberrant alpha heavy chain.

Autoimmune Hematologic Disorders

Various hematologic conditions can be caused by alloantibodies and autoantibodies. Examples of clinical syndromes caused by these antibodies are presented in Table 25-8.

Autoimmune Hemolytic Anemia

Autoimmune hemolytic anemia can be classified into four groups:

- Warm-reactive autoantibodies—the most common
- Cold-reactive autoantibodies—less than 20% of cases
- Paroxysmal cold hemoglobinuria—rare
- Drug-induced hemolysis—less than 20% of cases

Warm Autoimmune Hemolytic Anemia. Warm autoimmune hemolytic anemia is associated with antibodies reactive at warm temperatures (i.e., 37° C). In more than three fourths of cases, the erythrocytes are coated with both IgG and complement, although some may demonstrate coating with IgG alone or, more infrequently, with complement coating. In warm autoimmune hemolytic anemia very little serum autoantibody exists because the antibody reacts optimally at 37° C and is being continuously adsorbed by red cells in vivo. Elution of the antibody from the cells (mechanical removal of antibodies) can demonstrate an autoantibody, but testing for specificity is not routinely necessary.

TABLE 25-8	Immunohematologic Diseases
Category	**Examples**
Immune hemolysis	Warm autoimmune hemolytic anemia
	Cold agglutinin disease
	Paroxysmal cold hemoglobinuria
	Drug-induced hemolytic anemias
	Hemolytic disease of the newborn
Immune thrombocytopenia	Idiopathic (autoimmune) thrombocytopenic purpura
	Neonatal alloimmune thrombocytopenia
Immune neutropenia	Autoimmune neutropenia
Immune-mediated transfusion reactions	Acute hemolytic transfusion reaction
	Febrile reactions
	Pulmonary hypersensitivity reaction
	Allergic reactions
	IgA-deficient recipient
	Delayed hemolytic reactions
	Posttransfusion purpura
	Transfusion-associated graft-versus-host disease
Anemias	Pernicious anemia
Deficiency of hemostasis and coagulation	Autoimmune protein S deficiency

Cold Autoimmune Hemolytic Anemia. Cold hemagglutinin disease (CHAD), either in the acute or chronic form, is the most common type of hemolytic anemia associated with cold-reactive autoantibodies. The acute form is often secondary to *Mycoplasma pneumoniae* infection or lymphoproliferative disorders such as lymphoma. The chronic form is seen in older patients and produces a mild-to-moderate degree of hemolysis. In addition, Raynaud's phenomenon and hemoglobinuria occur in cold weather.

In cold hemagglutinin disease, a cold-reactive IgM autoantibody reacts with erythrocytes in the peripheral circulation when the body temperature falls to 32° C or below and binds complement to the cells. Hence complement is the only globulin detected on the erythrocytes. Elutions prepared from red cells collected at 37° C will not demonstrate antibody reactivity in the eluate.

Paroxysmal Cold Hemoglobinuria. Paroxysmal cold hemoglobinuria was previously associated with syphilis, but it is now more commonly seen as an acute transient condition secondary to viral infections, particularly in young children. It may also occur as an idiopathic chronic disease in older people.

The autoantibody is an IgG protein that reacts with red cells in colder parts of the body; this produces complement components C_3 and C_4 to bind irreversibly to the cells. At warmer temperatures, red cells are hemolyzed, and the antibody elutes from the cells. Eluates are also nonreactive. This IgG autoantibody, a biphasic hemolysin, can be demonstrated by performing the Donath-Landsteiner test. The autoantibody

TABLE 25-9 Drug-Induced Positive Direct Antiglobulin Test

	Drug Adsorption	Immune Complex	Membrane Modification	Autoantibody Formation
Common cause	IgG	Complement	Nonserologic	IgG
Antibody screening	Negative*	Positive†	Negative	Variable‡
Eluate reactivity with reagent red blood cells (RBCs)	Nonreactive	Nonreactive	Nonreactive	Reactive§
Penicillin-treated RBCs	Reactive with patient's serum and eluate	Nonreactive	Nonreactive	Nonreactive

*Unless irregular antibodies are present in the sample.
†If the drug and complement are present in the test system.
‡If the autoantibody is high enough in titer, screening tests may be positive with all cells tested.
§Will react with all normal cells tested, occasionally showing Rh like specificity.

has anti-p specificity and reacts with all except the rare p or p^k phenotypes. Exceptions that include examples with anti-IH specificity have been described.

Drug-Induced Hemolysis. Coating of red cells demonstrated by a positive direct antihuman globulin test (DAT) may be drug induced (Table 25-9) and accompanied by hemolysis. The mechanisms of reactivity have been described as being caused by four basic mechanisms:
- Drug adsorption
- Immune complex
- Membrane modification
- Autoantibody formation

Drug Adsorption. Penicillin is a representative example of a drug that displays drug adsorption. In this type of mechanism, the drug strongly binds to any protein, including red cell membrane proteins. This binding produces a drug-red-cell-hapten complex that can stimulate antibody formation. The antibody is specific for this complex, and no reactions will take place unless the drug is adsorbed on erythrocytes. Massive doses of intravenous penicillin are needed to coat sufficiently the erythrocytes for antibody attachment to occur.

Approximately 3% of affected patients will demonstrate a positive DAT, and less than 5% will develop hemolytic anemia because of the drug. The hemolysis of red cells is usually extravascular and occurs slowly. It is not life threatening and will abate when penicillin is discontinued. There appears to be no connection between this type of antibody production and allergic penicillin sensitivity caused by IgE production.

Other drugs that display drug adsorption are cephalothin derivatives (e.g., cephalothin [Keflin], quinidine).

Immune Complex. The mechanism of immune complexing is displayed by a variety of drugs, including phenacetin, quinine, rifampin, and stibophen. In this interaction the drug and antibody form a complex in the serum and attach nonspecifically to the red cells. Once attached, this complex initiates the complement cascade, which culminates in intravascular hemolysis. The immune complex may dissociate from the red cell membrane after complement activation and attach to another red cell. This action allows a small amount of drug to produce a severe anemia. When the offending drug is discontinued, the hemolytic process disappears quickly.

Membrane Modification Mechanism. Drugs of the cephalosporin type (e.g., cephalothin) occasionally cause a positive DAT with polyspecific and monospecific antihuman globulin antisera by membrane modification. In this type of mechanism, the drug alters the membrane so that there is nonspecific absorption of globulins, including IgG, IgM, IgA, and complement. Hemolysis is not a frequent complication in this type of membrane augmentation.

Autoantibody Formation. Drugs such as methyldopa (Aldomet), levodopa, and mefenamic acid (Ponstel) have been implicated in positive DATs caused by autoantibody formation. The autoantibody formed recognizes a part of the red cell and therefore reacts with most normal red cells. Some drug-induced autoantibodies have been shown to have specificities that appear to be of the Rh type, but most have no apparent specificity. Antibody production ceases with withdrawal of the drug.

Idiopathic Thrombocytopenia Purpura

Idiopathic thrombocytopenic purpura is now also known as immunologic thrombocytopenic purpura (ITP). Patients with ITP usually demonstrate petechiae, bruising, menorrhagia, and bleeding after minor trauma. ITP may be either acute or chronic. Children are most often afflicted with the acute type, while adults predominantly experience the chronic type. This common disorder may complicate other antibody-associated disorders such as SLE.

Although thrombocytopenia (a condition of absent or severely decreased platelets [below 10 to 20 × 10^9/L]) may result from a wide variety of conditions, such as occurs after the use of extracorporeal circulation in cardiac bypass surgery or from alcoholic liver disease, most thrombocytopenic conditions can be classified into three major categories:
- Decreased production of platelets
- Disorders of platelet distribution
- Increased destruction or use of platelets

Decreased production may result from invasion of the bone marrow by neoplastic cells and is usually not associated with an immunologic cause. Disorders of platelet distribution are associated with a sequestering of platelets in the spleen for a variety of nonimmunologic reasons. Increased destruction or use of platelets, however, is associated with immunologic mechanisms. These mechanisms of destruction are caused by antigens, antibodies, or complement.

Drugs or foreign substances including quinidine, sulfonamide derivatives, heroin, morphine, and snake venom can produce platelet destruction. Sulfonamide derivative reactions involve the interaction of platelet antigens with drug antibodies. Morphine reactions involve the activation of complement.

Bacterial sepsis causes increased destruction of platelets caused by the attachment of platelets to bacterial antigen-antibody immune complexes. Certain microbial antigens may initially attach to platelets, followed by specific antibodies to the microorganism. This mechanism has been reported to cause the thrombocytopenia that frequently complicates the *Plasmodium falciparum* type of malaria.

Antibodies of either autoimmune or isoimmune origin may produce increased destruction of platelets. Examples of thrombocytopenias of isoimmune origin include posttransfusion purpura and isoimmune neonatal thrombocytopenia. Neonatal autoimmune thrombocytopenia is a condition caused by immunization of a pregnant female by a fetal platelet antigen and by transplacental passage of maternal IgG platelet antibodies. The antigen is inherited by the fetus from the father and is absent on maternal platelets. Posttransfusion purpura is a rare form of isoimmune thrombocytopenia.

Pernicious Anemia

PA is a megaloblastic anemia characterized by a variety of hematologic and chemical manifestations (Table 25-10). It is caused by a deficiency of vitamin B_{12} that results from the patient's inability to secrete IF. In most cases of PA, antiintrinsic factors or antiparietal antibodies have been reported. Most authorities consider the demonstration of these antibodies to support the theory that pernicious anemia is an autoimmune disorder.

Assays for antiintrinsic factor measure antibodies to IF. The presence of IF-blocking antibodies is diagnostic of PA. Antibodies can be demonstrated in about 60% of cases. Antiparietal cell assays measure antibodies to parietal cells (large cells on the margin of the peptic glands of the stomach). Most (80%) patients with PA have parietal cell antibodies. In the presence of parietal cell antibodies, gastric biopsy almost always demonstrates gastritis. Low-antibody titers to parietal cells are often found with no clinical evidence of PA or atrophic gastritis, and are sometimes seen in older adult patients.

Neuromuscular Disorders

Several important neurologic disorders are related to the immune system. The immune system may play an important role in the pathogenesis and/or etiology of myasthenia gravis and multiple sclerosis. In addition, amyotrophic lateral sclerosis (ALS) has become one of the prime subjects of modern neurologic research.

Amyotrophic Lateral Sclerosis

Along with Alzheimer's disease and Parkinson's disease, ALS is one of the so-called degenerative diseases of the aging nervous system. The immune system has been implicated in ALS. Monoclonal paraproteinemia seems to be disproportionately frequent among patients with ALS. It has also been suggested that ALS patients have a higher incidence of lymphoproliferative disease-lymphoma, Waldenström's macroglobulinemia, and myeloma. There also seems to be an increased frequency of antibodies to a neuronal ganglioside, GM-1.

Inflammatory Polyneuropathies

This group of idiopathic disorders, which includes the acute disorder Guillain-Barré syndrome (GBS), is characterized clinically by the subacute onset of generally symmetric weakness ranging from modest lower-extremity weakness to total, life-threatening involvement of motor and even cranial nerves. Sensory symptoms are less prominent. Unstable blood pressure and potentially fatal arrhythmias have also been observed. Progression of GBS can be rapid; however, most patients do recover.

The etiology of GBS is unknown, but it is likely that an abnormal immune response against the peripheral nervous system (PNS) is involved. This may be triggered by an antecedent viral infection. There is infiltration of the PNS with lymphocytes and macrophages and patchy myelin destruction. Some patients display deposition of IgG, IgM, and IgA in PNS tissues. Markedly elevated Ig levels in the CSF, sometimes with oligoclonal bands, suggests locally altered immunoregulation. The antigenic targets of such Ig remain unknown.

Myasthenia Gravis

Myasthenia gravis is a disorder of the neuromuscular junction characterized by neurophysiologic and immunologic ab-

---

TABLE 25-10	Hematologic and Chemical Findings in Pernicious Anemia	
Hematologic manifestations	Hemoglobin	Severely decreased
	Hematocrit	Severely decreased
	Erythrocyte count	Decreased
	Leukocyte count	Slightly decreased
	Platelet count	Slightly decreased or normal
	Mean corpuscular volume	Increased
Chemical findings	Serum iron	Increased
	Total iron-binding capacity	Normal or decreased
	Percentage of Fe saturation	Increased
	Serum ferritin	Increased

normalities (Box 25-2). In this disease a postsynaptic defect is caused by a decrease in receptors for acetylcholine and frequently an anatomic defect in the neuromuscular junction plate. AcHR binding antibody is directed against acetylcholine receptors at neuromuscular junctions of skeletal muscle and AcHR-blocking antibodies. The ligand bungarotoxin or acetylcholine is important in producing a neuromuscular block. About one third of patients with myasthenia gravis demonstrate AcHR-blocking antibodies.

The role of these antibodies in producing disease is unclear. Complement-mediated, antibody-determined damage may be an important mechanism in myasthenia gravis because IgG, C3, and C9 can be demonstrated at the neuromuscular junction, and the motor endplate is often abnormal. This suggests that antibody to AcHR is capable of increasing the normal rate of degradation, resulting in fewer available receptors.

Multiple Sclerosis

Multiple sclerosis (MS) is a common demyelinating disease of the CNS related to abnormalities of the immune system. It is characterized by regions of demyelinization of varying size and age scattered throughout the white matter of the CNS. Demyelinization "plaques" have a propensity to form in the cerebrum, optic nerves, brainstem, spinal cord, and cerebellum.

Etiology. After a century of study, the cause of MS remains unknown. Although research studies support both genetic and environmental components of susceptibility. The findings of epidemiologic studies are most consistent with an environmental influence occurring with a background of genetic susceptibility as the cause of MS. There is little evidence for a single or unique environmental cause. Viral infection (e.g., human herpesvirus type 6 [HHV-6]) is highly suspected but unconfirmed. In addition, the EBV, which causes infectious mononucleosis and is associated with other diseases, may increase the risk of MS.

Epidemiology. The incidence, prevalence, and mortality rates of MS vary with latitude. MS is rare in tropical and subtropical areas. The higher risk for MS in Europeans and in relatives of patients with MS and the existence of MS-resistant ethnic groups (e.g., Eskimos, Norwegian Lapps, and Australian aborigines) support genetic predisposition to MS. A low prevalence of MS occurs in Africa, India, China, Japan, and Southeast Asia.

MS is the major acquired neurologic disease in young adults. Most patients develop symptoms between the ages of 18 and 50 years. Women are more often affected than men (2:1 ratio). Approximately 1 in 1000 persons of northern European origin who reside in temperate climates will develop prototypical MS in their lifetime. Up to 350,000 people in the United States have MS.

Pathophysiology. MS results from T-cell-dependent inflammatory demyelination of the CNS. Inflammatory demyelination caused by T lymphocytes induces B lymphocytes to produce antimyelin antibodies.

The ongoing pathologic process involves the formation of CNS lesions, called plaques, characterized by inflammation and demyelination. Plaques result from a localized inflammatory immune response, initiated by the entry of activated blood T cells into the CNS. These T cells cross the blood-brain barrier by binding to endothelial cells in blood vessels via reciprocal adhesion molecules. The release of enzymes, called matrix metalloproteinases, allows them to penetrate the basement membrane and extracellular matrix. At the same time, other blood immune system cells penetrate the CNS, causing additional local synthesis and release of damaging inflammatory mediators. The net result is destruction of myelin sheaths, injury to axons and glial cells, and formation of permanent scar tissue.

Research studies have demonstrated that osteopontin, which is known to play a role in enhancing inflammation, may play a critical role in the immune attack in MS and its progression. Osteopontin has been found to be very active in areas of myelin damage, both during relapse and remission, and both in myelin-making cells and in nerve cells. More research is required to determine the exact roles of this protein, as well as the therapeutic possibilities it presents.

Signs and Symptoms. MS begins as a relapsing illness with episodes of neurologic dysfunction lasting several weeks, followed by substantial or complete improvement (relapsing-remitting MS). Initial signs of MS are difficulty in walking, abnormal sensations (e.g., numbness, possible pain, and ineffective vision). Primary symptoms caused by demyelination include fatigue, bladder and bowel dysfunction, loss of balance, loss of memory, slurred speech, difficulty with swallowing, and seizures. Depression is a common symptom.

Relapsing MS is the most common form; 85% of patients are symptomatic at onset. The other forms of MS are:
- Primary progressive
- Secondary progressive
- Progressive relapsing

Primary progressive MS progresses insidiously from onset, with or without occasional plateaus and minor improvements. Secondary progressive MS develops in about half of relapsing MS patients about 10 years into the disease. Progressive relapsing is the rarest form of the disease. Patients begin with primary progression but subsequently experience one or more relapses.

Diagnostic Methods. Magnetic resonance imaging (MRI) is a key test in establishing a diagnosis of MS. No single laboratory test confirms a diagnosis, but appropriate laboratory tests must be evaluated carefully. Conditions that need to be excluded include collagen vascular disease, vitamin B_{12} deficiency, and endocrine disorders (e.g., thyroid and adrenal gland disease). It is also important to rule out infectious diseases (e.g., Lyme disease, syphilis, or infection with

---

Box 25-2	Abnormalities Associated With Myasthenia Gravis

- Thymic hyperplasia with germinal follicles
- Increase in thymic B cells
- Thymoma
- Expression of acetylcholine receptor (AcHR) binding antibody and AcHR blocking antibody
- Associated with other autoimmune diseases

Box 25-3	Immunologic Manifestation of Multiple Sclerosis

- Antimyelin antibodies
- Myelinotoxicity and glial toxicity of serum and cerebrospinal fluid in vitro
- In vitro cell-mediated immunity by blood and cerebrospinal fluid cells to myelin components
- Oligoclonal increase in cerebrospinal fluid immunoglobulin
- Increase in certain HLA and Ia antigens (HL-A A3, B7, DW2, and DRW2)

Box 25-4	Condition Associated With Oligoclonal Cerebrospinal Fluid Gammaglobulins

- Multiple sclerosis
- Neurosyphilis-paresthesia
- Paraneoplastic syndrome—subacute sclerosing panencephalitis
- Chronic mycobacterial and fungal meningitis
- Chronic viral meningitis and meningoencephalitis (uncommon)
- Acute viral meningitis (uncommon)
- Primary optic neuritis
- Acute disseminated encephalomyelitis
- Primary optic neuritis
- Peripheral neuropathy
- Guillain-Barré syndrome
- Burkitt's lymphoma
- Psychoneurosis
- Cerebral infarction

HTLV-1). Analysis of CSF may identify either of two immune abnormalities linked to the disease:
- An oligoclonal IgG band pattern
- Intrathecal IgG production

Immunologic Manifestations. The immunologic manifestations of this disease suggestive of its autoimmune nature are presented in Box 25-3. Antimyelin antibodies directed against components of the myelin sheath of nerves or myelin basic protein can be demonstrated in patients with MS or other neurologic diseases. However, myelin antibodies are not detectable in the CSF of MS patients.

Detection of Oligoclonal Bands. Oligoclonal Igs may be seen in both serum and CSF. An oligoclonal Ig pattern consists of multiple, homogeneous, narrow, and probably faint bands in the gamma zone on electrophoresis.

Electrophoresis on cellulose acetate will rarely resolve an oligoclonal pattern. Therefore electrophoretic media with greater resolution such as agar or agarose gel are required, and both require the use of concentrated CSF. It is important to perform electrophoresis a serum specimen concurrently with the CSF specimen to ensure that the demonstrated homogeneous bands are present only in the CSF, which implies endogenous synthesis rather than serum band that might appear secondarily in the CSF. Uncommonly, if a prominent CSF band is present, it may appear in the serum as a homogeneous band. This situation is most frequently encountered in subacute sclerosing panencephalitis.

High-resolution electrophoresis attempts to achieve better resolution of proteins beyond the classic five-band pattern. The primary reason for performing high-resolution protein electrophoresis is for the detection of oligoclonal bands in CSF to increase the diagnostic usefulness of protein patterns. About 80% of CSF proteins originate from the plasma. The electrophoretic pattern of normal CSF is similar to a normal serum protein pattern; however, several differences are detectable, including a prominent prealbumin band and two transferrin bands.

Immunofixation has been used in some research studies to show that the oligoclonal bands seen in CSF protein patterns are made up primarily of IgG. Although this may be of academic interest, characterization of the Ig bands does not significantly improve the diagnostic usefulness of the procedure. Isoelectric focusing, however, is becoming the method of choice for oligoclonal band detection.

Significance of Oligoclonal Bands. If oligoclonal bands are present in CSF but not in the serum, they are the result of increased production of IgG by the CNS. CNS production of

IgG occurs in the subarachnoid space of the brain in conjunction with the local accumulation of immunocytes. Each has its own specificity that gives rise to oligoclonal bands. Although the Ig is IgG, it is polyclonal in nature, with several groups of cells producing the Ig. Oligoclonal bands are therefore defined as discrete populations of IgG, with restricted heterogeneity demonstrated by electrophoresis.

One procedure for confirming local CNS production of oligoclonal IgG is to assay a matched serum specimen diluted 1:100 concurrently with an unconcentrated CSF sample. Oligoclonal bands present in CSF, but not in the serum, indicate CNS production. This matched sample procedure is especially useful if damage to the blood-brain barrier is suspected because of acute or chronic inflammations such as meningitis, intracranial tumor, or cerebral vascular disease.

Serum oligoclonal bands may represent immune complexes and are associated with diseases such as Hodgkin's or a nonspecific early immune response to a number of diseases (Box 25-4).

Findings in MS. Total CSF protein in patients with MS is usually normal or slightly elevated. In general, patients with no neurologic disease have IgG concentration of less than 10% of the total CSF proteins. Almost 70% of MS patients typically have IgG concentration of 11% to 35% of total CSF proteins.

Oligoclonal bands in serum are not absolutely indicative of MS, and their presence should be used in conjunction with other information available from clinical evaluation and other diagnostic procedures. Although oligoclonal bands can be present in more than 90% of MS patients at some time during the course of the disease, their presence does not correlate with the activity of the disease. The exact number of bands present in MS is variable. Some studies have demonstrated 7 to 15 bands.

Treatment. Corticosteroid therapy (e.g., methyl-prednisolone and prednisone) is a common symptomatic treatment for disease relapses. The relapsing form of MS can be treated with the immunomodulators: interferon beta-1b (Betaseron), interferon beta-1a (Avonex) and glatiramer acetate (Copaxone). All of these drugs are approved by the U.S. Food and Drug Administration for use in relapsing forms of MS. Possi-

TABLE 25-11 Neuropathy Syndromes Associated With Antibodies Directed Against Peripheral Nerve Components

Clinical Syndrome	Antibodies
Chronic sensorimotor demyelinating neuropathy	Antimyelin-associated glycoprotein
Chronic axonal sensory neuropathy	Antisulfatide or antichondroitin sulfate
Multifocal motor neuropathy	Anti-GM1 (IgM)
Acute axonal motor neuropathy	Anti-GM1 (IgG)
Fisher syndrome	Anti-GQ1b
Guillain-Barré syndrome	Anti-LM1, GD1b, GD1A, GT1b, sulfatide, B tubulin
Large fiber sensory neuropathy with ataxia	Anti-GQ1b, GD3, GD1b, GT1b
Subacute sensory neuropathy/encephalomyelitis	Antineuronal nuclear antibody type 1 (anti-Hu)

From Cohen B, Mitsumoto H: Neuropathy syndromes associated with antibodies against the peripheral nerve, *Lab Med* 26(7):459-463, 1995.

ble future therapeutic strategies may include combination therapies using existing therapies, standard immunosuppressive drugs, and new immunomodulating agents. Autologous bone-marrow transplantation, plasma exchange, T-cell receptor peptide vaccine, and gene therapy are also possibilities.

The Myeline Project Cell Culture Units at the University of Wisconsin-Madison and at Sweden's University of Lund are developing an immortal line of human cells, oligodendrocyte precursors, to repair myelin lesion in MS and the leukodystrophies. Studies have demonstrated that myelin produced as a result of transplantation is capable of restoring nerve conduction. The feasibility of transplanting glial cells derived from human tissue into the CNS is being explored.

In other research French researchers have demonstrated that progesterone promotes remyelination by activating genes that control the synthesis of important myelin proteins.

Neuropathies

A neuropathy is a derangement in the function and structure of peripheral motor, sensory, or autonomic neurons. Autoimmune disorders constitute one of the disease categories causing neuropathy. In many cases, evidence supports autoimmune pathogenesis. Demonstration of the relationships between specific neuropathy syndromes and antibodies directed against glycolipid and neural antigens are important recent scientific advances.

In the autoimmune neuropathies, antibodies directed against peripheral nerve components are associated with specific clinical syndromes (Table 25-11). Knowledge of these syndromes and antibody tests can be used to identify a treatable neuropathy. In addition, many autoimmune neuropathic syndromes are associated with malignancies, which they often precede. Recognition of these syndromes can lead to early identification and treatment.

Most antibodies implicated in the development of autoimmune-mediated neuropathies are directed against carbohydrate epitopes of glycoproteins or glycolipids. Glycolipids are concentrated in neural membranes where the lipid portion is immersed in the membrane bilayer and the carbohydrate portion is exposed extracellularly. The extracellular domain of the carbohydrate epitopes makes them vulnerable to antibody binding.

Systemic sclerosis, also known as scleroderma, is an autoimmune disease characterized by a wide spectrum of clini-

TABLE 25-12 Examples of the Relationship of Clinical Features and Antibodies

Clinical Features	Antibodies
SSc with diffuse cutaneous involvement (dcSsc)	Anti-RNA polymerase I, antitopoisomerase I
SSc with limited cutaneous involvement (lcSSc)	Anti-Th ribonucleoprotein anticentromere antibody
SSc-polymyositis overlap syndrome	Anti-PM-Scl

cal, pathologic, and serologic abnormalities. More that 90% of patients with systemic sclerosis spontaneously produce ANA. The structure and function of the intracellular antigens to which these ANAs are directed have been characterized. These serum autoantibodies are helpful markers because they correlate with certain clinical features of systemic sclerosis (Table 25-12). A new marker autoantibody, anti-RNA polymerase III antibody, has been identified in many patients who have systemic sclerosis with diffuse or extensive cutaneous involvement.

Renal Disorders

It is generally accepted that most immunologically mediated renal diseases fall into several categories (Box 25-5).

Renal Disease Associated With Circulating Immune Complexes

Renal diseases associated with circulating immune complexes are caused by nonrenal antigens and their corresponding antibodies (see Box 25-5). These complexes are deposited in one or more of several loci in the glomerulus. Deposition may be dependent on the size and other characteristics of the complex. Recent evidence suggests that potentially damaging immune complexes may be formed in situ and involve antigens already present or fixed in the glomerulus. In addition, immune complex activation of complement in the glomerular basement membrane may be augmented by the presence of cells with receptors for C3 located in that area. Activation probably releases biologically active products such as chemotactic substances and causes an inflammatory type of tissue injury. A renal complication of this type can be manifested in SLE.

Categories of Immunologic Renal Disease

ASSOCIATED WITH CIRCULATING IMMUNE COMPLEXES

Systemic lupus erythematosus
Certain vasculitis
Infections
Tumors (possibly)
Immunoglobulins and antiimmunoglobulins

MEMBRANOPROLIFERATIVE GLOMERULONEPHRITIS

Activation of the alternate complement pathway
Possible genetic factors

ASSOCIATED WITH ANTIGLOMERULAR BASEMENT MEMBRANE ANTIBODY

Most cases of Goodpasture's syndrome
Some rapidly progressive glomerulonephritis
Membrane altered by a virus or drugs (possibly)

TUBULOINTERSTITIAL NEPHRITIS

Associated with immune complex–mediated disease
Drugs and possibly infection
Involvement of transplanted kidneys

Membranoproliferative Glomerulonephritis

Another type of glomerular disease, membranoproliferative glomerulonephritis, is believed to be caused by nonimmunologically activated complement. Activation is thought to be analogous to the alternate pathway activation of C3 by certain bacterial products and polysaccharides.

Renal Disease Associated With Antiglomerular Basement Membrane Antibody

Glomerular basement membrane antibodies (anti-GBM) are directed against the glomerular basement membrane of the glomerulus of the kidney (Figure 25-3). These antibodies are induced in vivo against the basement membrane of the glomerulus and possibly the renal tubule or lung basement membrane. The factors that stimulate antibody production are not well defined, but it appears likely that binding of drugs such as methicillin, certain infectious agents, or renal damage caused by other immune mechanisms may lead to an immune antibody response. The end result may be direct damage to the bone marrow with or without complement activation. Production of antibone marrow antibodies, however, appears to be self-limited and lasts for several weeks to months after removal of the inciting agent (i.e., the kidney).

High-antibody titers of anti-GMB are suggestive of Goodpasture's disease, early SLE, or anti-GBM nephritis. The

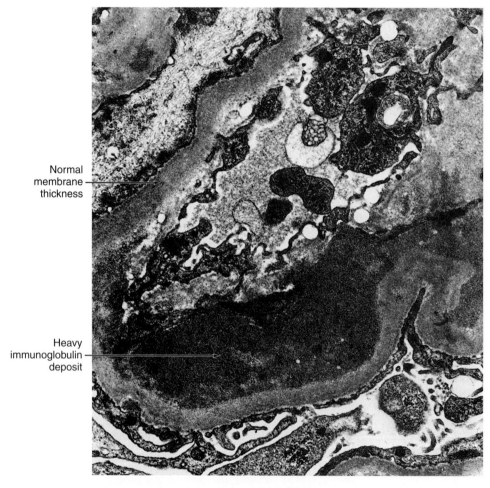

Normal membrane thickness

Heavy immunoglobulin deposit

Figure 25-3 An electron-photomicrograph demonstrating an immunoglobulin deposit in the basement membrane of a patient with systemic lupus erythematosus (SLE). (From Barrett JT: *Textbook of immunology,* ed 5, St Louis, 1988, Mosby.)

absence of antibodies, however, does not rule out Goodpasture's disease. This type of renal disease represents less than 5% of glomerular disorders.

Tubulointerstitial Nephritis

Tubulointerstitial nephritis involving the renal tubules has been associated with a variety of causes, including immune complex-mediated disease. Precipitating factors can include drugs and possibly infection, as well as the involvement of transplanted kidneys.

Skeletal Muscle Disorders

Inflammatory Myopathy

Polymyositis and dermatomyositis are the most common expressions of a group of chronic inflammatory disorders that can be subclassified into six categories: primary idiopathic polymyositis, primary idiopathic dermatomyositis, polymyositis or dermatomyositis associated with neoplasia, childhood polymyositis or dermatomyositis, dermatomyositis or polymyositis associated with collagen-vascular disease, and polymyositis or dermatomyositis associated with infections. All of these disorders have in common skeletal muscle damaged by a lymphocyte inflammatory process resulting in symmetric weakness, predominately of proximal muscles.

Polymyositis may be accompanied by inflammation at other sites, especially in the joints, lungs, and heart. The term *dermatomyositis* is used for the disorder when the clinical features of disease are accompanied by characteristic inflammatory manifestations in the skin.

The causes of these disorders remain unknown, but they may develop in genetically susceptible persons after exposure to environmental agents that induce immune activation and inflammation. Infection is the most likely initiating event. As part of the inflammatory response to the infection, susceptible individuals develop a persistent cell-mediated immune attack that continues to destroy muscle after the acute infection is eradicated.

Both polymyositis and dermatomyositis are more common in females, with peaks of occurrences in childhood and the fifth decade. Clinically these disorders present with proximal muscle weakness, sometimes associated with pain, fatigue, and low-grade fever, and lead to atrophy in progressive disease.

Evidence suggests the polymyositis and dermatomyositis result from immune destruction. Muscle biopsies in patients with dermatomyositis have shown vasculitis, with IgG and complement deposition in the vessel walls in children and infrequently in adults. There is a preponderance of B lymphocytes and increased CD4+:CD8+ T-cell ratio. An increased frequency of activated T cells has been noted in both polymyositis and dermatomyositis.

Patients with myositis have many immunologic abnormalities. One unique immunologic feature is the targeting by autoantibodies of certain cytoplasmic proteins and RNAs involved in the process of protein synthesis. These autoantibodies are found only in patients with myositis and are known as the myositis-specific autoantibodies (MSAs) (Box 25-6). The MSAs are antigen-driven, arise months before the onset of myositis, correlate in titer with disease activity, disappear after prolonged complete remission, and bind to and inhibit the function of targeted human autoantigenic enzymes in in vitro assays.

Skin Disorders (Bullous Disease and Other Conditions)

A wide variety of autoimmune disorders are associated with skin manifestations (Box 25-7).

Two immunologic assays that can be used in conjunction with other clinical information include measurement of antibodies to the basement membrane area of the skin and of antibodies to intercellular substance of the skin.

Antiskin (dermal-epidermal) antibodies are present in more than 80% of patients with bullous pemphigoid, but the absence of antibodies does not rule out the disorder. Antiskin (interepithelial) antibodies can be detected in most (90%) of patients with pemphigus. A rising antibody titer may indicate an impending relapse of pemphigus, and a falling titer is suggestive of effective control of the disease. The absence of demonstrable antibody usually excludes the diagnosis.

Box 25-6 Myositis-Specific Autoantibodies

ANTISYNTHETASES

Anti-Jo-1
Anti-PL-7
Anti-PL-12 (1)
Anti-PL-12 (II)
Anti-OJ
Anti-EJ

ANTI-SRP
ANTI-MI-2
OTHERS

Anti-FER
Anti-KJ
Anti-MAS

Box 25-7 Autoimmunity and the Skin

Discoid lupus
Bullous pemphigoid
Pemphigus group
Dermatitis herpetiformis
Skin may be involved in the autoimmune reaction in at least three ways:

1. Inflammatory involvement of cutaneous vessels with secondary effects (e.g., some lesions in systemic lupus erythematous, hypersensitivity angiitis, and the syndrome of urticaria and palpable purpura with or without mixed cryoglobulinemia)
2. Deposition of putative circulating immune complexes in the skin (e.g., systemic lupus erythematosus)
3. Localized autoreactivity against skin components (e.g., primary skin disorders)

Case Study

History and Physical Examination

Z.A. is a 50-year-old Caucasian woman, who visited her primary care provider because of extreme fatigue. She also reported experiencing a mild pain in her abdominal region. Physical examination revealed slight hepatomegaly. Her physician ordered a complete blood count and urinalysis.

Laboratory Data

Complete Blood Count	Patient's Results	Reference Range
Hemoglobin	6.2 g/dL	11.5-16.0 gm/dL
Hematocrit	0.22L/L	0.37-0.47 L/L
Red blood cell count	1.7×10^{12}/L	$4.2\text{-}5.4 \times 10^{12}$/L
White blood cell count	3.8×10^{9}/L	$4.5\text{-}11.0 \times 10^{9}$/L
Blood smear comments 3+ macrocytic red blood cells, polychromatophilia, a few nucleated red blood cells		
Red blood cells indices		
Mean corpuscular volume (MCV)	129.4 fL	80-96 fL
Mean corpuscular hemoglobin (MCH)	36.5 pg	27-32 pg
Mean corpuscular hemoglobin concentration (MCHC)	28%	32-36%

Questions and Discussion

1. What chemical and immunologic assays would be helpful in establishing a diagnosis for this patient?

    A vitamin B_{12} assay and a folic acid assay are essential chemical tests. The immunologic assays of value are: antiintrinsic factor and an antiparietal cell assay.
2. What is the prevalence of antiintrinsic factor in patients with pernicious anemia?

    About 60% of patients with pernicious anemia exhibit intrinsic factor antibodies.
3. What is the prevalence of parietal cell antibodies in patients with pernicious anemia?

    About 80% of patients with pernicious anemia exhibit parietal cell antibodies.

Diagnosis

Pernicious anemia

Case Study

History and Physical Examination

D.D. is a right-handed 25-year-old woman with no significant medical history. She came to the Emergency Department because of a sudden onset of slurred speech.

She reported being in excellent health until a month ago when she began to notice weakness and numbness in her right hand and leg. She felt unsteady when walking and experienced urinary urgency.

Physical examination revealed an overweight young female with a right facial droop. In addition, she staggered upon turning around, and had difficulty walking a straight line. A spinal tap and MRI were ordered.

Laboratory and Medical Imaging Data: Laboratory Findings

Cerebrospinal Fluid Examination

Assay	Patient Results	Reference Range
Color/clarity	Clear, colorless	Clear, colorless
Total cells	6	0-8
Nucleated cells	2	0-2
Differential, %		
Lymphocytes	75	40-60
CSF protein, mg/dL	125	20-40
CSF albumin		
CSF glucose, mg/dL	70	40-80
CSF IgG, mg/dL	8.5	0-33
Serum albumin, g/dL	4.2	3.5-5.0
Serum IgG, mg/dL	941	700-1450
CSF profile		
CSF:serum IgG index	1.2	0-0.7
CSF IgG:albumin ratio	0.28	0-0.23
Albumin index	7.38	0-7.0
CNS IgG synthesis rate, mg/dL	22.65	0-2.8

Additional Notes

CSF agarose electrophoresis: positive for oligoclonal bands (reference range negative)

CSF isoelectric focusing: positive for oligoclonal bands (reference range negative)

Serum protein electrophoresis interpretation: no apparent monoclonal peak (reference range no apparent monoclonal peak)

Serum immunofixation: no paraprotein detected (reference range no paraprotein detected)

Medical Imaging

0-0.6 RI scan revealed a masslike lesion in the region of the corpus callosum with extensions into the right and left hemispheres of the brain. The location of the lesion was consistent with the patient's presenting symptoms.

A follow-up biopsy of the brain was ordered. Histologically, a biopsy of white matter of the brain demonstrated sheets of macrophages, clumps of lymphocytes and plasma cells, and myelin debris.

Questions and Discussion

1. What is the etiology of the patient's symptoms?

   Symptoms such as the one's demonstrated by this patient are caused by the formation of demyelinating lesions in the white matter of the CNS. Lesions are associated with mononuclear infiltrates of macrophages and T lymphocytes. The severity of symptoms depends on the location of the lesions in the brain.

2. Does the patient's age provide a clue to the diagnosis?

   MS should be suspected in females aged 20 to 40 years who experience recurrent episodes of neurologic dysfunction (e.g., brain, spinal cord, optic nerve). MS is the most common, nontraumatic cause of neurologic disability in young and middle-age adults in the United States.

3. What is the significance of the laboratory analysis of the CSF?

   Laboratory analysis of intrathecal Ig synthesis is important in cases of suspected MS. Electrophoresis of CSF for detection of oligoclonal bands is a classic measurement to determine intrathecal IgG synthesis. Electrophoretic separation of paired CSF and serum samples for detection of oligoclonal bands in the gamma region.

   Laboratory analysis of CSF, patient history and physical examination, MRI examination, and electrophysiologic studies provide important information in establishing a clinical diagnosis of MS.

Follow-Up

Although the patient immediately began treatment with corticosteroid therapy and more recently Avonex, the patient has demonstrated worsening symptoms over the last 10 years.

Diagnosis

Multiple Sclerosis

CHAPTER HIGHLIGHTS

Autoimmunity represents a breakdown of the immune system in its ability to discriminate between self and nonself. The term *autoimmune disease* is used in those cases where demonstrable Igs, autoantibodies, or cytotoxic (T) cells display a specificity for self-antigens and contribute to the pathogenesis of the disease. Many disorders are believed to be related to immunologic abnormalities that manifest a full spectrum of tissue reactivity. At one extreme are organ-specific diseases such as Hashimoto's disease of the thyroid; at the other end of the spectrum are diseases that manifest themselves as organ-nonspecific diseases such as SLE and RA. In organ-specific diseases, both the lesions produced by

tissue damage and the autoantibodies are directed at a single target organ (e.g., the thyroid). Midspectrum disorders are characterized by localized lesions in a single organ and autoantibodies that are organ-nonspecific. Organ-nonspecific disorders are characterized by the presence of both lesions and autoantibodies not confined to any one organ.

The potential for autoimmunity, if given appropriate circumstances, is constantly present in every immunocompetent individual because lymphocytes that are potentially reactive with self-antigens exist in the body. Antibody expression appears to be regulated by a complex set of interacting factors including genetic factors, age, and exogenous factors. Autoimmune disease is usually prevented by the normal functioning of immunologic regulatory mechanisms. When these controls dysfunction, antibodies to self-antigens may be produced and bind to antigens in the circulation to form circulating immune complexes, or bind to antigens deposited in specific tissue sites. The mechanisms that govern the deposition in one organ or another are unknown; however, several mechanisms may be operative in a single disease. Wherever antigen-antibody complexes accumulate, complement can be activated, with the subsequent release of mediators of inflammation that increase vascular permeability, attract phagocytic cells to the reaction site, and cause local tissue damage. Alternatively, cytotoxic T cells can directly attack body cells bearing the target antigen, which releases mediators that amplify the inflammatory reaction.

Autoantibody and complement fragments coat cells bearing the target antigen, which leads to destruction by phagocytes or by antibody-seeking K-type lymphocytes.

An individual may develop an autoimmune response in a variety of immunogenic stimuli. These responses may be caused by antigens that do not normally circulate in the blood, altered antigens, a foreign antigen that is shared or cross-reactive with self-antigens or tissue components, mutation of immunocompetent cells to acquire a responsive to self-antigens, and loss of the immunoregulatory function by T-cell subsets. Self-recognition of membrane idiotypic receptors and the MHC antigens appear to be fundamental in facilitating the regulatory interactions between cells. Many of these interactions are mediated through the production of highly specific soluble fraction that contains Ia and idiotypic determinants and transmits signs from one cell to another. Whether the immunologic response to any given antigen will be expressed as immunity or tolerance is probably determined by a regulatory equilibrium, primarily established by the balance between helper and suppressor T cells. This equilibrium appears to be controlled by Ir genes linked to the MHC and expressed on the surface of lymphocytes and macrophages as the Ia antigens. In addition, aberrant Ia expression on inflamed cells may lead to inappropriate antigen presentation by these cells, immune cell activation, and ultimately, to organ-specific autoimmune disease.

Self-tolerance is induced by at least two mechanisms involving contact between antigen and immunocompetent cells: elimination of the small clone of immunocompetent cells programmed to react with the antigen (Burnet's clonal selection theory), or induction of unresponsiveness in the immunocompetent cells through excessive antigen binding to them and/or through triggering of a suppressor mechanism. The normal immune response is modulated by both antigen-specific and nonspecific suppressor cell activity. The major mechanism in antigen-specific suppression of antibody response appears related to an antiidiotypic immune response induced by the antigen-binding site (idiotype) unique for a particular antibody. In the opposite situation, prolonged antigen stimulation leads to polyclonal activation of the B-cell response with a resultant polyclonal hypergammaglobulinemia.

Major autoantibodies can be detected in different diseases. Many diagnostic laboratory tests are based on detecting these autoimmune responses. Commonly encountered autoantibodies include thyroid, gastric, adrenocortical, striated muscle, acetylcholine receptor, smooth muscle, salivary gland, mitochondrial, reticulin, myelin, islet cell, and skin antibodies. Antibodies to antinuclear antibodies include DNA, histone, and nonhistone protein antibodies.

REVIEW QUESTIONS

1. All of the following characteristics are common to organ-specific and nonorgan-specific disorders except:
   A. autoantibody tests are of diagnostic value
   B. antibodies may appear in each of the main immunoglobulin classes
   C. antigens are available to lymphoid system in low concentrations
   D. circulatory autoantibodies react with normal body constituents

2. Antibody expression in the development of autoimmunity is regulated by all of the following factors except:
   A. genetic predisposition
   B. increasing age
   C. environmental factors (e.g., UV radiation)
   D. active infectious disease

3. The mechanism responsible for autoimmune disease is:
   A. circulating immune complexes
   B. antigen excess
   C. antibody excess
   D. antigen deficiency

4. One of the mechanisms believed to induce self-tolerance is:
   A. induction of responsiveness in immunocompetent cells
   B. elimination of clone programmed to react with antigen
   C. decreased suppressor cell activity
   D. stimulation of clones of immunocompetent cells

Questions 5-8. Match the following (use an answer only once).

5. _____ Acetylcholine receptor-blocking antibodies

6. _____ Anticardiolipin antibody

7. _____ Anti-DNA antibodies

8. _____ Antiglomerular basement membrane antibodies
   A. helpful in monitoring Addison's disease
   B. found in one third of patients with myasthenia gravis
   C. useful in monitoring the activity and exacerbations of SLE

D. suggestive of Goodpasture's disease
E. present in SLE and associated with arterial and venous thrombosis

Questions 9-12. Match the following.

9. _____ Antinuclear ribonucleoprotein

10. _____ Anti-Scl

11. _____ Anti-Sm

12. _____ Antismooth muscle
    A. antibody to basic nonhistone nuclear protein, diagnostic of systemic sclerosis
    B. present in bullous pemphigoid
    C. presence of antibody confirms diagnosis of SLE
    D. seen in viral disorders
    E. characteristic of mixed connective tissue disease

Questions 13-15. Match the following.

13. _____ Anti SS-A

14. _____ Histone-reactive antinuclear antibody

15. _____ PM-I antibody
    A. detectable in patients with myasthenia gravis
    B. demonstrable in Sjögren's syndrome-sicca complex
    C. highly suggestive of drug-induced lupus erythematosus
    D. found in one third of patients with uncomplicated polymyositis and some patients with dermatomyositis
    E. found in majority of patients with polymyositis

16. The term *autoimmune disease* is used when:
    A. demonstrable immunoglobulins display specificity for self-antigens
    B. cytotoxic T cells display specificity for self-antigens
    C. cytotoxic T cells contribute to the pathogenesis of the disease
    D. all of the above

Questions 17-21. Indicate true statements with the letter "A," and false statements with the letter "B."

17. _____ The presence of autoantibodies are only associated with autoimmune disease.

18. _____ In organ-specific disorders, antigens are only available to the lymphoid system in low concentrations.

19. _____ There is a familial tendency to develop organ-specific disorders.

20. _____ In organ-specific disorders lesions are caused by deposition of antigen-antibody complexes.

21. _____ In organ-specific disorders a tendency to develop cancer exists.

22. Self-tolerance is induced by:
    A. Burnet's clonal selection theory.
    B. elimination of the small clone of immunocompetent cells programmed to react with the antigen.
    C. induction of unresponsiveness in the immunocompetent cells through excessive antigen binding.
    D. all of the above.

Questions 23-26. Match each term below with the correct description.

23. _____ acetylcholine receptor (AcHR)

24. _____ anticentromere antibody

25. _____ antiintrinsic factor antibody

26. _____ antimitochondrial antibody antibody
    A. strongly suggestive, in a high titer, of primary biliary binding antibody cirrhosis

B. useful in the diagnosis of myasthenia gravis
C. demonstrated in most patients with CREST syndrome
D. found in 60% of patients with pernicious anemia

Questions 27-30. Match each term below with the correct description.

27. _____ antimyelin antibody

28. _____ antimyocardial antibody

29. _____ antineutrophil antibody (C-ANCA)

30. _____ antinuclear antibody (ANA)
    A. associated with multiple myeloma
    B. marker for Wegener's granulomatosis
    C. characteristic of untreated systemic lupus erythematosus
    D. diagnostic of Dressler's syndrome or rheumatic fever

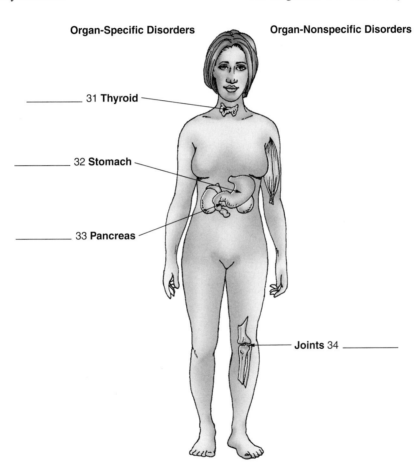

Organ-Specific Disorders   **Organ-Nonspecific Disorders**

_____ 31 **Thyroid**

_____ 32 **Stomach**

_____ 33 **Pancreas**

Joints 34 _____

Questions 31-34. Match each organ in the illustration with the appropriate disease.

Possible answers to question 31.
  A. Takayasu arteritis
  B. Behcet's disease
  C. Graves' disease
  D. scleroderma

Possible answers to question 32.
  A. eosinophilia-myalgia
  B. Hashimoto's thyroiditis
  C. Raynaud's phenomenon
  D. pernicious anemia

Possible answers to question 33.
  A. Addison's disease
  B. Sheehan's syndrome
  C. insulin-dependent diabetes
  D. Sjögren's syndrome

Possible answers to question 34.
  A. idiopathic biliary cirrhosis
  B. Crohn's disease
  C. rheumatoid arthritis
  D. multiple sclerosis

35. The immunologic manifestations of multiple sclerosis include all of the following except:
    A. antimyelin antibodies
    B. an oligoclonal increase in CSF immunoglobulin
    C. in vitro antibody-mediated immunity
    D. an increase in certain HLA and Ia antigens

36. Most immunologically mediated renal diseases fall into one of the following categories except:
    A. association with circulating immune complexes
    B. association with circulating antigen
    C. association with antiglomerular basement membrane antibody
    D. membranoproliferative glomerulonephritis

37. Polymyositis and dermatomyositis are the most common expressions of:
    A. rheumatoid heart disease.
    B. skeletal muscle disorders.
    C. rheumatoid arthritis.
    D. either A or B.

BIBLIOGRAPHY

Aahmed AE: Cellular immunology of autoimmune diseases, *Adv Med Lab Prof* 10:40-42, 1998.

Ascherio A: Epstein-Barr virus antibodies and risk of multiple sclerosis: a prospective study, *JAMA* 286(24):3083-3088, 2001.

Ashman RF: Rheumatic diseases. In Lawlor GJ, Fischer TJ, editors: *Manual of allergy and immunology,* ed 2, Boston, 1988, Little, Brown.

Barrett J: *Textbook of immunology,* ed 5, St Louis, 1988, Mosby.

Bottazzo GF, Doniach D: Autoimmune thyroid disease, *Annu Rev Med* 37:353-359, 1986.

Bridges AJ et al: Antinuclear antibody testing in a referral laboratory, *Lab Med* 24(6):345-349, 1993.

Caroscio JT: Quantitative CSF IgG measurements in multiple sclerosis and other neurologic diseases, *Arch Neurol* 40:409-413, 1983.

Chang A et al: Research results on myelin repair in long-standing MS brain, *N Engl J Med* 346(3):165-173, 2002.

Chaplin H: *Clinical usefulness of specific antiglobulin reagents in autoimmune hemolytic anemia,* vol 8, *Progress in hematology,* New York, 1973, Grune & Stratton.

Cohen B, Mitsumoto H: Neuropathy syndromes associated with antibodies against the peripheral nerve, *Lab Med* 26(7):459-463, 1995.

Coles AJ et al: Pulsed monoclonal antibody treatment and autoimmune thyroid disease in multiple sclerosis, *Lancet* 354:1691-1695, 1999.

Condemi JJ: The autoimmune diseases, *JAMA* 268(20):2888-2892, 1992.

D'Angelo A et al: Autoimmune protein S deficiency in a boy with severe thromboembolic disease, *N Engl J Med* 328(24):1753-1757, 1993.

Davies TF et al: Evidence of limited variability of antigen receptors on intrathyroidal T cells in autoimmune thyroid disease, *N Engl J Med* 325(4):238-244, 1991.

Eastwood A: Information resource center and library of the national MS Society, 2001 (www.nmss.org).

Flescher E, Talal N: Do viruses contribute to the development of Sjögren's syndrome? *Am J Med* 90:283-294, 1991.

Freedman J et al: Hemolytic warm IgM autoagglutinins in autoimmune hemolytic anemia, *Transfusion* 27(6):464-467, 1987.

Gerson B, Orr JD, Orr JM: Oligoclonal bands and quantitation of IgG in cerebrospinal fluid as indicators of multiple sclerosis, *Am J Clin Pathol* 75(1):87-91, 1980.

Hogancamp WE, Rodriguez M, Weinshenker BG: The epidemiology of multiple sclerosis, *Mayo Clin Proc* 72:871-878, 1997.

Kamb ML et al: Eosinophilia-myalgia syndrome in L-tryptophan-exposed patients, *JAMA* 267(1):77-82, 1992.

Keshgegian AA, editor: Oligoclonal immunoglobulins in cerebrospinal fluid in multiple sclerosis, *Clin Chem* 26(9):1340-1345, 1980.

Killingsworth LM: Clinical applications of protein determination in biological fluids other than blood, *Clin Chem* 28(5):1093-1258, 1982.

King D: Experts predict advances in autoimmune disease testing, *Adv Med Lab Prof* 13(4):8-11, 2001.

Lange LG, Schreiner GF: Immune mechanisms of cardiac disease, *N Engl J Med* 330(16):1129-1135, 1994.

Link H, Kostulas V: Utility of IEF of CSF and serum on agarose evaluated from neurological patients, *Clin Chem* 2915:810-815, 1983.

Malnick SDH, Sthoeger ZM: Autoimmune protein S deficiency, *N Engl J Med* 329(25):1898, 1993.

Mooney B: Diagnosing pediatric autoimmune diseases, *Adv Med Lab Prof* 4(5):13-14, 26, 2002.

Muliple Sclerosis Foundation: MS Information, 2002, Available on World Wide Web: www.msfacts.org.

Nakamura RM: Human autoimmune disease: progress in clinical laboratory tests, *Med Lab Observer* 32(10):32-47, 2000.

Miller FW: Myositis-specific autoantibodies, *JAMA* 270(15):1846-1849, 1993.

Noseworthy JH: Progress in determining the causes and treatment of multiple sclerosis, *Nature* 399(suppl):A40-A47, 1999.

Okano Y, Steen VD, Medsger TA: Autoantibody reactive with RNA polymerase III in system sclerosis, *Ann Intern Med* 119(10):1005-1013, 1993.

Oksenberk J: Immune protein may play role in MS attacks and progression, *Science* 294(5547):1613.2001.

Pagano JS: Amyotrophic lateral sclerosis and autoimmunity, *N Engl J Med* 327(4):1752-1753, 1992.

Papadopoulos NM et al: A unique protein in normal human cerebrospinal fluid, *Clin Chem* 29(10):1842-1844, 1983.

Pizarro TT, Kam L, Cominelli F: Interleukin-1 and interleukin-1 antagonism in inflammatory bowel disease, *Prog Inflamm Bowel Dis* 14(3):7-11, 1993.

Rees-Smith B: Autoantibodies to the thyrotropin receptor, *Endocr Rev* 9(1):106-121, 1988.

Robert C, Kupper TS: Inflammatory skin disease, T cells, and immune surveillance, *N Engl J Med* 341:1817-1827, 1999.

Roitt IM: *Essential immunology,* ed 5, Oxford, England, 1984, Blackwell Scientific Publications.

Rosenwasser LJ, Joseph BZ: Immunohematologic diseases, *JAMA* 268(20):2940-2945, 1992.

Salama AB et al: Immune complex-mediated intravascular hemolysis due to IgM cephalosporin-dependent antibody, *Transfusion* 27(6):460-463, 1987.

Scully RE et al: Case 3-1991, *N Engl J Med* 324(3):180-188, 1991.

Smiroldo J, Coyle PK: Advances in the treatment of multiple sclerosis, *Patient Care* 33(11):88-106, 1999.

Smith RG et al: Serum antibodies to L-type calcium channels in patients with amyotrophic lateral sclerosis, *N Engl J Med* 327(4):1721-1728, 1992.

Talal N: Clinical immunology. In Stein J, editor: *Internal medicine,* ed 4, Boston, 1994, Little, Brown.

Torassa U: Odd illnesses, strong clues—autoimmune woes target women, *San Francisco Chronicle,* Feb. 18, 2001, p. 69.

Troy JL: Eosinophilia-myalgia syndrome, *Mayo Clin Proc* 66:535-538, 1991.

Tsieh S et al: Synthesis of immunoglobulin within the central nervous system in multiple sclerosis and other neurological diseases, detection by analysis of CSF/serum IgG ratio, *Am J Clin Pathol* 76(4):458-461, 1981.

Turgeon ML: *Clinical hematology,* ed 3, Philadelphia, 1999, Lippincott-Williams & Wilkins.

Turgeon ML: *Fundamentals of immunohematology,* ed 2, Baltimore, 1995, Williams & Wilkins.

Utiger RD: The pathogenesis of autoimmune thyroid disease, *N Engl J Med* 325(4):278-280, 1991.

Voulgarelis M et al: Malignant lymphoma in primary Sjögren's syndrome, *Arthritis Rheum* 42:1765-1772, 1999.

Watanabe T et al: Anti-alpha-Fodrin antibodies in Sjögren syndrome and lupus erythematosus, *Arch Dermatol* 135:535-539, 1999.

Wright MZ, Dearing LD: The role of HLA testing in autoimmune disease, *Adv Med Lab Prof* 13:81-84, 2001.

Yorde L: Diagnosing thyroid disorder, *Adv Med Lab Prof* 12(12):17, 2000.

Zeher M et al: Correlation of increased susceptibility to apoptosis of CD4+ T cells with lymphocyte activation and activity of disease in patients with primary Sjögren's syndrome, *Arthritis Rheum* 42:1673-1681, 1999.

Chapter 26

Systemic Lupus Erythematosus

LEARNING OBJECTIVES

At the conclusion of this chapter, the reader should be able to:
- Describe the etiology, including factors such as hormones and drugs, that influence the development of systemic lupus erythematosus (SLE) and other forms of lupus.
- Explain the epidemiology and signs and symptoms of SLE.
- Describe the immunologic manifestations of SLE, including diagnostic evaluation.
- Discuss the laboratory evaluation of antinuclear antibodies.
- Analyze selected case studies.

Systemic lupus erythematosus (SLE) is the classic model of autoimmune disease. It is a systemic rheumatic disorder, the most commonly used term for the group of disorders that includes SLE and other abnormalities that involve multiple systems (e.g., joints, connective tissue, and the collagen-vascular system) in the disease process.

DIFFERENT FORMS OF LUPUS

There are several forms of lupus (Table 26-1): discoid, systemic, drug-induced, overlap syndrome or mixed connective tissue disease, and systemic.
- Discoid (cutaneous) lupus is always limited to the skin and is identified by a rash that may appear on the face,

TABLE 26-1	**American College of Rheumatology 1982 Revised Criteria for Classification of Systemic Lupus Erythematosus***

Criterion	Definition
1. Malar rash	Fixed erythema, flat or raised, over the malar eminences, tending to spare the nasolabial folds
2. Discoid rash	Erythematous raised patches with adherent keratotic scaling and follicular plugging; atrophic scarring may occur in older lesions
3. Photosensitivity	Skin rash as a result of unusual reaction to sunlight, by patient history or physician observation
4. Oral ulcers	Oral or nasopharyngeal ulceration, usually painless, observed by physician
5. Arthritis	Nonerosive arthritis involving two or more peripheral joints, characterized by tenderness, swelling, or effusion
6. Serositis	a. Pleuritis—convincing history of pleuritic pain or rubbing heard by a physician or evidence of pleural effusion OR b. Pericarditis—documented by ECG or rub or evidence of pericardial effusion
7. Renal disorder	a. Persistent proteinuria greater than 0.5 grams per day or greater than 3+ if quantitation not performed OR b. Cellular casts—may be red cell, hemoglobin, granular, tubular, or mixed
8. Neurologic disorder	a. Seizures—in the absence of offending drugs or known metabolic derangements (e.g., uremia, ketoacidosis, or electrolyte imbalance) OR b. Psychosis—in the absence of offending drugs or known metabolic derangements (e.g., uremia, ketoacidosis, or electrolyte imbalance)
9. Hematologic disorder	a. Hemolytic anemia—with reticulocytosis OR b. Leukopenia—<4000/mm^3 total on two or more occasions OR c. Lymphopenia—<1500/mm^3 on two or more occasions OR d. Thrombocytopenia—<100,000/mm^3 in the absence of offending drugs
10. Immunologic disorder	a. Positive LE cell preparation OR b. Anti-DNA: antibody to native DNA in abnormal titer OR c. Anti-Sm: presence of antibody to Sm nuclear antigen OR d. False-positive serologic test for syphilis known to be positive for at least 6 months and confirmed by *Treponema pallidum* immobilization or fluorescent treponemal antibody absorption test
11. Antinuclear antibody	An abnormal titer of antinuclear antibody by immunofluorescence or an equivalent assay at any point in time and in the absence of drugs known to be associated with "drug-induced lupus" syndrome

From Tan EM et al: The 1982 revised criteria for the classification of systemic lupus erythematosus, *Arthritis Rheum* 25:1271-1277, 1982.
*The proposed classification is based on 11 criteria. For the purpose of identifying patients in clinical studies, a person shall be said to have SLE if any 4 or more of the 11 criteria are present, serially or simultaneously, during any interval of observation.

neck, and scalp. Discoid lupus accounts for approximately 10% of all cases.

- Drug-induced lupus occurs after the use of certain prescribed drugs. The symptoms of drug-induced lupus are similar to those of systemic lupus.
- Mixed connective tissue disease affects approximately 10% of all lupus cases. These individuals will have symptoms and signs of more than one connective tissue disease, including lupus.
- Systemic lupus is usually more severe than discoid lupus, and can affect the skin, joints, and almost any organ

or system of the body, including the lungs, kidneys, heart, or brain. Approximately 70% of lupus cases are systemic. In about half of these cases, a major organ will be affected.

ETIOLOGY

The cause of SLE is unknown (idiopathic). Although no single etiologic agent has been identified, a primary defect in the regulation of the immune system is considered important in the pathogenesis of the disorder. Other influences include the effect of sex steroid hormones, genetic predisposition, and extraneous factors. A combination of these factors, however, may be synergistic.

Many of the clinical manifestations of SLE are a consequence of tissue damage from vasculopathy mediated by immune complexes. Other conditions (e.g., thrombocytopenia or the antiphospholipid syndrome) are the direct effects of antibodies to cell-surface molecules or serum components.

In addition to the antigenic specificity of autoantibodies, their other qualities are important determinants of the pathogenicity of the immune complexes that are formed in patients. Complexes composed of strongly complement-activating antibodies are more pathogenic than weaker complexes. Additional variables include the size of the immune complexes and the function of the complex clearing mechanisms.

Antibodies directed against T cells, including the membrane molecules that mediate their responses, are regularly detected in patients with SLE. Their role in the pathogenesis of autoimmunity is still unclear.

Hormonal Influences

Hormonal factors are considered to be significant contributors to SLE. A disproportionate number of females between puberty and menopause suffer from SLE. There is, in addition, a propensity for the disease to worsen during pregnancy and the immediate postpartum period. Strong evidence implicates sex steroid hormones (estrogens) in the pathogenesis of SLE. In addition, postmenopausal therapy is associated with an increased risk for developing SLE.

Genetic Predisposition

Evidence in humans points to a gene or genes linked to the HLA-DR and DQ loci in the class II immune-response complex as a genetic factor in the pathogenesis of spontaneous development of SLE.

Because there is an increased familial incidence of SLE, a primary genetic relationship to the disease is suspected. Although patients with SLE have an increased frequency of histocompatibility antigens HLA-B8, HLA-DRw2, HLA-DRw3, and of select B-cell alloantigens, as compared to the general population, none of these antigens is absolute for SLE. Therefore two or more of these genes may be involved in increased disease susceptibility, or these antigens may be associated with other specific disease-associated genes.

Environmental Factors

Various factors, including ultraviolet light and bacterial and viral infections, are capable of inducing or exacerbating the signs and symptoms of SLE. These factors may act in different ways. For example, ultraviolet light may cause DNA to form thymine dimmers, which significantly alters the antigenicity of DNA and could result in the formation of anti-DNA.

Drug-Induced Lupus

The symptoms of drug-induced lupus are similar to SLE. A reversible drug-induced lupus syndrome is caused by a number of chemically diverse drugs (Box 26-1). The most commonly implicated drugs are procainamide hydrochloride

---

| Box 26-1 | **Drugs That Can Produce Clinical and Serologic Features of Systemic Lupus Erythematosus** |

Antiarrhythmics
  Practolol
  Procainamide hydrochloride
Anticonvulsants
  Ethosuximide
  Mephenytoin trimethadione
  Phenytoin
  Primidone
Antihypertensives
  Hydralazine hydrochloride
  Methyldopa
Miscellaneous
  Chlorprothixene
  Chlorthalidone
  Chlorpromazine
  Isoniazid
  Methylthiouracil
  Penicillamine
  Penicillin
  Propylthiouracil
  Sulfonamides

(used to treat irregular heart rhythms), hydrazaline hydrochloride (used to treat high blood pressure or hypertension), chlorpromazine hydrochloride, and anticonvulsants. Some drugs (e.g., birth control pills and isoniazid) induce serum antinuclear antibodies (ANAs) without symptoms. The percentage of individuals using these drugs who develop drug-induced lupus is extremely small, and the symptoms usually fade when the medications are discontinued.

The physiologic mechanism of drug-induced lupus is unknown. Factors such as the rate of metabolism of the drug, the influence of the drug on immune regulation, and the host's genetic composition are all considered to influence pathogenesis.

Although drug-induced lupus resembles SLE, it is milder than idiopathic SLE. Patients with drug-related lupus suffer from a predominance of pulmonary and polyserositis signs and symptoms. There is no associated renal and central nervous system (CNS) disease in drug-induced lupus. In addition, lupus-inducing drugs do not appear to exacerbate idiopathic SLE.

Implicated drugs are capable of producing serologic abnormalities. The drugs procainamide hydrochloride and hydralazine hydrochloride are extremely potent inducers of ANA, antierythrocyte antibodies, and antilymphocyte antibodies. In these cases high antibody titers may exist for months without the development of any clinical symptoms. Even with discontinuation of the drug, antibody titers usually remain elevated for months or years.

Procainamide-induced disease does not induce antibodies to double-stranded (dsDNA). The ANAs in the drug-induced syndromes are histone-dependent, and they are never the only ANAs.

EPIDEMIOLOGY

The Lupus Foundation of America estimates that approximately 1,400,000 Americans have a form of lupus. The overall incidence of SLE is estimated to be 50 to 70 new cases per year per million of population.

Racial groups such as African-Americans, Native-Americans, Puerto Ricans, and Asians (particularly Chinese) demonstrate an increased frequency of SLE. Lupus is two to three times more prevalent among people of color.

The prevalence rate, based on a total population, is 1 in 2000, but it is 1 in 700 for women between 20 and 64 years old; 80% of those afflicted with systemic lupus develop it between the ages of 15 and 45 years. Lupus is most common in females during the reproductive years and may be present for years before diagnosis. The incidence of SLE in African-American women between the 20 and 64 years old is 1 in 245.

Survival is estimated to be greater than 90% at 10 years after diagnosis. The highest mortality rate is in patients with progressive renal involvement or CNS disease. The two most frequent causes of death are renal failure and infectious complications.

SIGNS AND SYMPTOMS

SLE is a disease of acute and chronic inflammation. Symptoms of SLE often mimic other less serious illnesses. Manifestations of the disease range from a typical mild illness limited to a photosensitive facial rash and transient diffuse arthritis to life-threatening involvement of the renal, cardiac, respiratory, or central nervous systems (Figure 26-1). In the early phases it is often difficult to distinguish SLE from several of the other systemic rheumatic disorders such as progressive systemic sclerosis (PSS), polymyositis, primary Sjögren's syndrome, primary Raynaud's phenomenon, and rheumatoid arthritis. Polyarthritis and dermatitis are the most common clinical manifestations.

The course of the disease is highly variable. It usually follows a chronic and irregular course with periods of exacerbations and remissions. Clinical signs and symptoms (Table 26-2) can include fever, weight loss, malaise, arthralgia (joint pain) and arthritis (inflammation of the joints), and the characteristic erythematous, maculopapular (butterfly) rash over the bridge of the nose. In addition, there is a tendency to increased susceptibility to common and opportunistic infections. Multiple organ systems may be affected simultaneously.

Cutaneous Features

Approximately 20% to 25% of patients with SLE develop dermal disorders as the initial manifestation of the disease. As many as 65% of patients will develop a cutaneous abnormality sometime during the course of the disease. The char-

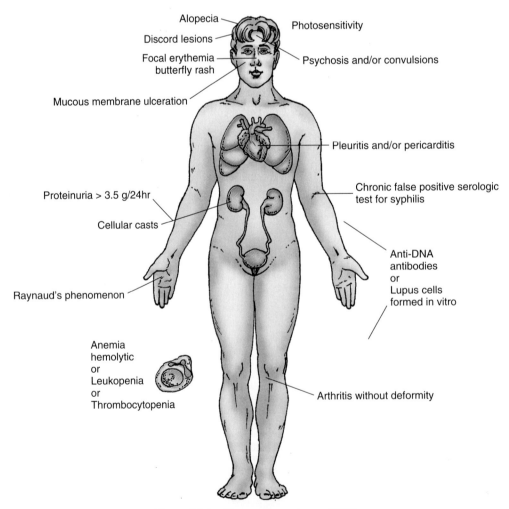

Figure 26-1 Signs and symptoms of SLE.

acteristic erythematous, maculopapular "butterfly rash" across the nose and upper cheeks is the cutaneous feature from which the disease gets its name, *lupus erythematosus,* the "red wolf" (Figure 26-2). This rash may also be observed on the arms and trunk of the body. Exposure to ultraviolet light will worsen erythematous, as well as other types of, cutaneous lesions.

The spectrum of cutaneous abnormalities includes urticaria, angioedema, nonthrombocytopenic purpura associated with the presence of cryoglobulins, scale formation, and ulcerations of oral and genital mucous membranes. Although neither the collection of immunoglobulins (Igs) and complement at the dermal-epidermal junction nor the presence of specific antibody nuclear ribonucleoprotein (RNP), Sm, native DNA, and single-stranded DNA appear to play a direct role in the pathogenesis of cutaneous lupus lesion, Ri (SS-A) and perhaps the La (SS-B) antibodies may be prominent factors.

Diffuse or patchy alopecia is also a common cutaneous manifestation. Hair loss is caused by pustular lesions of the scalp and is most often related to the stress of the disease process. Although the cause of pustular lesions is unknown, these inflammatory infiltrates are characterized by the presence of predominantly Ia-positive (activated) T lymphocytes with both CD4+ and CD8+ phenotypes.

Approximately 2% or 3% of SLE patients demonstrate lupus panniculitis. This condition is characterized by tender or nontender subcutaneous nodules that sometimes ulcerate and discharge a yellowish lipid material. In addition, various nonspecific skin changes are observable secondary to vascular insults. Raynaud's phenomenon is demonstrated by approximately one third of patients with SLE; this phenomenon appears to be increased in patients with SLE who have antibodies to nuclear RNP in their serum.

The presence of lesions, however, does not distinguish between the limited cutaneous (discoid lupus erythematosus) and the cutaneous manifestation of SLE. The term *discoid lupus* is used to differentiate the benign dermatitis of cutaneous lupus from the cutaneous involvement of SLE. In discoid lupus the round lesion is an erythematous, inflammatory dermatosis. These lesions are primarily located in light-exposed areas of the skin.

Renal Characteristics

Complement-mediated injury to the renal system is a usual consequence of the high levels of immune complexes in the blood that are deposited in tissues such as the kidneys. Renal disease progression is highly unpredictable. It may be acute, but more typically it progresses slowly. As the kidneys degenerate, the urinary sediment is typical of acute glomerulonephritis and later of chronic glomerulonephritis. Acute glomerulonephritis is characterized by the presence of erythrocytes, leukocytes, and granular and red blood cell casts in urinary sediment. The presence of proteinuria may lead to nephrotic syndrome. If end-stage renal failure occurs, it can be managed by dialysis or allograft transplantation.

The systemic necrotizing vasculitis of SLE involves small blood vessels and leads to renal involvement. The most common method of classification of the renal involvement of SLE is the World Health Organization system (Table 26-3), which is based on histopathologic criteria. The stages of renal disease range from the earliest and least severe form, class II, characterized by mesangial deposits of Ig and the C3 component of complement, to class V, the most severe form of involvement.

TABLE 26-2	Systemic Lupus Erythematosus Symptoms (Percentage of Cases)

Symptom	Percentage
Achy joints (arthralgia)	95
Frequent fevers of more than 37.8° C	90
Arthritis (swollen joints)	90
Prolonged or extreme fatigue	81
Skin rashes	74
Anemia	71
Kidney involvement	50
Pain in the chest on deep breathing (pleurisy)	45
Butterfly-shaped rash across the cheek and nose	42
Sun or light sensitivity (photosensitivity)	30
Hair loss	27
Abnormal blood clotting problems	20
Raynaud's phenomenon (fingers turning white and/or blue in the cold)	17
Seizures	15
Mouth or nose ulcers	12

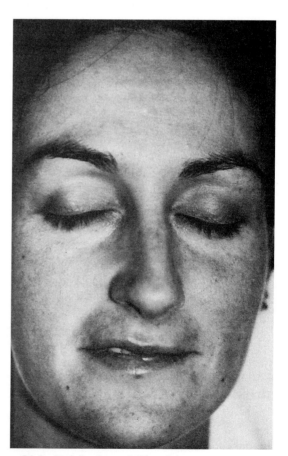

Figure 26-2 Facial rash over bridge of nose, upper lip, and chin in patient with active SLE. (From Kaye D, Rose LF: *Fundamentals of internal medicine,* St Louis, 1983, Mosby.)

TABLE 26-3	World Health Organization Classification System for Renal Involvement in Systemic Lupus Erythematosus					
Histologic Type	Class	Frequency (%)	Proteinuria	Nephrotic Syndrome	Death (%)	Uremic Death (%)
Normal	I	<5				
Mesangial	II	15	68	0	18	0
Focal proliferative	III	20	100	15	30	11
Diffuse proliferative	IV	50	100	87	58	36
Membranous	V	15	100	88	38	6

Lymphadenopathy

Enlargement of peripheral and axial lymph nodes and splenomegaly both occur in patients with SLE; however, these conditions are usually transient. Patients with SLE may be at a greater risk of developing lymphoma than the general population, especially if there is an associated secondary Sjögren's syndrome.

Serositis in Systemic Lupus Erythematosus

Serositis is an inflammation of the membrane consisting of mesothelium, a thin layer of connective tissue that lines enclosed body cavities. Mesothelium, a type of epithelium, is originally derived from the mesoderm lining the primitive embryonic body cavity. It becomes the covering of the serous membranes of the body surfaces such as the peritoneum, pleura, and pericardium. Inflammation of these serosal surfaces leads to sterile peritonitis, pleuritis, or pericarditis and is frequently accompanied by severe pain. In the presence of serositis, an increased frequency of thrombophlebitis is observed and may lead to pulmonary embolization.

Cardiopulmonary Characteristics

Inflammation of the myocardium in patients with SLE can produce persistent tachycardia and, occasionally, intractable congestive heart failure. Ischemic disease or, more commonly, atherosclerotic coronary disease may occur. Patients with severe nephrosis or those treated with corticosteroids for a prolonged time are at an increased risk for developing atherosclerosis.

Pulmonary function studies reveal occult diffusion and obstructive abnormalities in a high proportion of SLE patients, but clinical problems secondary to pulmonary involvement are unusual. Massive hemoptysis, however, may result from acute alveolar hemorrhage. This particular complication occurs in the absence of any detectable bleeding diathesis and is associated with a high rate of mortality.

Gastrointestinal Manifestations

Nonspecific gastrointestinal symptoms are relatively frequent in cases of SLE, but acute abdominal crises caused by visceral and peritoneal vasculitis are less common. However, infarction and perforation of the bowel and viscera, are associated with a high rate of mortality. Acute and chronic pancreatitis may also develop as a secondary complication of acute lupus or as a complication during therapy.

Musculoskeletal Features

A characteristic arthritis of SLE is a transient and peripheral polyarthritis with symmetric involvement of both small and large joints. Chronic arthritis can result in disability and deformity in SLE patients. Rheumatoid-like hand deformities develop in about 10% of patients. Osteonecrosis develops in one fourth of all SLE patients. Arthropathy of osteonecrosis, or avascular necrosis, is often initially detected in weight-bearing joints such as the hips and knees.

Neuropsychiatric Features

In SLE various kinds of neurologic and psychiatric manifestations develop secondarily to the involvement of the central and peripheral nervous systems. The most common abnormalities are disturbances of mental function, ranging from mild confusion, with memory deficiency and impairment of orientation and perception, to psychiatric disturbances such as hypomania, delirium, and schizophrenia. Seizures of the grand mal type may be the initial manifestation of SLE and may be present long before the multisystem disease develops. In addition, some patients may suffer from epilepsy and severe headaches.

Effects of Pregnancy

The incidences of premature delivery and spontaneous abortion are increased in pregnant women with SLE. Both the developing fetus and pregnant mother with lupus are at increased risk of various complications during and after pregnancy. Pregnant women are at an increased risk of disease flare-ups during pregnancy, as well as in the immediate postpartum period. Passive transfer of maternal antibodies across the placenta can produce transient abnormalities such as hepatosplenomegaly, cytopenia, and a photosensitive rash in the newborn. These conditions do resolve themselves in the newborn after the antibody titer declines.

Late-Onset Lupus

Lupus can occur at any age, in either sex, in any race. The average age of onset is 59 years; average age at diagnosis is

62 years. Late-onset lupus affects women eight times more often than men. Late-onset lupus is found primarily in Caucasians, but it occurs in all races.

Symptoms in most cases are relatively mild, but symptoms of lupus in older people can mimic other diseases (e.g., rheumatoid arthritis, Sjögren's syndrome, polymyalgia rheumatica). Distinguishing among these disorders can be difficult and may result in a delayed or missed diagnosis. Drug-induced lupus occurs more often in older people because they are more likely to have conditions (high blood pressure, heart disease) that require treatment that may cause the symptoms of lupus. Symptoms generally fade when the medication is discontinued. Patients with late-onset lupus have a good survival rate and rarely die of the disease or complications of therapy when treated conservatively.

IMMUNOLOGIC MANIFESTATIONS

Patients with SLE are known to produce multiple autoantibodies. There are two leading hypotheses as to why so many different antibodies develop. These hypotheses are not mutually exclusive. One hypothesis supports the belief that antibody-forming B lymphocytes are stimulated in a relatively nonspecific fashion, so-called polyclonal B-cell activation. The second hypothesis is that the immune response in SLE is specifically stimulated by antigens. The most compelling evidence in its favor is that the antibody molecules that are formed over time show evidence of gene rearrangement and somatic mutation that are characteristic of an antigen-driven response.

Laboratory features of SLE are the presence of ANAs, immune complexes, complement-level depression, tissue deposition of Igs and complement, circulating anticoagulants, and other autoantibodies.

Cellular Aspects

SLE is a disease that results from defects in the regulatory mechanism of the immune system. Studies of the immunopathogenesis of lupus nephritis have demonstrated a variety of aberrations in T-cell and B-cell function. It is uncertain, however, if the disease represents a primary dysfunction of T cells or B cells, but alterations in function do result. Lymphocyte subset abnormalities are a major immunologic feature of SLE. Among the T-cell subsets a lack of or reduced generalized suppressor T-cell function and/or hyperproduction of helper T cells occurs. The formation of lymphocytotoxic antibodies with a predominant specificity for T lymphocytes by patients with SLE at least partially explains the interference with certain functional activities of T lymphocytes manifested by the patient with SLE. Lymphocytotoxic antibodies are capable of both destroying T lymphocytes in the presence of complement and coating peripheral blood T cells.

The regulation of antibody production by B lymphocytes, ordinarily a function of the subpopulation of T suppressor cells, appears to be defective in patients with SLE. Although no single cause can be implicated in the pathogenesis of SLE, patients exhibit a state of spontaneous B-lymphocyte hyperactivity with ensuing uncontrolled production of a wide variety of antibodies to both host and exogenous antigens. Host response to some antigens, however, such as vaccination with influenza, is normal in many instances, and the patient manifests a specific well-controlled humoral immune response.

Humoral Aspects

Circulating immune complexes are the hallmark of SLE. Patients with SLE exhibit multiple serum antibodies that react with native or altered self-antigens. Demonstrable antibodies include antibodies to:
- Nuclear components
- Cell surface and cytoplasm antigens of polymorphonuclear and lymphocytic leukocytes, erythrocytes, platelets, and neuronal cells
- IgG

SLE is characterized by autoantibodies to almost any organ or tissue in the body. These antibodies may not be specifically diagnostic for SLE. In addition, some may have pathologic significance.

Antibodies to host antigens, particularly nuclear antigens such as DNA, are the principal type of antibody produced in SLE. ANAs are a heterogeneous group of antibodies produced against a variety of antigens within the cell nucleus. ANAs may be found in diseases other than SLE (e.g., other rheumatic and nonrheumatic diseases), as well as in some patients undergoing specific drug therapy and in healthy older individuals. The absence of ANAs virtually excludes the diagnosis of SLE unless the patient is being chemically immunosuppressed. ANA titers and specific anti-DNA fluctuate during the course of the disease. In some cases a rise in titer may forewarn of an impending disease flare-up.

Antigens to which antibodies are formed are present on nucleic acid molecules (DNA and RNA) or proteins (histones and nonhistones), and on determinants consisting of both nucleic acid and protein molecules. Drug-induced cases of lupus have a high incidence of antibodies to histones. Some of these antibodies are directed against the double-stranded helical DNA (native DNA or dsDNA). The presence of anti-native DNA (anti-nDNA) antibodies was reported in 1957. High titers of dsDNA are seen primarily in SLE and closely parallel disease activity. Most SLE patients simultaneously demonstrate antibodies to nucleoprotein and native DNA.

Other nuclear antibodies are directed at the determinants of single-stranded DNA (ssDNA). Antibody titers of 1:32 or greater indicate a substantial concentration of antibody in an autoimmune response. Antibody to the Smith (Sm) antigen, a nuclear acidic protein extractable by aqueous solution, is considered a marker for SLE because anti-Sm has been found almost exclusively in patients with SLE. The presence of anti-Sm is seen in 25% to 30% of patients with SLE, but it rarely occurs in other systemic rheumatic (collagen) diseases.

The antinuclear antibody (anti-DNP) gives rise to the LE cell, which is found in more than 90% of untreated patients with active SLE. SLE patients with serositis may form LE cells in vivo. The LE cell-testing procedure was the first method extensively developed to detect antibodies to nuclear antigens. LE cells have been shown to be an expression of the interaction between IgG antibodies and deoxyribonucleohistones (DNP). Anti-DNP is referred to as the LE serum factor.

Antibodies to the Robert (Ro) soluble substance-A (SS-A) nuclear antigens are associated with SLE skin disease and the neonatal SLE syndrome. Antibodies to the Lane soluble substance-B (SS-B) antigens are associated with SLE and primary (1°) form and secondary (2°) form Sjögren's syndrome (SS). Their presence with SS-A antigen in SLE indicates mild disease. When present as the only antibody, it is associated with 1° SS.

Autoantibodies to red blood cells result in hemolytic anemia and can be detected by the antihuman globulin test. Autoantibodies membrane-specific to neutrophils and platelets and autoantibodies to lymphocytes (cold-reactive type) are specific for SLE. Antibody titers correlate with disease activity.

Immunologic Consequences

Antibodies combine with their corresponding antigens to form immune complexes. When the mononuclear phagocytic system is unable to entirely eliminate these immune complexes, an accumulation of immune complexes results in the blood circulation. These circulating immune complexes are deposited in the subendothelial layers of the vascular basement membranes of multiple target organs, where they mediate inflammation. The sites of deposition are determined in part by the physiochemical properties of the particular antigens or antibodies involved. These properties include:

- Size
- Molecular configuration
- Ig class
- Complement-fixing ability

After deposition, the immune complexes seem to initiate a localized inflammatory response that stimulates neutrophils to the site of inflammation, activates complement, and results in the release of kinins and prostaglandins. These activities become the basis of antibody-dependent, cell-mediated tissue injury.

DIAGNOSTIC EVALUATION

The manifestations of SLE expressed in laboratory findings are numerous. Histologic, hematologic, and serologic abnormalities reflect the multisystem nature of this disease.

Histologic Changes

The earliest pathologic abnormalities are those of acute vasculitis. Supportive tissue becomes edematous, initially infiltrated with neutrophils and later with plasma cells and lymphocytes. Persistent inflammation results in local deposition of a cellular homogeneous material, histologically similar to fibrin. Nuclear debris from resulting cellular necrosis reacts with ANAs (discussed later in this section) to form hematoxylin bodies. The presence of Igs, predominantly IgM and IgG, in vascular lesions can be demonstrated by indirect immunofluorescence.

Renal pathology can also be observed in SLE. Two basic types of changes can be manifested. One type of change is proliferative glomerulonephritis, a condition that resembles the renal changes in immune complex nephritis. The other form of renal abnormality is membranous nephritis.

Hematologic and Hemostatic Manifestations

In SLE a moderate anemia (normocytic normochromic anemia) representing chronic disease is a consistent factor. Some patients display coating of erythrocytes, which can be demonstrated by a positive antihuman globulin (AHG), but actual hemolysis is infrequent. Lymphocytopenia is common and often reflects disease activity. Thrombocytopenia (50 to $100 \times 10^9/L$) may also be displayed.

Hemostatic Testing

Lupus anticoagulants, antiphospholipid antibodies, can be commonly seen in association with SLE. Antiphospholipid antibodies develop in up to 20% of patients with SLE. These form a group of antibodies detected by tests for lupus anticoagulant and anticardiolipin antibodies.

Circulating anticoagulants are believed to be associated with the presence of false-positive serologic test results for syphilis. Because of the presence of lupus anticoagulant, patients with SLE frequently demonstrate prolonged prothrombin and partial thromboplastin time results, but lupus anticoagulant rarely causes hemostatic problems. Inhibitors are not necessarily associated with bleeding unless some other defect is present. Because lupus anticoagulant is an inhibitor or a prothrombin activator, it is often associated with excessive thrombosis rather than with bleeding. Patients with SLE have a high incidence of thrombotic episodes. Although less common, specific coagulation factor antibodies directed against coagulation Factors VIII, IX, XI, and XII have been described. Thrombocytopenia can also occur because of removal of antiphospholipid antibody-coated platelets.

LE Cells

Previously the classic test for SLE was the LE cell test. Although this procedure is now obsolete, it is useful to understand the principles and conditions under which LE cells are formed. An LE cell is either a normal segmented neutrophil or other phagocytic cell (Figure 26-3) with the engulfed homogeneous and swollen nucleus of either a neutrophil or lymphocyte. The LE cell is formed when nuclei coated by antibodies to nucleoprotein are phagocytized by polymorphonuclear neutrophilic leukocytes.

Rosettes represent several phagocytic cells attempting to engulf one nucleus. Care must be taken to distinguish a "tart cell" from an LE cell. Tart cells usually represent monocytes that have phagocytized another whole cell or nucleus, often a lymphocyte. The ingested material is well preserved in contrast to the LE cell inclusion; it may even be found in normal persons. The significance of tart cells is unknown.

Cellular destruction within the marrow may lead to the phagocytosis of nuclear debris and, rarely, to the formation of in vivo LE cells. In patients with serositis, LE cells formed in vivo may be observed in aspirate fluid (e.g., pleural fluid).

Serologic Manifestations

Serologic testing frequently reveals high levels of anti-DNA antibodies, reduced complement levels, and the presence of complement breakdown products of C3 (C3d and C3c). In addition, cryoglobulins, which in some instances

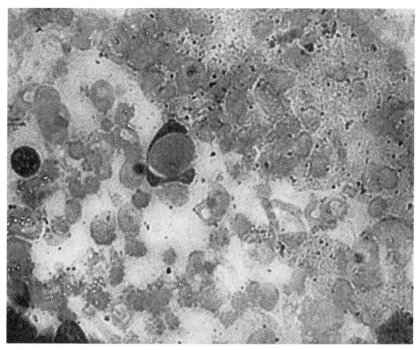

Figure 26-3   An LE cell in a peripheral blood specimen from a patient with systemic lupus erythematosus. (From Bauer JD: *Clinical laboratory methods,* ed 9, St Louis, 1982, Mosby.)

represent immune complexes, are frequently present in the serum of patients with SLE. Because monoclonal gammopathies have occasionally been described, a marked increase in gamma globulins may result in a hyperviscosity syndrome or renal tubular acidosis. Serum cryoglobulins of a mixed IgG-IgM type are found in patients with hypocomplementemia. The level of cryoglobulin correlates well with the severity of SLE. Procedural results helpful in assessing renal disease include:

- Antibody to double-stranded DNA
- Levels of C3, C4 (with C4 probably being the most sensitive)
- Cryoglobulin levels

A general correlation exists between abnormalities in each of these procedures and disease activity in many patients, but there is considerable disagreement about the usefulness of such measurements in predicting renal disease activity. The best laboratory procedures for monitoring the activity of renal disease are serum creatinine, urinary protein excretion, and careful examination of urinary sediment.

Complement

Inherited deficiencies of several complement components are associated with lupuslike illnesses. Some, but not all, deficiencies are coded for by autosomal recessive genes of the sixth chromosome, which are in linkage dysequilibrium with HLA-DRw2. It is possible that the association of complement deficiencies with SLE represents the fortuitous association of linked HLA-D region genes, rather than some unusual susceptibility induced by the complement deficiency.

Serum levels of complement are commonly reduced, particularly during states of active disease. Deficiencies in-

volving both the classic and alternative pathway complement components in patients with SLE have been noted as a result of consumption of components at the tissue sites of immune complex deposition and as a result of impaired synthesis, or from a combination of both. A depressed level of complement is not specific for the diagnosis of SLE, but it is a helpful guide in treating patients. Levels of complement (e.g., C3, and C4) are generally reduced in relationship to disease activity, and the fluctuation in these levels is often used to monitor disease activity. Patients with depressed levels are at risk for renal and CNS involvement. Deficiencies of C1, C3, and C4 are associated with SLE and other rheumatic diseases.

Antibodies

Nonspecific elevation in the levels of Igs, particularly IgM and IgG, are frequent in SLE. An actual deficiency of IgA appears to be more common in SLE than in normal individuals.

The ANA procedure (discussed in detail in the next section) is a valuable screening tool for SLE; it has virtually replaced the LE cell test because of its wider range of reactivity with nuclear antigens, as well as its greater sensitivity and quality-control characteristics.

Antinuclear Antibodies

Characteristics and Implications of ANAs. ANAs (Table 26-4) are a heterogeneous group of circulating Igs such as IgM, IgG, and IgA. These Igs react with the whole nucleus or nuclear components such as nuclear proteins, DNA, or histones in host tissues; therefore they are true autoantibodies. Generally, ANAs have no organ or species specificity and are capable of cross-reacting with nuclear ma-

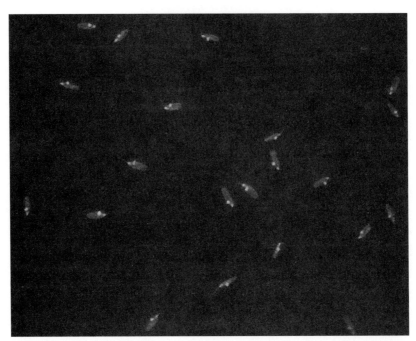

Figure 26-4 Anti-nDNA shown by indirect immunofluorescence. Staining of both the small kinetoplast and the adjacent larger nucleus of *Crithidia luciliae* occurs simultaneously. (From Bauer JD: *Clinical laboratory methods,* ed 9, St Louis, 1982, Mosby.)

TABLE 26-4	Antibodies in Systemic Rheumatic Diseases			
Systemic Lupus Erythematosus	**Progressive Systemic Sclerosis**	**Polymyositis**	**Rheumatoid Arthritis**
Antinuclear antibodies	Antinuclear antibodies	Antinuclear antibodies	Antinuclear antibodies
Antinative DNA	Anti-Scl-1	Anti-Jo-1	Rheumatoid factors
Anti-Sm			

terial from humans (e.g., human leukocytes) or various animal tissues (e.g., rat liver or mouse kidney).

Demonstration of ANAs in laboratory testing can indicate various systemic autoimmune connective tissue disorders. These disease states are characterized by antibodies that react with different nuclear components such as double-stranded DNA, single-stranded DNA, and Sm antigen. The presence of ANAs is the serologic hallmark of patients with SLE, which is considered to be the classic multisystem autoimmune disorder. Other disorders of this type include mixed connective tissue disease (MCTD), PSS or scleroderma, Sjögren's syndrome, polymyositis/dermatomyositis, and rheumatoid arthritis. A small percentage of patients with neoplastic diseases may also demonstrate the presence of ANAs.

However, ANAs can be exhibited by elderly individuals without disease and in a small percentage of healthy, nonelderly persons. These antibodies are also often detected in liver disease associated with autoimmunity such as chronic active hepatitis, primary biliary cirrhosis, and cryptogenic cirrhosis. In addition, varying levels of ANAs may be activated or induced by certain drugs, including procainamide hydrochloride, hydralazine hydrochloride, diphenylhydantoin, isoniazid, methyldopa, penicillin, tetracycline, strepto-

mycin, and oral contraceptives. The significance of the presence of ANAs in a patient must be assessed in regard to the patient's age, sex, clinical signs and symptoms, and other laboratory findings.

Systematic Classification of ANAs. It is possible to divide ANAs into different groups to provide a systematic classification. These groups are antibodies to DNA, antibodies to histone and nonhistone proteins, and antibodies to nuclear antigens.

Antibodies to DNA. Antibodies to DNA can be divided into two major groups: (1) antibodies that react with native (double-stranded) DNA, and (2) antibodies that recognize denatured (single-stranded) DNA only.

Antibodies that react with native DNA appear to interact with antigenic determinants present on the deoxyribose-phosphate backbone of the beta-helix of DNA. These autoantibodies characteristically stain the kinetoplast of the hemoflagellate, *Crithidia luciliae,* a substrate used to detect antinative DNA antibodies by indirect immunofluorescence (Figure 26-4). Antibodies reactive with denatured DNA probably react with the purine and pyrimidine bases of DNA. These bases are readily accessible on ssDNA; they are buried within the beta helix of dsDNA and are therefore inaccessible. Antidenatured DNA

TABLE 26-5	Antibodies to Nonhistone Proteins (Nhp) and Nhp-RNA Complexes in Systemic Rheumatic Diseases	
Antibody	**Disease**	**Incidence (%)**
Centromere/kinetochore	CREST variant of progressive systemic sclerosis (PSS)	70-90
	Diffuse scleroderma	10-20
Jo-I	Polymyositis	31
Ki antigen	Systemic lupus erythematosus (SLE)	20
Ku	Polymyositis/scleroderma overlap	55
Ma antigen	SLE	20
Mi-I	Dermatomyositis	11
NuMa (nuclear mitotic apparatus) antigen	Rheumatoid arthritis	
	Sjögren's syndrome	
	Carpal tunnel syndrome	
	SLE	3
Proliferating cell nuclear antigen (PCNA)	Rheumatoid arthritis	90
RANA (rheumatoid arthritis-associated nuclear antigen)	PSS	20
SCI-70	SLE	30
Sm (Smith)	Sjögren's syndrome	70
SS-A/Ro	SLE	50
	Other connective tissue diseases	
	Sjögren's syndrome	40-50
SS-B/la	SLE	15
	Mixed connective tissue disease	>95
UI-RNP	SLE	35

Modified from Reimer G, Tan E: Antinuclear antibodies. In Stein J, editor: *Internal medicine,* Boston, 1987, Little, Brown.
CREST, Calcinosis, Raynaud's phenomenon, esophageal motility abnormalities, sclerodactyly, and telangiectasia.

antibodies are unable to cross-react with native DNA. Conformational changes of the deoxyribose-phosphate backbone of denatured DNA appear to be important for antigenicity.

Antibodies to Histones. Antibodies to histones have been shown to react with all major classes of histones—H1, H2A, H2B, H3, and H4. Antihistone antibodies can be induced by drugs such as procainamide and hydralazine. Procainamide-induced lupus erythematosus is characterized by the IgG class of antibodies against the histone complex H2A-H2B in symptomatic cases of SLE. In asymptomatic cases the antibody may be restricted to the IgM class. Antibodies specific to other nuclear antigens are usually absent in drug-induced lupus, in contrast with cases of SLE, which have ANAs of multiple specificity. Therefore demonstration of only antihistone antibodies may be useful in distinguishing drug-induced lupus from SLE.

Antibodies to Nonhistone Proteins. Another primary class of ANAs in systemic autoimmune disorders is characterized by reactivity with soluble nonhistone nuclear protein and RNA-protein complexes. Clinically important antibodies that react with nuclear nonhistone proteins are listed in Table 26-5.

Antibodies to Nucleolar Antigens. The antibodies to nucleolar antigens are:
- U3-RNA-protein complex (the enzyme-transcribing ribosomal genes in the nucleolus)
- 7-2-RNP
- RNA polymerase I
- PM-Scl

These antinucleolar antibodies are primarily associated with polymyositis-scleroderma overlap, where they have the highest incidence and titers. However, they are rarely demonstrated in PSS, dermatomyositis, and scleroderma.

Laboratory Evaluation of Antinuclear Antibodies

The ANA method provides the laboratory with a simple and sensitive technique for detection and measurement of these antibodies. Indirect immunofluorescence is the preferred initial screening procedure. If the ANA method is positive, additional immunologic evaluation is necessary to determine the specificity of the reaction. These evaluations include double immunodiffusion, counterimmunoelectrophoresis, passive hemagglutination, enzyme-linked immunosorbent assay, radioimmunoassay, and identification of nuclear antigens by immunoprecipitation or immunoblotting. These evaluations may demonstrate that more than one ANA specificity is present in the serum. An LE cell preparation, however, has limited usefulness.

Indirect Immunofluorescent Technique

Detection of autoantibodies by immunofluorescence has become an extremely valuable tool. This method is extremely sensitive and may be positive in cases where procedures for ANAs, such as complement fixation or precipitation, are negative. At present the immunofluorescent method is the most widely used technique for ANA screening.

Principle of the Procedure. The antigen in the substrate tissue is fixed to a slide for testing. ANA is not specific for a particular organ; therefore any tissue containing nuclei may be used as substrate. The most commonly used tissues are rat or mouse liver or kidney, or cell-cultured fibroblasts grown on slides. If antibody is present in a patient's serum, the unlabeled antibody will attach to the nuclei in the substrate. After the substrate is washed in buffer, it is incubated with fluorescein-tagged goat AHG. If patient antibodies have affixed themselves to the nuclear antigens of the substrate, the fluorescein-tagged goat AHG will attach to these antibodies. When the slide is examined microscopically, fluorescence will be visible with ultraviolet light.

Interpretation of Staining Patterns. Because ANAs react with the whole nucleus or with nuclear components such as nuclear proteins, DNA, or histone, reaction patterns reflect the distribution of the various antigens within the nuclei. Several patterns of reactivity can be observed when a slide is examined in the ANA procedure.

Diffused or Homogeneous Pattern. The diffused or homogeneous pattern characterizes antideoxyribonucleic acid-nucleoprotein antibodies (i.e., antibodies to nDNA, dsDNA, ssDNA, DNP, or histones). Antibodies to DNP have been shown to have the same specificity as the LE factor. Although vacuoles may be seen, the whole nucleus fluoresces evenly. This pattern is typically seen in rheumatoid disorders. High titers of homogeneous ANA are suggestive of SLE, whereas low titers may be found in SLE, rheumatoid arthritis, Sjögren's syndrome, and MCTD.

Peripheral Pattern. The peripheral (marginal or rim) pattern results from antibodies to DNA (i.e., nDNA, dsDNA, or DNP). The central protein of the nucleus is only lightly stained or not stained at all, but the nuclear margins fluoresce strongly and appear to extend into the cytoplasm. This pattern is associated with SLE in the active stage of the disease and in Sjögren's syndrome.

Speckled Pattern. The speckled pattern occurs in the presence of antibody to any extractable nuclear antigen devoid of DNA or histone. The antibody is detected against the saline extractable nuclear antigens: anti-RNP and anti-Smith (Anti-Sm). A grainy pattern with numerous round dots of nuclear fluorescence, without staining of the nucleoli, is seen in this pattern type.

Antibodies to Sm antigen have been shown to be highly specific for patients with SLE and appear to be "marker" antibodies. Anti-RNP has been found in patients with a wide variety of rheumatic diseases including SLE, rheumatoid arthritis, Sjögren's syndrome, PSS, MCTD, and dermatomyositis.

Nucleolar Pattern. The nucleolar pattern reflects an antibody to nucleolar RNA (4-6S RNP). A few round, smooth nucleoli that vary in size will fluoresce when examined with ultraviolet light. The nucleolar pattern is present in about 50% of patients with scleroderma (PSS), Sjögren's syndrome, and in SLE. This pattern can also be observed in undiagnosed illnesses manifesting Raynaud's phenomenon.

Anticentromere Antibody. The anticentromere antibody reacts with centromeric chromatin of metaphase and interphase cells. The particular pattern on tissue culture cells is discrete and speckled. This antibody appears to be highly selective for the CREST variant of PSS. The CREST syndrome is a variant of systemic sclerosis characterized by the presence of calcinosis, Raynaud's phenomenon, esophageal motility abnormalities, sclerodactyly, and telangiectasia. This antibody is found infrequently in the serum of patients with SLE, MCTD, and PSS.

TREATMENT

For most patients with lupus, effective treatment and prevention methods can minimize symptoms, reduce inflammation, and maintain normal body functions. For photosensitive patients, avoidance of (excessive) sun exposure and/or the regular application of sunscreens will usually prevent rashes. Regular exercise helps prevent muscle weakness and fatigue. Immunization protects against specific infections. Support groups and counseling can help alleviate the effects of stress. Smoking, excessive consumption of alcohol, too much or too little prescribed medication, or postponing regular medical checkups are inadvisable behaviors.

Medications are often prescribed for people with lupus, depending on which organ(s) are involved, and the severity of involvement. Commonly prescribed medications include:

- Nonsteroidal antiinflammatory drugs (NSAIDs): These medications are prescribed for a variety of rheumatic diseases including lupus. Examples of such compounds include acetylsalicylic acid (aspirin), ibuprofen (Motrin), naproxen (Naprosyn), indomethacin (Indocin), nabumetone (Relafen), tolmetin (Tolectin), and others. These drugs are usually recommended for muscle and joint pain, and arthritis. Newer NSAIDs contain a prostaglandin in the same capsule (Arthrotec). The other NSAIDs work in the same way as aspirin, but may be more potent.
- Acetaminophen: Acetaminophen (e.g., Tylenol) is a mild analgesic that can often be used for pain. It has the advantage of causing less stomach irritation than aspirin, but it is not nearly as effective at suppressing inflammation as aspirin.
- Corticosteroids: Corticosteroids (steroids, e.g., prednisone) are used to reduce inflammation and suppress activity of the immune system. Side effects occur more frequently when steroids are taken over long periods of time at high doses (for example, 60 mg of prednisone taken daily for more than 1 month). Such side effects include weight gain, a round face, acne, easy bruising, "thinning" of the bones (osteoporosis), high blood pressure, cataracts, onset of diabetes, increased risk of infection, stomach ulcers, hyperactivity, and an increase of appetite.
- Antimalarials: Chloroquine (Aralen) or hydroxychloroquine (Plaquenil), commonly used in the treatment of malaria, may also be useful in some individuals with lupus. They are most often prescribed for skin and joint symptoms of lupus.
- Immunomodulating drugs: Azathioprine (Imuran) and cyclophosphamide (Cytoxan), cytotoxic drugs, act in a similar manner to the corticosteroid drugs in that they suppress inflammation and tend to suppress the immune system. Other agents (e.g., methotrexate and cyclosporin) can be used to control the symptoms of lupus. Some of these agents are used in conjunction with apheresis, a blood-filtering treatment. Apheresis has been tried by itself in an effort to remove specific anti-

TABLE 26-6	Examples of Drugs in Clinical Trials for SLE—Fall 2002		
Generic Name	**Trade Name**	**Phase**	**Manufacturer**
LJP-394	N/A	III	LaJolla Pharmaceutical
5G1.1	N/A	II	Alexion
N/A	LymphoStat-B	I	Human Genome Sciences
Prasterone—synthetic (dehydroepiandrosterone [DHEA])	Prestara	III	Gene Labs Technologies

bodies from the blood, but the results have not been promising.

Newer agents are directed toward specific cells of the immune system. These include agents that block the production of anti-DNA or agents that suppress the manufacture of antibodies through other mechanisms. Examples are intravenous Ig injections, which are given on a regular basis to increase platelet numbers.

- Anticoagulants: Anticoagulants range from aspirin at very low dose to heparin/coumadin. Generally, such therapy is lifelong in people with lupus and follows an actual episode of embolus or thromboses.

Clinical Trials

New drugs (Table 26-6) are being investigated as therapy for SLE. Another drug, Antova (generic name: anti CD-40 ligand antibody) has been discontinued by Biogen, Inc., the manufacturer. Gene Labs Technologies, the manufacturer of a fifth drug, Aslera (generic name: GL-701, prasterone), has been notified of nonapproval. However, the FDA issued an approval letter on August 28, 2002, for the company's new drug formula application for prasterone (PreStara), formerly known as GL701 (Aslera).

 Antinuclear Antibody Visible Method*

Principle

This is an indirect immunoenzyme method that uses tissue culture cells (human epithelial cells) as a substrate for the detection and titration of circulating antinuclear antibodies (ANAs) in human serum. Patient serum samples are diluted in buffer and added to microscope slide wells with HEp-2 (human epithelial) cells cultured in them. HEp-2 cells are characterized by extremely large nuclei and the presence of mitotic figures to aid in detection. If specific antibodies are present, stable antigen-antibody complexes are formed that bind antihuman globulin labeled with horseradish peroxidase (HRP). The presence of HRP is indicated by a reaction with 3, 3'-diaminobenzidine stain. The resulting dark brown to black staining patterns of the nuclei can be seen with a light microscope. The presence of one or more types of circulating autoantibodies is the hallmark of systemic rheumatic diseases.

Specimen Collection and Preparation

The patient should be in a fasting state before specimen collection. The patient must be positively identified when the specimen is collected, and the specimen is to be labeled at the bedside. Specimen labels must include the patient's full name, the date the specimen is collected, the patient's hospital identification number, and the phlebotomist's initials.

Blood should be drawn by an aseptic technique. A minimum of 5 to 8 mL of clotted blood (red top evacuated tube) is required. Allow the blood to clot at room temperature. The specimen should be centrifuged promptly, and the serum should be separated from the red cells immediately. Serum specimens may be stored at 2° to 8° C if tested within 24 to 48 hours. If the specimen cannot be tested within this period of time, it should be stored frozen at −20° C or below. Do not freeze and thaw sera more than once. Allow serum specimens to reach room temperature before testing. Avoid the use of sera exhibiting a high degree of lipemia, hemolysis, or microbial growth, as these characteristics may result in increased background staining, a decrease in titers, and/or unclear staining patterns.

Reagents, Supplies, and Equipment

WARNING: Sodium azide and thimerosol are used as preservatives. Sodium azide may react with lead and copper plumbing to form highly explosive metal azides. On disposal, flush with a large volume of water to prevent azide buildup. Sodium azide and thimerosol may be toxic if ingested.

1. The following reagents and controls are supplied in the Visible Test ANA System from ISOLAB, Akron, Ohio:
   a. Substrate slides. Each HEp-2 slide well contains HEp-2 cells grown and fixed on the slide. The slides are stable until the labeled expiration date when stored at −20° C. Do not handle the flat surface of the slide or the foil envelope. Protect the cells by handling the foil envelope by the edges.
   b. HRP lyophilized conjugate is stable before reconstitution until the labeled expiration date when stored at 2° to 8° C. The reconstituted conjugate is stable for 90 days when stored at 2° to 8° C.
   c. HRP stain reagent. Each vial contains 0.4% diaminobenzidine-HCl and phosphate buffer. Thimerosal is added as a preservative. Reconstitute the stain reagent with deionized water as directed on the label. Add the contents of one vial of 0.3% H_2O_2 immediately before

use. The unreconstituted stain reagent is stable until the labeled expiration date when stored at 2° to 8° C. CAUTION: Diaminobenzidine-HCl is a possible carcinogen. Avoid contact with the skin or ingestion.

   d. Hydrogen peroxide. Ready-to-use 0.3% hydrogen peroxide. The H_2O_2 is stable until the labeled expiration date when stored at 2° to 8° C.

   e. Phosphate-buffered saline (PBS). Each unit contains dry powder phosphate-buffered saline blend. Dissolve contents in distilled or deionized water as directed by the label and store at 2° to 8° C.

   f. Mounting medium. Ready-to-use. Contains phosphate-buffered glycerol. Thimerosal is added as a preservative.

2. 12- × 75-mm test tubes and rack
3. Pasteur and calibrated pipettes
4. Staining dish or Coplin jar
5. Moist chamber for incubation
6. Volumetric flask for PBS
7. Distilled or deionized water: CAP Type 1 or equivalent, pH 6.0-7.0
8. Forceps
9. Coverslips
10. Wash bottle
11. Blotting or bibulous paper
12. Light microscope

Quality Control

NOTE: These controls are commercially prepared by ISOLAB and included in the test kit.

Positive Control Serum

ANA- (homogeneous) positive control serum is a ready-to-use human serum in a dropper vial containing ANAs demonstrating a strong homogeneous staining reaction (1:40 dilution). Sodium azide (0.1% w/v) is added as a preservative. The positive control serum is stable until the labeled expiration date when stored at 2° to 8° C. The ANA-positive control should demonstrate homogeneous staining in the nuclei of the HEp-2 cells.

Negative Control Serum

This is a ready-to-use human serum in a dropper vial containing no detectable autoantibodies (1:40 dilution). Sodium azide (0.1% w/v) is added as a preservative. The negative control serum is stable until the labeled expiration date when stored at 2° to 8° C.

The ANA negative control serum should demonstrate little or no nuclear staining.

The control serums must be examined before any patient specimens are examined. The control results must provide the correct positive and negative reactions to validate procedural results. Controls that do not give expected reactions are considered unsatisfactory, and patient test results should not be reported. If the controls do not produce the expected results, the test procedure must be repeated.

CAUTION: Because the control serum is derived from human sources, it should be handled in the same manner as clinical serum specimens (see Universal Blood and Body Fluid Precautions in Chapter 6).

Procedure

Allow serum specimens to reach room temperature before testing. Do not interchange components from other sources.

1. Prepare sample by diluting each serum 1:40 in PBS. If a serum has previously tested positive, it should be titered to the end point.
2. Prepare slides by removing a sufficient number of slides from storage. Allow them to equilibrate to room temperature (15 to 30 minutes); remove from envelope and label. Handle envelope and slide by edges only.
3. Apply samples and controls. Use 1 drop of the screening dilution or titration dilution per well. Apply 1 drop of the positive control and 1 drop of the negative control to the appropriate wells on at least one slide of each test run. NOTE: From this step on, the slides must remain wet.
4. Incubate the slides in a covered moist chamber at room temperature for 30 minutes.
5. Remove the slides from the chamber and rinse briefly with a gentle stream of PBS. Direct the stream away from wells.
6. Place the slides in a Coplin or staining jar filled with PBS for 5 minutes to wash. Occasionally agitate the slides initially, at midpoint, and before removal. Repeat this wash process with fresh PBS.
7. Remove the slides one at a time from the wash solution; drain the excess PBS. If blotting is preferred, blot gently around slide periphery only, with the edge of blotting or bibulous paper. Do not blot directly over the wells. Return to moist chamber.
8. Apply conjugate by dispensing 1 drop (approximately 20 to 30 µL) of conjugate to each well on each slide used.
9. Incubate the slides in a moist chamber at room temperature for 30 minutes. Protect from excess light.
10. Remove the slides from the moist chamber and rinse briefly with a gentle stream of PBS. Direct the stream away from the wells.
11. Place the slides in a Coplin or staining jar filled with PBS to wash. Leave the slides in the PBS for 5 minutes with occasional agitation (initially, at midpoint, and before removing the slides from the wash). Repeat this washing process once with fresh PBS.
12. Reconstitute with 10 mL of distilled water. Add the contents of one vial of 0.3% H_2O_2 immediately before use. Mix well by gentle inversion or agitation.
13. Remove the slides from the wash buffer, drain the excess PBS, and return to the moist chamber. Flood the wells with the stain reagent. Do not allow wells to dry. Discard any unused reconstituted stain.
14. Incubate the slides for 15 minutes in a covered moist chamber at room temperature. Protect from light.
15. Remove the slides from the moist chamber and rinse with a gentle stream of PBS. Place the slides in a Coplin or staining jar filled with PBS for 10 minutes. Agitate at entry, midpoint, and before removal.

16. Remove the slides (one at a time) from the wash buffer and drain excess PBS by gently tapping the horizontal edge of the slide. If blotting is preferred, see directions in step 7.
17. Apply 1 small drop of mounting media in each specimen well. Gently apply coverslip without pressure.
18. Examine the slides with a light microscope using high (40×) magnification.

Reporting Results

Negative

No cytoplasmic or nuclear-specific stain is observed. The cells may be slightly colored due to some nonspecific reaction of the peroxidase stain reagent.

Positive

Serum is considered positive if the nuclei of the cells stain more intensely than the negative control well and there is a clearly discernible pattern of colorations.

A grading scale similar to the one shown in Box 26-2 may be helpful in establishing the criteria for each laboratory. Positive specimens should be confirmed by repeating the test with twofold dilutions of serum. All positive ANA patterns should be titered to endpoint dilution to detect possible mixed antinuclear reactions that may not be apparent when interpreting a single screening dilution. The end point titer is the last serial dilution in which a 1+ coloration with a clearly discernible pattern is detected.

Procedure Notes

The indirect immunofluorescence test and the immunoenzyme methods are probably the most practical ways of screening for ANA in the clinical laboratory. The peroxidase enzyme-conjugated antibody method, which is comparable in sensitivity and patterns of reactivity to fluorescent methods, has certain advantages. The HRP technique has the advantages of resulting in a permanent slide and requiring only a conventional light microscope with no special equipment.

Sources of Error

False-negative results can occur if the ANA happens to be specific for an antigen other than the one used in the procedure. False-negative results may also occur if the substrate is fixed in acetone and is inadequately washed. However, without fixation some soluble nuclear antigen may be lost. False-negative results may also be related to the binding of antinuclear factor to circulating immune complexes and to a low antibody titer.

False-positive interpretations may occur because of nonspecific staining, which may resemble a speckled pattern of reactivity. These staining reactions occur whenever the conjugate or the serum contains antibodies to other tissue antigens. Careful rinsing and removal of excess fluoresceinated conjugate minimizes the risk of some nonspecific staining reactions.

Clinical Applications

In the evaluation of patients with connective tissue disease, the ANA must be interpreted with caution. Under proper testing conditions, a negative ANA generally rules out SLE. A negative ANA result, however, can result from autoimmune disease in remission or nuclear autoantibodies not detectable with indirect immunofluorescent or peroxidase immunoenzyme procedures.

The significance of a positive ANA depends on the titer and to a lesser extent on the observed pattern (Table 26-7). There is no general agreement on the significance of the various patterns, and it should be noted that some patterns may mask other patterns in high concentration. Interpretation of ANA patterns, however, can provide additional information about the type of nuclear component reacting.

Because of the sensitivity of the HEp-2 cell substrate, some apparently normal individuals may show a low degree of staining at the 1:40 screening dilution. ANA titers of 1:10 to 1:80 usually have little significance but may be seen in patients with rheumatoid arthritis or scleroderma. Antinuclear antibodies are known to be sex and age dependent; therefore a positive low-titer result may be "normal" for certain individuals in the absence of other clinical signs and symptoms. If a specimen is positive at a 1:10 dilution, it should be retested at dilutions from 1:20 to 1:320. The higher the antibody titer, the more likely is the diagnosis of connective tissue disorder. Changes in the antibody titer can also be used to observe disease activity.

If the ANA test is positive, additional immunologic evaluation is necessary to determine the specificity of the reaction. These evaluations include double immunodiffusion, counterimmunoelectrophoresis, passive hemagglutination, radioimmunoassays, and identification of nuclear antigens by immunoprecipitation or immunoblotting. Such evaluations may demonstrate that more than one ANA specificity is present in the serum. An LE cell preparation is not useful because it is positive in only 75% of patients with confirmed SLE.

Limitations

No diagnosis should be based solely on the results of laboratory testing. Clinical data, antibody titers, and other laboratory findings should all be reviewed before a definitive diagnosis is established.

References

ISOLAB, Inc, Product Insert, 1985.

Box 26-2	Grading Reactions	
Negative	No cytoplasmic or nuclear specific stain observed. The cells may be slightly colored due to some nonspecific reaction of the peroxidase staining reagent.	
Borderline ±	Beige-specific stain	
Positive		
1+	Tan	
2+	Light brown	
3+	Medium brown	
4+	Dark chocolate brown to black	

TABLE 26-7 Antinuclear Antibody Patterns And Disorders

ANA Staining Pattern	Antibody Specificities	Related Disorders
Homogeneous	nDNA	Systemic lupus: erythematosus (SLE)
	dsDNA	
	ssDNA	Rheumatoid arthritis
	DNP	Sjögren's syndrome
	Histones	Mixed connective tissue diseases (MCTD)
Peripheral or rim	nDNA	Active SLE
	dsDNA	Sjögren's syndrome
	DNP	
Speckled	Smith (Sm)	SLE
	RNP	Rheumatoid arthritis
		Sjögren's syndrome
		Progressive systemic sclerosis (PSS)
		MCTD
Nucleolar	4-6S RNP	Scleroderma
		Sjögren's syndrome
		Undiagnosed illnesses manifesting
		Raynaud's phenomenon
Discrete, speckled	Centromere	CREST variant of PSS
	DNA, RNA, ENA	

CREST, Calcinosis, Raynaud's phenomenon, esophageal motility abnormalities, sclerodactyly, and telangiectasia.

Rapid Slide Test for Antinucleoprotein

Principle

SLE latex test provides a suspension of polystyrene latex particles that have been coated with deoxyribonucleoprotein (DNP). When the latex reagent is mixed with serum containing the ANAs, binding to the DNP-coated latex particles produces macroscopic agglutination. The procedure is positive in SLE and systemic rheumatic diseases (e.g., rheumatoid arthritis, scleroderma, Sjögren's syndrome, MCTD, and drug-induced lupus erythematosus).

Specimen Collection and Preparation

No special preparation of the patient is required before specimen collection. The patient must be positively identified when the specimen is collected, and the specimen is labeled at the bedside. Specimen labels must include the patient's full name, date the specimen is collected, patient's hospital identification number, and phlebotomist's initials.

Blood should be drawn by an aseptic technique. A minimum of 2 mL of clotted blood (red top evacuated tube) is required. The specimen should be centrifuged promptly and an aliquot of serum removed.

Use fresh serum. If the test cannot be performed immediately, refrigerate the specimen between 2° and 8° C for no longer than 72 hours after collection. Freeze the serum if testing is postponed for more than 72 hours.

Reagents, Supplies, and Equipment

Systemic Lupus Erythematosus (SLE) Test Kit (Product number 30D4 is available commercially from Wampole Laboratories, Princeton, NJ).

The following components are available in the kit:
1. SLE Reagent. Contains a suspension of deoxyribonucleoprotein extracted from calf thymus that is coated on polystyrene latex in a stabilized buffer. One 2.5-mL bottle. Refrigerate the latex reagent at 2° to 8° C. It is stable until the expiration date on the kit label. Do not use the reagent if it becomes grossly contaminated, or if evidence of freezing is apparent.
2. Disposable pipette/stir sticks.
3. Glass slide. It is essential that the glass slide is clean. Before use, wash it thoroughly with mild detergent, rinse several times with distilled water, and dry.

Additional required equipment: timer or stopwatch.

Quality Control

Positive Control (Human)

Must be tested with each set of tests. The positive control and SLE reagent should form a visible agglutination pattern distinctly different from the slight granularity that may be observed with the negative control. If agglutination is not visible with the positive control, the patient's test is invalid. Contains 0.1% sodium azide as a preservative.

Negative Control (Human)

The reaction between the negative control and SLE reagent should produce a smooth or slightly granular appearance at the end of 2 minutes of testing. If agglutination is observed, the patient's test is invalid. Contains 0.1% sodium azide as a preservative.

CAUTION: Because the control sera are derived from human sources, they should be handled in the same manner as clinical serum specimens (see Universal Blood and Body Fluid Precautions in Chapter 6).

WARNING: The latex reagent and controls contain 0.1% sodium azide as a preservative. Sodium azide may react with lead and copper plumbing to form highly explosive metal azides. On disposal, flush with a large volume of water to prevent azide buildup.

Procedure

NOTE: All reagents, controls, and test sera must be at room temperature before testing.

1. Check the slide for cleanliness.
2. Place one drop (50 μL) of the positive control onto the first field of the slide. Repeat this procedure for the negative control onto the second field and subsequent fields for patient specimens. Retain the pipette/stir stick for the mixing step.
3. Resuspend the latex reagent by gently mixing it. Add 1 drop of the SLE reagent to each of the divisions containing a serum specimen and the positive and negative controls. Using separate applicator sticks for each control or specimen, mix each control or specimen with the SLE reagent in a circular manner over the entire area within the division of the slide.
4. Slowly tilt the slide back and forth for 3 minutes. Observe for agglutination. Agglutination reactions with the SLE reagent are similar to those observed in blood grouping and typing reactions and should be read using a good source of indirect light.

Reporting Results

Positive = agglutination: proceed with the semiquantitative procedure if the patient result is positive.
Negative = no agglutination.

Procedure Notes

Sources of Error

Failure to observe the test mixture at the appropriate time can yield false results.

Clinical Applications

Sera from patients with SLE have been shown to contain several ANAs as determined by a wide variety of laboratory tests. A specific diagnosis depends on the evaluation of test results and clinical manifestations.

Limitations

No one test has been shown to be completely reliable for the diagnosis of SLE because many of the ANAs accompanying this disease are also demonstrated in other systemic rheumatic diseases such as rheumatoid arthritis, Sjögren's syndrome, and PSS.

Semiquantitative Procedure

1. Bring reagent and specimens to room temperature before use.
2. Using physiologic saline, dilute the patient specimens—1:2, 1:4, 1:8, 1:16, or more as needed.
3. Place one drop (50 μL) of each dilution onto successive fields of the slide.
4. Resuspend the latex reagent by gently mixing it. Add 1 drop of the SLE reagent to each of the divisions containing a serum specimen and the positive and negative controls. Using separate applicator sticks for each control or specimen, mix each control or specimen with the SLE reagent in a circular manner over the entire area within the division of the slide.
5. Slowly tilt the slide back and forth for 3 minutes. Observe for agglutination. Agglutination reactions with the SLE reagent are similar to those observed in blood grouping and typing reactions and should be read using a good source of indirect light.
6. Wash the glass slide thoroughly with mild detergent and rinse several times with distilled water.

References

SLE Latex Test Product Insert 30D4, 1995.

Case Study

This 39-year-old African-American woman with SLE was diagnosed with the illness 20 years ago. Her initial manifestations of illness developed during the postpartum period of her second pregnancy. The pregnancy had been complicated by proteinuria believed to be caused by toxemia of pregnancy.

She suffered from polyarthralgia, alopecia, and erythematous rashes of the face, arms, and legs. A renal biopsy was performed because her urinalysis revealed proteinuria and red blood cell casts. The renal biopsy revealed diffuse, proliferative glomerulonephritis. In addition to abnormal laboratory results related to renal function, she manifested antinuclear antibody (titer 1:1280) and antibodies to DNA and the C3 component of complement.

Questions and Discussion

1. Are the antibodies manifested by the patient typical of SLE?

Yes. Immunologic tests have a significant diagnostic impact. Systemic illnesses associated with ANAs, antibodies to DNA or ribonuclear proteins, and hypocomplementemia, irrespective of the clinical features, have come to be diagnosed as SLE. Also, this patient is more likely to suffer from SLE because the incidence of SLE in African-American women between the ages of 20 and 64 years is 1 in 245.

2. Do patients with SLE suffer from significant morbidity?

Yes. Several of the chronic manifestations of SLE may be responsible for significant morbidity. Discoid skin lesions can produce severe scarring and disfigurement. A rheumatoid arthropathy of the hands can develop. In addition, chronic scarring of the kidneys leads to renal failure. Infections resulting from compromised immune function secondary to SLE are responsible for significant morbidity and mortality.

Diagnosis

System Lupus Erythematosus

Case Study

History and Physical Examination

A 27-year-old female Caucasian seeks medical attention because of persisting pain in her wrists and ankles and an unexplained skin irritation on her face. On physical examination, swelling of the joints of the hands and ankles is evident, along with erythema of the skin over the bridge of the nose and the upper cheeks. The patient has a slightly elevated temperature.

Laboratory Data

The following laboratory tests are ordered: a complete blood count, urinalysis, and rheumatoid arthritis screening test. Results are:
- Hemoglobin and hematocrit: normal
- Total leukocyte count: 7.0×10^9/L
- Differential leucocyte count: normal
- Gross and microscopic urinalysis results: normal
- Rheumatoid arthritis screening test: positive

Follow-up

An ANA screening test is ordered. The results are positive.

Questions and Discussion

1. What is the most probable diagnosis in this case?

    The patient's symptoms are all highly suggestive of a collagen-type disease, such as one of the rheumatoid disorders. A positive ANA test result is highly suggestive of SLE.

    Manifestations of the disease range from a typical mild illness that is limited to a photosensitive facial rash and transient diffuse arthritis to life-threatening involvement of the renal, cardiac, respiratory, or CNS. In the early phases, it is often difficult to distinguish SLE from several of the other systemic rheumatic disorders, such as PSS, polymyositis, primary Sjögren's syndrome, primary Raynaud's phenomenon, and rheumatoid arthritis.
2. Does this patient fit into the general characteristics of patients with this disease?

    Yes, this disorder is approximately eight times more common in females than in males. It is most common in females during the reproductive years and may be present for years before diagnosis. The prevalence rate, based on a total population, is 1 in 2000, but it is 1 in 700 for women between 20 and 64 years old.

3. What is the principle of the ANA test?

    Antibodies to DNA with high titers of DS-DNA are seen primarily in SLE. ANA testing may be by fluorescent antibody technique or by radioimmunoassay. In the fluorescent technique, a substrate that contains only DS-DNA is used. Titers of 1:32 or greater indicate a substantial amount of antibody.

Diagnosis

Systemic Lupus Erythematosus

CHAPTER HIGHLIGHTS

SLE is the classic model of autoimmune disease. It is a systemic rheumatic disorder. Although no single cause of SLE has been identified, a primary defect in the regulation of the immune system is considered important in the pathogenesis of the disorder. Other influences include the affect of estrogens, genetic predisposition, and extraneous factors. A combination of these factors, however, may be synergistic.

SLE is a disease of acute and chronic inflammation. The manifestation of SLE results from defects in the regulatory mechanism of the immune system. Lymphocyte subset abnormalities are a major immunologic feature of SLE. The formation of lymphocytotoxic antibodies with a predominant specificity for T lymphocytes by SLE patients at least partially explains the interference with certain functional activities of T lymphocytes manifested by the patient with SLE. Regulation of antibody production of B lymphocytes, ordinarily a function of the subpopulation of T-suppressor cells, appears to be defective in SLE. Patients exhibit a state of spontaneous B lymphocyte hyperactivity with ensuing uncontrolled production of a wide variety of antibodies to both host and exogenous antigens. Host response to some antigens, however, is normal in many instances, and patients manifest a specific well-controlled humoral immune response.

Circulating immune complexes are the hallmark of SLE. Patients with SLE exhibit multiple serum antibodies that react with native or altered self-antigens. Demonstrable antibodies include antibodies to nuclear components; cell surface and cytoplasmic antigens of polymorphonuclear and lymphocytic leukocytes, erythrocytes, platelets, and neuronal cells; and IgG. The antinuclear antibody (anti-DNP) gives rise to the LE cell, which is found in the majority of untreated patients with active SLE. SLE patients with serositis may form LE cells in vivo. Antibodies also combine with their corresponding antigens to form immune complexes. When the mononuclear phagocytic system is unable to entirely eliminate these immune complexes, an accumulation of immune complexes results in the blood circulation. These circulating immune complexes are deposited in the subendothelial layers of the vascular basement membranes of multiple target organs, where they mediate inflammation. The sites of deposition are determined in part by the physiochemical properties of the particular antigens or antibodies involved.

The manifestations of SLE expressed in laboratory findings are numerous. Histologic, hematologic, and serologic abnormalities reflect the multisystem nature of this disease.

The ANA procedure is a valuable screening tool for SLE. It has replaced the LE cell test because of its wider range of reactivity with nuclear antigens and its greater sensitivity and quality control characteristics. ANA are a heterogeneous group of circulating Igs (e.g., IgM, IgG, and IgA). These Igs react with the whole nucleus or nuclear components such as nuclear proteins, DNA, or histones in host tissues; therefore, they are true autoantibodies. Generally, ANAs have no organ or species specificity and are capable of cross-reacting with nuclear material from humans (e.g., human leukocytes or various animal tissues). Demonstration of ANAs in laboratory testing can indicate various systemic autoimmune connective tissue disorders. These disease states are characterized by antibodies that react with different nuclear components such as double-stranded DNA, single-stranded DNA, and Sm antigen. ANAs can be found in SLE, MCTD, PSS (or scleroderma), Sjögren's syndrome, polymyositis/dermatomyositis, and rheumatoid arthritis. A small percentage of patients with neoplastic diseases may also demonstrate the presence of ANAs.

It is possible to divide ANAs into different groups to provide a systematic classification. These groups are antibodies to DNA, antibodies to histone and nonhistone proteins, and antibodies to nuclear antigens. Antibodies to DNA can be divided into two major groups: antibodies that react with native (double-stranded) DNA, and antibodies that recognize denatured (single-stranded) DNA only. Detection of autoantibodies by immunofluorescence has become an extremely valuable method. Immunofluorescence is extremely sensitive and may show positive results in cases where procedures for antinuclear antibodies, such as complement fixation or precipitation, give negative results. At present the immunofluorescent method is the most widely used technique for ANA screening.

REVIEW QUESTIONS

1. SLE is more common in:
   A. female infants
   B. male infants
   C. adolescent through middle-age women
   D. adolescent through middle-age men

2. One of the most potent inducers of abnormalities and clinical manifestations of SLE is:
   A. hydralazine
   B. procainamide
   C. isoniazid
   D. penicillin

3. The cellular aberrations in SLE include:
   A. B cell depletion
   B. deficiency of T-suppressor cell function
   C. hyperproduction of helper T cells
   D. both B and C

4. The principal demonstrable antibody in SLE is antibody to:
   A. nuclear antigen
   B. cell surface antigens of hematopoietic cells
   C. cell surface antigens to neuronal cells
   D. lymphocytic leukocytes

5. The sites of immune complex deposition in SLE are influenced by all of the following factors except:
   A. molecular size
   B. molecular configuration
   C. immune complex specificity
   D. immunoglobulin class

6. Renal disease secondary to SLE can be assessed by:
   A. antibody to native dsDNA
   B. levels of C3 and C4
   C. levels of ANA
   D. all of the above

7. SLE is a classic model of autoimmune disease and is:
   A. an abnormality of the joints
   B. a systemic rheumatoid disorder
   C. an abnormality of connective tissue
   D. all of the above

8. The overall incidence of SLE exists in an increased frequency among:
   A. American
   B. Native-Americans
   C. Puerto Ricans
   D. all of the above

9. Patients with SLE characteristically manifest:
   A. a butterfly rash over the bridge of the nose
   B. skin lesions on the arms and legs
   C. ulcerations on the trunk of the body
   D. photophobia

10. Laboratory features of SLE are:
    A. the presence of ANAs
    B. circulating anticoagulant and immune complexes
    C. decreased levels of complement
    D. all of the above

11. Laboratory procedures that are helpful in assessing renal disease include:
    A. antibody to double-stranded DNA
    B. levels of C3 and C4
    C. cryoglobulin assay
    D. all of the above

12. Antinuclear antibodies are always indicative of SLE.
    A. true
    B. false

Questions 13-16. Match the appropriate antibody and disease.

13. _____ Jo-1   A. systemic lupus erythematosus

14. _____ Mi-I   B. dermatomyositis
     C. progressive systemic

15. _____ SS-B/la   sclerosis
     D. polymyositis

16. _____ RANA

Questions 17 and 18. Match the interpretation of the ANA staining pattern to its respective antibody.

17. _____ diffuse or homogeneous pattern

18. _____ speckled pattern

A. anti-DNA-nucleoprotein antibody
B. antibody to nucleolar RNA
C. antibody to any extractable nuclear antigen devoid of DNA or histone
D. anti-centromere antibody

BIBLIOGRAPHY

Boumpas DT et al: Systematic lupus erythematosus: emerging concepts, *Ann Intern Med* 123(1): 42-53, July 1, 1995.

Bridges AJ et al: Antinuclear antibody testing in a referral laboratory, *Lab Med* 24(6):345-349, 1993.

CenterWatch Clinical Trials Listing Service, 2002, website: www.centerwatch.com.

Condemi JJ: The autoimmune diseases, *JAMA* 268(20):2882-2888, 1992.

Couser WG: Glomerular involvement in systemic diseases. In Stein J, editor: *Internal medicine,* ed 4, Boston, 1994, Little, Brown.

Fritzler MJ, Tan EM: Antibodies to histones in drug-induced and idiopathic lupus erythematosus, *J Clin Invest* 62:560, 1978.

Greenwals CA, Peebles CL, Nakamura RM: Laboratory tests for antinuclear antibody (ANA) in rheumatic disease, *Lab Med* 9:19-27, 1978.

Hammersburg G, Keren DF: Detection of antineutrophil cytoplasm antibodies in Wegener's granulomatosis, *Lab Med* 22(11):783-786, 1991.

Holborow EJ: Autoantibodies in rheumatic diseases. In Scott JT, editor: *Copeman's textbook of the rheumatic diseases,* ed 6, New York, 1986, Churchill Livingstone.

Hughes GVR: Systemic lupus erythematosus. In Scott JT, editor: *Copeman's textbook of the rheumatic diseases,* ed 6, New York, 1986, Churchill Livingstone.

Kallenberg C et al: Antineutrophil cytoplasmic antibodies: a still-growing class of autoantibodies in inflammatory disorders, *Am J Med* 93:675-682, 1992.

Karsh J et al: Anti-DNA, anti-deoxyribonucleoprotein and rheumatoid factor measured by ELISA in patients with systemic lupus erythematosus, Sjögren's syndrome and rheumatoid arthritis, *Int Arch Allergy Appl Immunol* 68:60, 1982.

Katan MB: Answers to the antiphospholipid antibody syndrome, *N Engl J Med* 33(15):1025, 1995.

Khamashta M et al: The management of thrombosis in the antiphospholipid-antibody syndrome, *N Engl J Med* 332(15):993-997, 1995.

Klippel JH: Systemic lupus erythematosus, *JAMA* 263(13):1812-1815, 1990.

Klippel JH, Decker JL: Systemic lupus erythematosus. In Stein JH, editor: *Internal medicine,* ed 4, Boston, 1994, Little, Brown.

Lockshin M: Therapy for systemic lupus erythematosus, *N Engl J Med* 324(3):189-192, 1991.

Lupus Foundation 2002, website: www.lupus.org.

Metzger AL et al, editors: In vivo LE cell formation in peritonitis due to systemic lupus erythematosus, *J Rheum* 1(1):130-133, 1974.

Mills JA: Systemic lupus erythematosus, *N Engl J Med* 330(26):1871-1879, 1994.

Pandya MR: In vivo L phenomenon in pleural fluid, *Arthritis Rheum* 19(5):962-963, 1976.

Persellin RH, Takeuchi A: Antinuclear antibody-negative systemic lupus erythematosus: loss in body fluids, *J Rheum* 7(4):547-550, 1980.

Provost TT, Alexander EL: Cutaneous manifestations of connective tissue disease. In Stein JH, editor: *Internal medicine,* ed 4, Boston, 1994, Little, Brown.

Sanchez-Guerrero J et al: Postmenopausal estrogen therapy and the risk for developing systemic lupus erythematosus, *Ann Intern Med* 122(6):430-433, 1995.

Steinberg AD: Systemic lupus erythematosus, *Ann Intern Med* 115(7):548-559, 1991.

Chapter 27

Rheumatoid Arthritis

LEARNING OBJECTIVES

At the conclusion of this chapter, the reader should be able to:
- Describe the etiology, epidemiology, and signs and symptoms of rheumatoid arthritis.
- Discuss the immunologic manifestations and diagnostic evaluation of rheumatoid arthritis.

- Briefly describe Felty's syndrome and juvenile rheumatoid arthritis.
- Explain diagnostic procedures used in the identification and evaluation of rheumatoid arthritis.
- Analyze representative case studies.

ETIOLOGY

The etiology of rheumatoid arthritis (RA) remains unknown. Genetic factors are important, as are hormonal and psychosomatic factors. Evidence exists that immunologic factors are involved in both the articular and extraarticular manifestations of the disease. RA may represent an unusual host response to one or perhaps many etiologic agents. An infectious etiology is possible, although it has not been established.

EPIDEMIOLOGY

Rheumatic diseases are among the oldest diseases recognized. Arthritis and osteoarthritis are among the most prevalent chronic conditions. Rheumatoid arthritis has an estimated incidence of 1% to 2% worldwide. The incidence of RA in the United States has an average of about 70 per 100,000 annually. RA affects all races.

This disease can begin at any age, but it initially occurs most frequently between the ages of 30 and 50 years. The incidence of rheumatoid arthritis is more than 10% in people older than 65 years. Older age and overweight are commonly recognized risk factors for arthritis. Analysis precludes determination of whether overweight precedes or results from arthritis; however, overweight has been established as a risk factor for osteoarthritis of the knee.

The female-male ratio of RA is 2.5:1. The National Health Interview Survey provides estimates of the prevalence and impact of arthritis among women 15 years old and over. For women over 45 years old, arthritis is the leading cause of activity limitation. An estimated 4.6 million (4.6%) women reported arthritis as a major or contributing cause of activity limitation from 1989 to 1991, and an estimated 22.8 million (22.7%) women self-reported arthritis from 1989 to 1991. The prevalence of self-reported arthritis increased directly with age and was 8.6% for women ages 15 to 44 years, 33.5% for women ages 45 to 64 years, and 55.8% for women ages 65 and over. Rates were higher for women who were overweight (28.9%), had 11 or fewer years of education (30.0%), and resided in households with an annual income of less than $20,000 (29.9%). Adjusted rates of activity limitation were higher for African-Americans and American Indians/Alaskan Native women than for Caucasian women.

RA occurs worldwide, but no definite geographic or climatic variation in incidence has been established. Although no specific genetic relationship has been established, a small increase in incidence has been noted in first-degree relatives of patients with RA. Persons with the HLA-DR4 haplotype do have a significantly higher incidence of RA.

Patients with RA have a shortened life span. The most frequent cause of death is cardiovascular disease. An increased prevalence of atherosclerosis in RA exists and is suspected to be related to: atherogenic side effects of some antirheumatic medications, the effects of chronic systemic inflammation on the vascular endothelium, or shared mechanisms between RA and atherosclerosis.

Complications resulting from an increased frequency of local or extraarticular infections in RA patients have been demonstrated. Mortality may result from conditions such as septicemia, pneumonia, lung abscess, or pyelonephritis. In the past decade the pharmacotherapy of RA has been improved by the development of more effective medications.

SIGNS AND SYMPTOMS

The term *rheumatic disease* does not have a clear boundary; more than 100 different conditions are labeled as rheumatic diseases, including rheumatoid arthritis, osteoarthritis, and autoimmune disorders (e.g., systemic lupus erythematosus [SLE] and scleroderma), osteoporosis, back pain, gout, fibromyalgia, and tendonitis.

RA is a chronic, multisystemic, autoimmune disorder and a progressive inflammatory disorder of the joints. It is, however, a highly variable disease that ranges from a mild illness of brief duration to a progressive, destructive polyarthritis associated with a systemic vasculitis (Figure 27-1).

The pathogenesis of the disorder has three distinct stages:
- Initiation of synovitis by the primary etiologic factor
- Subsequent immunologic events that perpetuate the initial inflammatory reaction
- Transition of an inflammatory reaction in the synovium to a proliferative destructive process of tissue

RA often begins with prodromal symptoms such as fatigue, anorexia, weakness, and generalized aching and stiffness not localized to articular structures. Joint symptoms

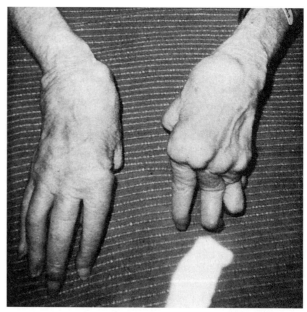

Figure 27-1 Swan-neck deformity, ulnar deviation, dorsal interosseous atrophy, and swelling of wrist—characteristics of rheumatoid arthritis. (From Kaye D, Rose LF: *Fundamentals of internal medicine,* St Louis, 1983, Mosby.)

Box 27-1	Extraarticular Manifestations of Rheumatoid Arthritis

Constitutional manifestations (e.g., weight loss and fatigue)
Subcutaneous rheumatoid nodules
Ocular abnormalities (e.g., inflammatory lesions of the episclera and sclera)
Vasculitis
Neuropathy (e.g., mononeuritis multiplex)
Myopathy
Cardiac manifestations (e.g., pericarditis)
Pulmonary manifestations (e.g., pleural effusion)
Osteoporosis
Felty's syndrome—a complex of chronic rheumatoid arthritis, splenomegaly, anemia, thrombocytopenia, and neutropenia

---

usually appear gradually over weeks to months. A wide variety of extraarticular manifestations (Box 27-1) can be manifested.

The revised American Rheumatism Association's criteria for diagnosis of RA are presented in Box 27-2. If these conditions are present for at least 6 weeks, the patient is designated as suffering from classic RA. Prognostic markers such as a persistently high number of swollen joints, high serum levels of acute-phase reactants of immunoglobulin (Ig)M rheumatoid factor, early radiographic and functional abnormalities, and the presence of certain HLA class II alleles may help identify patients with more severe RA who are still in the early stages of the disease.

<table>
<tr><td></td></tr>
</table>

| Box 27-2 | Classification of Rheumatoid Arthritis |

CRITERION

Four of the following must be present, with 1 through 4 present a minimum of 6 weeks.

1. Morning stiffness in and around the joints that lasts for at least 1 hour
2. Arthritis of 3 or more joint areas; at least 3 joints have soft tissue swelling or fluid. The 14 possible areas are right or left posterior interphalangeal (PIP), metacarpophalangeal (MCP), wrist, elbow, knee, ankle and metatarsophalangeal joints
3. Arthritis of wrist, MPC, or PIP joint
4. Symmetric involvement of joints; simultaneous involvement of the same joint areas as defined in No. 2 on both sides of the body
5. Rheumatoid nodules over bony prominences, or extensor surfaces, or in juxtaarticular regions
6. Positive serum rheumatoid factor
7. Radiographic changes, including erosions or bony decalcification localized in or adjacent to the involved joints

From Arnett FC et al: The American Rheumatism Association 1987 revised criteria for the classification of rheumatoid arthritis, *Arthritis Rheum* 31:315-324, 1988.

ANATOMY AND PHYSIOLOGY OF JOINTS

Diarthrodial joints are lined at their margins by a synovial membrane (synovium) with synovial cells lining this space. The lining cells synthesize protein as well as being phagocytic. Synovial (joint) fluid is a transparent, viscous fluid. Its function is to lubricate the joint space and transport nutrients to the articular cartilage. Mechanical, chemical, immunologic, or bacteriologic damage may alter the permeability of the membrane and capillaries to produce varying degrees of inflammatory response. In addition, inflammatory joint fluids contain lytic enzymes that produce depolymerization of hyaluronic acid, which greatly impairs the lubricating ability of the fluid.

A variety of disorders produces changes in the number and types of cells and chemical composition of the fluid. Analysis of synovial fluid plays a major role in the diagnosis of joint diseases. Arthrocentesis constitutes a liquid biopsy of the joint. It is a fundamental part of the clinical database together with the medical history, physical examination, and plain radiographic films. Analysis of aspirated synovial fluid is essential in the evaluation of any patient with joint disease because it is a better reflection of the events in the articular cavity than abnormal blood tests. For example, abnormal test results such as antinuclear antibody (ANA), increased erythrocyte sedimentation rate (ESR), elevated uric acid, and rheumatoid factor (RF) can be seen in normal individuals or in unrelated joint diseases.

Disorders such as gout, calcium pyrophosphate dihydrate deposition disease, and septic arthritis can be diagnosed definitively by synovial fluid analysis and may allow for consideration or exclusion of RA and SLE. Synovial fluid analysis can also support a diagnosis of diseases as disparate as amyloidosis, hypothyroidism, ochronosis, hemochromatosis, or even simple edema. In addition, arthrocentesis may alleviate elevated intraarticular pressure. Removal of fluid will relieve symptoms and potentially decrease joint damage. Removal of the products of inflammation is an important component in the treatment of infectious arthritis and may be beneficial in other forms of arthritis.

Routine analysis of synovial fluid should include wet preparation examination for cell count and differential, crystals, Gram stain, and microbiologic culture. Very turbid fluids, or if septic arthritis is considered for other reasons, should be sent for Gram stain and culture. A Gram stain is needed if a high likelihood of infection exists. Other observations and procedures can include volume and appearance, viscosity, mucin test, chemical analysis for protein, and glucose.

IMMUNOLOGIC MANIFESTATIONS

Two pathogenic mechanisms have been hypothesized in RA:

1. The extravascular immune complex hypothesis proposes an interaction of antigens and antibodies in synovial tissues and fluid. Antigens exist as complexes in collagen, cartilage, proteoglycans, fibrinogen or fibrin, partially digested IgG, and soluble nucleoproteins. These substances can be found in articular tissues or in byproducts of the inflammatory process. These complexes react with antibodies in joint tissues and initiate the complement cascade that generates various biologically active products. Subsequent initiation of phagocytosis, engulfment with the release of hydrolytic enzymes, and production of toxic O_2 and arachidonic acid metabolites are directly responsible for inflammation and tissue damage.
2. The alternate hypothesis is that RA results from cell-mediated damage because the accumulation of lymphocytes, primarily T cells, in the rheumatoid synovium resembles a delayed-type hypersensitivity reaction. The presence of lymphokines, which affect both articular inflammation and destruction, supports this hypothesis.

When the rheumatoid synovium is examined by the immunofluorescent technique, it can be seen to contain large amounts of IgG and IgM, alone or together. Igs can also be seen in synovial lining cells, blood vessels, and interstitial connective tissues. B cells make Ig in the synovium of patients with RA. As many as half of the plasma cells that can be located in the synovium secrete an IgG RF that combines in the cytoplasm with similar IgG molecules (self-associating IgG).

The leukotrienes play a major role in the inflammatory response to injury. This class of biologically active molecules has been implicated in the pathogenesis of RA as well as in other inflammatory diseases (e.g., asthma, psoriasis, and inflammatory bowel disease). Leukotrienes are major constituents of a group of oxygenated fatty acids that are synthesized de novo from membrane phospholipid through a cascade of enzymes known as the arachidonic acid cascade. Current research is focused on these molecules because leukotriene inhibitors and antagonists will probably become important agents in the group of antiinflammatory drugs.

DIAGNOSTIC EVALUATION

Low serum iron and a normal or low iron-binding capacity are common features. The ESR is elevated to a variable degree in most patients and roughly parallels the level of disease activity. Serum protein electrophoresis may demonstrate elevations in the alpha-2 and gamma globulin fractions, with a mild to moderate decrease in serum albumin. The gamma globulin increase is polyclonal.

Immunologic features of RA include RF, immune complexes, characteristic complement levels, and ANAs.

Rheumatoid Factor

RF belongs to a larger family of antiglobulins usually defined as antibodies with specificity for antigen determinants on the Fc fragment of human or certain animal IgG. RFs have been associated with three major Ig classes: IgM, IgG, and IgA. IgM and IgG RFs are the most common.

IgM RF is manifested in approximately 70% of adults, but it is not specific for RA. The determination of RF is important in the prognosis of RA. Being RF-positive correlates with:
- The severity of the disease (in general)
- Nodules
- Other organ system involvement (e.g., vasculitis, Felty's syndrome, Sjögren's syndrome).

Changes in the serologic activity in RA were initially observed in 1929 to 1931, when it was shown that sera from RA patients agglutinated various "coccal" organisms. In 1940 it was demonstrated that sera from RA patients agglutinated sheep cells "sensitized" with rabbit antibody against sheep cells. In 1953 it was found that Cohn fraction II, or gamma globulin in human sera, tended to inhibit the rheumatoid reaction. It was shown that tanned cells coated with human gamma globulin absorbed out all agglutinating activity from rheumatoid sera. This suggested that an antigen-antibody reaction occurred. It was later shown that the addition of latex particles coated with gamma globulin to sera caused flocculation with about 70% of rheumatoid sera. Agglutination tests for RF, such as the sensitized sheep cell test, latex agglutination, and bentonite flocculation, generally detect IgM RFs because these molecules are more potent than IgG in agglutinating appropriate antigen suspensions. Because conventional procedures are semiquantitative, they may be insensitive to changes in titer and may detect only those RFs that agglutinate. Newer, more sensitive methods such as nephelometric and turbidometric assays, radioimmunoassays, and enzyme-linked immunosorbent assays (ELISAs) have been developed.

RF has been associated with some bacterial and viral infections such as hepatitis and infectious mononucleois and some chronic infections such as tuberculosis, parasitic disease, subacute bacterial endocarditis, and cancer. Elevated values may also be observed in the normal elderly population.

Immune Complexes

Soluble, circulating immune complexes and cryoprecipitable proteins consisting of Igs, complement components, and RFs are demonstrable in the serum of some patients with RA. Antigamma globulins of the IgG and IgM classes are an integral part of these complexes.

The various vascular and parenchymal lesions of RA suggest that the lesions result from injury induced by immune complexes, especially those containing antibodies to IgG. Vasculitis is associated with complexes made up of IgG and 7S IgM RFs. A positive laboratory assay for mixed cryoglobulins indicates the presence of a large number of immune complexes and is associated with an increased incidence of extraarticular manifestations, particularly vasculitis.

Complement Levels

Serum complement levels are usually normal in patients with RA, except in those with vasculitis. Hemolytic complement levels are reduced in the serum of less than one third of patients, especially in patients with very high levels of RF and immune complexes. Levels of C4 and C2 are most profoundly depressed in these patients.

Antinuclear Antibodies

ANAs have been found in 14% to 28% of patients with RA. These patients usually suffer from advanced disease. However, disease manifestation is the same in both ANA-positive and ANA-negative patients.

FELTY'S SYNDROME

Felty's syndrome is the association of RA with splenomegaly and leukopenia. This syndrome almost always develops in patients with a high-titer RF assay, a positive ANA assay, and rheumatoid nodules. In addition, patients have a high titer of immune complex and low total serum complement levels.

HLA-DR4 is found in 95% of patients who have a propensity for bacterial infections.

JUVENILE RHEUMATOID ARTHRITIS

Etiology

Juvenile rheumatoid arthritis (JRA) is a condition of chronic synovitis beginning during childhood. The etiologic hypotheses are similar to those proposed for adult RA. The etiology is expected to be multiple and includes factors such as infection, autoimmunity, and trauma. Research done at Tulane University Medical Center suggests that JRA may be associated with a retroviral particle called human intracisternal A-type particle (HIAP). Antibodies to this particle have been found in a very high percentage of patients with JRA. These antibodies have also been found in a very high percentage of patients with three other autoimmune disorders: SLE, Sjögren's syndrome, and Graves' disease. Researchers believe that these four disorders may result from the presence of HIAP together with genetic factors and some internal or external stimulus, which all combine to dictate the specific symptomatology.

Epidemiology

The incidence of JRA in pediatric populations is between 0.1 and 1.1 per 1000 children in the United States.

Signs and Symptoms

Diagnostic criteria include onset before the age of 16 years, presence of arthritis (i.e., joint swelling for 6 consecutive

TABLE 27-1	Apparent Subgroups of JRA	
Subgroup	**Age at Onset**	**Immunologic Manifestations**
Systemic onset (Still's disease)	Any	ANA = negative RF = negative
RF-negative polyarthritis	Any	ANA = 25% positive RF = negative
RF-positive polyarthritis	Older	ANA = 50% positive RF = 100% positive HLA-DR4
Pauciarticular I	Younger	ANA = 60% positive HLA-DR5, HLA-DRw6, and HLA-DRw8
Pauciarticular II	Older	HLA-B27

References: Rheuma-Fac Rheumatoid Arthritis Test (Latex) Product Insert, Fountain Valley, Calif, July 1987, ICL Scientific (with permission); Sigma Diagnostics Product Brochure, Procedure No. SIA 107.

weeks or longer), and exclusion of other conditions known to cause or mimic childhood arthritis.

Several distinct subgroups of JRA (Table 27-1) vary in signs and symptoms and immunologic manifestations. These disorders include Still's disease, polyarticular onset, pauciarticular onset, and RA.

Still's Disease

One fifth of patients with juvenile RA suffer from Still's disease. These patients tend to be HLA-DR5 positive.

Systemic manifestations occur early and are present with a variety of signs and symptoms. These abnormalities include high intermittent fever with a rash, serositis, lymphadenopathy, hepatosplenomegaly, leukocytosis, and anemia. The diagnosis is frequently one of exclusion because polyarthritis and arthralgia are not prominent in the early stage. Arthritis occurs late in the course of the disease and rarely leads to chronic polyarthritis.

Polyarticular Onset

Polyarthritis begins in five or more joints and occurs in about 40% of patients. HLA-DRw6 has been correlated with this abnormality.

Pauciarticular Onset

Arthritis involving four or fewer joints occurs in 40% of patients. Two distinctive subgroups have been identified. The first group is populated by girls who are younger than 6 years old, are ANA positive, and have iridocyclitis. Iridocyclitis can lead to blindness. This subgroup is associated with HLA-Dw5 and HLA-DR5. The other subgroup is populated by boys younger than 6 years old with bilateral sacroiliitis. This subgroup is associated with HLA-B27.

Rheumatoid Arthritis

The remaining 20% of children meet the criteria for RA as defined by the American Rheumatism Association's criteria. Children in this group are HLA-DR4 positive.

Immunologic Manifestations

Immunologic features of JRA include RF, immune complexes, and ANAs.

Rheumatoid Factors

Approximately one fifth of children are positive for RF. Most patients who are positive for RF probably represent adult RA occurring in childhood. Detection of "hidden" RF can be detected in 65% of children with negative latex fixation tests. Children in this category do not develop the clinical manifestations of adults with RA.

Immune Complexes

Soluble immune complexes may be detected in patients with Still's disease and active synovitis. Monitoring of these complexes is not useful for diagnosis, prognosis, or monitoring of patients.

Antinuclear Antibodies

ANAs are detectable in very few patients with JRA. The exception is that most girls with pauciarthritis and chronic iritis demonstrate a positive test.

TREATMENT

The major goals of treatment of arthritis are to reduce pain and discomfort, prevent deformities and loss of joint function, and maintain a productive and active life. Inflammation must be suppressed and mechanical and structural abnormalities corrected or compensated for with assistive devices. Treatment options include reduction of joint stress, physical and occupational therapy, drug therapy, and surgical intervention.

Three general classes of drugs are commonly used in the treatment of RA: nonsteroidal antiinflammatory drugs (NSAIDs), corticosteroids, and remittive agents or disease-modifying antirheumatic drugs (DMARDs).

Nonsteroidal Antiinflammatory Drugs

Traditional treatment of RA consists of NSAIDs (e.g., salicylates, ibuprofen). The major effect of these agents is to reduce acute inflammation. Aspirin is the oldest drug of the nonsteroidal class, but the use of aspirin as the initial choice of drug therapy has largely been replaced by the newer NSAIDs.

Prostaglandins are a group of related compounds that are important mediators of a wide variety of physiologic processes, including immunomodulation. Prostaglandins are derived primarily from arachidonic acid via the cyclooxygenase enzymes (COX) pathway. NSAIDs inhibit prostaglandin synthesis by blocking two isoforms of COX: COX-1 and COX-2. Newer NSAID agents (e.g., Vioxx, Celebrex) selectively block the COX-2 enzyme that is primarily upregulated in response to tissue damage during inflammation but preserves COX-1 activity and enhances the safety profile.

Corticosteroids/Glucocorticoids

Corticosteroids (e.g., cortisone and prednisolone [prednisone]) have both antiinflammatory and immunoregulatory activity. Glucocorticosteroids pass through the cell membrane into the cytoplasm and activate the cytoplasmic glucocorticosteroid receptor, which represses gene expression through the transcriptional interference of activator protein 1 (AP-1) and nuclear factor kappa B. The proteins inhibited by glucocorticosteroids include IL-1, IL-2, IL-6, IL-8, tumor necrosis factor-alpha (TNF-α) and interferon gamma (IFN-γ). Glucocorticosteroids were the original selective COX-2 inhibitors.

Oral corticosteroids can produce a variety of complications, including high blood pressure, increased susceptibility to infection, and osteoporosis.

Disease Modifying Antirheumatic Drugs

Disease-modifying antirheumatic drugs (DMARDs) include leflunomide (Arava), soluble interleukin-1 (IL-1) receptor therapy, TNF inhibitors (Enbrel), infliximab (Remicade), antimalarials, methotrexate, intramuscular gold salts, hydroxychloroquine and sulfasalazine, d-penicillamine, immunosuppressive and other cytotoxic drugs (e.g., cyclosporin A, cyclophosphamide, and azathioprine).

Leflunomide (Arava)

Leflunomide was approved by the U.S. Food and Drug Administration (FDA) in October 1998. In a yearlong study, leflunomide was superior to methotrexate in preventing x-ray joint erosions. The mechanism of action is not fully understood but may be related to its ability to inhibit tyrosine kinase activity and de novo pyrimidine biosynthesis through the inhibition of the enzyme dihydroorotate dehydrogenase. In vitro studies have demonstrated the inhibition of mitogen and IL-2-stimulated T cells.

Soluble Interleukin-1 (IL-1)
Receptor IL-1Ra Product

IL-1Ra is a cytokine that has immune and proinflammatory actions and has the ability to regulate its own expression by autoinduction. Evidence supports the fact that the level of disease activity in RA, and progression of joint destruction, correlates with plasma and synovial fluid levels of IL-1. IL-1ra is an endogenous receptor antagonist.

Anakinra (Kineret)

Anakinra, a human recombinant IL-1 receptor antagonist (hu rIL-1Ra) was recently approved by the FDA for the reduction in signs and symptoms of moderately to severely active RA in patients 18 or older who have failed 1 or more DMARDS. Anakinra is the recombinant, nonglycosylated form of the human IL-1Ra. Anakinra blocks the biologic activity of IL-1 by binding to IL-1R type I.

Tumor Necrosis Factor Inhibitors

TNF-α is a proinflammatory cytokine produced by macrophages and lymphocytes. It is found in large quantities in the rheumatoid joint and is produced locally in the joint by synovial macrophages and lymphocytes infiltrating the joint synovium. The proinflammatory effects of TNF-α suggests that inhibition of TNF-α would be clinically useful in RA.

Etanercept (Enbrel)

Etanercept is a human fusion protein that combines two extracellular binding domains of the p75 form of the TNF receptor to the Fc portion of a human IgG$_1$ antibody molecule. The protein is entirely human and thus has a low potential for immunogenicity (anti-etanercept antibodies). A naturally occurring soluble form of the p75 TNF receptor is found in the circulation and may be part of a pathway to limit TNF activity in the inflammatory response to infection. The resultant fusion protein is a soluble molecule that binds TNF-α at high affinity. Similar to a monoclonal antibody, etanercept, when given as a therapeutic agent, binds TNF-α in the circulation, preventing interaction with the cell surface TNF-α receptors and clears TNF-α from the circulation. Etanercept inhibits TNF activity.

Etanercept, which was approved in 2002, is the first therapy approved for treatment of psoriatic arthritis. This medication can be used with or without methotrexate. Psoriatic arthritis is an often painful chronic inflammatory disease characterized by both joint and skin manifestations. Unlike other types of arthritis, patients with psoriatic arthritis often experience progressive joint pain and swelling, coupled with scaly red skin lesions. This form of arthritis typically begins with skin plaque symptoms and then progresses to joint involvement.

Infliximab (Remicade)

Infliximab, in combination with methotrexate, is indicated for reducing signs and symptoms and inhibiting the progression of structural damage in patients with moderately to severely active RA who have had an inadequate response to methotrexate. Infliximab is a chimeric monoclonal antibody that binds TNF-α with high affinity and specificity. During development infliximab was also called cA2. The antibody binding site for TNF is of mouse origin, with the remaining 75% of the infliximab antibody derived from a human IgG$_1$ antibody sequence. Infliximab, originally available for the treatment of refractory inflammatory bowel disease, is now approved by the FDA for use in RA. Infliximab is expected to bind TNF-α in the circulation, preventing its interaction with TNF-α receptors on the surface of inflammatory cells, and eventually clearing TNF-α from the circulation. Like etanercept, infliximab inhibits the activity of TNF.

Monoclonal antibody therapy has also been associated with "cytokine release syndrome" a clinical syndrome of fever, chills, and headache associated with the infusion of the antibody. The frequency of this syndrome has diminished with the use of chimeric and humanized antibodies that contain less mouse sequence and slower infusion rates.

Methotrexate (Rheumatrex, Trexall)

Methotrexate has become the most popular DMARD agent because of its early onset of action (4 to 6 weeks), good efficacy, and ease of administration and high patient tolerability. Methotrexate is a folic acid antagonist. The immunosuppressive and cytotoxic effects of methotrexate are due to the inhibition of dihydrofolate reductase.

Methotrexate is the only DMARD agent in which the majority of patients continue on therapy after 5 years. Methotrexate is best used in patients with persistent, active disease who may have poor prognostic factors such as the presence of RF, rheumatoid nodules, poor functional status, young age, or erosions on x-ray film.

Hydroxychloroquine (Plaquenil) or Sulfasalazine

These are generally the first DMARD agents used, particularly in patients with mild disease who are rheumatoid-factor negative. Either drug is often used in combination with an NSAID, corticosteroids, or other DMARD.

Intramuscular Gold (Myochrysine, Solganal)

Until recently, intramuscular gold salts were the most often used DMARD agents, but because of toxicity they are now used only after failure of methotrexate. A number of mechanisms have been postulated, but how gold works in patients with RA remains unknown.

d-Penicillamine

This also is a relatively toxic drug and is, like injectable gold, prescribed primarily for patients with persistent aggressive disease who have failed to achieve remission with less toxic agents.

Immunosuppressive and Other Cytotoxic Drugs

Immunosuppressive and other cytotoxic drugs, other than methotrexate (e.g., azathioprine, cyclophosphamide or cyclosporin A), are used only in patients who have aggressive disease or extraarticular manifestations such as systemic vasculitis. The most commonly used drugs are azathioprine (Imuran), cyclophosphamide (Cytoxan) and cyclosporin A. Because the potential of high toxicity, these agents are used for life-threatening extraarticular manifestations or severe articular disease refractory to other therapy.

- Azathioprine is a purine analog that can cause severe bone marrow suppression particularly in patients with renal insufficiency or when used concomitantly with allopurinol or angiotensin-converting enzyme inhibitors.
- Cyclophosphamide is an alkylating agent associated with serious toxicities including bone marrow suppression, hemorrhagic cystitis, premature ovarian failure, infection, and secondary malignancy particularly an increased risk of bladder cancer. For these reasons it is not used in the treatment of uncomplicated RA.
- Cyclosporine is an immunosuppressive agent approved for use in preventing renal and liver allograft rejection. Cyclosporine inhibits T-cell function by inhibiting transcription of IL-2.

Other Drugs

Antimalarial drugs are rapidly absorbed, relatively safe, well tolerated, and often effective remittive agents in the treatment of RA, particularly mild to moderate disease. The mechanism of action of antimalarial drugs in the treatment of patients with RA is unknown.

DIAGNOSTIC PROCEDURES

Rheumatoid factor assays

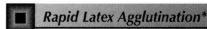

*Rapid Latex Agglutination**

Principle

The RA agglutination test is based on the reaction between patient antibodies in the serum, known as the "rheumatoid factor," and an antigen derived from human gamma globulin (IgG). Latex reagent consists of a stabilized latex suspension coated with albumin and chemically bonded with denatured human gamma globulin. This reagent serves as an antigen in the procedure. If RFs are present in the serum, macroscopic agglutination will be visible when the latex reagent is mixed with the serum. The determination of RFs is important in the prognosis and therapeutic management of rheumatoid arthritis; however, positive test results may be observed in a variety of disorders such as SLE, Sjögren's syndrome, syphilis, and hepatitis.

Specimen Collection and Preparation

No special preparation of the patient is required before specimen collection. The patient must be positively identified when the specimen is collected, and the specimen is to be labeled at the bedside. Specimen labels must include the patient's full name, the date the specimen is collected, the patient's hospital identification number, and the phlebotomist's initials.

Blood should be drawn by an aseptic technique. A minimum of 2 mL of clotted blood (red top evacuated tube) is required. The specimen should be centrifuged promptly and an aliquot of serum removed. No special preparation of the serum is required.

If the test cannot be performed immediately, the specimen should be refrigerated (2° to 8° C) for no longer than 24 hours. If additional delay occurs, the serum should be frozen at −20° C or below. Repeated freezing and thawing must be avoided. If turbidity is apparent upon thawing, the specimen should be clarified by centrifugation before use. WARNING: Do not use specimens showing gross hemolysis, lipemia, or turbidity.

Preliminary Patient Specimen Preparation

Dilute specimen 1:20 with the prepared diluent (e.g., 0.1 mL of serum and 1.9 mL of diluent) and thoroughly mix the tube contents.

Reagents, Supplies, and Equipment

The following components are commercially available in kit form (CDC Analyte Identifier Code: 5508).

*RHEUMATEX (a modification of the Singer and Plotz procedure) Wampole Laboratories (Cranbury, NJ).

1. RHEUMATEX: Latex reagent with dropper assembly. This is a suspension of latex particles sensitized with human IgG; contains buffer and preservative: sodium azide 0.1%. SHAKE WELL BEFORE USING.

   NOTE: Store at 2° to 8° C. Do not freeze latex reagent. Properly stored reagent is stable until expiration date indicated on the label. Do not use after the expiration date. Reagent that does not produce appropriate quality control results should be discarded after verification by repeat testing. The reagent should be a uniform, milky suspension of latex particles. If clumping cannot be removed after gentle vortex mixing, the reagent should be discarded.

2. Concentrated diluent 20× (Glycine-saline buffer); contains preservative: sodium azide 2.0%. Prepare a 1:20 dilution of the concentrated diluent by mixing the contents of the concentrated diluent vial with 190 mL of distilled water.

   NOTE: Store the prepared diluent at 2° to 8° C. Properly stored reagent is stable until expiration date indicated on the kit. Reagent that does not produce appropriate quality control results should be discarded after verification by repeat testing. Discard if contaminated (i.e., evidence of cloudiness or particulate material in solution).

   ADVISORY NOTE: Do not interchange reagents from different kits because the reagents from each kit have been assayed as a unit for proper sensitivity.

   The reagents in the kit contain sodium azide. See Material Safety Data Sheet (WM109ver.3 prepared 6/1/99) for identity, physical/chemical characteristics, fire and explosion hazard data, reactivity data, toxicology/health effects, first aid, precautions for safe handling, and control measures.

3. Glass slide

Additional Required Equipment and Supplies

1. Stopwatch or timer
2. 37° C water bath
3. 12- × 75-mm test tubes
4. Serologic pipettes (1-mL graduated) and safety pipette
5. Centrifuge capable 1000 μL × g
6. Light source
7. Capillary pipettes (50 μL)
8. Applicator sticks
9. Distilled water

Quality Control

A positive and negative control must be tested with each unknown patient specimen.

Positive Control

Rheumatoid Factor Positive Serum (Human); contains buffer, stabilizer and preservative: sodium azide 0.1%. This serum is provided in the RHEUMATEX kit. Store at 2° to 8° C.

NOTE: Failure to observe a positive reaction (agglutination) with this serum is indicative of deterioration of the latex reagent and/or positive control. The solution should be clear solutions—do not use if cloudy or obviously contaminated. Do not dilute the control. Observe results *immediately* at 1 minute. The positive control must show agglutination.

Negative Control

Rheumatoid Factor Negative Serum (Human); contains buffer, stabilizer and preservative: sodium azide 0.1%. This serum is provided in the RHEUMATEX kit. Store at 2° to 8° C.

NOTE: The solution should be clear solutions—do not use if cloudy or obviously contaminated. Do not dilute the control. Observe results *immediately* at 1 minute. If agglutination is exhibited with this control, the test should be repeated. If repeat testing produces the same results, the reagents should be replaced. The negative control should appear uniformly turbid.

CAUTION: Because the control sera are derived from human sources, they should be handled in the same manner as clinical serum specimens (see Universal Blood and Body Fluid Precautions in Chapter 6). Each donor unit used in the preparation of the POSITIVE and NEGATIVE CONTROLS and the Latex Reagent was tested for Hepatitis B Surface Antigen, HIV I/II and HCV by an FDA approved method and found to be nonreactive. However, handle all materials as if capable of transmitting disease (Biosafety Level 2).

Procedure

NOTE: All reagents and specimens must be at room temperature before testing.

Qualitative Slide Test

1. Prepare a 1:20 dilution of patient serum in with the prepared diluent.
2. Using a clean capillary pipette, place 1 free-falling drop of the diluted serum from the perpendicularly held pipette to the center of division of the slide.
3. Add 1 drop of positive control and 1 drop of negative control on either side section of the slide.
4. Mix the latex reagent and add 1 drop of reagent to the patient specimen and to each of the controls.
5. Mix each specimen with a separate applicator stick. All the contents of the mixtures are to spread evenly over the entire area of their respective divisions on the slide.
6. Tilt the slide back and forth, gently and evenly, for 1 minute, at a rate of 8 to 10 times per minute.
7. Observe for agglutination immediately at 1 minute, using an indirect oblique light source.
8. Positive sera exhibit readily visible agglutination. A weakly positive serum may exhibit very fine granulation or partial clumping. Negative sera appear uniformly turbid.

   WARNING: The latex reagent, controls, and buffer contain 0.1% sodium azide as a preservative. Sodium azide may react with lead and copper plumbing to form highly explosive metal azides. On disposal, flush with a large volume of water to prevent azide buildup.

Reporting Results

Positive reaction: positive sera exhibit readily visible agglutination. A weakly positive serum may exhibit very fine granulation or partial clumping.

Negative reaction: negative sera appear uniformly turbid.

Procedure Notes

Latex slide and tube tests demonstrate slightly greater sensitivity than sensitized sheep cells. The specificity of latex tube tests is comparable to sensitized sheep cell procedures.

Specimen collection and handling are important to the quality of the test. Strict adherence must be paid to technique, with a special emphasis on drop size, complete mixing, reaction time, and temperature of reagents.

The strength of a positive reaction may be graded as follows:

1+ Very small clumping with an opaque fluid background
2+ Small clumping with a slightly opaque fluid background
3+ Moderate clumping with a fairly clear fluid background
4+ Large clumping with a clear fluid background

Quantitative Slide Procedure

If a patient serum exhibits a positive reaction, it is recommended that a quantitative test be performed. The serum may be serially diluted with diluent to determine a quantitative estimate of the RA level.

1. Serum to be titrated should be serially diluted (e.g., 1:20, 1:40) with prepared diluent. At least 6 dilutions should be prepared.
2. Place 1 drop of each specimen dilution onto successive sections of the slide.
3. Test each specimen dilution as described under "Qualitative Slide Procedure" Steps 3 to 7.

Quantitative Tube Test

1. Label 11 12- × 75-mm test tubes (1 to 11) and place in a test tube rack.
2. Pipette 1.9 mL of prepared diluent into tube 1; 1.0 mL of prepared diluent into tubes 2 to 9; and 0.8 mL of prepared diluent into tubes 10 and 11.
3. Add 0.1 mL of specimen to tube 1. Mix the contents and transfer 1.0 mL of prepared diluent into tubes 2 to 9; and 0.8 mL of prepared diluent into tubes 10 and 11.
4. Pipette 0.2 mL of the positive control into tube 10 and 0.2 mL of the negative control into tube 11.

5. The concentrations of the dilutions are:

Tube Number	Dilution	Serum Concentration (IU/mL)
1	1:20	60
2	1:40	120
3	1:80	240
4	1:160	480
5	1:320	960
6	1:640	1920
7	1:1280	3840
8	1:2560	7680
9	1:5120	
10	Positive control	
11	Negative control	

6. To each tube add 1 drop of well-mixed latex reagent.
7. Shake all tubes thoroughly and incubate at 37° C for 15 minutes.
8. After incubation, centrifuge all tubes at 1000 × g for 2 minutes.
9. Gently shake each tube to resuspend the precipitate until an even suspension is achieved. Do not use automatic mixing devices.
10. Examine each tube for the presence of macroscopic agglutination by observing against a dark or black background under an oblique light.

Reporting Results

In the slide and tube quantitative procedures, the highest dilution at which agglutination can still be observed is considered the titer. If there is no agglutination at 1:20, the specimen is considered negative for RFs even if a subsequent dilution shows agglutination. When using RF latex tube titration procedures, a titer of 80 or greater is generally considered a positive reaction and titers of 20 or 40 are considered weakly positive reactions. The tube titration procedure is more sensitive than the slide procedure. Consequently, differences in the raw titers will be seen between the tube titration and slide procedures.

Sources of Error

False-positive results may be observed if:
- Serum specimens are lipemic, hemolyzed, or heavily contaminated with bacteria.
- The reaction time is longer than 2 minutes; a false-positive result may also be produced as a result of a drying effect.

Biologic false-positive results can be manifested by disorders such as systemic lupus erythematosus, Sjögren's syndrome, syphilis, and hepatitis. A low rate of positive reactions has been observed in abnormalities such as periarteritis nodosa, rheumatic fever, osteoarthritis, tuberculosis, cancer, some diseases of viral origin, osteoarthrosis, arthritis type undetermined, myositis, and polymyalgia rheumatica. Circulating RF appears to represent a phenomenon of aging independent of disease.

Clinical Applications

RF is present in the serum of approximately 70% to 80% of patients with clinically diagnosed RA. Nearly all patients with variants of RA (e.g., Felty's or Sjögren's syndrome) demonstrate positive results. The highest titers are often found in severe cases of RA. Although the latex agglutination procedure has a 95% correlation with a clinical diagnosis of probable or definite RA, RF is not exclusively limited to patients with RA.

In using latex tests for the detection of RF, a positive result can be expected in less than 5% of healthy individuals. In patients 60 years and older, as many as 30% may be seropositive.

Limitations

As in the case of other diagnostic procedures, the results obtained by this kit yield valuable data that must be evaluated as a component of the total clinical information obtained by the physician.

Approximately 25% of patients with definite RA may exhibit negative results for serum RF. Specimens from patients with JRA are usually negative for circulating RF.

The strength of the agglutination reaction in the qualitative procedure is not indicative of the actual titer. Weak reactions may occur with either slightly elevated or markedly elevated concentrations.

The RHEUMATEX test is classified as moderately complex under the CLIA'88 regulations.

References

Galen RS, Gambino SR: *Beyond normality: the predictive value and efficiency of medical diagnosis,* New York, 1975, John Wiley & Sons.

IgM RHEUMATEX, Wampole Laboratories (product insert), 1997, Dist. RHEUMATEX, 1997.

Jones WL, Wiggins GL: A study of rheumatoid arthritis latex kits, *Am J Clin Pathol* 60:703-706, 1973.

Mackay IR, Burnett FM, editors: *Autoimmune disease: serolgic reactions in rheumatoid arthritis,* Springfield, Ill, 1964, Charles C Thomas.

Singer JM, Plotz CM, Goldberg R: The detection of antiglobulin factors utilizing pre-coated latex particles, *Arthritis Rheum* 8:194-201, 1965.

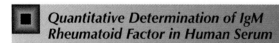

Quantitative Determination of IgM Rheumatoid Factor in Human Serum

Principle

The following procedure is an indirect enzyme-labeled immunoassay using microwells as a solid phase. Human IgG is coated onto wells of microplates. Diluted test samples are added to the coated wells and incubated. During incubation, rheumatoid factor IgM antibodies present in the sample will bind to the IgG-coated well. After a washing to remove unbound material, peroxidase conjugated goat antihuman IgM is added to the wells and the plate is incubated. The conjugate will react with antibody immobilize on the solid phase in the preceding step. The multiwells containing immobilized peroxidase conjugate are incubated with peroxidase substrate solution. Hydrolysis of the substrate produces a color change. After the reaction is stopped, the color intensity of the solution is measured photometrically. The color intensity of the solution is directly related to the antibody concentration in the test sample.

Establishing the presence of RF is useful in supporting the differential diagnosis of RA from other chronic inflammatory arthritis. The frequency of IgM RF is 70% to 80% in patients with clinical features of RA. Determination of RF is also important in the prognosis and therapeutic management of this disease. However, RF has been associated with some bacterial and viral infections such as hepatitis and infectious mononucleosis, and with some chronic infections such as tuberculosis, parasitic disease, subacute bacterial endocarditis, and cancer. Elevated values may also be observed in the normal elderly population.

Specimen Collection and Preparation

No special preparation of the patient is required before specimen collection. The patient must be positively identified when the specimen is collected, and the specimen is to be labeled at the bedside. Specimen labels must include the patient's full name, the date the specimen is collected, the patient's hospital identification number, and the phlebotomist's initials.

Blood should be drawn by an aseptic technique. A minimum of 2 mL of clotted blood (red top evacuated tube) is required. The specimen should be centrifuged promptly and an aliquot of serum removed.

If the test cannot be performed immediately, the specimen should be refrigerated (2° to 8° C) for no longer than 7 days. If additional delay occurs, the serum should be frozen at −20° C or below. Frozen serum should be thawed rapidly at 37° C. Specimens containing visible particulate matter should be clarified by centrifugation before testing. The serum sample should not be heat-inactivated before testing. Avoid multiple freeze/thaw cycles which may cause loss of antibody activity and give erroneous results.

Reagents, Supplies, and Equipment

Rheumatoid Factor EIA 507 Kit Reagents are available commercially from Sigma Chemical Co, St Louis, MO.

NOTE: Store reagents at 2° to 6° C. The reagents are stable until the expiration date on the label. The human IgG coated multiwell strips are stable for 60 days stored at 2° to 8° C. Wash Buffer and Stop Solution may be stored refrigerated or at room temperature.

1. Rheumatoid Factor ELISA plate. Microplate wells coated with human IgG. Store antigen wells with dessicant in the reusable plastic bag. Reseal the bag after opening.
2. Sample diluent. Green solution containing Tween-20, bovine serum albumin, and phosphate-buffered-saline (pH 7.2 ± 0.2). Ready to use.

Contains thimerosal 0.04%, which may be toxic if ingested.

3. Positive Control. Human serum containing IgM RF. Contains thimerosal 0.04%, which may be toxic if ingested.

4. Calibrator A, calibrator B, calibrator C, calibrator D. Contains thimerosal 0.04%, which may be toxic if ingested.

5. Negative Control. Human serum negative control. Contains thimerosal 0.04%, which may be toxic if ingested.

6. Conjugate. Horseradish peroxidase conjugated with goat antibodies to human IgM. Contains thimerosal 0.04%, which may be toxic if ingested.

7. TMB Substrate. Solution containing 3,3,5,t-tetramethylbenizidine (TMB) in dimethyl sulfoxide. Ready to use. TMB substrate is harmful. Irritating to eyes, respiratory system, and skin. Possible mutagen.

8. Wash buffer. Blue solution of phosphate-buffered-saline and Tween-20. Contains thimerosal 0.04%, which may be toxic if ingested. Wash buffer is an irritant to eyes, respiratory system, and skin. NOTE: after dilution 1X wash buffer is stable for 30 days refrigerated at 2 to 8° C or for 7 days at room temperature.

9. Stop solution. Solution containing sulfuric acid, 1 mol/L, and hydrochloric acid, 0.07 mol/L. Ready to use. The solution is toxic by inhalation. Causes burns and may cause cancer by inhalation.

NOTE: The kit also contains sample dilution plate (one 96-well plate for preparing serum dilutions), two mylar plate sealers, ELISA worksheet, and data sheet.

Additional Required Supplies and Equipment

1. Multiwell reader capable of accurately measuring absorbance at 450 nm
2. Pipetting device for the accurate delivery of volumes required for the assay 10 and 200 μL; adjustable multichannel pipette 50 to 200 μL for transferring diluted patient specimens or for dispensing conjugate, TMB Substance and Stop Solution; pipette tips.
3. Reagent reservoirs for multichannel pipettes
4. Timer
5. 1-L measuring cylinder
6. Squeeze bottle for dispensing wash solution
7. Distilled or deionized water
8. Disposal basin containing 10% bleach (0.5% sodium hypochlorite)
9. Serologic pipettes: 1, and 10 or 25 mL

Quality Control

Positive Control

Human serum containing IgM RF. Content (IU/mL) indicated on the label.

Negative Control

Human serum containing no detectable IgM RF.

CAUTION: Normal precautions exercised in handling laboratory reagents should be followed. Because the antigen wells and control and calibrator sera are derived from human sources, they should be handled in the same manner as clinical serum specimens (see Universal Blood and Body Fluid Precautions in Chapter 6).

Procedural Precautions

- Wipe bottom of plate clean.
- Do not dilute reagents.
- Do not use reagents from other sources unless common to another Sigma kit.
- Do not substitute reagents with different lot numbers.
- Never pipette by mouth.
- Avoid microbial and cross contamination of reagents and patient specimens.
- Do not use reagents that have turned a different color from the original color. Avoid strong light during storage.
- Use clean glassware.
- Wash plate carefully.
- Avoid splashing or generation of aerosols.
- Follow procedural directions carefully.
- Protect the conjugate from exposure to sodium azide.
- Do not expose any of the reactive reagents to bleach-containing solutions.

Procedure

Preparation of reagents
1. Dilute 1X wash buffer. Dilute the 100 mL of 10× concentrate with 900 mL of distilled or deionized water. Mix thoroughly to dissolve any crystals that may be present.
2. Calibrators, Sample Diluent, TMB Substrate, and Stop Solution are ready to use.
3. 1X Conjugate. Dilute the 10X conjugate 1:10 with the 1X Wash Buffer. Refer to Table 27-2 for the amount of conjugate needed for the number of tests to be run. Dilute only the amount of conjugate needed for the assay. Refrigerate remaining 10X conjugate at 2° to 8° C.

Test Procedure

1. Set-up assay.
2. Remove the individual kit components from storage and allow them to warm to room temperature (20° to 25° C). Determine the total number of calibrators, controls, and samples to be tested. The reagent blank, calibrators, negative control, and positive control must be included *each time* the assay is performed.
3. Determine the number of multiwells needed. After the strips and holder have warmed to room temperature, open the plastic bag, cut open the protective envelope, and remove the plate containing the antigen-coated multiwell strips. Unneeded strips should be returned to the pouch and plastic bag, and stored at 2° to 8° C.

TABLE 27-2   Preparation of 1X Conjugate

Number (Test)	Number (Strips)	10X Conjugate (mL)	1X Wash Buffer (mL)
8	1	0.1	0.9
9-16	2	0.2	1.8

Test Procedure

Setup of the Assay

NOTE: When using Sigma Diagnostics EIA Multi-well Plate or Strip Reader, the assay must be run as follows:

Blank	(A1)
Calibrator A	(B1)
Calibrator B	(C1)
Calibrator C	(D1)
Calibrator D	(E1)
Negative control	(F1)
Positive Control	(G1)

Controls and samples should be tested in duplicate until the laboratory becomes proficient with the test procedure. Each reagent blank, calibrators, controls, and sample requires one antigen coated multiwell.

Determine the number of multiwells needed. After the strips and holder have warmed to room temperature, open the plastic bag, cut open the protective envelope, and remove the plate containing the antigen coated multiwell strips. Strips that are not needed for the assay should be place in the pouch with dessicant and sealed. Return the pouch to the plastic bag and store at 2° to 8° C.

Prepare the 1X wash buffer according to the Preparation of Reagents section.

Serum Incubation

Prepare a 1:21 dilution of calibrators A, B, C, D, the negative and positive controls, and each patient serum as follows:

1. Add 10 μL of each sample to a separate well of the dilution plate provided. Add 200 μL of sample diluent to each well containing a sample.
2. Add 100 μL of sample diluent to well (A1) as a reagent blank. Using the multichannel pipette, transfer 100 μL of each diluted calibrator, control, and sample from the dilution plate to the test plate. Withdraw and expel several times before the final transfer to ensure that the samples are properly mixed. Use a different pipette tip for each sample.
3. Cover the wells with the plate sealer and incubate the plate at room temperature (20° to 25° C) for 20 to 22 minutes.
4. Wash the multiwell strips three times.
   a. Vigorously shake out the liquid from the wells.
   b. Fill each well with wash buffer. Make sure no air bubbles are trapped in the wells.
   c. Repeat steps (a) and (b) three times.
   d. Shake out the ash solution from all the wells. Invert the plate over a paper towel and tap firmly to remove any residual wash solution from the wells. Visually inspect the plate to ensure that no residual wash solution remains. Collect wash solution in a disposable basin

and treat with 0.5% sodium hypochlorite (bleach) at the end of the day's run.

NOTE: Auto Wash—set the dispensing volume to 300 to 350 μL/well. Set the wash cycle for three washes with no delay between washes. Remove plate from washer, invert plate over paper towel, and tap firmly to remove any residual wash solution from the well.

Conjugate Incubation

Add 100 μL of properly diluted conjugate solution (1×) to each well at the same rate and in the same order as the specimens were added.

Cover the plate with the plate sealer provided and incubate at room temperature (20° to 25° C) for 20 to 22 minutes.

Wash the plate by following the procedure in step 4 (a) through (d).

Substrate Incubation

1. Add 100 μL of TMB substrate to each well at the same rate and in the same order as the conjugate was added; 1 mL of TMB substrate is sufficient for 8 wells or 1 strip.
2. Incubate the plate at room temperature (20° to 25° C) for 10 to 12 minutes. Positive sample wells will turn blue.
3. Add 50 μL of stop solution to each well at the same rate and in the same order as the TMB substrate was added. Positive sample wells will turn from blue to yellow. After adding stop solution, tap the plate several times to ensure that samples are thoroughly mixed.
4. Set the EAI multiwell reader to read at a wavelength of 450 nm and measure the optical density (OD) of each well against the reagent blank. The plate should be read within 30 minutes after addition of the stop solution.

Quality Control

1. Each time the assay is run, a blank; calibrators A, B, C, and D; the positive control; and the negative control must be included.
2. Refer to the data sheet included with each kit. This sheet describes the lot-specific specification for each of the four calibrators. If any of the calibrators are out of range, the results are considered invalid, and patient results may not be reported.
3. The positive and negative controls must meet the following specifications: positive control must be >15 IU/mL; negative control must be <5 IU/mL.
   a. The OD value for the negative control divided by the mean OD of the positive control should be ≤0.9.
   b. If the above conditions are not met, the test should be considered invalid and should be repeated.

Interpretation of Results
Calculations
Calibrator. On the basis of testing of normal and disease-state specimens, and the World Health Organization international standard, a maximum normal IU value has been determined and correlated to the calibrators. The calibrators will allow you to determine the unit value of test samples. The unit values are determined for each lot of kit components and are printed on the data sheet.

Conversion of Optical Density to IU/mL
Optical density of the specimens are determined from the standard curve generated from the calibrators. A standard curve should be generated using the data points for each of the four calibrators (OD on the Y axis and corresponding IU/mL value on the X axis). Using the best fit, point to point curve, determine the IU/mL value by extrapolation for each of the specimens tested.

Interpretations
Negative	<6 IU/mL
Positive	≥6 IU/mL
Strongly reactive, indicative of rheumatoid arthritis	>25 IU/mL

Limitations
1. Tests result should be interpreted in conjunction with the clinical evaluation and the result of other diagnostic procedures.
2. A negative result does not exclude RA. Approximately 25% of patients with a diagnosed case of RA may present with a negative result for RF.
3. Certain nonrheumatoid conditions, connective tissue disorders, and a variety of other disease states (e.g., hepatitis) may elicit a positive RF test.
4. RF exists in three major Ig classes: IgA, IgG, and IgM. This test system will only detect IgM class RF antibodies.
5. Reproducible results with an ELISA system require careful pipetting, strict adherence to incubation periods and temperature requirements, as well as thorough washing of the test wells and thorough mixing of all solutions.
6. Hemolytic, icteric, or lipemic samples may interfere with this ELISA. These types of specimens should be avoided.

Clinical Applications
Determining the presence of RF is important to physicians in the diagnosis, prognosis, and therapeutic management of patients with RA.

Limitations
The results obtained with the assay should serve only as an aid to diagnosis and should not be interpreted as diagnostic in themselves.

References
Borque L et al: Turbidimetry of rheumatoid factor in serum with a centrifugal analyzer, *Clin Chem* 32:124, 1986.

Holborow EJ: Autoantibodies in the rheumatic diseases. In Scott JT, editor: *Copeman's textbook of the rheumatic diseases,* ed 6, New York, 1986, Churchill Livingstone.

Linker III JB, Williams RC Jr: Tests for detection of rheumatoid factors. In Rose NR, Friedman H, Fahey JL, editors: *Manual of clinical laboratory immunology,* ed 3, Washington, DC, 1986, American Society for Microbiology.

Sigma Diagnostics Product Brochure, SIA Rheumatoid Factor, St Louis, 1987.

Wernick R et al: IgG and IgM rheumatoid factors in rheumatoid arthritis: quantitative response to penicillamine therapy and relationship to disease activity, *Arthritis Rheum* 26:593, 1983.

Case Study

History and Physical Examination
A 62-year-old woman has been experiencing pain in her left knee unrelated to trauma. The pain occurs primarily with weight-bearing. She is currently being treated for hypertension, but is otherwise healthy.

She is obese. An examination of her knee shows tenderness over the medial epicondyle superior to the joint margin. There is a small effusion in her left knee.

Laboratory Data
Her laboratory data are normal, including RF assay, except for an elevated uric acid level. An x-ray film of her knee was read as normal.

Questions and Discussion
1. What is the cause of her painful knee?
    Because her serum uric acid is high, this patient is probably suffering from gouty arthritis rather than rheumatoid arthritis.
2. What might the effusion in her left knee demonstrate microscopically?
    Uric acid crystals might be seen.
3. Would a restricted diet be of value?
    Red meat should be restricted in patients suffering from gout.

Diagnosis
Arthritis

Case Study

A.D., age 31 years, was referred to a rheumatologist with increasing pain and stiffness in her fingers and wrists. Before her last pregnancy 3 years earlier, she had experienced similar symptoms but they had gone away. Since the birth of her last child, she has found it progressively more

TABLE 27-3 Case Study Laboratory Data	
Patient	**Result Reference Range**
Erythrocyte sedimentation rate	53 mm/hr
C- reactive protein	4+
IgM rheumatoid factor	Positive
ANA	Negative
Antibodies to extractable nuclear antigens	Negative
dsDNA binding activity	15%
Serum complement	
C3	1.1 (0. 75-1.65)
C4	0.4 (0.20-0.65)

awkward to carry out a variety of work tasks and hobbies such as needlepoint. The symptoms were worse in the morning. She did not have any trouble with her other joints.

Her family history revealed that her mother had RA. On physical examination the patient was pale. She had bilateral and symmetric tender and swelling of her wrists and proximal to the joints of her hands. She had normal range of movement. Her other body systems appeared to be within normal limits.

Laboratory Data

Laboratory assays were ordered (Table 27-3).

A diagnosis of early RA was made. The patient was advised to take one aspirin daily. This initially provided some relief of her symptoms. She returned to her doctor 4 months later with worsening symptoms in her hands, and pain in both knees. Synovial fluid was removed from her knees. A diagnosis of progressive RA was made.

Questions and Discussion

1. Do genetic associations exist with RA?
    RA is an autoimmune disease associated with the HLA-DR4 and DRI haplotypes.
2. Is RA more common in women?
    There is a 3:1 female-male ratio in cases of RA. Estrogens may play a role in the pathogenesis of RA. It is known that pregnancy produces a protective effect.
3. What is the immunopathogenesis of RA?
    The specificity of the T-cell response in RA is unknown. The antigen may be a self-antigen, a modified self-antigen, a foreign antigen or a superantigen. A high proportion (70% to 90%) of RA patients have antibodies to a protein from the Epstein-Barr virus (EBV). These antibodies, named rheumatoid arthritis precipitin, cross-react with a protein found in RA patients called rheumatoid arthritis nuclear antigen. RA patients also have elevated frequencies of EBV-infected B cells compared with normal subjects.
4. What is rheumatoid factor?
    RFs are autoantibodies that are able to bind IgG. RF exists in all five classes of Ig, although the best charac-

terized are IgG and IgM RF. Approximately 70% of RA patients are RF seropositive. This group tends to develop a more aggressive disease. RF appears to be a marker of disease activity with reduced levels associated with the remission of RA found during pregnancy.

Diagnosis

Rheumatoid arthritis

CHAPTER HIGHLIGHTS

Evidence exists that immunologic factors are involved in both the articular and extraarticular manifestations of RA. RA may represent an unusual host response to one or perhaps many etiologic agents. An infectious etiology is possible. RA is a chronic, usually progressive inflammatory disorder of the joints. It is, however, a highly variable disease that ranges from a mild illness of brief duration to a progressive, destructive polyarthritis associated with a systemic vasculitis.

Two pathogenic mechanisms have been hypothesized in RA. The extravascular immune complex hypothesis proposes an interaction of antigens and antibodies in synovial tissues and fluid. The alternate hypothesis is that RA results from cell-mediated damage because of the accumulation of lymphocytes, primarily T cells, in the rheumatoid synovium, resembling a delayed-type hypersensitivity reaction. The presence of cytokines, which effect both articular inflammation and destruction, supports this hypothesis.

If the rheumatoid synovium is examined by an immunofluorescent technique, it can be seen to contain large amounts of IgG and IgM, alone or together. Igs can also be observed in synovial lining cells, blood vessels, and in the interstitial connective tissues. B cells make Ig in the synovium of patients with RA. As many as half the plasma cells that can be located in the synovium secrete an IgG RF that combines in the cytoplasm with similar IgG molecules (self-associating IgG). The cause of the various vascular and parenchymal lesions of RA suggests that the lesions result from injury induced by immune complexes, especially those containing antibodies to IgG. The serum of most patients with RA has detectable soluble immune complexes. Antigamma globulins of the IgG and IgM classes are an integral part of these complexes. RF belongs to a larger family of antiglobulins usually defined as antibodies with specificity for antigen determinants on the Fc fragment of human or certain animal IgG. RFs have been associated with three major Ig: IgM, IgG, and IgA.

Felty's syndrome is the association of RA with splenomegaly and leukopenia. A high-titer RF assay, a positive ANA assay, and rheumatoid nodules are frequently found in patients with Felty's syndrome. Patients have a propensity for bacterial infections.

JRA is a condition of chronic synovitis, beginning during childhood. The etiologic hypotheses are similar to those proposed for adult RA. Subgroups of JRA include Still's disease, polyarticular onset, pauciarticular onset, and RA.

REVIEW QUESTIONS

1. Rheumatoid arthritis most frequently develops in:
   A. adolescent females
   B. adolescent males
   C. middle-age females
   D. middle-age males

2. In the United States, the incidence of rheumatoid arthritis is _____%.
   A. 1-2
   B. 2-4
   C. 5-10
   D. over 10

3. Women are _____ likely than men to develop rheumatoid arthritis.
   A. less
   B. equally
   C. two to three times more
   D. 10 to 20 times more

4. Rheumatoid factor is defined as:
   A. antigens with specificity for antibody determinants on the Fc fragment of human or certain animal IgG
   B. antibodies with specificity for antigen determinants on the Fc fragment of human or certain animal IgG
   C. antigens with specificity for antibody determinants on the Fc fragment of human or certain animal IgD
   D. antibodies with specificity for antigen determinants on the Fc fragment of human or certain animal IgD

Questions 5 and 6. The principle of the latex agglutination test is based on the reaction of patient _____ (5) and _____ (6) derived from gamma globulin.

5.
   A. antigen
   B. antibody
   C. complement levels
   D. leukocytes

6.
   A. antigen
   B. antibody
   C. complement levels
   D. leukocytes

Questions 7-9. Arrange the steps in the pathogenesis of rheumatoid arthritis in the proper order.

7. _____
8. _____
9. _____

   A. Immunologic events perpetuate the initial inflammatory reaction.
   B. The primary etiologic factor initiates synovitis.
   C. An inflammatory reaction in the synovium develops into a proliferative destructive process of tissue.

10. All of the following are criteria for rheumatoid arthritis except:
    A. morning stiffness
    B. evening stiffness
    C. rheumatoid nodules
    D. radiographic changes

11. RF correlates with all of the following except:
    A. the severity of the disease in general
    B. the presence of nodules
    C. other organ system involvement (i.e., vasculitis)
    D. age of the patient

12. In RA, vascular and parenchymal lesions suggest that lesions result from injury induced by immune complexes, especially those containing antibodies to:
    A. IgM
    B. IgG
    C. IgE
    D. IgD

13. Serum complement levels are usually _____ in patients with rheumatoid arthritis.
    A. normal
    B. decreased
    C. increased
    D. A or B

14. Still's disease occurs in _____% of patients with juvenile RA.
    A. 10
    B. 20
    C. 30
    D. 50

15. In the RF latex agglutination procedure, a false-negative result may be observed in undiluted serum specimens because of:
    A. complement interference
    B. high levels of C-reactive protein (CRP)
    C. antigen excess
    D. both B and C

16. In the indirect enzyme immunoassay (EIA) procedure for RF, biologic false-positive results can be caused by a variety of disorders including:
    A. infectious mononucleosis
    B. hepatitis
    C. systemic lupus erythematosus
    D. polymyositis

BIBLIOGRAPHY

American College of Rheumatology Ad Hoc Committee on Clinical Guidelines: Guidelines for the management of rheumatoid arthritis, *Arthritis Rheum* 39:713, 1996.

Anderson RJ: Principles in the diagnosis of rheumatic disease, *Int Rev Intern Med* 41:559-614, 1995.

Ashman RF: Rheumatic disease. In Lawlor GJ, Fischer TJ, editors: *Manual of allergy and immunology,* ed 2, Boston, 1988, Little, Brown.

Borque L et al: Turbidimetry of rheumatoid factor in serum with a centrifugal analyzer, *Clin Chem* 32:124, 1986.

Breedveld FD: New perspectives on treating rheumatoid arthritis, *N Engl J Med* 333(3):183, 1995.

Bridges AJ et al: Antinuclear antibody testing in a referral laboratory, *Lab Med* 24(6):345-349, 1993.

Cash JM, Klippel JH: Second-line drug therapy for rheumatoid arthritis, *N Engl J Med* 330(19):1368-1376, 1994.

Cohen MD: Update: treatment of rheumatoid arthritis, *Arthritis Care Res* 45:530-532, 2001.

Condemi JJ: The autoimmune diseases, *JAMA* 268(20):2885-2888, 1992.

Conn DL: Resolved: low-dose prednisone is indicated as a standard treatment in patients with rheumatoid arthritis, *Arthritis Care Res* 45:462-467, 2001.

Del Rincon I et al: High incidence of cardiovascular events in a rheumatoid arthritis cohort not explained by traditional cardiac risk factors, *Arthritis Rheum* 44(12):2737-2745, 2001.

Galen RS, Gambino SR: *Beyond normality: the predictive value and efficiency of medical diagnosis,* New York, 1975, John Wiley & Sons.

Henderson WR: The role of leukotrienes, *Ann Intern Med* 121 (9):684-696, 1994.

Holborow EJ: Autoantibodies in the rheumatic diseases. In Scott JT, editor: *Copeman's textbook of the rheumatic diseases,* ed 6, New York, 1986, Churchill Livingstone.

Jones WL, Wiggins GL: A study of rheumatoid arthritis latex kits, *Am J Clin Pathol* 60:703-706, 1973.

Liang H: Board review: rheumatology, *Int Rev Intern Med* 41:1467-1473, 1995.

Linker JB III, Williams RC Jr: Tests for detection of rheumatoid factors. In Rose NR, Friedman H, Fahey JL, editors: *Manual of clinical laboratory immunology,* ed 3, Washington, DC, 1986, American Society for Microbiology.

Mackay IR, Burnett FM, editors: *Autoimmune disease: serologic reactions in rheumatoid arthritis,* Springfield, Ill, 1964, Charles C Thomas.

Matsumoto AK: Rheumatoid arthritis-treatments, 2002, website: www.hopkins.som.jhmi.edu.

Prevalence and impact of arthritis among women—United States, 1989-1991, *MMWR* 44(17):329-334, 1995.

Pinals RS: Polyarthritis and fever, *N Engl J Med* 330(11):769-774, 1994.

Prevalence of arthritis, *MMWR* 43(17):305-309, 1994.

Sangha O: Epidemiology of rheumatic diseases, *Rheumatology* 39(suppl.2):3-12, 2000.

Singer JM, Plotz CM, Goldberg R: The detection of antiglobulin factors utilizing precoated latex particles, *Arthritis Rheum* 8:194-201, 1965.

Tive L: Celecoxib clinical profile, *Rheumatology* 39(suppl.2):21-28, 2000.

Turgeon ML: Synovial fluid. In *Clinical hematology,* ed 3, Philadelphia, 1993, Lippincott Williams & Wilkins.

Wernick R et al: IgG and IgM rheumatoid factors in rheumatoid arthritis: quantitative response to penicillamine therapy and relationship to disease activity, *Arthritis Rheum* 26:593, 1983.

Wong, JB, Ramey DR, Singh G: Long-term morbidity, mortality, and economics of rheumatoid arthritis, *Arthritis Rheum* 44(12):2746-2749, 2001.

Chapter 28

Solid Organ Transplantation

LEARNING OBJECTIVES

At the conclusion of this chapter, the reader should be able to:
- Name and describe the histocompatibility antigens.
- Explain the clinical applications of histocompatibility antigens and human leukocyte antigens.
- List frequently used terms in transplantation.
- Name various types of transplants.
- Define graft-versus-host disease.

- Explain the etiology, epidemiology, signs and symptoms, manifestations, diagnosis, and prevention of graft-versus-host disease.
- Describe the types of graft rejection.
- Briefly explain the mechanism of organ or tissue rejection.
- Name and explain some methods of immunosuppression.
- Analyze a representative transplantation case study.

INTRODUCTION

At present a variety of tissues and organs are transplanted in humans, including bone marrow, bone matrix, skin, kidneys, liver, cardiac valves, heart, pancreas, corneas, and lungs. Transplantation is one of the areas, in addition to hypersensitivity (see Chapter 23) and autoimmunity (see Chapter 25), in which the immune system functions in a detrimental way. Early in the history of transplantation, tissue antigens were recognized as important to successful grafting. If significantly different foreign antigens were introduced into an immunocompetent host, the transplanted tissue or organ would undoubtedly fail. Today tissue (histocompatibility) matching with concomitant immunosuppression of the host in many cases is used to enhance the probability of success in organ and tissue transplantation.

HISTOCOMPATIBILITY ANTIGENS

General Characteristics

All vertebrates capable of acute rejection of foreign skin grafts possess a localized complex involving many genes that exert major control over the organism's immune reactions. Some of these antigens are much more potent than others in provoking an immune response and are, therefore, called the major histocompatibility complex (MHC).

The MHC encodes the human leukocyte antigens (HLAs), which are the molecular basis for T-cell discrimination of self from nonself. The HLA complex on chromosome 6 contains over 200 genes, more than 40 of which encode leukocyte antigens, with the rest of them being an assortment of genes not directly related to the HLA genes. Many genes within this complex have nothing to do with immunity.

Structurally there are two classes of HLA molecules: class I and class II. Both classes are cell surface heterodimeric structures. Class I HLA molecules consist of an alpha chain, a highly polymorphic glycoprotein, encoded within the MHC on chromosome 6. This alpha chain noncovalently associates with beta 2 microglobulin, a nonpolymorphic glycoprotein, encoded by a non-HLA gene on chromosome 15. Class II HLA molecules are composed of alpha chains and beta chains that are encoded within the MHC. The conformation of class I and class II HLA molecules provides each with a groove in which linear peptides, consisting of 8 to 25 peptides, are displayed for recognition by the cell surface expression on lymphocytes of a transmembrane heterodimeric receptor. All nucleated cells of the body display transmembrane class I HLA molecules in association with the nontransmembrane beta 2 microglobulin molecule.

The MHC is divided into four major regions: D, B, C, and A. The A, B, and C regions are the classic or class Ia genes that code for class I molecules. The D region codes for class II molecules. Class I includes HLA-A, -B, and –C. The three principal loci (A, B, and C) and their respective antigens are numbered 1, 2, 3, etc. The class II gene region antigens are encoded in the HLA-D region and can be subdivided into three families, HLA-DR, HLA-DC (DQ), and HLA-SB (DP).

Multiple alleles occur at each locus and are followed by an Arabic number (e.g., HLA-A1 or HLA-B27). If there is not yet collective agreement, the number of the allele is preceded by a "w" (e.g., HLA-A2 [w69] or HLA-Cw7). Genes of class I, II, and III antigens at each locus are inherited as codominant alleles. Inheritance within families closely follows simple mendelian dominant characteristics. Conservation of entire haplotypes through generation after generation is the general rule. Very strong linkage disequilibrium is displayed between several HLA loci, creating super or extended haplotypes that may differ from race to race. For example, the most frequent Caucasoid superextended haplotype, AL, Xw7, BB, BfS, C2-1, C4AQOB1, DR3, is virtually absent in Orientals.

The class I major transplantation antigens have been serologically defined. Class I and class II antigens can be found on body cells (Table 28-1) and in body fluids. Class I and

TABLE 28-1	Expression of Human Leukocyte Antigens on Surface Membranes

Class I	
Not expressed	Erythrocytes, corneal endothelium, villus of trophoblast, exocrine pancreas, parotid acinar cells, and some duodenal Brunner's glands
Weakly expressed	Endocrine thyroid, parathyroid, pituitary, pancreatic islet cells, myocardial, skeletal muscle, gastric mucosa, and mature granulocytes
Variably expressed	Hepatocytes
Expressed	All other body cells
Class II	
Not expressed	Erythrocytes; all resting endocrine cells; hepatocytes and biliary epithelium, myocardial, skeletal, and smooth muscle cells; epithelial cells of the esophagus; stomach; Brunner's glands; colon and rectum; parotid acinar and ductal epithelium; spermatozoa; bladder; prostate and ureter epithelium; neurons; platelets; mature granulocytes; and resting T cells
Expressed	B cells, activated T cells, and immature granulocytes; epithelium of the epiglottis; trachea, tonsils, and epididymis; renal, glomeruli, and tubules; dura; Langerhans' cell; skin; dendritic cells; epithelial cells of the deeper layers of the duodenum, ileum, and appendix
HLA-DR expressed	Monocytes, macrophages, and vascular endothelial cells
HLA-DQ weakly expressed or absent	

From Thompson J: The human leukocyte antigen system. In Stein J, editor: *Internal medicine,* ed 2, Boston, 1987, Little, Brown.

class II molecules are surface membrane proteins. Class I molecules are transmembrane glycoproteins, but the class II dimer molecule differs from class I in that both dimers span the cell membrane. Class I and class II gene products are biochemically distinct, although they appear to be distantly related through evolution. Class III gene products such as C2, C4A, C4B, and Bf complement components are incomplete; but these structures are defined by genes lying between or very near the HLA-B and HLA-DR loci.

The Role of Major Histocompatibility Complex/Human Leukocyte Antigens

The histocompatibility complex that encodes cell surface antigens was first discovered in graft rejection experiments with mice. When the antigens were matched between donor and recipient, the ability of a graft to survive was remarkably improved. A comparable genetic system of alloantigens was subsequently identified in humans. The presence of HLA was first recognized when multiple-transfused patients experienced transfusion reactions despite proper cross-matching. It was discovered that these reactions resulted from leukocytes' antibodies rather than from antibodies directed against erythrocyte antigens. These same antibodies were subsequently discovered in the sera of multiparous women.

The MHC gene products have an important role in clinical immunology. For example, transplants are rejected if performed against MHC barriers; thus immunosuppressive therapy is required. These antigens are of primary importance and are second only to the ABO antigens in influencing the genetic basis of survival or rejection of transplanted organs.

Although HLA was originally identified by its role in transplant rejection, it is now recognized that the products of HLA genes play a crucial role in our immune system. T cells do not recognize antigens directly but do so when the antigen is presented on the surface of an antigen-presenting cell, the macrophage. In addition to presentation of the antigen, the macrophage must present another molecule for this response to occur. This molecule is a cell surface glycoprotein coded in each species by the MHC. T cells are able to interact with the histocompatibility molecules only if they are genetically identical (MHC restriction).

Both class I and class II antigens function as targets of T lymphocytes that regulate the immune response. Class I molecules regulate interaction between cytolytic T cells and target cells, and class II molecules restrict the activity of regulatory T cells (helper, suppressor, and amplifier subsets). Hence class II molecules regulate the interaction between helper T cells and antigen-presenting cells. Cytotoxic T cells directed against class I antigens are inhibited by CD8 cells; cytotoxic T cells directed against class II antigens are inhibited by CD4 cells. Many of the genes in both class I and class II gene families have no known functions.

Class III molecules bear no clear relation to class I and II molecules aside from their genetic linkage (the presence of the gene in or near the MHC complex). Class III molecules are involved in immunologic phenomenon because they represent components of the complement pathways.

Human Leukocyte Antigen Applications

HLA matching is of value in organ transplantation, as well as in the transplantation of bone marrow. In kidney allo-

grafts, the method of organ preservation, the time elapsed between harvesting and transplanting, the number of pretransplantation blood transfusions, the recipient's age, and the primary cause for kidney failure are all important determinants of early transplant success or failure. HLA compatibility, however, exerts the strongest influence on long-term kidney survival. The 1-year survival for kidneys transplanted from an HLA-identical sibling approaches 95%. Approximately 50% to 65% of cadaver kidneys mismatched for all four HLA-A and B antigens function for 6 months but deteriorate thereafter with time. Only 15% to 25% of these mismatched cadaver kidneys remain functioning 4 years after transplantation.

It is obligatory to select HLA-identical donors for bone marrow transplantation to reduce the frequency of graft-versus-host disease (GVHD) (discussed later in this chapter). A new method, however, that depletes donor marrow T cells capable of recognizing foreign host antigens has markedly reduced the incidence of GVHD.

HLA-matched platelets are useful to patients who are refractory to treatment with random donor platelets. In paternity testing, HLA typing, along with the determination of ABO, Rh, MNSs, Kell, Duffy, and Kidd erythrocyte antigen, is used. In the past, most laboratories involved in testing individuals in disputed parentage cases used only the ABO, Rh, and MNSs systems. The chances of identifying a falsely accused man with these tests was 58%. Additional testing for Kell, Duffy, and Kidd erythrocyte antigens and for HLA typing offers an exclusion rate estimated at 92%.

HLA typing is also useful in forensic medicine, anthropology, and basic research in immunology. In studies of racial ancestry and migration, some antigens are virtually excluded or confirmed to a race (e.g., A1 and B8 are rarely detected in Mongoloids, and Bw57 is uncommon in Caucasians and African-Americans). These distinctions allow for precise conclusions to be drawn regarding origin and ancestry.

HLA testing is increasingly being used as a diagnostic and genetic counseling tool. Knowledge of HLA antigens and their linkage is becoming important because of the recognized association of certain antigens (Box 28-1) with distinct immunologic-mediated reactions, autoimmune diseases, some neoplasms, and other disorders; these disorders, although nonimmunologic, are influenced by non-HLA genes also located within the major MHC region.

Box 28-1	Relationship of Certain Human Leukocyte Antigens and Diseases	
Ankylosing spondylitis	B27
Reiter's syndrome	B27
Psoriasis vulgaris	Cw6
Rheumatoid arthritis	DR4
Behçet's disease	B5 (Bw51)
Type I diabetes	DR3
Gold-induced nephropathy	DR5
Congenital adrenal hyperplasia	B47
Chronic lymphatic leukemia	DR5
Kaposi's sarcoma (Mediterranean)	DR5

The estimated relative risks or chances of developing a disease if a given antigen is present (Table 28-2) may be elevated in individuals bearing certain HLA antigens compared to individuals who lack the antigen. The HLA-B27 antigen, however, is the only HLA antigen with a disease association strong enough to be useful in differential diagnosis. Although the degree of association between HLA antigens and other diseases may be statistically significant, it is not strong enough to be of diagnostic or prognostic value.

Although only 8% of normal Caucasians carry HLA-B27 antigen, 90% of patients with either ankylosing spondylitis (AS) or spondylitis in association with Reiter's syndrome are positive for the antigen. An elevated percentage of HLA-B27-positive patients is also observed in juvenile chronic arthritis with spinal involvement. Therefore the major indication for screening for HLA-B27 test is to rule out AS when back pain develops in relatives of patients with the disease and to help to distinguish incomplete Reiter's syndrome from gonococcal arthritis, or chronic or atypical Reiter's syndrome from rheumatoid arthritis. A negative test for HLA-B27, however, does not exclude the diagnosis of AS or Reiter's syndrome.

Methods of Detection

Because different individuals in a species carry different HLA antigens on their cell surfaces, introduction of foreign antigens can stimulate T cells. These T cells are prominently implicated in graft rejection, and they can also stimulate antibody formation under certain circumstances. Human sera containing these antibodies can be obtained from some multiple-transfused patients or multiparous women for use as reagents to detect different HLA antigens.

Class I antigens are determined by several techniques; the most popular and reproducible method is the lymphocyte microcytotoxicity method (complement-mediated cytotoxicity). With this technique, a battery of reagent antisera and isolated target cells are incubated with a source of complement under oil to prevent evaporation. If a specific alloantibody and cell membrane antigen combine, complement-mediated damage to

TABLE 28-2 Relationship of Human Leukocyte Antigens to Risk of Disease

Antigen Present	Related Disease	Increased Risk of Developing the Disease Over a Lifetime
B27	Ankylosing spondylitis	100×*
	Reiter's syndrome	40×
	Anterior uveitis	25×
	Arthritic infection with *Yersinia* or *Salmonella*	20×
	Psoriatic arthritis with spinal involvement	11×
	Spondylitis associated with inflammatory bowel disease	9×
	Juvenile chronic arthritis with spinal involvement	5×
B8	Celiac disease	9×
	Addison's disease	6×
	Myasthenia gravis	5×
	Dermatitis herpetiformis	4×
	Chronic active hepatitis	4×
	Sjögren's syndrome	3×
	Diabetes mellitus (insulin-dependent)	2×
	Thyrotoxicosis	2×
B5	Behçet's syndrome	6×
BW38	Psoriatic arthritis	7×
BW15	Diabetes mellitus (insulin-dependent)	3×
DR2	Goodpasture's syndrome	16×
	Multiple sclerosis	4×
DR3	Gluten-sensitive enteropathy	21×
	Dermatitis herpetiformis	14×
	Subacute cutaneous lupus erythematosus	12×
	Addison's disease	11×
	Sjögren's syndrome (primary)	10×
DR4	Pemphigus†	32×
	Giant-cell arthritis	8×
	Rheumatoid arthritis	6×
	Juvenile diabetes mellitus	5×
DR5	Pauciarticular juvenile arthritis	5×
	Scleroderma	5×
	Hashimoto's thyroiditis	3×

From Ashman RF: Rheumatic diseases. In Lawlor GJ, Fischer TJ, editors: *Manual of allergy and immunology,* ed 2, Boston, 1998, Little, Brown.
*Varies with ethnic group (e.g., 3× for Pima Indians and 300× for Japanese).
†Jewish persons.

the cell wall allows for penetration of a vital dye, and the cells are killed. Cell death is determined by staining. A stain such as trypan blue will penetrate dead cells but not living ones. Unaffected cells remain brilliantly refractile when observed microscopically. Other methods of analysis include leukocyte agglutination and complement fixation on platelets in suspension.

Class II HLA-DR and HLA-DQ specificities are also recognized by similar serologic methods, except that isolated B cells are the usual target cells because their surface is rich in these molecules, as well as in class I determinants. At present, HLA-Dw and HLA-DP cannot be serologically defined, and their detection relies on the ability of these molecules to stimulate newly synthesized DNA when added to primary mixed lymphocyte (HLA-Dw) or when readded to secondary primary lymphocyte (HLA-DP) in vitro cultures. Class III complement specificities are recognized by the availability of diagnostic reagents, but reagents remain scarce.

FACTS ABOUT SOLID ORGAN TRANSPLANTATION

Each day in the United States 13 people die while waiting for an organ transplant. If donor organs had been readily available, 4000 patients on organ waiting lists in the United States alone could be saved in 1 year. Organ transplantation is widely viewed as the preferred treatment for end-stage organ failure because of the quality of life the treatment offers for patients and because of the long-term cost benefits. The increased demand for organ transplantation is fueled by the transplant success rate. Worldwide, the demand for transplant operations is increasing by about 15% per year, but the number of donated organs has remained static.

The first successful transplant, a kidney transplant, was in 1954. In 1984, the U.S. Congress passed the National Organ Transplant Act. The goal of this legislation is to match a low supply of organs with the most critically ill patients no matter where they reside in the country. On April 12, 2002, the United Network for Organ Sharing patient waiting list for an organ transplant contained 79,368 names. The list continues to grow because of the scarcity of organs (Box 28-2). Most of these registrants (51,753) were waiting for a kidney transplant. The next two highest groups of registrants were waiting for a liver (17,607) or heart (4149) transplant. The distribution of other transplant registrants was for lung (3811), kidney and pancreas (1,529), pancreas (1252), pancreas islet cell (287), heart and lung (206), and intestine (179). Approximately 25% of patients waiting for a liver transplant are children under 10 years old.

The most common causes for the need of solid organ transplant vary by the type of organ. Kidney recipients usually suffer from diabetes, glomerulonephritis, hypertensive nephrosclerosis, or polycystic kidneys. Liver recipient transplant patients ordinarily suffer from noncholestatic cirrhosis, cholestatic liver disease, biliary atresia, or acute hepatic necrosis. Patients suffering from cardiomyopathy, congenital heart disease, valvular heart disease, or coronary artery disease are the most frequent heart transplant recipients. In 2000 kidney transplants led the list of transplanted organs with 13,372 transplants. Of these kidney transplants 5293 were living donors.

Overall 1-year graft and patient survival rates for most organs, except heart-lung transplants, improved between 1990 and 1998 (Figure 28-1). The greatest improvements in graft

Box 28-2	Some Factors Contributing to the Scarcity of Organs

- Demand for transplantation has increased because more patients are considered eligible.
- Age limits for heart and liver transplants eligibility have increased.
- Diabetes is no longer an absolute contraindication for transplant eligibility.
- The number of donors has shown little growth.

Source: website: www.upenn.edu/ldi/issuebrief2_5.html.

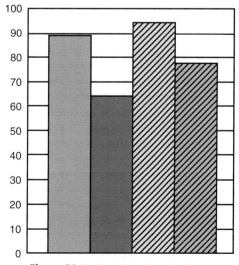

- Kidney 1 = cadaver kidney 1 yr after transplant

- Kidney 2 = cadaver kidney 5 yrs after transplant

- Kidney 3 = living donor 1 yr after transplant

- Kidney 4 = living donor 5 yrs after transplant

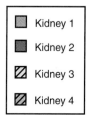

Kidney 1
Kidney 2
Kidney 3
Kidney 4

Figure 28-1   Renal graft survival.

TABLE 28-3	**Transplantation Terms**

Term	Definition
Autograft	Graft transferred from one position to another in the same individual (e.g., skin, hair, bone)
Syngraft	Graft transplanted between different but identical recipient and donor (e.g., kidney transplant between monozygous twins)
Allograft (homograft)	Graft between genetically different recipient and donor of the same species; the grafted donor tissue or organ contains antigens not present in the recipient
Xenograft (heterograft)	Graft between individuals of different species (e.g., a pig heart valve to a human heart)

survival were seen for pancreas transplants, and for kidney and pancreas grafts from kidney-pancreas transplants. Patient survival rates for kidney and pancreas transplantation were much higher because of the availability of dialysis and insulin. One-year graft survival for kidney and heart transplantation at major transplant centers is now greater than 90%, with acute rejection rates less than 30%.

TRANSPLANTATION TERMINOLOGY

The transplanting or grafting of an organ or tissue ranges from self-transplantation (such as skin grafts from one part of the body to another to correct burn injuries, or hair transplants from one area of the scalp to another to correct patterned balding) to the grafting of a body component from one species to another, such as the transplanting of a pig's heart valve to a human. The most recent terms used in transplantation are presented in Table 28-3.

TYPES OF TRANSPLANTS

Eleven different organs or human body parts can be transplanted. These are corneas, middle ear, lung, heart, blood vessels, liver, pancreas, kidneys, bone, bone marrow, and skin. Successful organ transplants have increased since the advent of the immunosuppressive drug, cyclosporine.

Living donor transplants have attracted significant media attention in the last few years. According to the United Network for Organ Sharing and the Health Resources and Services Administration of the U.S. Department of Health and Human Services, the number of living donor transplants increased 16.5% between 1999 and 2000, the largest ever 1-year increase. A living donor may donate a single kidney, segment of the liver, portion of the pancreas, or the lobe of a lung.

Kidney

The first successful human kidney transplant was performed in 1954 between monozygotic twins. Induction of tolerance

(discussed later in this chapter) was attempted through the use of sublethal total body irradiation and allogeneic bone marrow transplantation, followed by renal transplantation. By 1960 renal transplantation was firmly established as a viable treatment for end-stage renal disease. Because of the continuing problems associated with total body irradiation, chemical immunosuppression became the mode of treatment. The criteria for recipients of renal allografts generally exclude elderly patients and those with a history of malignancy. In addition, patients with active sepsis or patients in whom chronic infection may be reactivated by treatment with steroids or immunosuppressive therapy are also not considered transplant candidates.

Kidney donations are not accepted from individuals over 65 years old because of a decreased likelihood of recipient survival. Donors are excluded if chronic renal disease or sepsis is present. Donations are additionally not accepted from individuals with generalized or systemic diseases such as diabetes mellitus, hypertension, and tuberculosis. Young trauma victims are the most desirable source of cadaver organ transplants, including the kidneys. Cadaver organs are not accepted from donors with a history of any malignancy other than that involving the central nervous system.

In addition to compatibility of ABO blood group systems, newer methods of harvesting kidneys have reduced the sensitizing effect related to "passenger" leukocytes against transplantation antigens borne on these cells. HLA-A and HLA-B loci matches have the best chance for long-term survival of the graft and the recipient. The increased survival rate with HLA-A and HLA-B matches is determined not as much by class I compatibility as by the HLA-D region-related antigens associated with these regions. The strongest association between transplant survival and tissue antigens is with the D region-related antigens (-DR, -MB, -MT). Lewis antigens on the erythrocytes and H-Y antigens associated with X and Y chromosomes are among the other antigen systems that demonstrate a reasonably significant association with graft survival.

Heart Valves

Xenogenic valve replacements are a standard modality for the treatment of aortic and mitral valve defects. Sources of these xenogenic valves are either bovine (cow) or porcine (pig), and the valves are chemically or physically modified to reduce antigenicity.

Patients receiving xenoallografts of heart valves are not immunosuppressed after surgery because only minimal or nonexistent graft rejection reactions take place in these modified valves.

Heart

The first successful allograft cardiac transplant was performed in 1967 by Dr. Christian Barnard in Cape Town, South Africa. The criteria for selecting the donor and recipient combination for cardiac transplantation are essentially the same as those used for cadaver renal transplantation. The most significant exclusion for cardiac transplantation, however, is the presence of an active infection. Cardiac transplantation donors must have sustained irreversible brain death, but nearly normal cardiac function must be maintained. Prophylactic antibiotics and cytotoxic drugs are given to the donor just before harvesting of the heart. Because of the urgency of most situations, most grafts are performed despite multiple HLA incompatibilities. Transplantation recipients are maintained on immunosuppressive therapy, anticoagulants, and antithrombotic agents, as well as on low-lipid diets.

Cornea

Corneal transplants have been a common form of therapy for many years. The first human corneal eye bank was established in New York City in 1944. This type of transplantation has an extremely high success rate because of the ease in obtaining and storing viable corneas.

Corneal grafts are generally performed to replace nonhealing corneal ulcerations. Because of the avascularity (lack of blood vessels) of this tissue, a reasonably low concentration of class I transplantation antigens, and an essential absence of class II antigens, graft rejection is minimal. To prevent rejection, grafts are made as small as possible and are placed centrally to avoid contact with the highly vascularized limbic region. Eccentrically placed grafts are subject to a high rate of immunologic failure because vascularity will allow for lymphocyte contact. Immunosuppression is not routinely administered.

Skin

The development of nonimmunogenic skin replacement materials has lowered the demand for allografts of skin. Skin allografts elicit the rejection phenomenon because skin has an extremely high density of class I histocompatibility antigens. Therefore sensitization and recognition of antigenic differences are very likely, with resultant rejection of the grafted skin. If done, skin allografts are performed and supported with immunosuppressive therapy.

Liver

Potential liver transplant recipients must have no extrahepatic disease or infection present. The largest group of transplant recipients has been those suffering from congenital biliary atresia. Patients with cirrhosis may also be good candidates. HLA cross-matching appears to increase the rate of graft survival, but the influence of tissue typing is somewhat unclear. Immunosuppressive regimens such as azathioprine and corticosteroids or cyclosporin A increase survival. Major complications of this procedure have been biliary tract fistulae or leaks, which have occurred in 30% to 50% of patients.

Lung

Successful lung transplants have been difficult to achieve because of technical, logistic, and immunologic problems. Technically, lung donor and recipient must have essentially identical bronchial circumferences to obtain a good match. An additional technical problem is that the lungs are extremely sensitive to ischemic damage, and successful preservation after harvesting has been unsuccessful. Occasional lung and heart combination transplants have been attempted. The combined procedure is less difficult than single organ transplant.

The lungs are susceptible to infection; sepsis is very common among potential donors. Severe rejection is common because of the high density of Ia-positive cells in the vasculature and the high concentration of passenger leukocytes trapped in the alveoli and blood vessels. Intensive immunosuppressive therapy is needed to maintain the graft. Many lung recipients have died from massive infection and sepsis.

Pancreas

New modes of transplantation include full pancreatic or isolated islet cell transplantation. Pancreatic grafts have been successful for only a short period because of a high rate of technical failure or irreversible rejection. Transplantation of small quantities of isolated islet cells into the retroperitoneal space, however, has demonstrated a reasonably good success rate.

Bone

Bone matrix autografts or allografts are common. Transplantation of bone matrix is used after certain limb-sparing tumor resections and to correct congenital bone abnormalities. The major criteria for bone donation are a lack of infection, no history of IV drug use, and no history of prolonged steroid therapy or human growth hormone treatment. Bone can be easily harvested and frozen. Freezing not only preserves the bone but offers the additional benefit of concomitant diminution of histocompatibility antigens.

The major technical requirement for allograft transplantation is maintaining the periosteal sheath of the recipient bone in order to strip the donor bone completely of all periosteal elements. Transplantation of bone is an easy procedure. Processed bone lacks significant quantities of immunogenic substances; therefore the need for immunosuppression is almost completely eliminated.

Stem Cells

The possibility exists for manipulation of brains and spinal cords into repairing trauma from stroke or other disease through the use of stem cell transplantation. Experiments on rats demonstrated that stem cells developed into neurons and other mature brain tissue when transplanted into normal and stroke-damaged adult rats. Blood vessels were also seen growing to nourish the transplanted cells.

GRAFT-VERSUS-HOST DISEASE

Graft-versus-host disease (GVHD) can be an unintentional consequence of blood transfusion or transplantation in severely immunocompromised or immunosuppressed patients. The degree of immunodeficiency in the host, rather than the number of transfused immunocompetent lymphocytes, determines whether or not GVHD will occur.

Etiology

When immunocompetent T lymphocytes are transfused from a donor to an immunodeficient or immunosuppressed recipient, the transfused or grafted lymphocytes recognize that the antigens of the host are foreign and react immunologically

TABLE 28-4	Requirements for Potential Graft-vs-Host Disease

Factor	Comments
1. A source of immunocompetent lymphocytes	Blood products, bone marrow transplant, organ transplant
2. Human leukocyte antigen differences between patient and recipient	Differences at human leukocyte antigen or H-2 can be fatal; the stronger the antigen difference, the more severe the reaction
3. Inability to reject donor cells	Patients are severely immunocompromised or immunosuppressed

against them (Table 28-4). Instead of the usual transplantation reaction of host against graft, the reverse graft-versus-host reaction occurs and produces an inflammatory response.

In a normal lymphocyte transfer reaction, the results of a GVHD are usually not serious, as the recipient is capable of destroying the foreign lymphocytes. However, engraftment and multiplication of donor lymphocytes in an immunosuppressed recipient are a real possibility because lymphocytes capable of mitosis can be found in stored blood products. If the recipient cannot reject the transfused lymphocytes, the grafted lymphocytes may cause uncontrolled destruction of the host's tissues and eventually death. A patient can develop acute or chronic GVHD. Where the donor and recipient differ at HLA or H-2 loci, the reaction can be fatal. The stronger the antigen difference, the more severe the reaction.

Epidemiology

It is now accepted that GVHD can occur whenever immunologically competent allogeneic lymphocytes are transfused into a severely immunocompromised host. Patients at risk include those who are immunodeficient or immunosuppressed with severe lymphocytopenia and bone marrow suppression. Despite chemotherapy at the time of bone marrow transplantation, 20% to 50% of patients will develop acute GVHD, and 20% to 40% of these patients will die of GVHD or associated infections.

Chronic GVHD affects 20% to 40% of patients within 6 months after transplantation. Two factors closely associated with the development of chronic GVHD are increasing age and a preceding episode of acute GVHD.

Cases of transfusion-related GVHD have increased significantly in the past two decades. This reaction has been reported subsequent to blood transfusion in bone marrow transplant recipients after total body irradiation, and in adults receiving intensive chemotherapy for hematologic malignancies. GVHD has also occurred in infants with severe congenital immunodeficiency and in those who have received intrauterine transfusions followed by exchange transfusion. Nearly 90% of patients with posttransfusion GVHD will die of acute complications of the disease. The usual cause of death is generalized infection.

Signs and Symptoms

GVHD causes an inflammatory response. Posttransfusion symptoms begin within 3 to 30 days after transfusion. Because of lymphocytic infiltration of the intestine, skin, and liver, mucosal destruction (including ulcerative skin and mouth lesions, diarrhea, and liver destruction) results. Other clinical symptoms include jaundice, fever, anemia, weight loss, skin rash, and splenomegaly.

In bone marrow transplant patients, acute GVHD develops within the first 3 months of transplantation. The initial manifestations are lesions of the skin, liver, and gastrointestinal tract. An erythematous maculopapular skin rash, particularly on the palms and soles, is usually the first sign of GVHD. Disease progression is characterized by diarrhea, often with abdominal pain, and liver disease. Other signs and symptoms of complications related to therapy include fever, granulocytopenia, and bacteremia. Interstitial pneumonia, frequently associated with cytomegalovirus (CMV), can also occur.

Chronic GVHD resembles a collagen vascular disease with skin changes such as erythema and cutaneous ulcers, and a liver dysfunction characterized by bile duct degeneration and cholestasis. Patients with chronic GVHD are susceptible to bacterial infections. For example, increasing age and preexisting lung disease increase the incidence of interstitial pneumonia.

Immunologic Manifestation

In immunocompromised patients the transfused or grafted lymphocytes recognize the antigens of the host as foreign and react immunologically against them. Instead of the usual transplantation reaction of host against graft, the reverse GVHD occurs.

In a normal lymphocyte-transfer reaction, the results of GVHD are usually not serious because the recipient is capable of destroying the foreign lymphocytes. If the recipient cannot reject the transfused lymphocytes, however, the grafted lymphocytes may cause uncontrolled destruction of the host's tissues and then death.

Diagnostic Evaluation

Laboratory evidence of immunosuppression or immunodeficiency, such as a decreased total lymphocyte concentration, suggests that a patient may develop GVHD. Evidence of inflammation such as an increased C-reactive protein, elevated leukocyte count with granulocytosis, and increased erythrocyte sedimentation rate may suggest that GVHD has developed in GVHD candidates. Complications of anemia and liver disease, characterized by increased bilirubin and blood enzymes (such as transaminases and alkaline phosphatase) and the presence of opportunistic pathogens (e.g., CMV) can further support the diagnosis.

Pathologic features include lymphocytic and monocytic infiltration into perivascular spaces in the dermis and dermoepidermal junction of the skin and into the epithelium of the oropharynx, tongue, and esophagus. Infiltration can also be observed into the base of the intestinal crypts of the small and large bowel and into the periportal area of the liver, with secondary necrosis of cells in infiltrated tissues.

Prevention

Although a minimal number of bone marrow transplant recipients actually develop GVHD disease, the incidence of GVHD can be minimized by depletion of mature lymphocytes from the marrow by using monoclonal antibodies or physical methods. The risk of GVHD, however, can be minimized if not eliminated by irradiation of the marrow transplant or blood products. Blood product irradiation is believed to be the most efficient and probably the most economical method available for prevention of posttransfusion GVHD. No cases of posttransfusion GVHD have been reported after administration of blood products irradiated with at least 1500 rad. The recommended radiation dose ranges from a minimum of 1500 to 3000 rad as an effective and appropriate radiation dose.

Several categories of patients possess the clinical indications for irradiated products.

High-Risk Patients

Patients at the highest risk with an absolute need for irradiated blood products include:

- Recipients of autologous or allogeneic bone marrow grafts. Recipients of autologous bone marrow may be expected to have the same risk of posttransfusion GVHD as patients receiving allogeneic bone marrow.
- Children with severe congenital immune deficiency syndromes involving T lymphocytes. The degree of immunodeficiency in the host, rather than the number of transfused immunocompetent cells, determines whether GVHD will occur.

Intermediate-Risk Patients

Patients considered to be at less of a risk of developing GVHD include:

- Infants receiving intrauterine transfusions followed by exchange transfusions, and possibly infants receiving only exchange transfusions. The immune mechanism of the fetus and newborn infant may not be sufficiently mature to reject foreign lymphocytes, and prior transfusions may induce a state of immune tolerance in the newborn. Transfused lymphocytes may continue to circulate for a prolonged time in some immunologically tolerant hosts without the development of GVHD. There is insufficient evidence to recommend irradiation of blood given to all premature infants.
- Patients receiving total body radiation or immunosuppressive therapy for disorders such as lymphoma and acute leukemia. Although routine irradiation of blood products given to these patients can be justified, it cannot be regarded as absolutely indicated, as the risk of developing GVHD is so small. Blood product irradiation, however, is advised for selected patients with hematologic malignancies, especially when transfusions are given in or near the time of sustained and severe therapy-induced immunosuppression.

Low-Risk Patients

Patients also at risk but considered the least susceptible include:

- Patients with solid tumors. The incidence of the development of GVHD is difficult to determine. However, in nonhematologic malignancies such as neuroblastoma, the disease has developed. In one case the disease developed after the infusion of a single unit of packed red cells.
- Patients with aplastic anemia receiving antithymocyte globulin theoretically may be at increased risk of posttransfusion GVHD during therapy-induced periods of lymphocytopenia.
- Although a theoretical risk of posttransfusion GVHD may exist in patients with acquired immunodeficiency syndrome (AIDS), the disease has not actually been observed in this disorder. The routine use of irradiated blood is not recommended.

Effects of Radiation on Specific Cellular Components

Lymphocytes. Ionizing radiation is known to inhibit lymphocyte mitotic activity and blast transformation. Irradiation of normal donor lymphocytes with 1500 rad from a cesium-137 source results in a 90% reduction in mitogen-stimulated ^{14}C-thymidine incorporation. An 85% reduction in mitogen-induced blast transformation after exposure to 1500 rad and a 97% to 98.5% reduction in mitogenic response have been noted after exposure to 5000 rads.

Granulocytes. Ionizing radiation may impair granulocyte function; this impairment is dose dependent. The degree of actual damage to granulocytes is controversial. Chemotactic activity decreased linearly with increasing doses of irradiation from 500 to 120,000 rads, but the reduction only reached statistical significance at 10,000 rad. A linear dose-response curve demonstrates that granulocyte locomotion is affected by very small doses of irradiation. A dose of 2000 rads is likely to eliminate lymphocytic mitotic activity and to prevent GVHD without causing significant damage to granulocytes or altering their chemotactic or bactericidal ability. Irradiation before transfusion has been demonstrated to contribute to defective oxidative metabolism, but this effect is highly variable.

Mature Red Blood Cells. Mature red cells appear to be highly resistant to radiation damage. After red cells were exposed to 10,000 rad, ^{52}Cr-labeled in vivo red cell survival was the same as that of untreated controls. It has been shown that stored erythrocytes could be treated with up to 20,000 rads without changing their viability or in vitro properties, including adenosine triphosphate and 2,3 diphosphoglycerate levels, plasma hemoglobin, and potassium ions.

Platelets. Ionizing radiation may impair platelet function. Although this impairment is dose dependent, the effects of irradiation on platelets have been difficult to characterize. Several studies have demonstrated unchanged in vivo platelet survival after exposure to 5000 to 75,000 rad. A 33% decrease in the expected platelet count increase was noted after transfusion of platelets exposed to 5000 rad, and similarly irradiated autologous platelets had a diminished ability to correct the bleeding times in a small number of volunteers who had consumed aspirin. In one study, platelet aggregation was not affected by exposure to 5000 rad, but an impaired response to collagen was noted.

FACTORS IN GRAFT REJECTION

Organs vary with respect to their susceptibility to rejection based on inherent immunogenicity (Box 28-3), which is influenced by factors such as vascularity.

Types of Graft Rejection

The role of sensitized lymphocytes and antibodies in graft rejection differs and is influenced by the type of organ transplanted. Lymphocytes, particularly recirculating small lymphocytes, are effective in shortening graft survival. Cell-mediated immunity is responsible for the rejection of skin and solid tumors. However, humoral antibodies can also be involved in the rejection process. The complexity of the action and interaction of cellular and humoral factors in grafts is considerable. Five possible categories of graft rejection (Table 28-5) have been demonstrated in human kidney transplant rejection: hyperacute, accelerated, acute, chronic, and immunopathologic.

First- and Second-Set Rejection

Skin transplantation (Figure 28-2) is the most common experimental model for transplantation research. Rejection of skin and solid tumors can be divided into first- and second-set rejection. Activation of cellular immunity by T cells is the predominant cause of the first-set allograft rejection. Lymphocytes can directly attack cellular antigens to which they are sensitized by previous exposure or by cytotoxic lymphokines. The primary role of lymphocytes in first-set rejection is consistent with the histology of early reaction and shows infiltration by mononuclear cells with very few polymorphonuclear leukocytes or plasma cells. Sensitization occurs within the first few days of transplantation, and the tissue is lost in 10 to 20 days.

When sensitized lymphocytes are already present as the result of prior graft rejection, an accelerated rejection of tissue results from regrafting second-set rejection. Lymphocytes from a sensitized animal transferred to a first-graft recipient will accelerate rejection of the graft. Graft rejection is primarily a T-cell function, with some assistance from antibodies.

Hyperacute Rejection

Hyperacute reactions are caused entirely by the presence within the host of preformed humoral antibodies, which react with donor tissue cellular antigens. These antibodies are usually anti-A–related or anti-B–related to the ABO blood group systems or antibodies to class I MHC antigens (hypersensitivity type II). Potential recipients harboring antibodies to HLA-A, HLA-B, and HLA-C (class I) but not HLA-DR (class II) antigens are at high risk for this process.

The interaction of cellular antigens with antibodies activates the complement system and leads to grafted cell lysis and clotting within the grafted tissue. Kidney allografts can be rejected by the hyperacute rejection process within minutes of transplantation. The irreversible kidney damage of hyperacute rejection is characterized by sludging of erythrocytes, development of microthrombi in the small arterioles and glomerular capillaries, and infiltration of phagocytic cells.

It could be as little as 2 years before genetically altered pig organs are available for transplantation into humans, but it is likely to be at least 5 years before full-scale studies can get underway. Future xenotransplantation will depend on overcoming problems of hyperacute rejection. In hyperacute rejection, the recipient of the organ produces xenoreactive antibodies, which lodge on the cells lining the blood vessels of the new organ and trigger the release of complement. This release triggers inflammation, swelling, and ultimately blockage of the blood vessels, leading to death of the organ.

Accelerated Rejection

Accelerated rejection is comparable to the second-set rejection phenomenon observed in animal models. In these cases, retransplantation is less severe than hyperacute rejection and is considered to be accelerated rejection. Accelerated rejection is due to activation of the T-cell-mediated response.

Box 28-3	Examples of the Immunogenicity of Different Transplant Tissues	
Most immunogenic		Bone marrow
		Skin
		Islets of Langerhans
		Heart
		Kidney
		Liver
		Bone
		Xenogeneic valve replacements
Least immunogenic		Cornea

TABLE 28-5 Categories and Characteristics of Graft Rejection Based on Immune Destruction of Kidney Grafts

Type	Time of Tissue Damage	Predominant Mechanism	Cause
Hyperacute	Within minutes	Humoral	Preformed cytotoxic antibodies to donor antigens
Accelerated	2 to 5 days	Cell-mediated	Previous sensitization to donor antigens
Acute	7 to 21 days	Cell-mediated (possibly antibody cell-mediated cytotoxicity)	Development of allogeneic reaction to donor antigens
Chronic	Later than 3 months	Cell-mediated	Disturbance of host/graft tolerance
Immunopathologic damage to the new organ	Later than 3 months	1. Immune complex disorder 2. Complex formation with soluble antigens	Immunopathologic mechanisms related to circumstances necessitating transplant

Acute Rejection

Acute rejection can result after the first exposure to alloantigens. In this reaction, donor antigens select reactive T-cell clones and initiate visible manifestation of rejection within 6 to 14 days. The early processes in acute rejection appear to be T-cell mediated; however, later aspects may involve antibodies and complement.

Acute rejection is equivalent to a first-set allograft rejection in experimental animals, and an accelerated rejection is equivalent to second-set rejection. Both are primarily mediated by cells. Immunopathologic changes include the presence of immune complex deposition and other hypersensitivity reactions already present in the recipient.

Acute early rejection, which occurs up to about 10 days after transplantation, is histologically characterized by dense cellular infiltration and rupture of peritubular capillaries. It appears to be a cell-mediated hypersensitivity reaction involving T cells. In comparison, acute-late rejection occurs 11 days or more after transplantation in patients suppressed with prednisone and azathioprine. In kidney allografts, acute-late rejection is probably caused by the binding of immunoglobulin (Ig), presumably antibody and complement, to the arterioles and glomerular capillaries, where they can be visualized by immunofluorescent techniques. These Ig deposits on the vessel walls include platelet aggregates in glomerular capillaries, which cause acute renal shutdown. The possibility of damage to antibody-coated cells through antibody-dependent, cell-mediated cytotoxicity (ADCC) may also take place.

Chronic Rejection

Chronic rejection occurs in most graft recipients. The process results in a slow but continual loss of organ function over months or years. However, chronic rejection is often responsive to various immunosuppressive therapies.

In kidney allografts this insidious rejection is associated with subendothelial deposits of Ig and the C3 component of complement on the glomerular basement membranes. This may occasionally be an expression of an underlying immune complex disorder that may have originally necessitated the transplant, or it may result from complex formation with soluble antigens derived from the grafted kidney.

Immunologic Tolerance

The importance of tolerance to self-antigens was recognized very early in the study of immunology. Immunologic tolerance is the acquisition of nonreactivity toward particular antigens. Self-tolerance is a critical process, and the failure to recognize self-antigens can result in autoimmune disease (see Chapter 25).

Various pathways to immunologic tolerance have been recognized. It has been suggested that both T and B cells are affected independently and differently and may be tolerated under certain circumstances. Several mechanisms may operate simultaneously in a single host. During fetal development of the immune system and during the first few weeks of neonatal life, none of the cells of the immune system has reached maturity. For this reason, the entire immune system

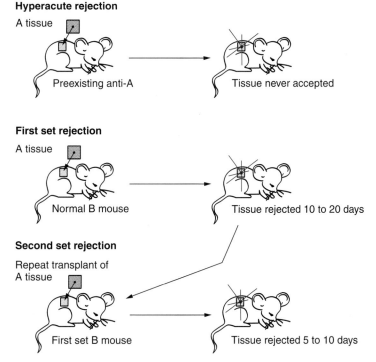

Figure 28-2   Hyperacute rejection results from placement of tissue in an animal already possessing antibodies to antigens of grafted tissue. Second-set rejection is an accelerated first-set reaction and is seen in animals that have already rejected tissue at least once. (Redrawn from Barrett JT: *Textbook of immunology,* ed 5, St Louis, 1988, Mosby.)

is particularly susceptible to tolerance induction at this stage of development.

T-Cell Tolerance

T cells do not show a marked difference in tolerance at different stages of maturation. The antigen required to produce tolerance and the circumstance of its presentation are specific for each individual T-cell subset. At least three pathways have been recognized for T-cell tolerance:

- Clonal abortion. Immature T-cell clones may be aborted in a manner similar to B cells.
- Functional deletion. The subsets of a mature T cell may be individually deleted, leading to the loss of only one of the functions of the T-cell group.
- T-cell suppression. T-cell suppressors actively suppress the actions of other T-cell subsets or B cells.

B-Cell Tolerance

As a B cell matures, it becomes less susceptible to tolerization. In addition, during B-cell maturation the forms of antigen presentation that will produce tolerance also vary. Four pathways have been established for the induction of B-cell tolerance. The mode of tolerance, therefore, is dependent on the maturity of the cell, the antigen, and the manner of antigen presentation to the immune system.

The pathways of B-cell tolerance are:

- Clonal abortion. A low concentration of multivalent antigen may cause the immature clone to abort. Tolerance of immature B cells by this mechanism is high.
- Clonal exhaustion. Repeated antigen challenge with a T-independent antigen may remove all mature functional B-cell clones. Tolerance of mature B cells is moderate.
- Functional deletion. The combined absence of the T-helper subset and presence of T-dependent antigen (or with T-suppressor cells), or an excess of T-independent antigen, prevent mature B cells from functioning normally. The ability to tolerize B cells by this mechanism is moderate.
- Antibody-forming cell blockade. An excess of T-independent antigen interferes with the secretion of antibody by antibody-forming cells. B-cell tolerance by this mechanism is low.

Immune Response Gene-Associated Antigens

The specific immune responses to a variety of antigenic substances are now known to be regulated by an immune response (Ir) gene. Ir gene control is considered genetically dominant. The homology of the HLA-D region with the animal I region suggests that the human Ir gene might be linked to the HLA complex. Evidence for the existence of the Ir gene is obtained from family and population studies. Additional evidence for the presence of Ir genes comes from HLA-linked disease susceptibility genes and HLA-disease associations. It is believed that individuals who lack that gene are unresponsive.

The generally accepted concept is that the Ir gene is responsible for the interaction of T cells with both B cells and macrophages, which are necessary for T-cell activation. Activation of T cells is necessary for:

- Conversion to active helper function
- Production of lymphokines

Mediation of delayed and contact hypersensitivity, as the proliferative response to antigen depends on the interaction of T cell with an antigen-presenting cell, usually macrophage-monocytes. Helper function also depends on T-cell interaction with precursors of antibody-secreting cells. T cells interact with these cells by recognizing specific antigen bound to macrophages or to B cells and the I region gene products expressed on the surface of these cells. T cells are able to recognize the precise details of antigen structure and distinguish between two closely related immune response gene-associated molecules expressed on the surface of these antigen-presenting cells or on the B cell.

MECHANISMS OF REJECTION

General Characteristics

Variations in the expression of class II histocompatibility antigens by different tissues and the presence of antigen-presenting cells in some tissues highly influence the success of a transplant. Antigen-presenting cells that enter the graft through the donor's circulation are very likely to elicit graft rejection. If these "passenger lymphocytes" leave the graft after transplantation and enter the draining lymphatic system, they are particularly effective in sensitizing the host.

Rejection of a graft displays the two key features of adaptive immunity:

- Memory
- Specificity

Only sites accessible to the immune system in the recipient are susceptible to graft rejection. Certain "privileged" sites in the body allow allogeneic grafts to survive indefinitely.

The Role of T Cells

Graft rejection is primarily regulated by the interaction of the host's T cells with the antigens of the graft. Unmodified rejection, however, results from the destructive effects of cytotoxic T cells, activated macrophages, and antibody.

In tissue transplants the graft consists of tissue cells that carry class I antigens (HLA-A, HLA-B, and HLA-C) and of lymphocytes that carry both class I and class II antigens (HLA-D and related antigens of the associated immune response gene). Activated T cells specific for class I antigens have the potential to express cytotoxic activity, which damages both the endothelium and the parenchymal cells of the graft. Binding of these cells to the class I antigens on target cells of the donor organ triggers the release of lymphokines and subsequently activates a nonspecific inflammatory response in the allograft.

T cells specific for class II antigens of the donor tissue are unable to react directly with the parenchymal cells of the graft not expressing class II antigens. However, these cells can activate lymphocytes in the transplant through lymphokine release. Therefore damage to the graft can result from a cytotoxic reaction directed against cells of the transplanted organ or from a severe nonspecific inflammatory response, or both.

Activation of T-helper cells by class II antigens such as HLA-DR probably stimulates the release of interleukin-1 (IL-1). IL-1 subsequently stimulates the release of various lymphokines from helper T cells, which in turn activate macrophages, cytotoxic T cells, and antibody-releasing B cells, as well as increase the immunogenicity of the graft. In addition, macrophages and other accessory cells are subsequently stimulated by T-cell products and release IL-1, which in turn stimulates formation of interleukin-2 (IL-2) receptors, as well as the release of IL-2 by T-helper cells. IL-2 interacts with specific IL-2 receptors expressed on activated helper and cytotoxic T cells. This interaction stimulates the initiation of DNA synthesis and the eventual clonal proliferation of IL-2 receptor-bearing cells. IL-2 also causes the release of gamma-interferon, which activates macrophages and stimulates the release of B cell differentiation factors required for the proliferation of antigen-activated B cells. The release of IL-2-dependent gamma-interferon by activated T cells may initiate a vicious circle, as gamma-interferon induces the expression of class II molecules on endothelial cells, as well as the expression of certain class II negative macrophages.

Histologic examination of an allogenic skin graft during the process of rejection demonstrates that the dermis becomes infiltrated by mononuclear cells, many of which are small lymphocytes. This accumulation of lymphocytes precedes the destruction of the graft by several days. Although this graft rejection process is caused by cytotoxic T cells, in some cases the helper cells are also elicited by MHC gene differences. Graft rejection may be a special form of response related to delayed hypersensitivity reactions, in which case the ultimate effectors of graft destruction are the monocytes and macrophages recruited to the site. It is debatable whether the macrophages seen in grafts are effectors of graft destruction or just arrive as a consequence of the inflammatory process and cell damage.

Antibody Effects

Cell-mediated immunity is the major effector mechanism in graft rejection. Antibodies, however, can also be involved in graft rejection. Antibodies can cause rapid (hyperacute) graft rejection, but they are usually less significant than cell-mediated immunity. Exceptions include cases where the recipient has been previously sensitized to a particular antigen, where there are reactions to hematopoietic cells, and where the graft is directly connected to the host's blood circulation (e.g., a kidney allograft).

In dispersed cellular grafts such as infusion of erythrocytes, leukocytes, and platelets, antibodies (humoral immunity) may dominate the rejection process because antigens are fully exposed to a preexisting or a developing antibody response. Cells are highly susceptible to complement-activated membrane damage. If cytolysis does not occur immediately, antibodies may function as opsonins to encourage phagocytic destruction of transfused cells.

Humoral immunity is suspected of playing a major role in the rejection of xenografts. Xenografts possess a large number of antigens shared between donor and recipient. One species can possess agglutinins for cells of distantly related species, which can attack the xenogenic tissue as soon as it is transplanted.

Immunologic Evaluation of Potential Transplant Recipients

Systems developed to ascertain compatibility between donor and recipient include screening the potential recipient's serum for the presence of a positive lymphocytotoxic cross-match, which is associated with hyperacute or accelerated rejection in kidney allografts. ADCC is another sensitive method for the detection of antibodies important in graft rejection. The target cells from the donor are incubated with serum from the recipient to detect donor-specific antibodies. Graft failure is correlated with the presence of a positive ADCC cross-match.

Immunosuppression

Immunosuppression is usually necessary to modify or suppress immune responses to allow the recipient to accept an allogenic graft. Immunosuppression may be a component of induction therapy preoperatively or as maintenance therapy after transplant. Forms of immunosuppression can or have included chemical immunosuppression (Box 28-4), biologic immunosuppression, or irradiation of the lymphoid system or the donated organ. The immunosuppressive activities of therapeutic agents used in transplantation directly interfere with the allograft rejection response. The problem arising from all immunosuppressive techniques is that the individual is more susceptible to infection. If infection occurs, immunosuppression must be suspended, at which time allogeneic reactions frequently develop.

Immunosuppressive measures may be antigen specific or antigen nonspecific (Table 28-6). Antigen-nonspecific immunosuppression includes drugs and other methods of specifically altering T-cell function. Many cytotoxic drugs are primarily active against dividing cells and therefore have some functional specificity for any cells activated to divide by donor antigens. The use of these drugs is limited by the toxic effects they may have on other dividing cells or on the physiologic functioning of organs such as the liver.

Box 28-4	Immunosuppression in Organ Transplantation
1945-1955	Research on antimetabolites, including 6-mercaptopurine azothioprine and corticosteroids used to improve kidney graft survival
Late 1960s	Antilymphocyte globulin proved successful
1976	Cyclosporine developed
1983	Cyclosporine approved by FDA
1984	OKT3 (Muromonab CD 3) approved by FDA
1987	Tacrolimus (FK 506) and rapamycin (1989) investigated
1994	Tacrolimus (FK 506) approved by FDA
1995	Mycophenolic acid approved by FDA (almost 30 years after development)
1996	Cyclosporine microemulsion (Neoral) approved by FDA
1997	Dacliximab (Zenapax) approved by FDA
1999	Sirolimus (Rapamune) approved by FDA

FDA, U.S. Food and Drug Administration.

Antigen-specific immunosuppression is an ideal form of immunosuppression. Antigen-specific tolerance is that induced by the infusion of donor cells. This is generally impractical in transplantation, but it may be useful in the phenomenon of immunologic enhancement. Enhancement of tolerance has been attempted in renal allograft patients. In a donor-specific blood transfusion program, the patient is transfused several times before elective transplantation with blood from the prospective kidney donor. The overall effect of these transfusions appears to be a tolerance of the recipient to donor transplantation antigens other than those in the HLA-linked regions, such as minor histocompatibility loci, red blood cell loci, and leukocyte surface antigens. This treatment has prolonged graft survival markedly in these patients.

Cytotoxic Drugs

Cytotoxic drugs are the most common form of therapy and most frequently include alkylating agents (Figure 28-3), purine and pyrimidine analogs (Figure 28-4), folic acid analogs (Figure 28-5), or the alkaloids. The drugs of choice, excluding alkylating drugs, are azathioprine, 6-mercaptopurine, 6-thioguanine, 5-fluorouracil, cytosine arabinoside, methotrexate and aminopterin, and vinblastine and vincristine.

Most immunosuppressive drugs administered alone, however, cannot produce antigen-specific tolerance because they act equally on all susceptible clones. With the exception of certain drugs (e.g., cyclosporin A) most immunosuppressive drugs can only be rendered antigen specific by including an antigen-specific element in the tolerizing regimen. In these

TABLE 28-6	Types of Immunosuppressive Treatments	
Drugs	**Antigen-Nonspecific**	**Antigen-Specific**
	Azathioprine	Neonatal tolerization
	Steroids	
	Cyclosporine	
	Antilymphocyte globulin	Enhancing (antiallogenic) antibodies
	Radiation	Antiidiotype antibodies to receptors on T cells
		Blood transfusion in human kidney transplant

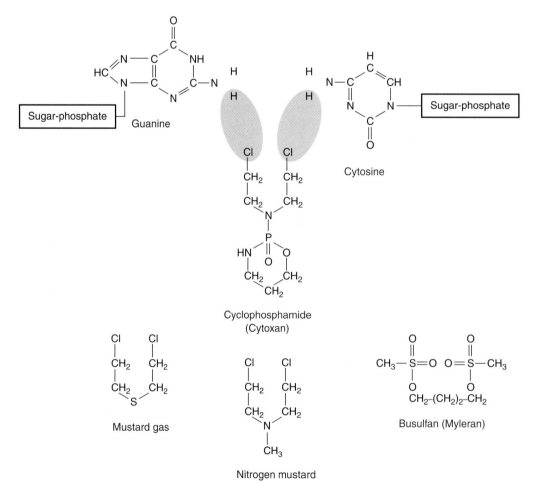

Figure 28-3 Structures of cyclophosphamide and busulfan, which are alkylating immunosuppressants, clearly are related to the structure of mustard gas. The alkylating reaction of cyclophosphamide with nucleic acids also is illustrated. (Redrawn from Barrett JT: *Textbook of immunology,* ed 5, St Louis, 1988, Mosby.)

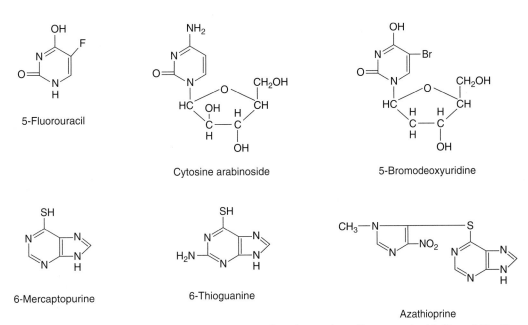

Figure 28-4 Pyrimidine analogs *(upper row)* and purine analogs *(lower row)* with B- and T-cell-suppressing activity. A large number of similar compounds are available for human use. (Redrawn from Barrett JT: *Textbook of immunology,* ed 5, St Louis, 1988, Mosby.)

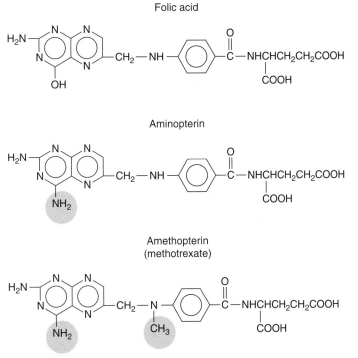

Figure 28-5 Structural analogs of folic acid-aminopterine and methotrexate differ from the vitamin by the substituents in the stippled circles. These differences confer an immunosuppressant function on the analogs. (Redrawn from Barrett JT: *Textbook of immunology,* ed 5, St Louis, 1988, Mosby.)

cases the drugs act as cofactors in tolerogenesis. Experimental evidence suggests that these regimens may act as follows:
- Lowering the threshold for tolerance induction
- Blocking the differentiation sequence in cells triggered by antigen

Azathioprine

Since its introduction in 1961, azathioprine, an oral purine analog that is an antimetabolite with multiple activities, has been the mainstay of antirejection therapy. Azathioprine requires activation to 6-mercatopurine, which is further metabolized to active 6-thioguanine nucleotides. Metabolites of azathioprine, such as the in vivo metabolite, 6-mercaptopurine, are incorporated into cellular DNA. This inhibits purine nucleotide synthesis and metabolism and alters the synthesis and function of RNA. Therefore azathioprine acts at an early stage in either T- or B-cell activation during the proliferative cycle of effector lymphocyte clones. Azathioprine is useful in preventing acute rejection because it inhibits the primary immune response; however, it has little or no effect on secondary responses. Adverse effects include bone marrow suppression, myopathy, alopecia, pancreatitis, and hepatitis. A drug interaction can occur with allopurinol.

Corticosteroids

Corticosteroids can be used in conjunction with azathioprine or another immunosuppressant such as cyclosporine. Corticosteroids directly inhibit antigen-driven T-cell proliferation. Steroids (Figure 28-6) do not directly act on the IL-2-producing T cell. They do, however, inhibit production of lymphokines by preventing monocytes from releasing IL-1, thereby blocking IL-1–dependent release of IL-2 from antigen-activated T cells. Other activities of monocytes, such as inhibition of chemotaxis, are also likely to be important in the immunosuppressive process.

High doses of corticosteroids are used to treat acute rejection. In addition, steroids probably reverse in vivo rejection episodes by preventing the production of IL-2, which would inhibit activated T cells as an essential trophic factor.

Cyclosporin (Cyclosporin A)

Cyclosporin, isolated in 1971 from the fungus *Tolypocladium inflatum,* has become the mainstay of immunosuppressive therapy in transplantation. Cyclosporin affects T cells preferentially by inhibiting the induction of cytotoxic T cells. Unlike corticosteroids, cyclosporin does not inhibit the capacity of all accessory cells to release IL-1. Cyclosporin blocks calcineurin to the IL-2 gene transcription pathway and the release of certain other lymphokines, such as gamma-interferon. Cyclosporin binds to cyclophilin, and the complex binds to and inhibits calcineurin (a protein phosphatase). This prevents activation of transcription factor.

The secretion of B-cell growth and differentiation factors by activated T cells is also inhibited by cyclosporin. Therefore, under the influence of cyclosporin, helper T-cell–dependent B cells are not fully activated because of a lack of necessary helper T-cell stimulation. In pharmacologic doses, however, cyclosporin does not grossly interfere with the activation and proliferation of suppressor T cells. Recent data indicate prolonged renal allograft survival with the use of cyclosporin despite potential mismatches of the HLA system. Adverse effects of corticosteroids include fluid retention, electrolyte abnormalities, hyperglycemia, hypertension, peptic ulcer disease, osteoporosis, and adrenal insufficiency. Hepatotoxicity has been observed in 4% to 7% of patients. Drug interactions can occur with grapefruit juice, erythromycin, oral contraceptives, and a variety of other drugs. Drug monitoring is critical because of the narrow therapeutic range.

A newer cyclosporin microemulsion offers the advantage of improved trough measurement correlation with the actual patient circulating concentration.

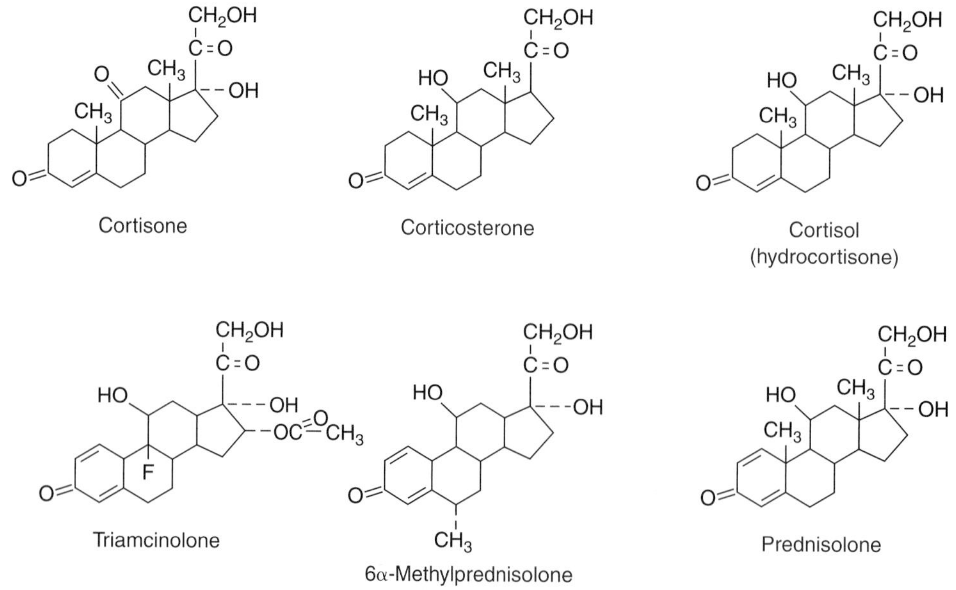

Figure 28-6 Chemical structures of some steroidal immunosuppressants. The differences in structure reside primarily in the side chains and the oxidation state of carbon 11 in the C ring. (Redrawn from Barrett JT: *Textbook of immunology,* ed 5, St Louis, 1988, Mosby.)

Tacrolimus

Tacrolimus (FK 506), a macrolide with mechanisms similar to that of cyclosporine, is derived from a fungus, *Streptomyces tsukub,* found in soil samples in Japan. FK-506 is 50 to 100 times more powerful than cyclosporine. Its primary target appears to be the helper T lymphocytes, with little effect on other aspects of the immune response. FK-506 acts early in the process of T-cell activation and inhibits the production of IL-2. As a result, T lymphocytes do not proliferate, secretion of gamma-interferon is inhibited, MHC class II antigens are not induced, and further activation of macrophages does not occur.

Because FK-506 is a more potent immune suppressant than cyclosporine, patient recovery time is faster. FK 506 has higher toxicity compared to cyclosporine. Nephrotoxicity, hyperkalemia, hypokalemia, hypomagnesemia, hypertension, and other side effects may occur, but FK-506 causes no serious side effects (e.g., kidney damage, elevated blood pressure, or mood swings). Patients receiving FK-506 have increased susceptibility to infections (e.g., CMV) and an increased risk of developing lymphoma or posttransplant lymphoproliferative diseases. Inhibitors and inducers of p450 3A4 may demonstrate an altered rate of metabolism that requires an adjustment in the dose of the drug.

Sirolimus

Sirolimus (Rapamune), previously referred to as rapamycin, has been under development for more than 20 years before gaining approval by the U.S. Food and Drug Administration (FDA). Sirolimus is derived from the fungi, *Streptomyces hygroscopicus,* from the soil of Easter Island. Structurally, sirolimus resembles tacrolimus and has the same intracellular binding protein or immunophilin known as FKBP-12 but has a novel mechanism of action. Sirolimus is a substrate for p450 3A4 and inhibits the activation and proliferation of T lymphocytes and subsequent production of IL-2, IL-4, and IL-15. Sirolimus also inhibits antibody production. Sirolimus is approved as an adjunctive agent (in combination with steroids) for the prevention of acute renal allograft rejections. The main side effects include increased risk of infections and lymphoma, hypercholesterolemia and hypertriglyceridemia, interstitial pneumonitis, insomnia and tremor, and thrombocytopenia.

Mycophenolate Mofetil

Mycophenolate mofetil (RS-61443) inhibits de novo guanosine synthesis by inhibiting inosine monophosphate dehydrogenase. This drug inhibits T- and B-lymphocyte proliferation and antibody formation by B lymphocytes and has been efficacious as both prophylactic and rescue therapy in refractory renal allograft rejection in clinical trials. Findings suggest that mycophenolate is effective in preventing acute rejection and may also slow the progression to chronic rejection. Possible toxic effects of drug therapy can include nausea and vomiting, abdominal pain, gastrointestinal hemorrhage, anemia, and neutropenia.

Antilymphocyte Globulin

Other immunosuppressive measures directed at T cells include the use of antilymphocyte globulin (ATG), an IgG polyclonal antibody, at the time of transplantation and of lymphoid irradiation before transplantation. Use of ATG in preventing or reversing rejection in renal allograft recipients is well established. Adverse side effects can include complement-mediated lysis of lymphocytes, serum sickness, leukopenia, and thrombocytopenia.

Monoclonal Antibodies

Monoclonal antibody (OKT3) is used because the CD3 surface membrane marker is found on all mature postthymic T cells. Interaction between OKT3 and the surface of mature T lymphocytes produces T-cell depletion. The use of OKT3 reverses almost all acute renal transplant rejection and is indicated for treatment of steroid-resistant rejection. A side effects of this drug is cytokine-release syndrome, which is a condition with flulike symptoms, dyspnea, aseptic meningitis, and pulmonary edema.

Dacliximab (Zenapax) is a recently approved humanized monoclonal antibody to the alpha subunit of the IL-2 receptor. A decreased incidence of renal allograft rejection has been observed with triple and/or double immunosuppressive regimens.

Immunosuppressive Protocols

Protocols for immunosuppression (Box 28-5) of transplant recipients vary widely depending on the transplant center, type of organ transplanted, after transplantation, underlying etiology of organ failure, and preexisting conditions. Protocols are becoming more complex because of the choice of more immunosuppressive drug choices. In general, protocols include:
- Lymphokine synthesis inhibitors (e.g., cyclosporine, tacrolimus)
- Nucleoside syntheses inhibitors (e.g., azathioprine, mycophenolate mofetil)
- Steroids (e.g., prednisone).
- Induction or pretransplant therapy may include antithymocyte globulin, OKT3, or dacliximab)

New Approaches in Immunosuppression

New suggested strategies include:
- Cellular transplants
- Transgenic organs
- Development of chimerism
- Localized immunosuppression
- Prevention of chronic rejection

Box 28-5	Example Protocol (Liver)
Intra-op	Methylprednisolone 1g ×1
Day 0	Methylprednisolone 1g ×1
Day 1	Prednisolone 200 mg/day (qid)
Day 2	Taper
Day 0-5	Antilymphocyte globulin ATG 15 mg/kg IV; given until adequate cyclosporin A levels obtained
Day 0-5	Azathioprine 1 mg/kg per day IV
Day 6	Azathioprine 2 mg/kg per day po
Day ?	CyA 10-15 mg/kg per day (bid); adjust to level

From Tsunoda S: *Update on immunosuppression,* Boston, Mass, 2000, Tufts University School of Medicine Transplant Teleconference Series.

Postorgan Transplant Complications

Complications are associated with transplantation. Early diagnosis and treatment of complications are essential. The primary risks of transplantation are rejection and infection. Infections can be viral (CMV 80%, Epstein-Barr virus 20% to 30%, hepatitis B, or hepatitis C). Other pathogens can include *Pneumocyctis carini,* and *Aspergillus.* Organisms associated with central nervous system infection in renal transplant recipients in decreasing order of frequency are *Listeria, Cryptococcus, Mycobacteria, Nocardia, Aspergillus, Mucor, Toxoplasma,* and *Strongyloides.* Recently published guidelines attempt to minimize transplant risk. According to the guidelines, transplant teams should:

- Screen for infectious disease agents in both donors and recipients before transplantation
- Culture and identify known and novel pathogens in recipients after transplantation
- Archive serologic samples before transplantation for identification of new infections later

Five other major complications of organ transplantation are cancer, osteoporosis, diabetes, hypertension, and hypercholesterolemia.

Cancer

Organ transplant recipients have a 20% greater risk of the development of cancer. The incidence of non-Hodgkin's lymphoma is increased by 40%. The greatest risk for lymphoma is within the first 6 to 12 months posttransplant. Transplant recipients also run a greater risk of skin cancer and a slightly increased risk of cervical cancer.

Osteoporosis

In the general population osteoporosis afflicts 1 in 4 women and 1 in 8 men. The general risk factors for the disorder are age, postmenopausal state, sedentary lifestyle, and inadequate calcium intake. Transplant recipients are at an increased risk of developing osteoporosis because of pretransplant immobility and the long-term effects of steroid therapy. Regular bone density scanning should be a routine component of posttransplant care.

Diabetes

The threat of diabetes can develop in two risk groups: patients with preexisting diabetes (25%) and the development of diabetes after transplantation (20%). Patients with preexisting diabetes may require increased doses of insulin until stabilized on medications. Posttransplant steroid-induced hyperglycemia can produced physiologic conditions that negatively affect a graft. Steroid medication might aggravate a familial tendency towards diabetes. Steroids produce decreased use of insulin by peripheral tissues, eventual insulin resistance with decreasing receptor sites, reduction in insulin production, and accelerated glycogenolysis by the liver to assist in glucose availability. These metabolic activities perpetuate hyperglycemia. In addition to threatening graft survival, diabetes can produce other negative health consequences: adult blindness, vasculopathy, neuropathy, retinopathy, bladder infections, and a shortened life span.

Hypertension

An abnormal increase in blood pressure is usually a preexisting medical condition in transplant recipients. This condition is commonly associated with renal failure. Hypertension can negatively affect the patient's general health and graft survival.

Hypercholesterolemia

Increased blood cholesterol is a serious posttransplant concern because of long-term vascular effects to the patient and engrafted organ. Hypercholesterolemia can be the consequence of the return of the patient's appetite and the lifting of dietary restrictions.

Xenotranplantation

Xenotransplantation is the logical next step (Box 28-6) in transplantation. There is a worldwide shortage of organs for clinical transplantation. Pigs' heart valves are already used to repair human hearts and porcine pancreatic islet cells are used to treat diabetes, so it is not a big leap to envision transspecies, whole-organ transplants. Pigs are considered the most likely organ transplant donors into humans because their organs are similar in size to human organs, they are easy to breed, and the extensive biologic differences between pigs and human beings make it unlikely for infectious diseases in pigs to infect human beings. Another application of cross-species organ use was successfully demonstrated in a Phase I clinical trial that used transgenic pig livers as an ex vivo (outside the body) support system for patients with acute liver failure. The pig liver was used to bridge the gap between organ failure and obtaining an appropriate human liver for transplantation in these patients. New protocols are being developed for a Phase I in vivo (inside the body) clinical trial.

Other procedures, some of which are in early clinical trials, aim to use cells or tissues from other species to treat life-threatening illnesses such as cancer, AIDS, diabetes, liver failure, and Parkinson's disease. Even if whole organs are not transplanted, animal cells or tissues will likely be used to treat many diseases including Parkinson's disease. In 1995 doctors in California transplanted bone marrow from a baboon into an AIDS patient in a highly controversial procedure that prompted the creation of strict guidelines for transplantation by the FDA, the National Institutes of Health, and the Centers for Disease Control and Prevention.

Box 28-6	Milestones in Xenotransplantation
1963-1964	Chimpanzee-to-human renal transplants
1964	Pig heart valve transplant
1968	Sheep heart transplant
1984	"Baby Fae" transplanted with a baboon heart
1992	Baboon-to-human liver transplant
1994	Pig pancreatic islets transplanted to insulin-dependent patients
1995	Neuronal cells from a fetal pig transplanted to patients with Parkinson's disease
1996	Baboon bone marrow transplanted to AIDS patient

Modified from Wilde M: Rejection: retroviruses major barriers to xenotransplantation, *Adv Med Lab Prof* 21:11, 1997.

Ethical and medical concerns surround xenotransplantation. One very real risk is that the transplanted tissue may carry unknown latent infections that, once introduced into the recipient, could be activated and give rise to infection. In addition, an optimal antirejection drug protocol is not yet known.

Case Study

Forty-year-old C.G. was seen by her family physician after several episodes of painless hematuria. On direct questioning she complained of worsening malaise and swelling of her legs and hands over the previous 2 weeks. She also reported that despite a high fluid intake she was urinating far less frequently than normal. She had no significant medical history.

On examination, the patient was pale and had generalized swelling of her extremities. Her temperature was 38.5° C, and her blood pressure was 160/110 mm Hg. She had no palpable masses or hepatosplenomegaly.

A diagnosis of idiopathic and rapidly progressive glomerulonephritis was made. She was given antihypertensive agents, corticosteroids, and azathioprine for 2 weeks, but her renal function deteriorated and end-stage renal failure was diagnosed. Hemodialysis was initiated.

In preparation for a possible renal transplant, she was tissue typed for major histocompatibility antigens (MHC) using anti-HLA antibodies. She was found to be HLA-A10, -A28, -B7, -Bw52, -Cw2, -Cw6, -DR2, -DRw10, and blood group B positive. A suitable cadaveric kidney was found from a donor of HLA type-A9, -A28, -B7, -B17, -Cw2, -Cw6, -DR2, -DR4, and also blood group B positive. A cross-match of the patient's serum with donor lymphocytes was satisfactory.

She underwent successful kidney transplantation. Her posttransplant treatment was a combined triple immunosuppressive regimen of prednisolone, cyclosporin A, and azathioprine. She progressed well immediately after transplant.

Twelve days after engraftment, the patient developed a fever and was noted to be lethargic. Physical examination revealed generalized edema. Her blood pressure was 165/110 mm Hg. Her urine output had dropped significantly. A renal biopsy was performed. Histologic examination demonstrated significant interstitial mononuclear cell infiltration. This finding was consistent with the diagnosis of acute graft rejection. She was immediately treated with parenteral methylprednisolone. This treatment failed to improve her renal function and an antilymphocyte monoclonal antibody was administered. Her renal function improved and she was eventually discharged on cyclosporin A treatment.

Questions and Discussion

1. What factors are important in matching donor to recipient in renal transplantation?

   Two groups of antigens are important in renal transplantation: the ABO blood group system and the MHC/ HLA system. It is essential that the ABO grouping is compatible between the donor and recipient. Donor and recipient must be HLA compatible. Donor lymphocytes are incubated with recipient serum to detect antibodies to MHC I and II molecules. HLA matching is carried out with a focus on MHC II molecules.

2. How does this patient's graft rejection compare with other types of graft rejection?

   Renal transplant rejection is classified according to the timing of the episode. Hyperacute rejection occurs minutes to hours after transplantation. It occurs because the patient has antibodies to either MHC class I or ABO blood group antigens, both of which are expressed on the renal epithelium. Blood transfusions, previous transplantation, or pregnancy can presensitize a patient. Accelerated rejection occurs 3 to 5 days after transplantation. Presensitized cytotoxic T lymphocytes or noncomplement-binding antibodies may be responsible. The latter mediate an antibody-dependent, cell-mediated, cytotoxic reaction against the graft by binding to Ec receptors. Vascular endothelium is often targeted because it expresses MHC I and II molecules. Histologically, the graft is infiltrated with mononuclear cells. Immunosuppressive agents may save the graft.

   Acute rejection, which takes place 7 days to 3 months after transplantation, accounts for 85% of all rejection episodes. Cellular rejection is a T-cell–mediated (type IV) phenomenon characterized histologically by edema and cellular infiltration. In addition, varying degrees of vascular rejection are present, initiated by IgG or IgM antibodies to vascular wall components (a type II reaction). Grafts may be saved with high-dose methylprednisolone or, as in this case, by the use of ATG therapy.

   Chronic rejection manifests itself from several months to years after transplantation. It appears to be an immune complex-mediated phenomenon. Immunosuppressive therapy is usually ineffective.

CHAPTER HIGHLIGHTS

All vertebrates capable of acute rejection of foreign skin grafts possess a localized complex involving many genes that exert major control over the organism's immune reactions. Many nucleated cells possess cell-surface-protein antigens, which are part of this complex that readily provokes an immune response if transferred into an allogeneic individual of the same species. Some of these antigens are much more potent than others in provoking an immune response and therefore are called the MHC. In humans the MHC is referred to as HLA. It is the most complex immunogenetic system presently known in humans and is controlled by an MHC, or supergene, which includes several loci closely linked on the short arm of chromosome 6. The MHC is divided into four major regions: D, B, C, and A. The A, B, and C regions code for class I molecules, whereas the D region codes for class II molecules. Class I and class II antigens can be found on surface membrane proteins of body cells and in body fluids.

The presence of HLA was first recognized when multiple-transfused patients experienced transfusion reactions despite proper cross-matching. It was discovered that these reactions resulted from leukocyte antibodies rather than from antibodies directed against erythrocyte antigens. The MHC gene products have an important role in clinical immunology. For example, transplants are rejected if performed against MHC barriers; thus immunosuppressive therapy is required. These antigens are of primary importance in influencing the genetic basis of survival or rejection of transplanted organs.

Although HLA was originally identified by its role in transplant rejection, it is now recognized that the products of HLA genes play a crucial role in our immune system. T cells do not recognize antigens directly but do so when the antigen is presented on the surface of an antigen-presenting cell, the macrophage. In addition to presenting the antigen, the macrophage must present another molecule for this response to occur. This molecule is a cell surface glycoprotein coded in each species by the MHC. T cells are able to interact with the histocompatibility molecules only if they are genetically identical (MHC restriction). Both class I and class II antigens function as targets of T lymphocytes that regulate the immune response. Class I molecules regulate interaction between cytolytic T cells and target cells, and class II molecules restrict the activity of regulatory T cells (helper, suppressor, and amplifier subsets). Hence class II molecules regulate the interaction between helper T cells and antigen-presenting cells. HLA matching is of value in organ transplantation, as well as in the transplantation of bone marrow. HLA-matched platelets are useful to patients who are refractile to random donor platelets. In paternity testing, HLA typing and selected erythrocyte antigens are used. HLA testing is also increasingly being used as a diagnostic and genetic counseling tool. Knowledge of HLA antigens and their linkage is becoming important because of the recognized association of certain antigens with distinct immunologic-mediated reactions, autoimmune diseases, some neoplasms, and other disorders, which, although nonimmunologic, are influenced by non-HLA genes also located within the major MHC region.

Various tissues and organs are transplanted in humans. Transplantation is one of the areas (in addition to hypersensitivity and autoimmunity) in which the immune system functions in a detrimental way. The transplanting or grafting of an organ or tissue ranges from self-transplantation to the grafting of a body component from one species to another. Tissues and organs transplanted include bone marrow, bone matrix, skin, kidneys, liver, cardiac valves, heart, pancreas, corneas, and lungs.

In instances such as bone marrow transplantation, host immunity to the donor can cause GVHD. This condition is believed to result from the patient being sensitized to unshared HLA antigens before transplantation or transfusion. When allogenic T lymphocytes are transfused from donor to recipient with a graft or blood transfusion, the patient can develop acute or chronic GVHD. Engraftment and multiplication of donor lymphocytes can also be caused by transfused blood because lymphocytes capable of mitosis can be found in stored blood products. Where the donor and recipient differ at HLA or H-2 loci, the reaction can be fatal. It is now accepted that GVHD can occur whenever immunologically competent allogeneic lymphocytes are transfused into a severely immunocompromised host. Patients at risk include those who are immunodeficient or immunosuppressed with severe lymphocytopenia and bone marrow suppression. In bone mar-row transplant patients, acute GVHD develops within the first 3 months after transplantation. Chronic GVHD resembles a collagen vascular disease with skin changes such as erythema and cutaneous ulcers, and liver dysfunction characterized by bile duct degeneration and cholestasis. Patients with chronic GVHD are susceptible to bacterial infections. In immunocompromised patients, the transfused or grafted lymphocytes recognize the antigens of the host as foreign and react immunologically against them. Instead of the usual transplantation reaction of host against graft, the reverse GVHD occurs. The risk of graft-versus-host disease, however, can be minimized if not eliminated by irradiation of the marrow or blood products. Radiation has an effect on specific cellular components such as lymphocytes. In these cells, ionizing radiation is known to inhibit lymphocyte mitotic activity and blast transformation.

The role of sensitized lymphocytes and antibodies in graft rejection differs and is influenced by the type of organ transplanted. Lymphocytes, particularly recirculating small lymphocytes, are effective in shortening graft survival. Cell-mediated immunity is responsible for the rejection of skin and solid tumors. Humoral antibodies, however, can also be involved in the rejection process. The complexity of the action and interaction of cellular and humoral factors in grafts is considerable. Five possible categories of graft rejection have been demonstrated in human kidney transplant rejection: hyperacute, accelerated, acute, chronic, and immunopathologic.

The importance of tolerance to self-antigens was recognized early in the study of immunology. Immunologic tolerance is the acquisition of nonreactivity toward particular antigens. Self-tolerance is a critical process, and the failure to recognize self-antigens can result in autoimmune disease. The specific immune responses to a variety of antigenic substances are now known to be regulated by an immune response (Ir) gene. Ir gene control is considered to be genetically dominant. The homology of the HLA-D region with the animal I region suggests that the human Ir gene might be linked to the HLA complex.

Immunosuppressive measures may be antigen specific or antigen nonspecific. Antigen-nonspecific immunosuppression includes drugs and other methods of specifically altering T-cell function. Many cytotoxic drugs are primarily active against dividing cells and therefore have some functional specificity for any cells activated to divide by donor antigens. Other immunosuppressive measures directed at T cells include the use of ATG at the time of transplantation and of lymphoid irradiation before transplantation.

REVIEW QUESTIONS

Questions 1-4. Match the following items.

1._____ Autograft

2._____ Syngraft

3._____ Allograft (hemograft)

4._____ Xenograft

A. graft transplanted between different but identical recipient and donor

B. graft transferred from one position to another in the same individual

C. graft between genetically different recipient and donor of the same species

D. graft between individuals of different species

5. Graft-versus-host disease is most frequently associated with which transplant?
   A. corneal
   B. bone marrow
   C. bone matrix
   D. lung

Questions 6-9. Match the following types of graft rejection.

6. _____ Hyperacute
7. _____ Accelerated
8. _____ Acute
9. _____ Chronic

A. caused by preformed cytotoxic antibodies
B. an immunopathologic mechanism
C. caused by previous sensitization to donor antigens
D. disturbance of host/graft tolerance
E. development of allogeneic reaction to donor antigens

10. The immune system functions in a detrimental way in:
    A. hypersensitivity reactions
    B. autoimmunity
    C. transplantation
    D. all of the above

11. The probability of success in organ and tissue transplantation increases as a result of:
    A. histocompatibility testing
    B. immunosuppression
    C. surgical technique
    D. both A and B

12. The D region of the major histocompatibility complex (MHC) codes for class _____ molecules.
    A. I
    B. II
    C. III
    D. IV

13. Class I includes HLA- _____ antigens.
    A. A, B, and C
    B. B, C, and D
    C. DR, DC(DQ), and A
    D. DR, DC(DQ) and SB

14. Class I molecules:
    A. regulate interaction between cytolytic T cells and target cells
    B. restrict activity of regulatory T cells and target cells
    C. regulate interaction between helper T cells and antigen-presenting cells
    D. represent components of the complement pathways

15. The 1-year survival for kidney transplantation from HLA-identical siblings approaches _____ %.
    A. 50
    B. 75
    C. 95
    D. 100

Questions 16-19. Match the following to show the relationship between certain HLA antigens and diseases.

16. _____ ankylosing spondylitis
17. _____ type I diabetes
18. _____ myasthenia gravis
19. _____ multiple sclerosis

A. B8
B. B 27
C. DR2
D. DR3

20. The most common form of bone marrow transplant is (are):
    A. allogeneic
    B. autologous
    C. xenografts
    D. syngrafts

21. Potential GVHD has all of the following characteristics except:
    A. source of immunocompetent T lymphocytes
    B. source of immunocompetent B lymphocytes
    C. HLA differences between patient and recipient
    D. inability to reject donor cells

22. In GVHD post-transfusion, symptoms begin within _____ day(s) after transfusion.
    A. 1
    B. 2 to 4
    C. 3 to 5
    D. 3 to 30

23. GVHD can be prevented by:
    A. irradiating the patient pretransfusion.
    B. irradiating the blood component pretransfusion.
    C. administering antibiotics pretransfusion.
    D. administering steroids posttransfusion.

24. The mainstay of immunosuppression therapy in transplantation is:
    A. azathioprine
    B. corticosteroids
    C. cyclosporin
    D. antilymphocyte globulin

BIBLIOGRAPHY

Allen KA: Cytodiagnostic urinalysis effective in detecting transplant rejection, *Adv Med Lab Prof* 7(15):8-9, 1995.

Bennett WM, Norman DJ: Action and toxicity of cyclosporine, *Annu Rev Med* 37:215-224, 1986.

Bonnem EM: Alpha interferon: combinations with other antineoplastic modalities, *Semin Oncol* 14(2):48-60, 1987.

Bronsther O et al: Prioritization and organ distribution for liver transplantation, *JAMA* 271(2):140-143, 1994.

Burckart G: Overview of organ transplantation, May 15, 2002, website: www.pitt.edu.

Caplan A: Organ procurement and transplantation: ethical and practical issues, September 1995, Issue Brief (2)5, website: www.upenn.edu.

Chang N et al: Laboratory of molecular immunology, *Guthrie J* 63 (2):59-60, 1994.

Clinical Clips: Cell transplants help brain repair after stroke, *Adv Med Lab Prof* 13:35, 2001.

Hardy MA, Goodman ER: Transplantation, *JAMA* 270(2):262-264, 1993.

Ichida T et al: Living related-donor liver transplantation from adult to adult for primary biliary cirrhosis, *Ann Intern Med* 122(4): 275-276, 1995.

Janin A et al: Fasciitis in chronic graft-versus-host disease, *Ann Intern Med* 120(12):993-998, 1994.

Kirkpatrick CH, Rowlands DT Jr: Transplantation immunology, *JAMA* 268(20):2952-2958, 1992.

Kobashigawa JA et al: Effect of pravastatin on outcomes after cardiac transplantation, *N Engl J Med* 333(10):621-633, 1995.

Kuruga D, Eisenbrey AB: Role of molecular tools in tissue transplantation, *Lab Med* 24(9):589-595, 1993.

Markin RS, McPherson, RA: Laboratory support for organ transplantation: part II, *Lab Med* 22(5):319-324, 1991.

Marks DI et al: Allogeneic bone marrow transplantation for chronic myeloid leukemia using sibling and volunteer unrelated donors, *Ann Intern Med* 119(3):207-214, 1993.

McPherson RA, Markin RS: Laboratory support for organ transplantation: Part I, *Lab Med* 22(4):243-252, 1991.

Mehltretter S: Clinical cytogenetics, *Adv Med Lab Prof* 7(13):6-9, 20, 1995.

Ndimbie OK, Riddle PB: Serological assessment of the prospective organ donor, *Lab Med* 24(2):103-108, 1993.

Nehlsen-Cannarella SL: HLA and disease, *Complements* 3(1):2, 1983.

Opelz G, Wujciak T: The influence of HLA compatibility on graft survival after heart transplantation, *N Engl J Med* 330(12):816-817, 1994.

Roitt IM: *Essential immunology,* ed 5, Oxford, England, 1984, Blackwell Scientific Publications.

Russell PS, Colvin RB, Cosimi AB: Monoclonal antibodies for the diagnosis and treatment of transplant rejection, *Annu Rev Med* 37:63-79, 1986.

Schwartz RS: Jumping genes and the immunoglobulin V gene system, *N Engl J Med* 333(1):42-44, 1995.

Shelton C: Post organ transplantation complications, Toronto, Canada (workshop handout) 1999.

Solinger AM: Organ transplantation and the immune response gene. Symposium on clinical immunology I, *Med Clin North Am* 69(3):565-577, 1985.

Starzl TE, Fung JJ: Transplantation, *JAMA* 263(19):2686-2687, 1990.

Starzl TE et al: Kidney transplantation under FK 506, *JAMA* 264(1):63-67, 1990.

Starzl TE et al: Chimerism after liver transplantation for type IV glycogen storage disease and type 1 Gaucher's disease, *N Engl J Med* 328(11):745-749, 1993.

Stein JH: *Internal medicine,* ed 4, Boston, 1994, Little, Brown.

Takemoto S et al: Survival of nationally shared, HLA-matched kidney transplants from cadaveric donors, *N Engl J Med* 327(12): 834-839, 1992.

Terasaki PI et al: High survival rates of kidney transplants from spousal and living unrelated donors, *N Engl J Med* 333(6):333-336, 1995.

Thompson J: The human leukocyte antigen system. In Stein J, editor: *Internal medicine,* ed 2, Boston, 1987, Little, Brown.

Tsunoda SM: *Update on immunosuppression,* Boston, Mass, 2000, Tufts University School of Medicine Transplant Teleconference Series.

Turgeon ML: *Fundamentals of immunohematology,* ed 2, Baltimore, 1995, Williams, & Wilkins.

United Network for Organ Sharing: Critical data: U.S. facts about transplantation, May 15, 2002, website: www.unos.org/Newsroom/critdata_main.htm.

Upton H: Origin of durgs in current use: the cyclosporin story, October 28, 2002, website: www.oldkingdom.org.

Valantine HA, Schroeder JS: Recent advances in cardiac transplantation, *N Engl J Med* 333(10):660-661, 1995.

Van Twuyver E et al: Pretransplantation blood transfusion revisited, revisited, *N Engl J Med* 325 (17):1210-1213, 1991.

Venkataramanan R et al: Clinical utility of monitoring tacrolimus concentrations in liver transplant patient, *J Clin Pharmacol* 10:51, 2001.

Wilde M: Rejection, retroviruses major barriers to xenotransplantation, *Adv Med Lab Prof* 9:14-19, 1997.

Chapter 29

Bone Marrow Transplantation

LEARNING OBJECTIVES

At the conclusion of the chapter, the student should be able to:
- Name and discuss various types of cancer treated with progenitor cell transplants.
- Define the term, progenitor cell.
- Name three types of stem cell transplants.
- Discuss available treatment options for cancer.
- Name and discuss the evaluation of candidates for transplant.
- Describe the process of obtaining blood stem cells.

- Discuss the transplantation protocol, related complications, manipulation and storage of the graft, and infusion of cells.
- Compare at least three current directions in bone marrow transplantation.
- Name and discuss four future directions in bone marrow transplantation.
- Analyze laboratory and clinical data of the stated case study and apply these concepts to the field of bone marrow transplantation.

INTRODUCTION

Stem cell transplantation is currently being used to treat patients with malignant and nonmalignant diseases (e.g., chronic myelogenous leukemia, severe combined immunodeficiency disorder, non-Hodgkin's lymphoma). The goals of transplanting bone marrow or peripheral blood progenitor cells are to achieve a potential cure or to help patients recover from high-dose chemotherapy that has destroyed stem or marrow cells, a condition known as myeloablation.

CANCERS TREATED WITH PROGENITOR CELL TRANSPLANTS

Leukemia

In most types of leukemia, the body produces large numbers of immature white blood cells that do not function properly. Under appropriate conditions, bone marrow transplantation may be useful in treating certain types of leukemia (Box 29-1).

Acute lymphoblastic leukemia is the most common type of leukemia in young children, but may also affect adults,

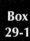

Box 29-1 — Diseases Treatable by Stem Cell Transplantation

ACUTE LEUKEMIA

Acute lymphoblastic leukemia
Acute myelogenous leukemia

CHRONIC LEUKEMIAS

Chronic myelogenous leukemia
Chronic lymphocytic leukemia

MYELODYSPLASTIC SYNDROMES

Refractory anemia
Refractory anemia with ringed sideroblasts
Refractory anemia with excess blasts
Chronic myelomonocytic leukemia

STEM CELL DISORDERS

Aplastic anemia
Fanconi anemia
Paroxysmal nocturnal hemoglobinuria

MYELOPROLIFERATIVE DISORDERS

Acute myelofibrosis
Polycythemia vera

LYMPHOPROLIFERATIVE DISORDERS

Non-Hodgkin's lymphoma
Hodgkin's disease

PHAGOCYTE DISORDERS

Chédiak-Higashi syndrome
Chronic granulomatous disease

IMMUNODEFICIENCIES

Severe combined immunodeficiency

INHERITED PLATELET ABNORMALITIES

Congenital thrombocytopenia

PLASMA CELL DISORDERS

Multiple myeloma
Plasma cell leukemia
Waldenström's macroglobulinemia

OTHER MALIGNANCIES

Breast cancer
Ewing sarcoma
Neuroblastoma
Renal cell carcinoma

INHERITED ERYTHROCYTE ABNORMALITIES

Beta thalassemia major
Pure red cell aplasia
Sickle cell disease

LIPOSOMAL STORAGE DISEASES

Mucopolysaccharidoses
Hurler's syndrome
Gaucher's disease
Niemann-Pick disease

---

especially those age 65 and older. It is a rapidly progressive malignant disorder involving the production of immature white blood cells (blasts), which often results in the replacement of normal bone marrow with blast cells. Acute myeloid leukemia, also referred to as nonlymphoblastic leukemia, occurs in both adults and children.

Although chronic lymphocytic leukemia most often affects adults over the age of 55 years and sometimes occurs in younger adults, it rarely affects children. Chronic myeloid leukemia occurs mainly in adults with a very small number of children developing this disease.

Non-Hodgkin's and Hodgkin's Lymphoma

In Hodgkin's disease and non-Hodgkin's lymphoma, cells in the lymphatic system become abnormal. They divide too rapidly and grow without any order or control, and old cells do not die as cells normally do. Because lymphatic tissue is present in many parts of the body, Hodgkin's disease and non-Hodgkin's lymphoma can start almost anywhere. These diseases may occur in a single lymph node, a group of lymph nodes, or, sometimes, in other parts of the lymphatic system (e.g., bone marrow or spleen).

For patients with lymphoma, chances of survival depend on the grade and stage of cancer, overall health, and response to treatment. Hodgkin's lymphoma is one of the most curable forms of cancer. Patients diagnosed with stage I disease have more than a 90% chance of living 10 years or more. Of interest, higher-grade aggressive types are more likely to be cured with chemotherapy. Lower-grade lymphoma often can have longer average survival times with a mean survival time of 10 years in some cases. Most children respond well to treatment, even though children tend to have the higher grade types of lymphoma. As many as 70% to 90% of these children survive 5 years or more (Table 29-1).

WHAT ARE PROGENITOR BLOOD CELLS?

Progenitor cells are said to be pluripotent because they have the ability to evolve into different types of cells. Bone marrow and peripheral blood progenitor cells are capable of reconstituting a person's immune system because they contain the precursor to the cells that make up the blood: lymphocytes, granulocytes, macrophages, and platelets. Some progenitor cells circulate in the bloodstream and are called peripheral blood stem cells (PBSCs). PBSCs are found in much smaller quantities in the circulating blood than in the bone marrow.

TABLE 29-1	Estimated 5-Year Survival Rates After Transplantation	
Disease	**Allogeneic (%)**	**Autologous (%)**
Severe combined immunodeficiency	90	N/A
Aplastic anemia	90	N/A
Thalassemia	90	N/A
Acute myeloid leukemia		
First remission	55-60	50
Second remission	40	30
Acute lymphocytic leukemia		
First remission	50	40
Second remission	40	30
Chronic myeloid leukemia		
Chronic phase	70	ID
Blast crisis	15	ID
Chronic lymphocytic leukemia	50	ID
Myelodysplasia	45	ID
Multiple myeloma	30	35
Non-Hodgkin's lymphoma		
First relapse/second remission	40	40
Hodgkin's disease		
First relapse/second remission	40	50

These estimates based on data reported by the International Bone Marrow Transplant Registry.
N/A, Not applicable; *ID,* insufficient data.

The hematopoietic stem cell population is not fully characterized, but the CD34 antigen identifies a population of stem cells that can reconstitute hematopoiesis after *myeloablative* chemotherapy. The required minimal dose of CD34+ cells is difficult to define, but most transplant centers will infuse a minimal dose of 2×10^6 CD34+ cells/kg of the patient's weight in the autologous and allogeneic PBSC setting.

Historically the dose of bone marrow has been based on the nucleated cell (NC) count (i.e., 2 to 4×10^8 NC/kg recipient weight). There is no established amount of CD 34+ bone marrow stem cells to infuse because there may be more primitive cells, thus likely to be CD34−, in the marrow that are capable of reconstituting the recipient's marrow.

TYPES OF TRANSPLANTS

There are three major types of transplants: allogeneic, syngeneic, and autologous. In an allogeneic setting, a person receives bone marrow or PBSC from a related or unrelated donor depending on the availability of a good human leukocyte antigen (HLA) match. Because HLA tissue types are inherited, patients are more likely to find a matched donor from within their own family, racial, or ethnic groups. In syngeneic transplants, patients receive stem cells from their identical twin. Patients who undergo an autologous transplant have donated their own cells after mobilization with granulocyte colony stimulating factor (G-CSF) or granulocyte-macrophage colony stimulating factor (GM-CSF) mobilized PBSCs.

TRADITIONAL TREATMENT OPTIONS

To understand why bone marrow and PBSCs are used and how they work, it is helpful to understand how chemotherapy and radiation therapies affect these cells. Chemotherapy and radiation target rapidly dividing cells. These therapies are used to treat cancers because cancer cells divide more rapidly than healthy cells. Bone marrow cells also divide at a rapid rate and can be severely damaged or destroyed by high-dose treatments. Without healthy bone marrow, the patient cannot make the blood cells that are able to fight off infections, carry oxygen, or prevent bleeding. Bone marrow and PBSC transplants can replace abnormal as well as normal blood cells that were destroyed during treatment.

Treatment for cancer can include chemotherapy, radiation therapy, surgery, hormone therapy, or immunotherapy. These therapies may be administered alone or in combination with each other to effectively eliminate malignant cells.

Chemotherapy

Chemotherapy may involve one drug, or a combination of two or more drugs, depending on the type of cancer and its rate of progression.

It is possible to divide chemotherapeutic drugs into those that are active on both dividing and nondividing cells, those that are active on dividing cells and affect a very particular phase of cell division, and those that affect all or most of the phases of the cell cycle (Table 29-2). Whatever the mode of action of these drugs, an important finding is that they destroy malignant cells according to first-order kinetics. In other words, the same proportion of cells is killed for each dose of chemotherapeutic agent.

Alkylating Agents, Antimetabolites, and Alkaloids

The first chemotherapeutic agents to be used in bone marrow transplant were alkylating agents such as cyclophosphamide and busulfan. The common mechanism of action for these drugs is that on entering the cells, the alkyl groups bind to

TABLE 29-2	Commonly Used Cancer Chemotherapy Agents

Direct DNA-Interacting Agents	Indirect DNA-Interacting Agents
Alkylators	**Antimetabolites**
Cyclophosphamide	Deoxycoformycin
Chlorambucil	6-Mercaptopurine
Melphalan	2-Chlorodeoxyaden-
BCNU*	osine
CCNU†	Hydroxyurea
Ifosfamide	Methotrexate
Procarbazine	5-Fluorouracil (5-FU)
Cisplatin	Cytosine arabinoside
Carboplatin	(ARA-C)
	Gemcitabine
Antitumor Antibiotics	Fludarabine phosphate
Bleomycin	Asparaginase
Actinomycin D	
Mithramycin	**Antimitotic Agents**
Mitomycin C	Vincristine
Etoposide (VP16)	Vinblastine
Topotecan	Paclitaxel
Doxorubicin and daunorubicin	Estramustine phosphate
Idarubicin	
Mitoxantrone	

*BCNU, proprietary name US brand name (Sterile Carmustine, Bristol Myers Squibb).
†CCNU, Lomustine (generic name).

the electrophilic sites in DNA and other biologically active molecules. This bifunctional alkylation of DNA results in efficient cross-linking of the DNA, leading to strand breakage and ultimately cell death.

Antimetabolites such as 5-fluorouracil, cytarabine, and fludarabine induce cytotoxicity by serving as false substrates in biochemical pathways. Many are nucleoside analogs that are incorporated into DNA and RNA and therefore inhibit nucleic acid synthesis. They are cell-cycle active and are specific mainly for cells in S phase.

The vinca alkaloids, vincristine and vinblastine, which were isolated from the periwinkle plant, inhibit microtubule assembly by binding to tubulin. This microtubule stabilization prevents the cells from dividing and thus are cytotoxic predominantly during the M phase of the cell cycle. Bleomycin, an antitumor antibiotic, induces single strand and double strand breaks through free radical generation and is cytotoxic mainly during the G2 and M phases of the cell cycle.

Radiotherapy

Radiotherapy uses large doses of high-energy beams or particles to destroy cancer cells in a specifically targeted area. Radiation damages DNA and keeps the cells from dividing. Radiotherapy is most commonly used on localized solid tumors and on cancers such as leukemia and lymphoma that affect the bloodstream. More than 50% of patients with cancer undergo radiation therapy; for some it will be the only cancer treatment they need. Radiation is often used in combination with other treatments to shrink the tumor or to make surgery or chemotherapy more effective. Used after chemotherapy or surgery, it destroys any cancer cells that might remain. Normal cells that may be affected by radiotherapy will usually repair themselves.

EVALUATION OF CANDIDATES FOR PBSC/BONE MARROW TRANSPLANT

Factors that influence the eligibility for a bone marrow transplant include age, disease status, performance status for the recipient, organ function (i.e., heart, lung, liver, kidney function), infectious disease status, compatibility of the donor and recipient, and psychosocial status. Patients who undergo high-dose chemotherapy and hematopoietic stem cell transplantation require a careful evaluation of all body systems to ensure they are able to tolerate the aggressive therapy and also the isolation that occurs during their hospital stay, which can be anywhere from days to months.

Pretransplant evaluation and testing may include: HLA tissue typing, bone marrow biopsy and aspiration, electrocardiogram (ECG), echocardiogram, complete history and physical examination, chest x-ray study, pulmonary function tests, dental cleaning, blood tests such as complete blood count, blood chemistries, and screening for viruses (e.g., hepatitis, human T-lymphotropic virus I/II, cytomegalovirus [CMV], herpes, and human immunodeficiency virus) (Figure 29-1).

At some point before transplant, a central venous catheter is usually placed in a large vein to help in drawing blood samples, infusing medications during and after the transplant, and the actual infusion of bone marrow or PBSC.

OBTAINING CELLS FOR TRANSPLANT

Bone Marrow

In the procedure for "harvesting" bone marrow, the donor is given general or regional anesthesia, and marrow is usually aspirated with large needles from the posterior iliac crest; the anterior crest can also be used in certain cases (Figure 29-2). The goal of the procedure is to collect 10 to 15 mL of marrow per kilogram of recipient weight. Approximately 600 to 900 mL of marrow is collected. The aspirated marrow is collected in bags containing a buffered isotonic solution and heparin to prevent coagulation. After the marrow has been collected, it is filtered to remove any bone chips, fat, and clots that may have been collected or formed during the procedure. The bone marrow is frequently processed to remove undesired volume and/or cells. If the marrow is matched and no further manipulation is needed, it is transfused within 12 to 24 hours after collection, depending on the location of the recipient. If it is not transfused within 24 hours, it is cryopreserved.

Peripheral Blood Progenitor Cells

Peripheral blood progenitor cells are increasingly being used in place of bone marrow as a source of stem cells for allogeneic transplants. Reasons for this trend are the large amount of hematopoietic stem cells that can be collected, more rapid hematologic recovery, elimination of the surgical procedure and anesthesia risk for the donor, and reduced

**Pre-Transplant Checklist for
Allogeneic Donor**

Name:_____   Medical Record #:_____

Date of Collection:_____   Pre-Test:_____ Where:_____

Contact:_____   Phone:_____ Fax:_____

Protocol:_____

HLA Typing performed by _____   Date of repeat HLA at Hospital:_____

Name of Recipient:_____   Medical Record #:_____

Type of Collection (circle):   Marrow/PBSC   Syngeneic/Related/Unrelated

Test	Required (√)	Date Ordered	Date Report Received	Eligibility Criteria	Meets Eligibility (√)
History and Physical	√				
Transfusion History	√				
Vaccination History	√				
Chest x-ray	√				
EKG	√				
Laboratory Tests					
ABO group / Rh type	√				
HLA Typing	√				
Confirmatory HLA	√				
Toxoplasma Antibody	√				
CMV	√				
HSV I and II	√				
Infectious Disease Markers					
HIV consent obtained	√	Date:			
Anti-HIV 1 / 2	√			negative	
HIV-1-Ag	√			negative	
Anti-HTLV	√				
HBsAg	√				
Anti-HBc	√				
HCV	√				
RPR	√				
CBC with Differential	√				
Electrolytes	√				
BUN	√				
Creatinine	√				

Originated: 11/99
Revised:

Form 9929

Figure 29-1   Pretransplant checklist for allogeneic donor.

Continued

Pre-Transplant Checklist for
Allogeneic Donor

Test	Required (√)	Date Performed	Date Report Received	Eligibility Criteria	Meets Eligibility (√)
Beta HCG - **females only**				negative	
Liver Function Tests					
SGOT	√				
SGPT	√				
LDH	√				
Alkaline Phosphatase.					
Total Bilirubin	√				
Chimerism - Peripheral Blood					
Urinalysis	√				
PT	√				
PTT	√				

High risk behavior yes no	Comments:

Additional Testing:

ABO Compatibility	Donor ABO/Rh _____ Recipient ABO/Rh _____ compatible _____ major incompatibility _____ minor incompatibility _____
CMV Compatible yes no	Donor _____ Recipient _____
OR Date _____	
Autologous Blood Stored yes no	No. of units _____

PBSC donors

Sent to Blood Bank for donor evaluation	Date: _____ Cleared by Blood Bank yes no If no, comments _____

Request for Hematopoietic Progenitor Cell Product Collection Form #9904 completed	Date:
Informed Consent obtained and donor given opportunity to ask questions.	Date:

The above results have been reviewed, and the donor meets all eligibility criteria for donation of PBSC/Bone Marrow. Any abnormal results have been discussed with the donor.

Attending Physician

_____   _____
Signature   Date

Originated: 11/99   Form 9929
Revised:

Figure 29-1, cont'd   Pretransplant checklist for allogeneic donor.

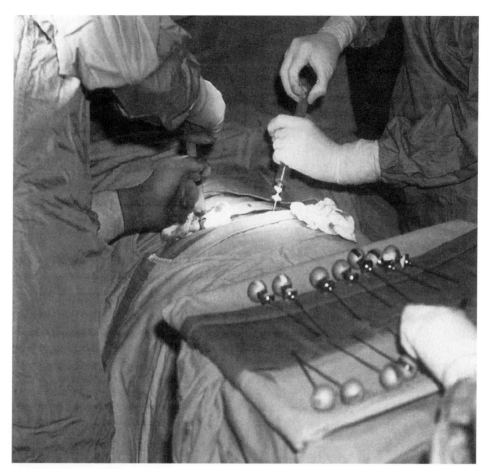

Figure 29-2 Bone marrow harvest from posterior iliac crest. (Courtesy Bone Marrow Transplant Unit, Massachusetts General Hospital, Boston, MA.)

transplant costs. But a patient who receives allogeneic peripheral blood progenitor cells may be at a greater risk for chronic graft-versus-host disease (GVHD) possibly as a result of the high amount of lymphocytes that are contained in the product. Up to a log increase in lymphocytes is collected in a peripheral blood stem cell collection compared to a bone marrow. Conversely, this increase in lymphocytes could aid in the patient's immune reconstitution and also impart a graft versus leukemia effect.

Peripheral blood progenitor cells are obtained for transplant by a procedure called apheresis or leukapheresis. For 4 or 5 days before apheresis, normal donors are given G-CSF that increases the amount of stem cells released into the bloodstream. Typically, in the autologous setting, the patient is "mobilized" whereby G-CSF is given for 7 to 10 days after myelosuppressive chemotherapy. Disease status and prior treatment influence the ability to mobilize autologous PBSCs. The levels of hematopoietic stem cells rise up to 50-fold in the recovery phase after myelosuppressive chemotherapy and/or administration of G-CSF.

In apheresis, the blood is removed through a central venous catheter or vein in the arm. The blood goes through a continuous flow apheresis machine where mononuclear cells (presumably including the desired stem cells) are separated from the red blood cell and plasma fractions by centrifugation and the latter two components are returned to the donor

during the procedure. The process usually takes one or two sessions of 3 to 5 hours per collection. The collected cells are then cryopreserved (i.e., frozen) in liquid nitrogen for later use or transplanted into the recipient.

TRANSPLANTATION

The high-dose chemotherapy given before transplant leads to prolonged cytopenias, which account for much of the morbidity and mortality associated with the procedure. After the bone marrow or PBSCs are transplanted into the recipient via a central catheter, the cells migrate to the bone marrow, whereby they begin to produce new blood cells in a process known as engraftment. The primary measure of hematopoietic recovery, or engraftment, is when the neutrophil count reaches at least 0.5×10^9/L for three consecutive days and a platelet count of 20×10^9/L is maintained without platelet transfusion. Engraftment usually occurs within 2 to 4 weeks after infusion of stem cells. The type of transplant, source, and dose of stem cells are factors with engraftment times. Complete recovery of immune function takes much longer, up to several months for autologous transplant recipients and 1 to 2 years for allogeneic transplant recipients. Recent data have shown that patients receiving allogeneic PBSCs compared to bone marrow were less likely to get infections following transplantation.

Transplant-Related Complications

Complications after transplantation of bone marrow or PBSCs can range from death, infection, GVHD, rejection, and organ damage to infertility. Early complications usually occur within the first 100 days after transplantation. After an allogeneic transplant, rejection rates can range between 1% and 2% in HLA-matched recipients and 5% to 10% in the mismatched recipients. The occurrence of GVHD can be attributed to many factors: HLA mismatch between donor and recipient, conditioning regimen, viral exposure of donor and recipient, and the dose of T cells infused into the patient. Acute GVDH occurs within the first weeks after transplantation, is the result of complex interactions between the donor T cells, and involves the recognition of MHC antigens on the recipient's organs (i.e., liver, gastrointestinal tract, skin and mucosal membranes). Chronic GVHD occurs later and is defined as the presence or persistence of GVHD beyond 100 days since transplantation. GVHD can be prevented or controlled by corticosteroids, calcineurin inhibitors (e.g., cyclosporin-A and tacrolimus), and T-cell depletion of the graft.

Manipulation and Storage of the Graft

The processing of bone marrow and PBSCs varies from laboratory to laboratory, so there are various techniques to accomplish the same result. A bone marrow harvest results in the collection of a large volume of marrow that contains progenitor blood cells. Therefore it is desirable to concentrate the marrow both in the autologous and allogeneic setting. The purpose is twofold: to reduce the volume and remove red blood cells.

ABO incompatibility between donor and recipient is encountered in 23% to 30% of all hematopoietic cell transplants. A major incompatibility exists between donor and recipient when the recipient possesses antibodies against the red blood cell antigens of the donor, which would result in lysis of the transfused donor cells (e.g., group A donor and group O recipient).

It has been shown that differences between donor and recipient's ABO or Rh blood groups have no effect on marrow engraftment, rejection, or GVHD. As long as the transplant recipient has antibodies against the red blood cells of the donor, red cells will be destroyed inside the marrow at an early stage. This could result in a state of "pure red cell aplasia" that can last for 4 to 6 weeks after the marrow infusion, but durations of up to 8 months have been reported.

To prevent acute hemolysis, the main objective of the laboratory is to remove as many red blood cells while preserving the hematopoietic progenitor cells to ensure timely engraftment. This can be accomplished mainly by automated means, but manual methods are still used. Low-speed centrifugation sediments the cellular elements of the marrow so the plasma and collection media can be removed and the white cell rich buffy coat can be expressed into a separate container while the red cells are retained in the original container. This manual method has an increased risk of contamination of the graft, is dependent on the technique of the technologist for good recovery of the cells, and is labor intensive.

Automated procedures involving apheresis equipment; such as the COBE Spectra and Fenwall CS-3000 PLUS, use a closed, sterile system that rapidly recovers the desired mononuclear cells (Figure 29-3). The Fenwall CS-3000 PLUS cell separator recovers mononuclear bone marrow cells in a

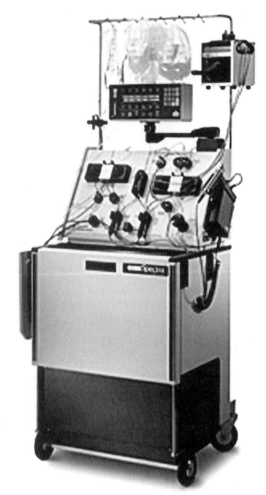

Figure 29-3 COBE Spectra Apheresis System GambroBCT. (Courtesy Gambro BCT, Lakewood, CO.)

200-mL volume with greater than 95% reduction in contaminating red blood cells and minimal granulocyte contamination.

Minor ABO mismatches are present in 15% to 20% of HLA-matched donor-recipient pairs. Patients who receive hematopoietic progenitor cells from a minor ABO-incompatible donor are at risk of developing immediate immune hemolysis caused by isohemagglutinins infused with the marrow or PBSC or delayed hemolysis caused by isohemagglutinins produced by the donor lymphocytes (i.e., B cells). Immediate hemolysis can be avoided by simple removal of plasma from the graft before infusion. However, delayed hemolysis caused by antibody production from donor-derived B lymphocytes requires the ex vivo removal of lymphocytes or suppression of T-lymphocyte function by cyclosporine.

Removal of the plasma from the graft is used to minimize the risk of immediate hemolysis. This is accomplished by placing the marrow or PBSCs into standard blood transfer bags, centrifuging and removing supernatant plasma. Normal saline or other media can be added to the product in a volume equivalent to about half of the volume of the discarded plasma to dilute the remaining donor antibody and lower the hematocrit for easier infusion.

With the development of monoclonal antibodies, there has been an increase in stem cell selection (e.g., CD34+ cells) and purging of grafts (e.g., CD19+/CD20+ B cells). These techniques have resulted in decreased tumor reinfusion into

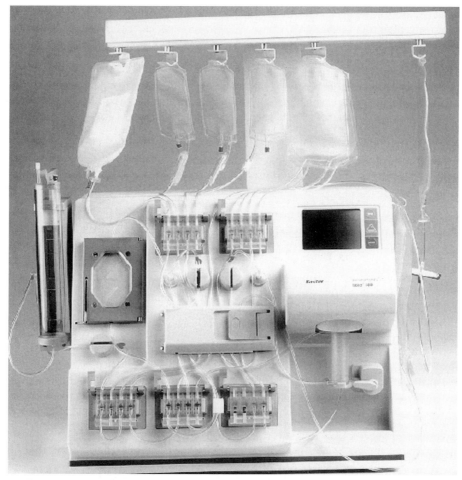

Figure 29-4   Baxter Isolex 300i Magnetic Cell Selector. (Courtesy Baxter, Deerfield, IL.)

autologous recipients and decreases in the amount of T cells infused in allogeneic recipients. The Isolex 300i Magnetic Cell Selection system (Figure 29-4) has been shown to effect an approximate 4 log depletion of T cells, resulting in most situations in a residual T-cell content of $\leq 1 \times 10^5$/kg recipient weight.

The cryopreservation of the product is usually accomplished by the addition of 10% dimethylsulfoxide (DMSO) and autologous plasma or 5% DMSO with 6% pentastarch, and 4% human albumin. DMSO and pentastarch are thought to keep the cells from "dehydrating" during the freezing process, which would cause them to lyse. The product is then frozen in a controlled rate freezer, which reduces the temperature of the product by 1° to 3° C a minute or by "dump" freezing in a $-80°$ C freezer. After the product is frozen, it is kept in a liquid nitrogen freezer, either vapor or liquid phase, until the time of transplant.

Infusion of the Cells

At the time of transplant, the product is thawed in a 37° C water bath in the laboratory or at the patient's bedside and is then infused without a filter through a central line. Toxicities and side effects have been associated with the infusion of cryopreserved products, mainly from the DMSO and volume overload. Most common symptoms are mild nausea, vomiting, and hypertension. Side effects of the infusion are rare and often mild. DMSO can cause patients to experience an immediate garlic-like taste. Sucking on hard candies during and after the infusion may help. Most patients undergoing allogeneic or syngeneic transplants do not experience this problem, as the cells most likely were not mixed with DMSO or cryopreserved.

TRANSPLANTS FROM UNRELATED DONORS

The National Marrow Donor Program (NMDP) is a nonprofit organization that facilitates unrelated marrow and blood stem cell transplants for patients who do not have matching donors in their families. This program has facilitated approximately 12,000 unrelated transplants. Through a network of national and international affiliates, the program aids in more than 130 transplants each month. Approximately 40% of the transplants facilitated by the NMDP involve a U.S. patient receiving stem cells from an international donor or an international patient receiving stem cells from a U.S. donor.

CURRENT DIRECTIONS

Research in techniques of gene transfer, gene expression, and hematopoietic stem cell manipulation remain under development and need to be improved before these techniques are able to change the course of diseases (e.g., cancer and AIDS). Recently there has been promising gene therapy work done in the field of bone marrow transplant and controlling GVHD in vivo. The use of donor T cells expressing the herpes simplex virus thymidine kinase gene ("suicide gene") followed by ganciclovir treatment could allow for specific modulation of the alloreactivity occurring after transplantation.

Donor and recipient matching is a significant factor in graft survival, but identification of minor HLA antigens and their significance in rejection might be of value in transplantation.

Donor leukocyte infusions are used for a graft versus lymphoma or leukemia (GVL) effect in the transplant setting. This treatment may kill any residual cancer cells, but has the potential to simultaneously cause GVHD. The ability to control the life-threatening GVHD while still having the desired GVL effect from the T cells is being researched.

FUTURE DIRECTIONS

The following initiatives should be explored:
- Develop methods to deliver specific cell populations through positive or negative selection, activation, and possible expansion.
- Create and test new immunosuppressive drugs that are more effective in controlling rejection, less costly, and not as immunosuppressive as traditional agents.
- Focus new treatment programs on using highly specific monoclonal antibodies directed at antigens present on lymphoma cells.
- Institute a nonmyeloablative approach to chemotherapy with bone marrow transplantation because it is less toxic to the patient and may result in mixed chimerism.

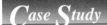

History and Physical

M.C. is an obese 46-year-old Caucasian woman with diabetes. She came to the Emergency Department with complaints of rectal bleeding and a feeling of significant fatigue.

Medical History

The patient has a long-standing history of infected foot ulcerations that are not secondary to vascular insufficiency or diabetes. She received a prolonged course of chloramphenicol for the foot infections in Brazil. After treatment, she was found to be pancytopenic and required transfusions of packed red blood cells and platelets on a regular basis.

Her medical history also includes a history of a positive PPD test for which she received antituberculosis therapy for 4 months. She received facial fractures in a car accident several years ago.

Medications

The patient takes Rifampin (300 mg by mouth daily), INH (300 mg by mouth daily), pyridoxine (50 mg by mouth daily), cyclosporine (Sandimmune), insulin morning and evening, and metformin (Glucophage).

Social History

Mrs. M.C. is a citizen of Brazil. Her husband died several years ago. She has three children, one living in the United States and two living in Brazil.

Allergies

She has no known allergies.

Family History

The patient's father died of heart disease at age 63; her mother died of cancer at age 48. The patient has nine siblings; six of them live in Brazil, and three live in the United States. One sister, age 42, lives in United States and is HLA matched.

Physical Examination

The patient weighs 233 lb; her blood pressure is 120/70 mm Hg, and her pulse 66 beats/min and regular.

Her temperature is 37.1° C. She has ecchymoses and petechiae of the skin with mild bruising on her left shoulder. She has multiple scars on her feet and legs. There are no other abnormal physical findings.

Laboratory Data

	Patient Results	Reference Range	
WBC	2.1 × 10⁹L	4.5-11 × 10⁹/L	
HCT	20.4%	36%-46%	
HGB	6.9 g/dL	12-16 g/dL	
RBC	1.83 × 10¹²L	4-5.20 × 10¹²/L	
PLT	49 × 10⁹/L	150-350 × 10⁹/L	Post-transfusion
MCV	112 fLl	80-100 fL	
RDW	20.2%	11.5%-14.5%	
Reticulocyte count	1.5%	0.5%-1.9%	

Leukocyte Differential

Segmented neutrophils	27%	40%-70%
Lymphocytes	57%	22%-44%
Monocytes	13%	4%-11%
Eosinophils	0%	0%-8%
Basophils	0%	0%-3%

Remarks

Variant lymphocytes 3%
Anisocytosis 2+
Hypochromia 1+
Macrocytes 3+

Blood Chemistry

Electrolytes: within normal limits
Liver function tests:

Alkaline phosphatase	131 IU/L	30-100 IU/L
Transaminase-SGPT	167 IU/L	7-30 IU/L
Transaminase-SGOT	56 IU/L	9-25 IU/L
Lactic dehydrogenase	266 IU/L	110-210 IU/L
Plasma glucose	123 mg/dL	70-110 mg/dL

Immunologic studies:
Hepatitis A antigen = positive
Hepatitis B and hepatitis C screening tests = negative

Follow-Up Evaluation

A bone marrow biopsy was performed. Histologic study of the aspirate and clot revealed a hypocellular marrow with trilineage hematopoiesis and dyserythropoiesis. Cytogenetic studies were normal (karyotype: 46,XX). Flow cytometry revealed polyclonal (kappa+ and lambda+) CD19+ B cells, CD4+ and CD8+ T-cells. The iron stains was normal.

HLA typing:

Patient: A 11, 68	B18, 52	DR4, 15	DQ3, 6
Donor: A11, 28	B18, 52	DR4, 15	DQ3, 6

3-Month Follow-Up Evaluation

The patient is feeling well. The pain and swelling in her right arm has resolved. She has had no fever, nausea, vomiting, diarrhea, rash, chest pain, shortness of breath, dysuria, hematuria, headache, or edema.

Medications

The patient was receiving the following medications: fluconazole (Diflucan 200 mg/day), ursodiol (Actigall 300 mg/day), valganciclovir (Valcyte 450 mg twice daily), cyclosporine (110 mg twice daily), sulfamethoxazole (Bactrim DS, 1 tablet by mouth Monday, Wednesday, and Friday), magnesium oxide (twice daily), norgestimate/ethinyl estradiol (Ortho Tri-Cyclen once daily).

Physical Examination

The patient now weighs 152.6 pounds, her blood pressure is 139/93 mm Hg, temperature 35.9° C, and pulse is 69 beats/min and regular. She has no skin rash.

Her eyes and mouth are without scleral icterus or mucositis and the lungs are clear. Her heart beat has a regular rate and rhythm. Her abdomen is soft and nontender without masses or organomegaly. Extremities are without edema. Her neurologic examination revealed no tremors.

Laboratory Data

Assay		Reference Range
Sodium	139 mEq/L	135-145 mEq/L
K+	4.7 mEq/L	3.5-5 mmEq/L
Magnesium	1.6 mEq/L	1.4-2 mEq/L
BUN	28 mg/dL	8-25 mg/dL
Creatinine	1.8 mg/dL	0.6-1.5 mg/dL
Total bilirubin	0.2 mg/dL	0-1 mg/dL
Direct bilirubin	0.1 mg/dL	0-0.4 mg/dL
Alkaline phosphatase	99 IU/L	30-100 IU/L
SGOT	16	9-25 IU/L
LDH	208 IU/L	100-210 IU/L
White blood count	3.7×10^9/L	$4.5\text{-}11 \times 10^9$/L
Hematocrit	39%	36%-46%
Platelet count	173,000	$200\text{-}400 \times 10^{12}$/L

Impressions

1. Day +88 after HLA-matched donor stem cell transplantation for severe aplastic anemia: stable trilineage hematopoiesis. Mild leukopenia is probably a result of valganciclovir and/or sulfamethoxazole.
2. Right arm cellulitis: resolved.
3. Renal insufficiency secondary to focal glomerulosclerosis: persistent proteinuria (1.4 g per 24 hr) and elevated BUN/creatinine (despite a low therapeutic cyclosporin level).

Treatment Plan

1. Check cyclosporin level today and adjust dose accordingly.
2. Refill norgestimate/ethinyl estradiol.
3. Continue sulfamethoxadole DS for PCP prophylaxis and valganciclovir for previous CMV infection.

Questions and Discussion

1. What is the etiology of this patient's aplastic anemia?

    Extended treatment with high doses of chloramphenicol is notorious for causing aplastic anemia.
2. Did the patient have any other treatment options?

    No. The patient had completed the normal course of treatment (e.g., cyclosporin and ATC) for aplastic anemia. It was unsuccessful. Because aplastic anemia is a life-threatening condition, the only remaining treatment option was a bone marrow transplant.
3. What are the risks involved in bone marrow transplant?

    A patient faces the risk of bone marrow rejection and GVHD. In addition, because of the induced immunosuppression, patients run the risk of developing a CMV infection, which is commonly a reactivation of the disease. In addition bacterial and particularly fungal infections are serious health threats.
4. What drug is highly effective in preventing rejection?

    The drug that produced a significant breakthrough in transplantation survival is cyclosporine.

Diagnosis

Bone marrow transplantation due to drug-induced aplastic anemia

CHAPTER HIGHLIGHTS

The goals of transplanting bone marrow or peripheral blood progenitor cells are to achieve a potential cure or to help patients recover from high-dose chemotherapy that has destroyed healthy stem cells or marrow cells.

Bone marrow and peripheral blood progenitor cells are capable of reconstituting a patient's immune system because they contain the precursor to the cells that make up the blood. Some stem cells circulate in the bloodstream and are called

PBSCs. There are three major types of transplants: allogeneic, syngeneic, and autologous.

Chemotherapy and radiation target rapidly dividing cells. These therapies are used to treat cancers because cancer cells divide more rapidly than healthy cells. Bone marrow cells also divide at a rapid rate and can be severely damaged or destroyed by high-dose treatments. Without healthy bone marrow, a patient cannot make the blood cells that are needed to fight off infections, carry oxygen, or prevent bleeding. Bone marrow and PBSC transplants can replace both the normal and abnormal cells that were destroyed during treatment.

Factors that influence the eligibility for a bone marrow transplant include age, disease status, performance status for the recipient, organ function, infectious disease status, compatibility of the donor and recipient, and psychosocial status.

The procedure for obtaining or "harvesting" bone marrow is the same for all types of transplants. The goal of the harvest procedure is to collect 10 to 15 mL of bone marrow per kilogram recipient weight.

Complications that develop from transplantation of bone marrow or PBSCs can range from death, infection, GVHD, rejection, and organ damage to infertility.

REVIEW QUESTIONS

1. The following diseases are treatable by stem cell transplantation:
   A. acute lymphoblastic leukemia and acute myelogenous leukemia
   B. aplastic anemia and non-Hodgkin's lymphoma
   C. severe combined immunodeficiency disorder and chronic myeloid leukemia
   D. all of the above

2. Progenitor blood cells are:
   A. pluripotent
   B. are found only in bone marrow
   C. are *not* useful in reconstituting a person's immune system
   D. determined by the exact number of CD34 and stem cells

Questions 3-5. Match the following transplants:

3. _____ allogeneic   A. stem cells from identical twins
               B. marrow from a related or
4. _____ autologous   unrelated donor
               C. transplant of own cells
5. _____ syngeneic

6. Radiotherapy is most commonly used for:
   A. myelodysplastic syndrome
   B. localized solid tumors
   C. Hodgkin's disease
   D. both B and C

7. Pretransplant evaluator includes:
   A. HLA tissue typing and hepatitis screening
   B. ECG and complete blood count (CBC)
   C. bone marrow biopsy and complete history of physical examination
   D. all of the above

8. Bone marrow is usually aspirated from:
   A. sterum
   B. anterior iliac crest
   C. posterior iliac crest
   D. vertebrae

9. PBSCs are obtained by:
   A. phlebotomy
   B. apheresis
   C. leukapheresis
   D. both B and C

10. Engraftment of bone marrow or PBSCs is the:
    A. production of cells in the bone marrow
    B. matching donor and patient
    C. measured by the number of lymphocytes in circulation
    D. antibody production

11. Complications of bone marrow or PBSC transplantation can include:
    A. infection or graft-versus-host disease
    B. acute rejection or organ damage
    C. chronic rejection or death
    D. all of the above

12. Differences between donor and recipient's ABO or Rh blood groups have _____ effect on marrow engraftment.
    A. no
    B. some
    C. a major
    D. a total

13. Stem cell selection can be improved using the CD _____ cell surface marker.
    A. 4+
    B. 8+
    C. 34+
    D. 56+

14. Increased cell selection and purging of grafts using cell surface membrane markers has resulted in:
    A. decreased risk of tumor reinfusion
    B. lesser GVHD
    C. transfusing fewer erythrocytes as contaminants
    D. all of the above

15. Toxicity associated with infusion of cryopreserved products are mainly due to:
    A. dimethylsulfoxide (DMSO)
    B. pentastarch
    C. human albumin
    D. glycerol

BIBLIOGRAPHY

Anderson KC: The role of the blood bank in hematopoietic stem cell transplantation, *Transfusion* 32:272-285, 1992.

Antin J et al: Peripheral blood stem cells for allogenic transplantation: a review, *Stem Cells* 19:108-117, 2001.

Areman EM et al: Automated processing of human bone marrow can result in a population of mononuclear cells capable of achieving engraftment following transplantation, *Transfusion* 31:724-730, 1991.

Areman EM et al: Use of a licensed electrolyte solution as an alternative to tissue culture medium for bone marrow collection, *Transfusion* 33:562-566, 1993.

Barrett AJ: Mechanisms of graft-versus-leukemia reaction, *Stem Cells* 15:248-258, 1997.

Bensinger W et al: Factors that influence collection and engraftment of autologous peripheral-blood stem cells, *J Clin Oncol* 13:2547-2555, 1995.

Bensinger W et al: Transplantation of bone marrow as compared with peripheral blood cells from HLA-identical relatives in patients with hematologic cancers, *N Engl J Med* 344:175-181, 2001.

Blume KG et al: A review of autologous hematopoietic cell transplantation, *Biol Blood Marrow Transplant* 6:1-12, 2000.

Braziel RM et al: The Burkitt-like lymphomas: a Southwest Oncology group study delineating phenotypic, genotypic and clinical features, *Blood* 97:3713-3720, 2001.

Brecher ME, Lasky LC, Sacher RA, Issitt LA: *Hematopoietic progenitor cells: processing, standards and practice,* Bethesda, Md, 1995, American Association of Blood Banks.

Chabner BA, Longo DL, editors: *Cancer chemotherapy and biotherapy: principles and practice,* ed 3, Philadelphia, 2001, Lippincott Williams & Wilkins.

Contassot E et al: Ganciclovir-sensitive acute graft-versus-host disease in mice receiving herpes simplex virus-thymidine kinase expressing donor T-cells in a bone marrow transplantation setting, *Transplantation* 4:503-508, 2000.

Davies SM et al: Engraftment and survival after unrelated-donor bone marrow transplantation: a report from the National Marrow Donor Program, *Blood* 96:4096-4103, 2000.

Erslev AJ: Pure red cell aplasia. In Beutler E, Lichtman MA, Coller BS, Kipps TJ, editors: *Williams hematology,* New York, 1995, McGraw-Hill.

Franks LM, Teich NM: *Introduction to the cellular and molecular biology of cancer,* ed 3, New York, 1999, Oxford University Press.

Johnston LJ, Horning SJ: Autologous hematopoietic cell transplantation in Hodgkin's disease, *Biol Blood Marrow Transplant* 6:289-300, 2000.

Krause D et al: Isolation and flow cytometric analysis of T-cell-depleted CD34+ PBPCs, *Transfusion* 40:1475-1481, 2000.

Lasky LC, Warkentin PI: Marrow and stem cell processing for transplantation, Bethesda, Md, 1995, American Association of Blood Banks.

Leukemia and Lymphoma Society: website: www.lymphoma.org.

Martin-Henao GA et al: Isolation of CD34+ progenitor cells from peripheral blood by use of an automated immunomagnetic selection system: factors affecting the results, *Transfusion* 40:35-43, 2000.

National Marrow Donor Program, 2001, website: www.nmdp.org.

Nikolic B et al: A novel application of cyclosporin A in nonmyeloablative pretransplant host conditioning for allogeneic BMT, *Blood* 96:1166-1172, 2000.

Ross DW: *Introduction to oncogenes and molecular cancer medicine,* New York, 1998, Springer.

Sacher RA, AuBuchon JP: Marrow transplantation: practical and technical aspects of stem cell reconstitution, Bethesda, Md, 1992, American Association of Blood Banks.

Sacher RA, McCarthy LJ, Sibinga CS: Processing of bone marrow for transplantation, Arlington, Va, 1990, American Association of Blood Banks.

Serody JS et al: Comparison of granulocyte colony-stimulating factor (G-CSF)-mobilized peripheral blood progenitor cells and G-CSF-stimulated bone marrow as a source of stem cells in HLA-matched sibling transplantation, *Biol Blood Marrow Transplant* 6:434-440, 2000.

Solano C et al: Chronic graft-versus-host disease after allogeneic peripheral blood progenitor cell or bone marrow transplantation from matched related donors: a case-control study. Spanish Group of Allo-PBT, *Bone Marrow Transplant* 12:1129-1135, 1998.

Spitzer TR, McAfee SL: Bone marrow transplantation. In Ginns LC, Cosimi AB, Morris PJ, editors: *Transplantation,* Cambridge, 1999, Blackwell Science.

Spitzer TR et al: Intentional induction of mixed chimerism and achievement of antitumor response after nonmyeloablative conditioning therapy and HLA-matched donor bone marrow transplantation for refractory hematologic malignancies, *Biol Blood Marrow Transplant* 6:309-320, 2000.

Spitzer TR: Nonmyeloablative allogeneic stem cell transplant strategies and the role of mixed chimerism, *Oncologist* 5:215-223, 2000.

Standards for hematopoietic progenitor cell services, ed 2, Bethesda, Md, 2000, American Association of Blood Banks.

Storek J et al: Immune reconstitution after allogeneic marrow transplantation compared with blood stem cell transplantation, *Blood* 97:3380-3389, 2001.

Sutherland R et al: The CD 34 antigen: structure, biology and potential clinical applications, *J Hematotherapy* 1:115-129, 1992.

Sykes M et al: Mixed lymphohaemopoietic chimerism and graft-versus-lymphoma effects after non-myeloablative therapy and HLA-mismatched bone marrow transplantation, *Lancet* 353:1755-1759, 1999.

Zambelli A et al: Clinical toxicity of cryopreserved circulating progenitor cells infusion, *Anticancer Res* 18:4705-4708, 1998.

Chapter 30

Tumor Immunology

LEARNING OBJECTIVES

At the conclusion of this chapter, the reader should be able to:
- Compare the characteristics of benign and malignant tumors.
- Describe the epidemiology of cancer in adults and children.
- Explain the characteristics of the three major etiologic factors in human cancer.
- Compare the stages of carcinogenesis.
- Describe the aspects of cancer-related genes.

- Define and give examples of proto-oncogenes.
- Describe the role of oncogenes.
- Name and describe the characteristics of the major body defenses against cancer.
- Name and explain the characteristics of tumor markers.
- Compare various modalities for treating cancer.
- Analyze representative case studies.

INTRODUCTION

Oncology is that branch of medicine devoted to the study and treatment of tumors. The term *tumor* is commonly used to describe a proliferation of cells that produces a mass rather than a reaction or inflammatory condition. Tumors are neoplasms and are described as benign or malignant. Most tumors are of epithelial origin (ectoderm, endoderm, or mesoderm); the remaining tumors are of connective tissue origin (Figure 30-1). The key distinction between benign and malignant tumors is the capacity of malignant tumors to invade normal tissue and to metastasize to other secondary sites.

Benign Tumors

Benign tumors are commonly named by adding the suffix "oma" to the cell type (e.g., lipoma), but there are exceptions (e.g., lymphomas, melanomas, hepatomas). Benign tumors arising from glands are called adenomas; those from epithelial surfaces are named polyps or papillomas.

Benign tumors are characterized as:
- Commonly being encapsulated
- Growing slowly
- Usually being nonspreading
- Having minimal mitotic activity
- Resembling the parent tissue

Other types of tumors include non-neoplastic lesions associated with an overgrowth of tissue that is normally present in the organ (e.g., hyperplastic tissue) and choristomas, normal tissue in a foreign location (e.g., pancreatic tissue in the stomach).

Malignant Tumors

A malignant neoplasm of epithelial origin is referred to as carcinoma or cancer. Those arising from squamous epithelium (e.g., esophagus, lung) are called squamous cell carcinoma; those arising from glandular epithelium (e.g., stomach, colon, pancreas) are called adenocarcinomas, and those arising from transitional epithelium in the urinary system are called transitional cell carcinomas.

Other kinds of malignant tumors include amine precursor uptake and decarboxylational tumors. These are neuroendocrine tumors that commonly develop from neural crest and neural ectoderm, (e.g., small-cell carcinoma of lung). Sarcomas, malignant tumors of connective tissue origin (e.g., fibrosarcoma), and teratomas are derived from all three germ cell layers (e.g., teratoma of the ovary or testis).

Malignant tumors are characterized by:
- Increase in the number of cells that accumulate
- Usually invasion of tissues
- Dissemination by lymphatic spread or by seeding within a body cavity
- Metastasis
- Characteristic nuclear cellular features
- Receptors for integrin molecules (e.g., fibronectin), which help malignant cells to adhere to extracellular matrix; type IV collagenases, which dissolve basement membranes; and proteases
- Secretion of transforming growth factor alpha and beta to promote angiogenesis and collagen deposition
- Often recurrence after attempts to eradicate it by surgery, radiation, or chemotherapy

EPIDEMIOLOGY

Lung, colorectal, and breast cancer are the leading causes of cancer deaths in the United States. The types of cancer that are increasing in incidence are cancer of the lung, breast, prostate, pancreas, multiple myeloma, malignant melanoma, and Hodgkin's lymphoma. The types of cancer that are decreasing in incidence are cancer of the stomach, cervix, and endometrium.

Cancer in Adults

The lifetime probability of developing cancer is higher in men than in women. The three most common cancers in men are prostate, lung, and colorectal; the three most common

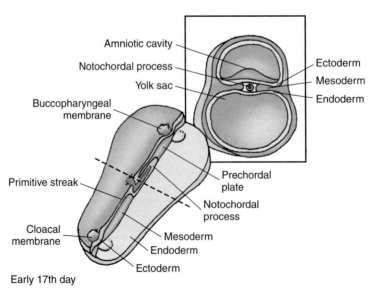

Figure 30-1 Embryonic primary germ layers. (Redrawn from Larsen WJ: *Human embryology*, ed 3, Philadelphia, 2001, Churchill Livingstone.)

cancers in women are breast, lung, and colorectal. Leukemia is the most common cause of cancer death among men under age 40 years and women under age 20 years. For all sites combined, age-adjusted cancer incidence rates declined an average of 1.3% per year from 1992 to 1997, reversing increasing trends in earlier years. Despite reductions in age-adjusted rates of cancer death, the total number of recorded cancer deaths in the United States continues to increase as a result of an aging and expanding population.

Cancer in Children

Cancer is the second leading cause of death among children between 1 and 14 years old in the United States. Acute lymphoblastic leukemia continues to be the most common cause of pediatric cancer deaths followed by tumors of the central and sympathetic nervous system, malignant lymphoma, soft tissue sarcomas, and renal tumors. From 1974 to 1976 and 1989 to 1996, 5-year relative survival rates among children for all cancer sites combined improved from 56% to 75%.

Risk factors are important in specific cancers. Smoking is responsible for one third of cancers. Other risk factors include a high-fat, low-fiber diet, obesity, and a sedentary lifestyle. Certain types of cancer are more prevalent in specific populations. For example, African-Americans have a 20% greater prevalence of cancer than Caucasians. The risk of breast cancer increases with age, and deaths are related to geography. In breast cancer a family history, particularly breast cancer in a first-degree relative; first pregnancy after age 30 years; the presence of fibrocystic disease; probably the use of oral contraceptives or hormone replacement therapy; prior breast or chest wall radiation; prior breast cancer; and ethanol consumption are all considered to be risk factors.

ETIOLOGIC FACTORS IN HUMAN CANCER

Factors that cause the majority of neoplasms are unknown. Etiologic factors can be classified into environmental associations (e.g., chemical and radiation), host factors and disease associations, and viruses.

Environmental Factors

The incidence of cancer has been correlated with certain environmental factors. Environmental factors, such as aerosols and industrial pollutants, and drugs that have been definitely linked with cancer are cited in Table 30-1. Radiation exposure is also known to be associated with specific types of cancer (e.g., acute leukemia, thyroid cancer, sarcomas, breast cancer). Women concerned about possible organochlorine (e.g., polychlorinated biphenyls [PCBs], dioxins, and organochlorine pesticides [DDT]) can be reassured that available evidence does not suggest an association between these chemicals and breast cancer.

Most chemical carcinogens are inactive in their native state and must be activated by enzymes in the cytochrome p450 or other enzymes systems (e.g., bacterial enzymes or enzymes induced by alcohol).

In radiation carcinogenesis, ionizing particles (e.g., alpha and beta particles, gamma rays, and x-rays) hydrolyze water into free radicals, which are mutagenic to DNA by activating protooncogenes. Ultraviolet (UV) light, especially UVB induces the formation of thymidine dimers, which distort the DNA molecule leading to skin cancers (e.g., basal cell carcinoma or malignant melanomas).

TABLE 30-1 Selected Environmental Factors Associated With Cancer

	Factor	Type of Cancer
Aerosol and/or industrial pollutants	Asbestos (silica)	Mesothelioma
	Lead, copper, zinc, arsenic, cyclic aromatics, tobacco	Lung cancer
	Vinyl chloride	Liver angiosarcoma
	Benzene	Leukemia
	Aniline dyes, coal	Skin and bladder carcinoma
Drugs	Androgenic steroids	Hepatocellular carcinoma
	Stilbestrol (prenatal)	Vaginal adenocarcinoma
	Estrogen (postmenopausal)	Endometrial carcinoma
	Hydantoins	Lymphoma
	Chloramphenicol, alkylating agents	Leukemias, lymphomas
Infectious agents	Epstein-Barr virus	Burkitt's lymphoma, nasopharyngeal cancer,? Hodgkin's disease
	Human papilloma virus	Cervical cancer
	Herpes virus, type 2	Cervical cancer
	Human immunodeficiency virus (HTLV-III)	Kaposi's sarcoma, non-Hodgkin's lymphoma, primary lymphoma of the brain, bladder cancer
	HTLV-I	Non-Hodgkin's lymphoma
	Hepatitis B	Hepatocellular carcinoma

Modified from Zeltzer PM: The immune system and neoplasia. In Lawlor GI, Fischer TJ, editors: *Manual of allergy and immunology,* ed 2, Boston, 1988, Little, Brown.
HTLV, Human T cell leukemia virus.

Box 30-1   **Cancer-Related Conditions**

DISEASE	RELATED CANCER
Paget's disease	Osteogenic sarcoma
Cryptorchidism	Testicular cancer
Neurofibromatosis	Brain tumors, sarcoma
Esophageal webbing	Esophageal carcinoma
Achlorhydria and pernicious anemia	Gastric carcinoma
Cirrhosis	Hepatoma
Cholelithiasis	Gallbladder cancer
Chronic inflammatory bowel disease	Colon cancer
Migratory thrombophlebitis	Adenocarcinoma, especially pancreatic
Myasthenia gravis, pure red cell aplasia, T cell	Thymoma
Nephrotic syndrome	Membranous carcinomas
	Lymphomas, especially Hodgkin's

Host Factors and Disease Associations

A variety of host factors have been linked to a higher-than-expected incidence of cancer. For example, the presence of certain genetic disorders (e.g., Down syndrome) is associated with an increased incidence of leukemia. The link between certain genetic abnormalities and leukemia is consistent with a germinal or somatic mutation in a stem cell line.

Familial clustering of germ-cell tumors, malignant tumors arising in the testis, has been observed, particularly among siblings. Cryptorchidism and Klinefelter's syndrome are predisposing factors in the development of germ-cell tumors arising from the testis and mediastinum, respectively.

The incidence of cancer is extremely increased (10,000 times greater than expected) in patients suffering from immunodeficiency syndromes. The increased incidence of lymphomas in congenital, acquired, and drug-induced immunosuppression is consistent with the failure of normal immune mechanisms or antigen overstimulation with a loss of normal feedback control. Other cancer-related conditions are shown in Box 30-1.

Viruses

Viral causes of some cancers are known. Viruses associated with specific cancers are listed in Table 30-1. Nonpermissive cells that prevent an oncogenic RNA or DNA virus from completing its replication cycle often produce changes in the genome that result in activation of proto-oncogenes or inactivation of suppressor genes.

STAGES OF CARCINOGENESIS

Some precancerous conditions progress through a series of growth alterations before becoming cancerous. For example, cervical cancer progresses from squamous metaplasia to squamous dysplasia to carcinoma in situ and finally to invasive cancer. Endometrial cancer progresses from endometrial hyperplasia to atypical endometrial hyperplasia to carcinoma in situ and finally to invasive cancer.

Box 30-2   **The Process of Cancer**

Cancer is a multistep process involving:
- Initiation (irreversible mutations involving proto-oncogenes)
- Promotion (growth enhancement to pass on the mutation to other cells), and
- Progression (e.g., development of tumor heterogeneity for metastasis, drug resistance)

Cancer (Box 30-2) results from a series of genetic alterations that can include:
- Activation of oncogenes that promote cell growth
- Loss of tumor suppressor gene activity, which inhibits cell growth

Mutation or overexpression of oncogenes produces proteins that can stimulate uncontrolled cell growth, whereas mutation or deletion of tumor suppressor genes results in the production of nonfunctional proteins that can no longer control cell proliferation. The mutant cell multiplies and the succeeding generations of cells aggregate to form a malignant tumor.

Interleukin-24 (IL-24), initially named MOB-5, is a protein that is usually secreted by immune system cells in response to injury or infection. New research on colon cancer cells has demonstrated that IL-24 in conjunction with its receptors appears to give a cancer cell the ability to fuel its own growth. The secreted proteins are released from one cell to transmit a signal to grow, migrate, or survive to another cell. These proteins cannot act alone and must act through a receptor or receptors on the receiving cell.

CANCER-PREDISPOSING GENES

Cancer-predisposing genes may act in several ways:
- They may affect the rate at which exogenous precarcinogens are metabolized to actively carcinogenic forms that can damage the cellular genome directly.
- They may affect a host's ability to repair resulting damage to DNA.
- They may alter the immune ability of the body to recognize and eradicate incipient tumors.
- They may affect the function of the apparatus responsible for the regulation of normal cell growth and associated proliferation of tissue.

Relatively few cancer-predisposing genes have been described. An absence of functional alleles at specific loci, however, allows the genesis of the malignant process (Table 30-2). For example, individuals with certain mutations in the gene BRCA2 are at a very high (up to 85%) risk for developing breast cancer and other cancers (e.g., ovarian) because a DNA repair path cannot properly repair ongoing wear and tear to the DNA.

Recently researchers may have found that a mutation in a gene thought to be responsible for colon cancer may initially cause it. This gene, APC, normally limits the expression of a protein, survivin. When APC is altered, survivin works overtime and instead of dying, stem cells in the colon overpopulate, resulting in cancer. Survivin is overexpressed in colon cancer. Survivin prevents programmed cell death, or apoptosis, the process by which cells normally die. Rather than dy-

TABLE 30-2	Examples of Tumors Associated With Homozygous Loss of Specific Chromosomal Loci

Tumor Type	Chromosomal Linkage
Multiple endocrine neoplasia, type 2	1
Renal cell carcinoma	3
Lung carcinoma	3
Colon carcinoma, familial polyposis	5
Multiple endocrine neoplasia, type 2a	10
Wilms' tumor, hepatoblastoma, rhabdomyosarcoma	11
Retinoblastoma	13
Ductal breast carcinoma	13
Colon carcinoma	17
Acoustic neuroma, meningioma	22

ing on schedule, cancer cells are instead growing out of control. The APC gene controls the amount of survivin by shutting down its production.

PROTO-ONCOGENES

Proto-oncogenes act as central regulators of the growth in normal cells that code for proteins involved in growth and repair processes in the body. They are antecedents of oncogenes or genes that produce cancer. Activation of proto-oncogenes (e.g., *ras*) that are involved in the growth process or inactivation of suppressor genes (e.g., p53), which keeps growth in check by binding and activating genes that put the brakes on cell division, is responsible for neoplastic transformation of a cell. Defects in the gene for p53 cause about half of all cancers.

However, not one of the proto-oncogenes has yet been linked to genes thought to increase the risk of cancer. The rare involvement of these genes in the cancer process is a consequence of somatic mutation that takes place in specific target tissues with conversion of these genes into oncogenic alleles. Because oncogene alleles arise somatically, they cannot be used to explain genetic susceptibilities to cancer that exist at the moment of conception.

THE ROLE OF ONCOGENES

The genetic targets of carcinogens are oncogenes. Oncogenes have been associated with various tumor types (e.g., HER-2/*neu* oncogene association with breast, kidney, and ovarian cancer. Oncogenes are considered altered versions of normal genes. Over a lifetime a variety of mutations can convert a normal gene into a malignant oncogene. Once an oncogene is activated by mutation, it promotes excessive or inappropriate cell proliferation. Oncogenes have been detected in about 15% to 20% of a variety of human tumors and appear to be responsible for specifying many of the malignant traits of these cells. More than 30 distinct oncogenes, some of which are associated with specific tumor

Box 30-3	Examples of Oncogenes Formed by Somatic Mutation of Normal Genetic Loci

ONCOGENE	DISORDER
ab1	Chronic myelogonous leukemia
myc	Burkitt's lymphoma
N-*myc*	Neuroblastoma
EGFR, HER-2	Mammary carcinoma
Ras type	Wide variety of tumors

types, have been identified (Box 30-3). Each gene has the ability to evoke many of the phenotypes characteristic of cancer cells.

Major classes of oncogene products involved in the normal growth process of cells are:
- Growth factors (e.g., *sis* oncogene)
- Epidermal growth factor receptors (EGFR)
- Membrane-associated protein kinases (e.g., *src* oncogene)
- Membrane-related guanine triphosphate-binding proteins (e.g., *ras* oncogenes)
- Cytoplasmic protein kinases (e.g., *ras* oncogene)
- Transcription regulators located in the nucleus (e.g., *c-myc* oncogene)

In addition, tumor suppressor genes (antioncogenes) are guardians of unregulated cell growth (e.g., p53, Rb oncogenes).

Mechanisms of Activation

Point mutations, translocations (e.g., t8; 142 in Burkitt's lymphoma) and gene amplification (multiple copies of the gene with overexpression of products) are mechanisms of activation.
- Overexpression of the c-erbB-2 (HER-2/*neu*) oncogene is noted in up to 34% of patients with invasive ductal breast carcinoma and predicts poor survival.
- Activation of the *ras* proto-oncogene (point mutation) is associated with about 30% of all human cancers. About 25% of patients with acute myelogenous leukemia display this point mutation. *Ras* is mutated frequently in colon and pancreatic cancers; it appears that *ras* activation leads to unregulated expression of IL-24 and its receptors.
- Translocation of the *abl* proto-oncogene from chromosome 9 to chromosome 22 with formation of a large *bcr-abl* hybrid gene on chromosome 22 (Philadelphia chromosome) results in chronic myelogenous leukemia.
- Inactivation of suppressor genes (point mutations) leads to unrestricted cell division, elgl inactivation of each of the RB1 suppressor genes on chromosome 13 is associated with malignant retinoblastoma in children; inactivation of the p53 suppressor gene on chromosome 17 accounts for one fourth to one half of all malignancies involving the colon, breast, lung, and central nervous system.

Viral Oncogenes

Various RNA and DNA viruses have been associated with human malignancies (Box 30-4). Some viral agents have a clear causative role, such as the Epstein-Barr virus and

Box 30-4	Oncogenic Viruses

Ribonucleic acid: leukemia, carcinoma viruses, mammary tumor viruses

Deoxyribonucleic acid: herpesviruses, adenoviruses, papilloma viruses

---

certain papilloma viruses that are the etiologic agents in Burkitt's lymphoma and cervical carcinoma, respectively.

Viruses carry viral oncogenes into target cells, where they become firmly established. Clonal descendants then carry the viral genes, which maintain the malignant phenotype of the cell clones.

Tumor-Suppressing Genes

A very different class of cancer genes has recently been discovered. These tumor-suppressing genes in normal cells appear to regulate the proliferation of cell growth. When this type of gene is inactivated, a block to proliferation is removed and cells begin a program of deregulated growth, or the genetically depleted cell itself may proliferate uncontrollably. Thus tumor-suppressing genes are referred to as antioncogenes. In time their discovery will lead to the reformulation of ideas about how the growth of normal cells is regulated.

Much speculation exists concerning the operation of tumor-suppressing genes in normal tissue. It is known that normal cells exert a negative growth influence on each other within a tissue. Normal cells also secrete factors that are negative regulators of their own growth and that of adjacent cells. Diffusible factors may also be released by normal cells to induce the end-stage differentiation of other cells in the immediate environment. Examples of such factors include:

- Interferon-beta
- Tumor growth factor
- Tumor necrosis factor (TNF)

Normal gene products appear to prevent malignant transformation in some way. It is speculated that normal cells must have receptors that detect the presence of these growth-inhibiting and differentiation-inducing factors, which allow them to process the signals of negative growth and respond with appropriate modulation of growth. Genes may specify proteins necessary to detect and respond to the negative regulators of growth. If this process becomes dysfunctional as a result of inactivation or the absence of a critical component such as the loss of chromosomal loci, a cell may continue to respond to mitogenic stimulation but lose its ability to respond to negative feedback to cease proliferation. Animal experiments suggest that humans carry a repertoire of genes, each of which is involved in the negative regulation of the growth of specific cell types. Somatic inactivation of these genes may be involved in the initiation of tumor cell growth or the transformation of benign tumors into malignant ones. Therefore the somatic inactivation of tumor-suppressing genes may be as important to carcinogenesis as the somatic activation of oncogenes.

BODY DEFENSES AGAINST CANCER

Although no single satisfactory explanation exists for the success of tumors in escaping the immune rejection process, it is believed that early clones of neoplastic cells are eliminated by the immune response. The growth of malignant tumors is primarily determined by the proliferative capacity of the tumor cells and by the ability of these cells to invade host tissues and metastasize to distant sites. It is believed that malignant tumors are able to evade or overcome the mechanisms of host defenses.

Tumor immunity has these general features:

- Tumors express antigens that are recognized as foreign by the immune system of the tumor-bearing host
- The normal immune response frequently fails to prevent the growth of tumors
- The immune system can be stimulated to kill tumor cells and rid the host of the tumor

Host defense mechanisms against tumors are both humoral and cellular. Effector mechanisms can include:

- T lymphocytes
- Natural killer cells
- Macrophages
- Antibodies

T Lymphocytes

Cytolytic T lymphocytes (CTLs) provide effective antitumor immunity in vivo. CTL-mediated rejection of transplanted tumors is the only established example of completely effective specific antitumor immunity in vivo. Mononuclear cells derived from the inflammatory infiltrate in human solid tumors, called tumor-infiltrating lymphocytes also include CTLs with the capacity to lyse the tumor from which they were derived. CD4+ T cells may play a role in antitumor responses by providing cytokines for effective CTL development.

Natural Killer Cells

Natural killer (NK) cells can be activated by direct recognition of tumors or as a consequence of cytokines produced by tumor-specific T lymphocytes. These cells use the same lytic mechanisms as CTLs to kill cells, but they do not express T-cell antigen receptors and they have a broad range of specificities. Research is also focused on the role of IL-2-activated NK cells in tumor killing. These cells, referred to as lymphokine-activated killer cells, are derived in vitro by culture of peripheral blood cells or tumor-infiltrating lymphocytes from tumor patients with high doses of IL-2.

NK cells may play a role in immunosurveillance against developing tumors, especially those expressing viral antigens.

Macrophages

Activated macrophages produce the cytokine, TNF. As the name implies, the factor can kill tumors but not normal cells. TNF kills tumors by direct toxic effects and indirectly by effects on tumor vasculature.

Antibodies

Antibodies are probably less important than T lymphocytes in mediating the effect of antitumor immune responses, but

TABLE 30-3   Examples of Non-Neoplastic Conditions in Which Elevated Serum/Plasma Concentrations of Tumor Markers Occur

Tumor Marker	Concentration in Normal Serum	Non-Neoplastic Conditions
Carcinoembryonic antigen	<2.5 ng/mL	Inflammatory bowel disease, pancreatitis, gastritis, smoker's chronic bronchitis, alcoholic liver disease, hepatitis
Alpha-fetoprotein	<40 ng/mL	Pregnancy, regenerating liver tissue after viral hepatitis, chemically induced liver necrosis, partial hepatectomy, cystic fibrosis, ataxia-telangiectasia, premature infants, and tyrosinemia
Beta subunit of human chorionic gonadotropin (β-hCG)	Negative	Pregnancy
Serum acid phosphatase	Negative	Pregnancy
Placental alkaline phosphatase	Negative	Pregnancy

tumor-bearing hosts do produce antibodies against various tumor antigens. These serve as tumor markers.

Although malignant tumors may express protein antigens that are recognized as foreign by the tumor host, and despite the fact that immunosurveillance may limit the outgrowth of some tumors, the immune system often does not prevent the occurrence of cancer. The simplest explanation is that the rapid growth and spread of a tumor overwhelm the effector mechanisms of immune response.

TUMOR MARKERS

In tumor immunology a fundamental tenet is that when a normal cell is transformed into a malignant cell, it develops unique antigens not normally present on the mature normal cell. Tumors frequently produce tumor-specific antigens (TSAs) to which the host may develop antibodies. Virus-induced cancers are the most antigenic; chemical-induced antigens are the least antigenic.

A tumor marker (e.g., hormone, enzyme) is a substance present in or produced by a tumor itself, or produced by the host in response to a tumor that can be used to differentiate a tumor from normal tissue or to determine the presence of a tumor. Non-neoplastic conditions can also exhibit tumor marker activity (Table 30-3). Some tumor markers are used to screen for cancer, but markers are more commonly used to monitor recurrence of cancer or to determine the degree of tumor burden in the patient. To be of any practical use, the tumor marker must be able to reveal the presence of the tumor while it is still susceptible to destructive treatment by surgical or other means. Tumor markers can be measured quantitatively in tissues and body fluids using biochemical, immunochemical, or molecular tests (Table 30-4).

The search for tumor markers goes back more than 150 years. The earliest identified tumor marker was Bence-Jones protein, a light chain immunoglobulin, found in patients with multiple myeloma (see Chapter 24). Over the last decade the use of tumor markers in the United States has risen dramatically. Tumor markers play an especially important role in the diagnosis and monitoring of patients with prostate, breast, and bladder cancers. At Memorial Sloan-Kettering Cancer Center in New York, the three tu-

TABLE 30-4   Tumor Markers in Neoplasms

Tumor Markers	Clinical Value
Carcinoembryonic antigen	Monitors response to therapy of patients with various types of cancer
Alpha₁-fetoprotein	Diagnosis of germ cell and hepatic tumors
CA 125	Diagnosis of ovarian cancer
Beta subunit of chorionic gonadotropin (β-hCG)	Diagnosis of germ cell tumors
Prostate acid phosphatase	Diagnosis of prostate cancer

mor markers with the greatest increase in testing are carcinoembryonic antigen (CEA), prostate specific antigen (PSA), and CA 15-3.

Older, well-established markers include alkaline phosphatase and collagen-type markers in bone cancer, immunoglobulins in myeloma, catecholamines and their derivatives in neuroblastoma and pheochromocytoma, and serotonin metabolites in carcinoid. In addition, there are many breast tissue prognostic markers (e.g., hormone receptors, cathepsin-D, HER/neu oncogenes, plasminogen receptors and inhibitors). The list of FDA-approved tumor markers continues to grow (Table 30-5). Multiple marker combinations (Table 30-6) are useful in the management of some cancers, but the use of more than two markers is questionable.

Categories of Tumor Antigens

Tumor cells manifest tumor antigens, as well as self-HLA antigens. The four types of identified tumor antigens are:

- Tumor-specific antigens on chemically induced tumors
- Tumor-associated antigens on virally induced tumors
- Carcinofetal antigens
- Spontaneous tumor antigens

TABLE 30-5   Examples of Serum Markers

Type of Cancer	Alpha-Fetoprotein	Carcinoembryonic Antigen	Beta Subunit of Human Chorionic Gonadotropin	Neuronal Enolase	Other Hormones
Adrenocortical	—	—	—	—	+
Breast	—	+	—	—	—
Choriocarcinoma	—	—	+	—	+
Colorectal	Rare	+	—	—	—
Esophageal	—	+	—	—	+
Gastric	Rare	+	—	—	—
Ovarian	—	Rare	—	—	+
Pancreatic	Rare	+	—	—	Rare
Parathyroid	—	—	—	+	+
Pheochromocytoma	—	—	—	+	+
Pulmonary (oat-cell)	—	—	+	+	+
Pulmonary (squamous)	—	+	+	—	+
Seminoma	—	—	—	—	—
Teratocarcinoma	+	—	+	—	—
Thyroid (colloid)	—	—	—	—	+
Thyroid (medullary)	—	—	—	+	+

TABLE 30-6   Applications of Tumor Markers

Markers	Comments
AFP and β-hCG	Valuable combination in therapy and follow-up in patients with germ cell tumors of the testes
CEA, AFP, and LDH	Combination seems to help differentiate primary liver cancer from liver metastases related to another organ
Ratio of free to total PSA	The ratio may distinguish benign prostatic hypertrophy from prostate cancer
CEA and numerous mucin type markers	Combinations are being evaluated and compared for breast cancer applications (the markers are not necessarily useful as adjuncts to therapy, but may complement each other)
TAG-72, CEA, and CA 19-9	Evaluated for use in gastric cancer, but the combination offered no improvement in sensitivity over TAG-72 alone
Serial assays of CA-125	Serial assays over a finite period of time may aid in initial diagnosis in ovarian cancer

From Schwartz MK: New approaches to tumor marker testing. In *Tumor markers: challenges and solutions,* Washington DC, 1998, American Association for Clinical Chemistry.
AFP, Alpha fetoprotein; *β-hCG,* beta subunit of chorionic gonadotropin; *CEA,* carcinoembryonic antigen; *LDH,* lactate dehydrogenase; *PSA,* prostate specific antigen.

Tumor-Specific Antigens

Chemically induced tumors are known to develop antigens called TSAs, which are uniquely associated with each tumor. These antigens are not found in normal cells. They demonstrate little or no cross-reactivity between different tumors caused by the same carcinogen, perhaps because every tumor caused by chemical agents has unique surface characteristics.

Tumor-Associated Antigens

Tumor-associated antigens (TAAs) are cell surface molecules coded for by tumorogenic viruses. These antigens are not expressed on the virion but are synthesized by the host cell. In contrast to TSAs, TAAs are virus specific. Therefore each specific virus induces the same antigens irrespective of the tissue of origin or the animal species.

Carcinofetal Antigens

Well-differentiated tissue produces and secretes little or no fetal gene products. The abnormal behavior of malignant cells is believed to derepress genes normally only expressed during fetal life. Because the products of these fetally active genes are recognized as self, they do not elicit either humoral or cell-mediated responses.

During malignant transformation, however, gene derepression is responsible for the production of increased concentrations of these gene products, which are known as oncofetal proteins. CEA is an example of a carcinofetal antigen.

Spontaneous Tumor Antigens

Tumors caused by no known mechanism are thought to produce antigens. Disagreement exists regarding whether these tumors are similar to those produced experimentally by chemical, viral, or physical agents. Although substantial evidence supports the contention that these tumors do not produce unique antigens, some evidence refutes this contention. The importance of these findings remains unclear.

Specific Tumor Markers

Specific tumor markers include:
- Alpha-fetoprotein (AFP)
- Beta subunit of human chorionic gonadotropin (β-hCG)
- CA 15-3
- CA 19-9
- CA 27.29
- CA 125
- CEA
- PSA and prostatic acid phosphatase
- Miscellaneous enzyme markers
- Miscellaneous hormone markers

Alpha-Fetoprotein

AFP is normally synthesized by the fetal liver and yolk sac. It is secreted in the serum in nanogram to milligram quantities in the following conditions: hepatocarcinoma, endodermal sinus tumors, nonseminomatous testicular cancer, teratocarcinoma of the testis or ovary, and malignant tumors of the mediastinum and sacrococcyx. In addition, a small percentage of patients with gastric and pancreatic cancer with liver metastasis may have elevated AFP levels. Both AFP and β-hCG should be quantitated initially in all patients with teratocarcinoma because one or both markers may be secreted in 85% of patients. The concentration of AFP may be elevated in nonneoplastic conditions such as hepatitis and cystic fibrosis.

AFP is a reliable marker for following a patient's response to chemotherapy and radiation therapy. Levels should be obtained every 2 to 4 weeks (metabolic half-life in vivo is 4 days).

Beta Subunit of Human Chorionic Gonadotropin

β-hCG, an ectopic protein, is a sensitive tumor marker with a metabolic half-life in vivo of 16 hours. A serum level of β-hCG greater than 1 ng/mL is strongly suggestive of pregnancy or a malignant tumor such as endodermal sinus tumor, teratocarcinoma, choriocarcinoma, molar pregnancy, testicular embryonal carcinoma, or oat cell carcinoma of the lung.

CA 15-3

CA 15-3 is a high-molecular-weight glycoprotein coded by the MUC-II gene and expressed on the ductal cell surface of most glandular epithelial cells. The main purpose of the assay is to monitor patients after mastectomy. Using a cut-off of 25 U/mL for CA 15-3, the detection rate is only 5% for stage I breast cancer. The sensitivity is much better in higher-stage disease, which makes it a good measure of tumor burden. CA 15-3 is positive in other conditions, including patients with liver disease, some inflammatory conditions, and other carcinomas. A change in the CA 15-3 concentration is more pre-dictive than the absolute concentration. Over time, tumor markers exhibit a steady state in the body, a balance between antigen production by the tumor and degradation and excretion. Changes in tumor burden are reflected by changes in the tumor marker concentration.

CA 19-9

CA 19-9 is a glycolipid Lewis blood group carbohydrate. Elevated levels have been found in patients with pancreatic, hepatobiliary, colorectal, gastric, hepatocellular, pancreatic, and breast cancers. Its main use is as a marker for colorectal and pancreatic carcinoma. This marker has greater specificity for pancreatic cancers than CEA. CA19-9 is also known as gastrointestinal cancer-associated antigen.

CA 27.29 (Breast Carcinoma-Associated Antigen)

Carcinoma of the breast often produces mucinous antigens that are high-molecular-weight glycoproteins with O-linked oligosaccharide chains. Monoclonal antibodies directed against breast carcinoma-associated antigen (CA 27.29) are available to quantitate the levels of this antigen in serum. The antibodies recognize epitopes of a breast cancer-associated antigen encoded by the human MUC1 gene, which is also referred to as MAM6, milk mucin antigen, CA 27.29, and CA 15-3. This tumor marker may be useful in conjunction with other clinical methods for predicting early recurrence of breast cancer. It is not recommended as a breast cancer screening assay. Increased levels of CA 27.29 (>38 U/mL) may indicate recurrent disease in a woman with treated breast carcinoma and may indicate the need for additional testing or procedures. Some clinical investigators do not endorse the routine use of this new marker.

CA 125

CA 125, a mucinlike glycoprotein, is expressed on the surface of coelomic epithelium and human ovarian carcinoma cells. CA 125 is relatively more sensitive in low state ovarian cancer. It reacts against a monoclonal antibody developed against a cell line from one patient's ovarian cystadenocarcinoma. It is elevated in carcinomas and benign disease of various organs (e.g. pelvic inflammatory disease and endometriosis), but it is most useful in ovarian and endometrial carcinomas.

Carcinoembryonic Antigen

CEA is a cell surface protein found predominantly on normal fetal endocrine tissues in the second trimester of gestation. If CEA is detected in mature individuals, it is of limited diagnostic value, but it is helpful in differentiating between benign and malignant pleural and ascites effusions. CEA was first described in 1965 as a tumor marker specifically elevated in patients with colon cancer; it was later found to be elevated in patients with others cancers (e.g., breast, lung, liver, pancreas). Plasma levels greater than 12 ng/mL are strongly correlated with malignancy. Elevated neoplastic states frequently associated with an increased CEA level are endodermally derived gastrointestinal neoplasms and neck and breast carcinomas. Also, 20% of smokers and 7% of former smokers have elevated CEA levels.

CEA is used clinically to monitor tumor progress in patients who have diagnosed cancer with a high blood CEA level. If treatment leads to a decline to normal levels (<2.5 ng/mL), a rise in CEA may indicate a cancer recurrence to the clinician. A persistent elevation is indicative of residual disease or poor therapeutic response. In patients who have undergone colon cancer resection surgery, the rate of clearance of CEA levels usually return to normal within 1 month but may take as long as 4 months. Blood specimens should be obtained 2 to 4 weeks apart to detect a trend.

Prostate-Specific Antigen and Prostatic Acid Phosphatase

Prostate cancer is a leading cause of cancer death in American men. There are two tumor markers for cancer of the prostate: PSA and prostatic acid phosphatase. PSA is a marker that is prostate tissue-specific, but not prostate cancer-specific. PSA is a protease enzyme secreted almost exclusively by prostatic epithelial cells. Blood levels of PSA are increased when normal glandular structure is disrupted by benign or malignant tumor inflammation. Serum PSA is directly proportional to tumor volume, with a greater increase per unit volume of cancer compared with benign hyperplasia. Free PSA assists in distinguishing cancer of the prostate from benign prostatic hypertrophy. Prostate-specific antigen levels appear useful for monitoring progression and response to treatment among patients with prostate cancer.

Other techniques that have been in detection of prostate cancer include PSA velocity (the incremental increase of PSA over time), PSA density (the ratio of serum PSA to prostate volume), age-adjusted PSA (PSA increasing with age), biostatistically derived algorithms, free and total PSA, complexed PSA, and most recently, human kallikrein II, a molecule similar, but not identical, to PSA.

Prostatic acid phosphatase is another marker for prostate cancer. It is a serum enzyme exclusively diagnostic of prostatic carcinoma.

Miscellaneous Enzyme Markers

Lactic dehydrogenase (LDH) is the very commonly measured enzyme of the glycolytic pathway. LDH is elevated in a wide variety of malignancies and other medical disorders. The level of LDH has been shown to correlate to tumor mass in solid tumors so it can be used to monitor progression of these tumors.

Neuron-specific enolase is an isoenzyme specific for all tumor cells derived from the neural crest. An enzyme increase has been detected in neuroblastoma, pheochromocytoma, oat cell carcinomas, medullary thyroid and C cell parathyroid carcinomas, and other neural crest-derived cancers. Serum levels are frequently elevated in disseminated disease.

Placental alkaline phosphatase can be detected during pregnancy. It is also associated with the neoplastic conditions of seminoma and ovarian cancer.

Miscellaneous Hormone Markers

Elevated or inappropriate serum levels of hormones can function as tumor markers. Adrenocorticotropic hormone (ACTH), calcitonin, and catecholamines may be secreted by differentiated tumors of endocrine organs and squamous cell lung tumors. Oat cell carcinomas may produce β-hCG, antidiuretic hormone, serotonin, calcitonin, parathyroid hormone, and ACTH. These hormones can be used to follow a patient's response to therapy.

In addition, some breast cancers demonstrate progesterone and/or estradiol (estrogen) receptors, which are strongly correlated with a positive response to antihormone therapy. Patients with neuroblastomas and pheochromocytomas secrete catecholamine metabolites that can be detected in the urine. Neuroblastomas also release neuron-specific enolase and ferritin; these markers can be used for diagnosis and prognosis.

Breast, Ovarian, and Cervical Cancer Markers

For more than a decade, circulating beast cancer antigens have been used to monitor therapy and evaluate recurrence of the cancer. Estrogen and progesterone receptors are universally accepted as both prognostic markers and therapeutic choice indicators. A relatively new approach has been the use of the oncogene HER-2/*neu* as a prognostic indicator and a marker related to the choice of therapy. This is particularly useful, as the introduction of Herceptin as a chemotherapeutic agent that targets the HER-2/*neu* receptor. Breast cancer patients who express HER-2 in their cancers have a poor prognosis with shorter disease-free and overall survival than patients who do not express HER-2/*neu*. The evaluation of HER-2/*neu* has two clinical functions:

1. A predictive marker for response to Herceptin (trastuzumab) therapy.
2. A prognostic marker.

A new and more powerful predictor of the outcome of primary breast cancer in young women recently was reported. Microarray analysis of a previously established 70-gene profile demonstrated that a good-prognosis gene-expression signature was a strongly independent factor in predicting disease outcome.

Epidermal Growth Factor Receptor

Epidermal growth factor receptor (EGFR) and human epidermal growth factor receptor-2 (HER-2, HER-2/neu, or c-erB-2) are both transmembrane tyrosine kinase receptors expressed on normal epithelial cells but overexpressed in some cancer cells. A portion of both receptors have been shown to be released from the cell surface and have been found to circulate in normal people and in abnormally high levels in cancer patients. The shed portions can be measured in serum or plasma using antibody-based immunoassays that allow real-time assessment of the patient's HER-2/*neu* or EGFR status, allow repeat testing for patient monitoring, and can be performed in a standardized and quantitative manner.

HER-2 and EGFR have been the targets of considerable pharmaceutical activity to develop therapies that will interfere with the oncogenic potential of these growth factor receptors. The therapies include small molecule inhibitors that are designed to target and block the function of HER-2 protein overexpression. One drug, trastuzumab (Herceptin) is a humanized antibody that targets cells that overexpress the HER-2/*neu* and has been successfully used in combination with chemotherapy to increase the efficacy of the antibody-based treatment. An anti-ECFR antibody known as IMC-225 is directed against cells that overexpress the EGFR oncoprotein.

Molecular Diagnosis of Breast Cancer

The assessment of DNA content (aneuploid, diploid) and cell cycle analysis (G_0G_1, S and G_2M) can be of prognostic use in certain solid tumors (e.g., breast cancer). Cell cycle analysis can be performed on fresh or frozen tissue. In breast cancer, research indicates that low S-phase and diploid DNA content are associated with a relatively good prognosis; a high S-phase number of cells and aneuploid DNA content have a tendency to indicate a worse prognosis. The DNA content of a tumor is classified in order of worsening prognosis from diploid, near-diploid, tetraploid, aneuploid, hypertetraploid, and hypoploid. The ratio of tumor G_0G_1 DNA content to normal G_0G_1 DNA content is called the DNA index. Ploidy status and S-phase fraction should be combined with other indicators (e.g., hormone receptor status) to evaluate treatment options and prognosis.

Bladder Cancer

Bladder cancer tumor markers for the management of patients with bladder cancer have been actively investigated. Several assays have been approved for clinical use including:
- Matritech Nuclear matrix protein (NMP-22)
- Bard's BTA test.

Nearly all human tumors contain telomerase, a growth enzyme that promotes the malignant proliferation of cancer. Normal cells usually do not have the enzyme, but telomerase renews the DNA of tumor cells and permits indefinite replication.

Telomerase was first observed in ovarian cancer cells and its presence was later established in virtually all cancers. It is not clear whether other vital cells need telomerase to function. For example, telomerase inhibition could adversely affect stem cells, which help produce blood cells and lymphocytes and may need the enzyme to function. Second, telomerase inhibition has not been proved or tested physiologically in the human system where it would come into play. Finally, a drug based on

telomerase would have to reduce that ability of the cancer to spread. Screening for telomerase inhibitors and plans for future studies to discover and develop chemicals that block the action of telomerase may suggest a design of more effective anticancer drugs.

MODALITIES FOR TREATING CANCER

Until recently three modalities were used to treat cancer: surgery, radiation, and chemotherapy. The biologic response modifiers such as interferon (IFN) are a newer modality. Many different modes of therapy, including angiogenesis inhibitors, which keep tumors from building new blood vessels to supply themselves with food and oxygen, have demonstrated effectiveness in the treatment of cancer (Table 30-7); however, drug-induced immunosuppression and IFN therapy alone or in combination with drugs are the most frequent forms after surgery or in cases where surgery is not appropriate (e.g., hematologic disorders).

Chemotherapeutic Agents

Drugs are used in cancer therapy for curing, palliation, and research to develop more effective therapy. The mechanisms of drug action are linked to the mitotic cell cycle, as such antitumor drugs may be placed into three classes:
- Cell cycle active, phase specific
- Cell cycle active, phase nonspecific
- Noncell cycle active

Cell Cycle Active, Phase Specific

Drugs in this category act on the S, G2, or M phase of mitosis.

S phase active drugs are divided into antimetabolites, antifols, and synthetic enzyme inhibitors. Antimetabolites act through the incorporation of nucleotide analog into DNA, resulting in an abnormal nucleic acid (e.g., 5-fluorouracil, 6-mercaptopurine, 6-thioguanine, or fludarabine). The antifols act as competitive inhibitors of the enzyme dihydrofolate

TABLE 30-7	Immunotherapy in Malignant Disease		
Approach		**Agent**	**Proposed Mechanism**
Active			
Specific		Modified or unmodified tumor cells, cell extract	Cellular and/or humoral response
Nonspecific systemic		Calmette-Guérin bacillus (BCG)	General immunocompetence
		Methanol-extracted residue of mycobacterial skeletal wall, *Corynebacterium parvum*, *Pseudomonas* vaccine	Increased mononuclear phagocyte system activity
		Levamisole, interferon	Restores immunocompetence
Local		BCG	Macrophage activation; killing of tumor with bystander effect
		Virus, hapten, dinitrochlorobenzene	
Passive			
Adoptive specific		Allogeneic organogenesis antibody	Removes soluble antigen or directly kills target cell
		Targeted monoclonal antibody	Conjugated with antitumor drug or radioisotope
		Lymphocytes, lymphocyte extract (i.e., immune RNA transfer factor)	Transfer of immunity
		Lymphokine-activated killer cells	Cytolysis of tumor cells

reductase, which is necessary for the generation of CH3 groups required for thymidine synthesis (e.g., methotrexate). Synthetic enzyme inhibitors include DNA polymerase inhibitor (cytosine arabinoside) and nucleotide reductase inhibitor (hydroxyurea).

G2 phase active drugs include bleomycin, which is thought to cause fragmentation of DNA, and etoposide (Eposin, Etopophos, Vepesid, VP-16), which is thought to cause double-stranded breaks in DNA by complexing with topoisomerase.

M phase active drugs include vinca alkaloids (e.g., vincristine and vinblastine), which are thought to inhibit mitotic spindle apparatus, and paclitaxel (Taxol), which stablilizes microtubules.

Cell Cycle Active, Phase Nonspecific

Drugs in this category are either intercalating agents, alkylating agents, or 5-fluorouracil. Examples of intercalating agents are anthracyclines (Adriamycin, Daunomycin, Idarubicin, Mitoxantrone) and actinomycin D (Dactinomycin-D and Cosmegan Lyovac). The alkylating agents in this category include cyclophosphamide and ifosfamide. These drugs act by distorting normal DNA through the insertion of flat, aromatic ring systems between the levels of base pairs into the DNA double helix.

Noncell Cycle Active

Drugs in this category can be divided into five types: alkylating agents, L-asparaginase, corticosteroids, hormone antagonists, and miscellaneous. Alkylating agents (e.g., nitrogen mustard and mustard derivatives: mechlorethamine [Mustargen], cyclophosphamide [Cytoxan], chlorambucil [Leukeran], and melphalan [Alkeran]) act by interstrand cross-linking of DNA, thereby preventing normal DNA replication. This interference is not only cytotoxic, but also potentially mutagenic and carcinogenic. Asparaginase inhibits protein synthesis.

Glucocorticosteroids are the most commonly used steroids. Steroids control the damaging inflammatory immune response. The target cells are monocytes and T lymphocytes. Monocytes block IL-1 production, block TNF-γ and reduce chemotaxis. The consequences are inhibition of T-cell activation, activation and recruitment of monocytes and neutrophils, and inhibition of the migration of cells to the site of inflammation. The steroids used in cancer oncology include glucocorticoids (prednisone), estrogens (diethylstilbestrol), androgens (testosterone proprionate), and progestational agents (medroxyprogesterone, megestrol acetate).

Hormone antagonists (e.g., tamoxifen) competitively bind to specific cytoplasmic receptors.

Cytokines

Cytokines (discussed in detail in Chapter 5) (e.g., IFN, IL-2, and colony-stimulating factors) constitute another group of cancer chemotherapy drugs. IFN, IL-2, and colony-stimulating factors are being used to treat certain types of cancer in patients. Currently IFNs are being used to treat patients with hairy cell leukemia, chromic myelogenous leukemia, and multiple myeloma. IL-2 is being used in the treatment of renal cell carcinoma and melanoma. Colony-stimulating factors decrease the duration of chemotherapy-induced neutropenia and may permit more dose-intensive therapy.

Interferon

The clinical development of recombinant IFN-α represents the most rapid development of any antineoplastic drug in the United States. IFN was first recognized as a naturally occurring antiviral substance in 1957 and identified for its antineoplastic properties. In 1981 large amounts of highly purified IFN-α became available because of recombinant DNA technology. Before that time, IFN preparations were produced by purification of supernatants harvested from virally stimulated leukocytes. The Food and Drug Administration approved IFN for clinical use in the United States in June, 1986, without the benefit of animal studies. Research scientists were unable to study IFN in animal models because it is a species-specific molecule.

IFN-α appears to have activity in a wide range of malignancies. Beginning in 1982, IFN-α was demonstrated to inhibit tumor growth in the absence of effector cells such as monocytes or lymphocytes. The most notable responses to IFN have been in certain hematologic malignancies, including diseases of presumptive B-cell, T-cell, and myeloid origin. High rates of activity have also been seen in patients with Kaposi's sarcoma associated with acquired immunodeficiency syndrome. However, the response of most solid tumors has not been as dramatic.

IFN has been used as a sole therapeutic agent, but it has been clearly demonstrated that an additive effect or synergy in various cell lines can occur with several cytotoxic drugs and different forms of interferons. For example, patients with malignant hematologic disease who had demonstrated resistance to standard agents have had positive responses to simultaneous or sequential treatments with IFN-α and the cytotoxic agent to which resistance had occurred.

The ultimate role of IFNs in the management of malignant disease has not yet been fully explored. IFN alone or in combination with cytotoxic agents, radiation therapy, or other lymphokines may prove to be the most effective form of therapy for many patients with malignancies.

The Effects of Drug-Induced Immunosuppression

Drugs used to treat malignancies such as solid tumors or leukemia have profoundly suppressive effects on the inflammatory response, delayed hypersensitivity, and/or specific antibody production (Table 30-8). Examples of the immune depression induced by drugs include depletion of T cells by corticosteroids because of the blocking of egress from the bone marrow into the circulation, and dysfunction of the antibody response caused by folate antagonists and purine analogs. For this reason, infection secondary to immune suppression is a major cause of death in cancer patients beginning therapy and those who are in clinical remission.

Recent Advances

Immunotherapy for tumors can take the form of active or passive therapy. Active host immune responses may be achieved by:

- Vaccination with killed tumor cells, or tumor antigens or peptides
- Enhancement of cell-mediated immunity to tumors by expressing costimulators and cytokines and treating with cytokines that stimulate the proliferation and differentiation of T lymphocytes and NK cells

TABLE 30-8	Examples of the Effects of Chemotherapy on the Immune Response			
	Antibody		**Delayed Hypersensitivity**	
	Primary Response	**Secondary Response**	**Primary Response (Initial)**	**Secondary Response (Recall)**
Corticosteroid	0	0	++	+
Methotrexate	++	+	+	0
6-Mercaptopurine	0	+	+	0
Azathioprine	0	+	+	0
6-Thioguanine	0	+	+	0
Cytosine arabinoside	+	++	0	0
Cyclophosphamide	++	0	+	0
L-asparaginase	+	0	0	0
Daunomycin	+	0	+	0

TABLE 30-9	Examples of New Therapeutic Agents	
Drug	**Mode of Action**	**Application**
Herceptin	Antigrowth latches on to HER-2 receptor	Breast cancer
Rituxan	Monoclonal antibody targeted cell membrane protein	Non-Hodgkin's lymphoma
Campath	Targeted celled destruction	Chronic lymphocytic leukemia
Gleevec	Antigrowth	Chronic myelogenous leukemia

- Nonspecific stimulation of the immune system by the local administration of inflammatory substances or by systemic treatment with agents that function as polyclonal activators of lymphocytes

Passive immunotherapy consists of:

- Adoptive cellular therapy by transferring cultured immune cells with antitumor reactivity into a tumor-bearing host
- Administration of tumor-specific monoclonal antibodies for specific tumor immunotherapy

One new approach to cancer therapy is augmentation of the natural immune response in the body to improve surveillance and remove abnormal cells (e.g., IFN, bacille Calmette-Guérin [BCG] vaccine for tuberculosis). BCG promotes the movement of macrophages and T lymphocytes to the site, where they may destroy the tumor cell. This is not first-line treatment presently.

What's New in Drug Therapy?

The list of drugs used for cancer therapy continues to grow. The website, www.phrma.org, lists 402 experimental drugs. The new therapeutics target various modes of action and applications (Table 30-9).

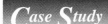

History and Physical Examination

LL, a 59-year-old Caucasian man, visited his primary care provider because of the need to urinate frequently and urgently. Over the last several years, his urine output had been in small volumes with a decreasing flow rate over the past several years.

On physical examination, he noted that the patient had an enlarged prostate with a smooth uniform surface. A PSA assay was ordered.

Laboratory Data

PSA Assay	Patient's Results	Reference Range
Current, ng/mL	5.5	0-3.5
1 year ago, ng/mL	2.3	0-3.5

Questions and Discussion

1. Is the change in the patient's PSA results in 1 year significant?

   The reference range of PSA increases with age and is age-dependent. In this case, the patient's results were within range 1 year ago but are above the reference range currently. The current results suggest the presence of a prostatic tumor.

2. What is the clinical significance of the patient's results?

   The annual increase of PSA is defined as the PSA velocity. A rise in the PSA value greater than 0.7 ng/mL per year or an increase of greater than 20% per year is indicative of cancer (Rittenhouse-Diakun).

   Some scientists believe that PSA results between 2 ng/mL and 10 ng/mL are too insensitive and nonspecific to distinguish between benign prostatic hypertrophy and prostate cancer, does not diagnose prostate cancer, and cannot distinguish between indolent and aggressive prostate cancer.

A number of new assays have been introduced to aid in the interpretation of PSA results between 4 and 10 ng/mL to assist in determining whether a biopsy of the prostate should be performed. Free-PSA and complexed PSA are two such assays. Free-PSA:PSA ratio can be determined. Other suggested biomarkers are isoforms of PSA and (-2)pPSA. Genomic and proteonomic include transcriptional profiling on microarrays (O'Kane).

3. What is the expected follow-up regimen for a patient with this profile?

A biopsy of multiple sites of the prostate would be a common follow-up procedure. In this case, specimens were obtained from six sites. Three of these sites revealed prostatic adenocarcinoma. A bone scan also was performed. No metastasis to the bone was seen. The patient subsequently underwent a radical prostatectomy.

4. After a radical prostatectomy, what PSA values would be expected?

No prostate tissue should remain after a radical prostatectomy. Because no PSA is produced after a radical prostatectomy, the laboratory results of a PSA assay should be 0 ng/mL. If the patient's postoperative PSA is above 0.1 ng/mL, this is considered to be reliable evident of the persistence of the malignant tumor.

Diagnosis

Prostatic adenocarcinoma

Bibliography

Rittenhouse-Diakun K: Clinical immunology No. CI-4 2000, Tech Sample, *Am Soc Clin Pathol* :23-27, 2000.
O'Kane DJ: Biomarkers for prostate cancer, *Adv Med Lab Prof* 14(12)18-20, 2002.

Case Study

History and Physical Examination

M.S., a 65-year-old African-American woman, visited her primary care provider for an annual examination, including a routine pelvic examination. Although she had gained some weight since her last examination, she reported that her general health was good, but she reported that she had been experiencing some gastrointestinal problems over the last 6 weeks.

A palpable mass was discovered during her pelvic examination. A CA 125 assay and a transvaginal ultrasound examination were ordered.

Laboratory Data and Diagnostic Imaging Findings

The patient's CA 125 was 425 U/mL (reference range, <35 U/mL). The presence of a mass in the right side of the abdomen and abdominal ascites were confirmed.

Follow-Up

The patient had a total abdominal hysterectomy with bilateral salpingo-oophrectomy; 4 weeks after operation she began a chemotherapy series. The patient was judged to be in remission for 6 months when recurrence of the tumor was noted with diagnostic imaging. Subsequent chemotherapy was ineffective and the patient died 8 months later.

Questions and Discussion

1. Is CA125 an effective diagnostic blood serum tumor marker?

CA 125 is considered to be the best serum marker for ovarian cancer. About 50% of women in the earliest localized stage (stage I) of the disease exhibit an elevated level of this cancer antigen. The majority of patients with advanced ovarian cancer demonstrate elevated levels of CA 125.

2. Is CA 125 a specific tumor marker for ovarian cancer?

CA 125 is a useful component in the initial preoperative diagnosis of ovarian cancer, but it is not specific for ovarian cancer. Elevated levels can be demonstrated in various malignancies:
   - Breast
   - Lung
   - Colon
   - Pancreas
   - Liver

Elevated levels of CA 125 can be observed in benign gynecologic conditions:
   - Uterine fibroids
   - Ovarian cysts
   - Endometriosis

3. What is the major clinical use of CA 125?

The major clinical application of CA 125 is in postoperative monitoring of patients with a confirmed diagnosis of ovarian cancer. Declining levels correlate well with a positive response to chemotherapy and accompanying reduction in tumor mass. A rise in the level of CA 125 is a reliable indicator of disease recurrence.

Diagnosis

Ovarian Cancer

CHAPTER HIGHLIGHTS

Tumors are neoplasms described as benign or malignant. A benign neoplasm is a nonspreading tumor; a malignant neoplasm is a growth that infiltrates tissues, metastasizes, and often recurs after attempts to remove it surgically. The presence of a malignant neoplasm can be referred to as carcinoma or cancer. The factors that cause the majority of neoplasms are unknown. The incidence of cancer, however, has been correlated with certain environmental factors such as occupational exposure to known carcinogenic agents and to host susceptibility considerations such as heredity, sex, or age.

Malignant proliferation of cells is also related to genes. Cancer often begins when a carcinogenic agent damages the DNA of a critical gene in a cell. The mutant cell multiplies, and the succeeding generations of cells aggregate to form a malignant tumor. Proto-oncogenes act as central regulators of the growth in normal cells and are antecedents of oncogenes. The genetic targets of carcinogens are known to be oncogenes. Oncogenes have been associated with various tumor types that stem in large part from preexisting genes present in the normal human genome. Therefore oncogenes are considered altered versions of normal genes. Over a lifetime, a variety of mutations can convert a normal gene into a malignant oncogene. Once an oncogene is activated by mutation, it promotes excessive or inappropriate cell proliferation. Various RNA and DNA viruses have been associated with human malignancies. Some viral agents have a clear causative role, such as the Epstein-Barr virus and certain papilloma viruses that are the etiologic agents in Burkitt's lymphoma and cervical carcinoma, respectively.

Viruses carry viral oncogenes into target cells, where they become firmly established. Clonal descendants then carry the viral genes, which maintain the malignant phenotype of the cell clones. A very different class of cancer genes has been recently discovered. These tumor-suppressing genes in normal cells appear to regulate the proliferation of cell growth. When this type of gene is inactivated, a block to proliferation is removed and cells begin a program of deregulated growth, or the genetically depleted cell itself may proliferate uncontrollably. Thus tumor-suppressing genes are referred to as antioncogenes; their discovery will probably lead to the reformulation of ideas about how the growth of normal cells is regulated.

Although no single satisfactory explanation exists for the success of tumors in escaping the immune rejection process, it is believed that early clones of neoplastic cells are eliminated by the immune response. Cells such as the large granular lymphocytes, antibody-dependent cell-mediated cytotoxicity reaction effector cells, and cytotoxic T cells dominate the rejection process that leads to the elimination of foreign tissue; therefore cells rather than immunoglobulins are believed to dominate tumor immunity. Tumor cells manifest tumor antigens, as well as self-HLA antigens. The four types of identified tumor antigens are tumor-specific antigens on chemically induced tumors, tumor-associated antigens on virally induced tumors, carcinofetal antigens, and spontaneous tumor antigens. A tumor marker is a characteristic of a neoplastic cell that can be detected in plasma or serum. Although these markers are not tumor specific and may be detected in non-neoplastic conditions, markers may be useful in diagnosis and selection of different treatment approaches, monitoring therapies, or prognoses. Tumor markers include CEA, AFP, β-hCG, neuron-specific enolase, prostatic acid phosphatase, and placental alkaline phosphatase.

Until recently, three modalities were used to treat cancer—surgery, radiation, and chemotherapy. The biologic response modifiers such as IFN are now the newest or fourth modality. Many different modes of therapy have been demonstrated in the treatment of cancer; however, drug-induced immunosuppression and IFN therapy alone or in combination with drugs are the most frequent forms of therapy after surgery or in cases where surgery is not appropriate (e.g., hematologic disorders).

REVIEW QUESTIONS

1. Benign tumors are characterized as:
   A. growing slowly
   B. resembling the parent tissue
   C. usually invades tissues (metastasizes)
   D. both A and B

2-5. Match the following:

2. _____ benign tumor arising from glands

3. _____ benign tumor arising from epithelial surfaces

4. _____ malignant tumor of connective tissue

5. _____ malignant tumor of glandular epithelium (e.g., colon)
   A. sarcoma
   B. adenoma
   C. adenocarcinoma
   D. papillomas

6. Which of the following factors is *not* a risk factor in the development of cancer?
   A. smoking
   B. low-fat diet
   C. obesity
   D. sedentary lifestyle

7. Risk factors associated with breast cancer are:
   A. first-degree family history of breast cancer
   B. pregnancy after 30 years of age
   C. use of estrogen (oral contraceptives or hormone replacement)
   D. all of the above

8-10. True or False A = True; B = False

8. _____ Antibodies dominate body defenses against cancer.

9. _____ Tumors express antigens that can be recognized as foreign by the immune system of the tumor-bearing host.

10. _____ The normal immune response frequently fails to prevent the growth of tumors.

11. The cells involved in the immune response to tumors are:
    A. T lymphocytes, B lymphocytes, macrophages
    B. cytotoxic T lymphocytes, NK cells, macrophages
    C. neutrophils, lymphocytes, monocytes
    D. CD8+ lymphocytes, monocytes, basophils

12. Which of the following is *not* an environmental factor associated with carcinogenesis?
    A. ultraviolet light
    B. organically grown herbs
    C. benzene
    D. asbestos

13. The risk factor associated with the development of basal cell carcinoma or malignant melanoma is:
    A. infrared light
    B. sunless tanning lotions
    C. ultraviolet light
    D. strobe lights

14. Patients with Down syndrome have a higher incidence of:
    A. leukemia
    B. breast cancer
    C. prostate cancer
    D. teratomas

15. Tumor cells typically carry _____ genetic change(s).
    A. one
    B. two
    C. three to six
    D. multiple

16. Cancer predisposing genes may:
    A. affect a host's ability to repair damage to DNA
    B. increase cell cohesiveness
    C. decrease cell motility
    D. enhance the host's immune ability to recognize and eradicate incipient tumors

17. Oncogenes are:
    A. genetic targets of carcinogens
    B. altered versions of normal genes
    C. detectable in 15% to 20% of a variety of human tumors
    D. all of the above

18-19. Match the following definitions:

18. _____ mutation or overexpression of oncogenes

19. _____ mutation or overexpression of tumor suppressor genes
    A. results in the production of nonfunctional proteins that can no longer control cell proliferation
    B. produces proteins that can stimulate uncontrolled cell growth

20. A tumor marker might be used:
    A. to screen patients for malignancies
    B. to monitor a cancer patient for disease recurrence
    C. to determine the degree of tumor burden
    D. all of the above

21-23. Match the following:

21. _____ tumor-specific antigens

22. _____ tumor-associated antigens

23. _____ carcinofetal antigens
    A. cell surface molecules coded for by tumorogenic viruses
    B. gene products resulting from gene derepression
    C. antigens uniquely related to each tumor
    D. probably do not produce unique antigens

24. Carcinoembryonic antigen is:
    A. an oncofetal protein, elevated in some types of cancer, found on normal fetal endocrine tissue in the last trimester of gestation
    B. strongly correlated with various malignancies, found on normal fetal endocrine tissue in the second trimester of gestation, an oncofetal protein
    C. used clinically to monitor tumor progress in some type of patients, persistently elevated even in residual disease or poor therapeutic response
    D. elevated in 20% of smokers, an alpha-fetoprotein, a cell surface protein found on normal epithelial tissue

25. Alpha-fetoprotein (AFP):
    A. is synthesized by the fetal liver and yolk sac
    B. can be elevated in some non-neoplastic conditions
    C. is a very reliable marker for monitoring a patient's response to chemotherapy and radiation therapy
    D. all of the above

26. β-hCG is *not*:
    A. elevated in normal pregnancy
    B. a sensitive tumor marker
    C. elevated in squamous cell carcinoma of the lung
    D. elevated in teratocarcinoma and choriocarcinoma

27. Prostate-specific antigen is:
    A. prostate tissue–specific
    B. prostate cancer–specific
    C. not useful for monitoring response to therapy among patients with prostate cancer
    D. not proportional to tumor volume directly in prostate malignancies

28-32. Match the following tumor marker and application.

28. _____ CEA

29. _____ AFP

30. _____ CA 125

31. _____ CA 19-9

32. _____ CA 27-29
    A. frequently elevated in endometrially derived gastrointestinal neoplasms
    B. most useful in ovarian and endometrial carcinomas
    C. increased levels may indicate recurrent breast carcinoma
    D. may be elevated in patients with gastrointestinal malignancies
    E. should be quantitated with β-hCG initially in all patients with teratocarcinoma

33-36. Match an example of a therapeutic intervention with the appropriate mode of action (an answer may be used more than once).

33. _____ 6-mercaptopurine

34. _____ corticosteroids

35. _____ alkylating agents or 5-fluorouracil

36. _____ vinca alkaloids
    A. cell cycle active, phase specific
    B. cell cycle active, phase nonspecific
    C. noncell cycle active
    D. hormone antagonist

37. Tamoxifen acts as a _____ pharmaceutical agent.
    A. cell cycle active, phase specific
    B. cell cycle active, phase nonspecific
    C. noncell cycle active
    D. estrogen receptor blocking

38. Active host immunotherapy responses may be achieved by:
    A. transferring immune cells into host
    B. vaccination with killed tumor cells
    C. administration of tumor-specific monoclonal antibodies
    D. administration of IFN-alpha

39-43. Match the selected environmental factor and an associated cancer.

39. _____ benzene

40. _____ estrogen

41. _____ Epstein-Barr virus

42. _____ Hepatitis B

43. _____ asbestos

A. endometrial cancer
B. hepatocellular carcinomas
C. Burkitt's lymphoma
D. leukemia
E. mesothelioma

BIBLIOGRAPHY

Ahern H: Tumor marker measurement aids in cancer diagnosis therapy, *Adv Med Lab Prof* 9(10):12-15, 1995.

American Association of Clinical Chemistry. Use of tumor markers in cancer patients leads to better detection, decreasing mortality, 2001.

Bosl GJ, Motzer RJ: Testicular germ-cell cancer, *N Engl J Med* 337:242-250, 1997.

Calle EE et al: Organochlorines and breast cancer risk, *CA A Cancer Journal for Clinicians,* 52:301-307, 2002.

Cannistra SA: Cancer of the ovary, *N Engl J Med* 329(21):1550-1559, 1993.

Carney WP, Williams J: HER-*2/neu* and EGFR oncoprotein expression in breast, ovarian and cervical cancers, *Adv Med Lab Prof* 13(13):18-20, 2001.

Cattral MS, Levy GA: Progress in colon cancer—do molecular markers matter? *N Engl J Med* 331(4):267-269, 1994.

Chang N et al: Laboratory of molecular immunology, *Guthrie J* 63(2):59-60, 1994.

Coffman NB: Practical parameters for tumor markers, *Adv Med Lab Prof* 11:32-41, 1999.

Come SE: Selected topics in oncology, *Int Rev Intern Med* 499-525, 1995.

Delgado JC et al: Standardization of carcinoembryonic antigen testing in the setting of clinical laboratory consolidation, *Lab Med* 32:2, 2001.

Eyre HJ, editor: News Briefs, *CA Cancer J Clin* 52(5):248-251, 2002.

Friend SH, Dryja TP, Weinberg RA: Oncogenes and tumor-suppressing genes, *N Engl J Med* 318(10):618-623, 1988.

Gann PH, Hennekens CH, Stampfer MJ: A prospective evaluation of plasma prostate-specific antigen for detection of prostatic cancer, *JAMA* 273(4):289-294, 1995.

George H: Tumor immunology: tumor markers and their significance, *Can J Med Lab Sci* 61:166, 1999.

Goljan EF: *Pathology review,* Philadelphia,1998, WB Saunders.

Herberman RB: Tumor immunology, *JAMA* 268(20):2935-2939, 1992.

Holloway TL: Protein sustains cancer cells, *Adv Med Lab Prof* 14(8):12, 2002.

Holloway TL: Clinical clips: scientists find possible origin of colon cancer, *Adv Med Lab Prof* 14(1):9, 2002.

Howlett NG et al: *Science,* June 13, 2002, (10.1126/science. 1073834)

Jen J et al: Allelic loss of chromosome 18q and prognosis in colorectal cancer, *N Engl J Med* 331(4): 213-221, 1994.

Karp JE, Broder S: Oncology, *JAMA* 270(2):237-240, 1993.

Krontiris TG: Molecular medicine: oncogenes, *N Engl J Med* 333(5):303-306, 1995.

Leavelle DE: *Interpretive data for diagnostic laboratory tests,* Rochester, Minn, 1997, Mayo Medical Laboratories.

Mehltretter S: Clinical cytogenetics, *Adv Med Lab Prof* 7(13):6-9, 20, 1995.

Mishra R: Boston researchers find 6 breast cancer risk genes, website: www.boston.com, June 14, 2002.

Pennisi E: Tumor suppressor's structure revealed, *Sci News* 146(3):36, 1994.

Roitt IM: *Essential immunology,* ed 5, Oxford, England, 1984, Blackwell Scientific Publications.

Schwartz RS: Jumping genes and the immunoglobulin V gene system, *N Engl J Med* 333(1):42-44, 1995.

Turgeon ML: *Fundamentals of immunohematology,* ed 3, Baltimore, 1999, Williams, & Wilkins.

vandeVijuer MJ et al: A gene-expression signature as a predictor of survival in breast cancer, *N Engl J Med* 347:1999-2009, 2002.

Weiss RL, editor: *Guide to molecular diagnostics clinical laboratory testing,* Salt Lake City, 2001, ARUP.

Witt E, Ashworth A: D-Day for BRCA2, Sciencexpress, website: www.sciencexpress.org/13June2002/page2/10.1126/science. 1074482.

Wittliff JL: Prognostic factors in managing breast carcinoma, *Adv Med Lab Prof* 10:20, 1998.

Answers to Review Questions

CHAPTER 1

1. E	9. C	17. D	25. B
2. A	10. B	18. C	26. B
3. B	11. C	19. B	27. A
4. C	12. A	20. A	28. A
5. D	13. B	21. A	29. C
6. A	14. D	22. A	30. A
7. D	15. B	23. B	31. B
8. E	16. C	24. B	32. D

CHAPTER 2

1. B	14. D	27. D	40. B
2. A	15. C	28. B	41. A
3. D	16. B	29. D	42. D
4. D	17. A	30. B	43. C
5. D	18. C	31. D	44. A
6. C	19. B	32. B	45. B
7. A	20. C	33. C	46. D
8. D	21. A	34. A	47. C
9. B	22. D	35. A	48. D
10. E	23. D	36. E	49. B
11. B	24. B	37. C	50. D
12. E	25. C	38. B	
13. A	26. A	39. D	

CHAPTER 3

1. C	11. B	21. B	31. D
2. D	12. C	22. A	32. C
3. A	13. B	23. C	33. B
4. B	14. D	24. D	34. B
5. D	15. C	25. B	35. D
6. D	16. A	26. D	36. A
7. A	17. A	27. A	37. B
8. D	18. C	28. C	38. D
9. A	19. A	29. C	39. A
10. E	20. B	30. C	40. C

CHAPTER 4

1. B	15. D	29. D	43. A
2. C	16. A	30. B	44. D
3. D	17. C	31. D	45. C
4. B	18. C	32. D	46. B
5. D	19. C	33. B	47. A
6. A	20. D	34. D	48. B
7. C	21. B	35. A	49. B
8. B	22. B	36. B	50. B
9. C	23. C	37. B	51. C
10. A	24. A	38. A	52. A
11. C	25. C	39. C	53. D
12. A	26. C	40. D	
13. D	27. D	41. C	
14. B	28. B	42. B	

CHAPTER 5

1. D	20. C	38. C	56. A
2. D	21. D	39. D	57. B
3. A	22. A	40. D	58. D
4. A	23. D	41. A	59. C
5. B	24. B	42. C	60. A
6. A	25. A	43. B	61. A
7. C	26. C	44. C	62. B
8. D	27. D	45. A	63. A
9. B	28. B	46. B	64. B
10. C	29. A	47. D	65. C
11. A	30. D	48. A	66. A
12. B	31. C	49. D	67. D
13. A	32. C	50. C	68. D
14. C	33. D	51. B	69. B
15. A	34. B	52. D	70. D
16. A	35. A	53. A	71. B
17. A	36. B	54. B	72. A
18. A	36. B	54. B	73. C
19. B	37. A	55. C	

CHAPTER 6

1. D	13. A	25. B	37. B
2. C	14. B	26. B	38. D
3. D	15. A	27. B	39. D
4. C	16. A	28. D	40. C
5. A	17. B	29. B	41. C
6. D	18. A	30. A	42. A
7. D	19. B	31. C	43. D
8. B	20. B	32. C	44. B
9. B	21. A	33. A	45. D
10. D	22. A	34. C	
11. D	23. A	35. A	
12. D	24. D	36. D	

CHAPTER 7

1. D	9. D	17. D	25. B
2. C	10. C	18. D	26. D
3. D	11. A	19. B	27. C
4. B	12. C	20. A	28. A
5. B	13. B	21. D	29. B
6. C	14. A	22. C	30. A
7. C	15. C	23. D	31. C
8. B	16. E	24. A	

CHAPTER 8

1. C	5. A	9. B	13. D
2. D	6. B	10. D	14. A
3. C	7. A	11. D	15. D
4. B	8. A	12. C	16. A

CHAPTER 9

1. D	5. A	9. A	13. A
2. A	6. B	10. C	14. B
3. B	7. B	11. B	15. C
4. D. All of the above	8. C	12. A	16. D

CHAPTER 10

1. B	3. C	5. C	7. D
2. A	4. D	6. B	8. D

CHAPTER 11

1. A	4. D	7. A	10. B
2. D	5. A	8. C	11. B
3. C	6. B	9. A	12. B

CHAPTER 12

1. D	5. C	9. A	13. B
2. D	6. D	10. B	14. B
3. B	7. D	11. C	15. C
4. D	8. C	12. A	16. B

CHAPTER 13

1. D	7. C	13. A	19. C
2. B	8. D	14. D	20. A
3. D	9. C	15. C	21. B
4. A	10. B	16. D	22. C
5. C	11. C	17. D	23. A
6. A	12. A	18. A	24. B

CHAPTER 14

1. B	7. d	13. B	19. B
2. A	8. A	14. B	20. B
3. D	9. B	15. A	21. C
4. B	10. D	16. A	
5. A	11. C	17. C	
6. B	12. A	18. B	

CHAPTER 15

1. B	7. A	13. B	19. B
2. D	8. B	14. B	20. C
3. A	9. B	15. D	21. C
4. C	10. B	16. B	22. D
5. C	11. A	17. B	23. D
6. E	12. A	18. B	24. A

CHAPTER 16

1. D	9. B	17. C	25. B
2. D	10. B	18. D	26. C
3. B	11. C	19. A	27. C
4. C	12. D	20. C	28. A
5. B	13. D	21. C	29. D
6. B	14. A	22. A	30. A
7. A	15. B	23. C	
8. B	16. D	24. B	

CHAPTER 17

1. C	4. B	7. B
2. D	5. B	8. C
3. D	6. A	9. A

CHAPTER 18

1. D	8. C	15. A	22. A
2. D	9. B	16. B	23. A
3. B	10. A	17. C	24. B
4. D	11. D	18. C	25. A
5. B	12. B	19. C	26. D
6. C	13. C	20. B	27. B
7. A	14. A	21. D	

CHAPTER 19

1. D	5. D	9. C	13. C
2. B	6. D	10. C	14. C
3. C	7. D	11. B	15. A
4. D	8. A	12. C	16. B

CHAPTER 20

1. B	15. A	29. B	43. A
2. A	16. E	30. A	44. D
3. C	17. C	31. B	45. C
4. D	18. B	32. D	46. D
5. D	19. D	33. C	47. B
6. A	20. B	34. B	48. A
7. C	21. D	35. A	49. B
8. B	22. C	36. C	50. C
9. A	23. A	37. A	51. A
10. D	24. B	38. A	52. D
11. B	25. D	39. A	53. C
12. C	26. B	40. A	
13. D	27. A	41. B	
14. B	28. B	42. B	

CHAPTER 21

1. C	5. B	9. D	13. B
2. A	6. C	10. A	14. A
3. D	7. C	11. B	15. B
4. A	8. D	12. A	16. D

CHAPTER 22

1. B	8. D	15. E	22. B
2. B	9. C	16. B	23. C
3. D	10. C	17. C	24. D
4. D	11. A	18. C	25. B
5. C	12. B	19. A	26. C
6. B	13. D	20. B	27. B
7. C	14. A	21. D	28. A

CHAPTER 23

1. D	8. D	15. D	22. D
2. A	9. B	16. B	23. D
3. C	10. B	17. C	24. D
4. B	11. C	18. A	25. D
5. D	12. A	19. D	
6. D	13. B	20. D	
7. D	14. A	21. B	

CHAPTER 24

1. C	5. C	9. D	13. A
2. D	6. D	10. C	14. B
3. D	7. D	11. A	15. A
4. D	8. C	12. D	16. B

CHAPTER 25

1. C	11. C	21. A	31. C
2. D	12. D	22. D	32. D
3. A	13. B	23. B	33. C
4. B	14. C	24. C	34. C
5. B	15. E	25. D	35. C
6. E	16. D	26. A	36. B
7. C	17. B	27. A	37. B
8. D	18. A	28. D	
9. E	19. A	29. B	
10. A	20. B	30. C	

CHAPTER 26

1. C	6. D	11. D	16. C
2. B	7. D	12. B	17. A
3. D	8. D	13. D	18. C
4. A	9. A	14. B	
5. C	10. D	15. A	

CHAPTER 27

1. C	5. B	9. C	13. A
2. A	6. A	10. B	14. B
3. C	7. B	11. D	15. D
4. B	8. A	12. B	16. C

CHAPTER 28

1. B	7. C	13. A	19. C
2. A	8. E	14. A	20. B
3. C	9. D	15. C	21. B
4. D	10. D	16. B	22. D
5. B	11. D	17. D	23. B
6. A	12. B	18. A	24. C

CHAPTER 29

1. D	5. C	9. D	13. C
2. A	6. B	10. A	14. A
3. B	7. D	11. D	15. A
4. A	8. C	12. A	

CHAPTER 30

1. D	12. B	23. B	34. C
2. B	13. C	24. B	35. B
3. D	14. A	25. D	36. A
4. A	15. D	26. C	37. D
5. C	16. A	27. A	38. B
6. B	17. B	28. A	39. D
7. D	18. A	29. E	40. A
8. B	19. B	30. B	41. C
9. A	20. D	31. D	42. B
10. A	21. C	32. C	43. E
11. B	22. A	33. A	

APPENDIX A

1. B
2. B
3. A

APPENDIX B

1. C	22. B	43. A	64. A
2. A	23. C	44. B	65. A
3. B	24. D	45. B	66. D
4. D	25. D	46. C	67. B
5. B	26. C	47. D	68. C
6. C	27. B	48. A	69. D
7. A	28. A	49. A	70. C
8. D	29. A	50. B	71. B
9. A	30. C	51. D	72. A
10. B	31. B	52. C	73. B
11. C	32. D	53. D	74. A
12. D	33. C	54. C	75. D
13. C	34. D	55. B	76. C
14. D	35. A	56. A	77. C
15. A	36. B	57. B	78. D
16. B	37. D	58. A	79. B
17. B	38. C	59. D	80. A
18. C	39. B	60. C	81. A
19. D	40. A	61. C	82. D
20. A	41. C	62. D	83. B
21. A	42. D	63. B	84. C

Appendix A

Preparing Dilutions and Serial Dilutions

Serum may need to be diluted in a single sample or as a serial dilution if it contains a concentrated amount of antibody. A dilution involves two components: the solute, the material being diluted, and the diluent, the medium constituting the rest of the solution. The relationship between the solute and solvent is expressed as a fraction. For example, if a 1:10 dilution is required, it is prepared with 1 part of solute and 9 parts of (solvent) diluent.

The denominator is the total volume. The total volume represents the volume of solute + solvent.

$$\frac{1}{\text{Dilution}} = \frac{\text{Amounts of Solute}}{\text{Total Volume}}$$

EXAMPLE
If 5 mL of a 1:10 dilution is required for a serologic procedure, an algebraic equation can be set up to determine the amount of solute and the amount of solvent (diluent) needed to make a dilution. For example:

$$\frac{1}{10} = \frac{x}{5 \text{ mL}}$$

NOTE: 10 represents the total number of parts in the solution; 5 mL represents the total volume.

Solving this equation for x yields 0.5 mL for the amount of serum required to prepare this dilution. The volume of diluent is obtained by subtracting 0.5 mL from 5 mL. = 4.5 mL.

Alternate Situation:
If the amount of serum available is known, the amount of diluent can be determined.

EXAMPLE
A 1:5 dilution of patient serum is required. There is 0.1 mL of serum available. What is the necessary amount of diluent?

Using the basic equation, the necessary amount of diluent = x

$$\frac{1}{5} = \frac{0.1 \text{ mL}}{x}$$

The total volume (x) is 0.5 mL. To obtain the total volume, the amount of diluent would be 0.4 mL or 1 part of solute + 4 parts of solvent.

SERIAL DILUTIONS

When a serial dilution is to be prepared, the first step is to plan the number of dilutions (tubes) and the sizes of simple dilutions required to reach the desired end point. A 1:64 dilution can be prepared in a serial dilution by preparing successive 1:2 dilutions. Although any volume can be used, it is easier to think of the following table as 1-mL quantities.

Solute (serum)	Solvent (diluent/saline)	Total Volume	Final Dilution
1 mL	1 mL	2 mL	1:2
1 mL (1:2)	1 mL	2 mL	1:4
1 mL (1:4)	1 mL	2 mL	1:8
1 mL (1:8)	1 mL	2 mL	1:16
1 mL (1:16)	1 mL	2 mL	1:32
1 mL (1:32)	1 mL	2 mL	1:64

PRACTICE PROBLEMS

1. How many parts of diluent are there in a 2:8 dilution?
   A. 2   C. 6
   B. 4   D. 8

2. How much diluent needs to be added to 0.2 mL of serum to make a 1:10 dilution?
   A. 0.8 mL   C. 10.8 mL
   B. 2 mL   D. 19.8 mL

3. A volume of 5 mL of a 1:50 dilution is required for a serologic procedure. How much serum is required to prepare a minimum quantity of this dilution?
   A. 0.10 mL   C. 2.50 mL
   B. 0.49 mL   D. 4.9 mL

Appendix B

Review Questions

Define the terms used in immunology. The terms are clustered in groups using answers A-D for each group.

1. _____ acquired
2. _____ acute
3. _____ adenopathy
4. _____ affinity

A. sudden or short duration
B. swelling or enlargement of the lymph nodes
C. not inherited
D. the bond between a single antigenic determinant and an individual combining site

5. _____ agglutination
6. _____ agglutinin
7. _____ alloantibodies
8. _____ allograft

A. immunoglobulins produced in response to exposure of foreign antigen of the same species
B. clumping or aggregation of particles
C. antibody
D. transfer of tissue from a genetically different member of the same species

9. _____ anamnestic response
10. _____ anaphylactic shock

A. memory response
B. a severe allergic reaction
C. lacking a yellow color
D. marked deviation from normal

11. _____ anicteric

12. _____ anomaly

13. _____ antenatal
14. _____ anticore window
15. _____ antigenicity
16. _____ antineutrophil antibody

A. ability of an antigen to stimulate an immune response
B. antibody divided into c-ANCA or p-ANCA
C. before birth
D. antigen cannot be detected

17. _____ arthralgia
18. _____ arthritis
19. _____ asymptomatic
20. _____ atrophy

A. wasting or lack of growth of tissues or organs
B. pain in a joint
C. inflammation of a joint
D. no symptoms

21. _____ autologous
22. _____ avidity
23. _____ bacteremia
24. _____ carrier state

A. self or part of the same individual
B. strength of a multivalent antigen and antibody bond
C. infection of the blood
D. condition of harboring an infectious organism

25. _____ colony-stimulating factors
26. _____ convalescent period
27. _____ cosmopolitan distribution
28. _____ cytokines

A. polypeptide products of activated cells that control a variety of cellular responses and thereby regulate the immune system
B. widely distributed
C. time of recovery
D. molecular substances that stimulate hematopoietic progenitor cells to form an identical group of cells

29. _____ diagnosis
30. _____ disease
31. _____ dysplastic
32. _____ endemic

A. determination of the nature of a disorder
B. abnormal development of body tissue
C. a pathologic condition characterized by a specific and unique set of signs and symptoms
D. present at all times

33. _____ erythema
34. _____ etiology
35. _____ fulminant
36. _____ genome

A. occur suddenly with great intensity
B. complete set of hereditary factors
C. redness
D. study of or cause of a disease

37. _____ grafting
38. _____ hapten
39. _____ hemolysis
40. _____ hemostatic

A. stoppage of bleeding
B. rupturing of a cell with subsequent dumping of cytoplasmic contents
C. very small molecules that can bind to a larger carrier molecule and behave as an antigen
D. transfer of cells or organs from one individual to another or from one site to another in the same individual

41. _____ heterogeneous
42. _____ homogeneous
43. _____ humoral
44. _____ hybridoma

A. any fluid or semifluid in the body
B. formed by fusion of a lymphocyte or plasma cell and a tumor cell
C. different
D. the same

45. _____ immune complex
46. _____ immunity
47. _____ immunology
48. _____ inflammation

A. tissue reaction to injury
B. noncovalent combination of an antigen with its specific antibody
C. process of being protected against foreign antigens
D. study of body defenses

49. _____ in vitro
50. _____ in vivo
51. _____ jaundice
52. _____ latent

A. in the test tube
B. in the body
C. hidden or inactive
D. yellow appearance

53. _____ leukotriene
54. _____ ligand
55. _____ localized
56. _____ lymphokine

A. soluble mediator released by sensitized lymphocytes on contact with an antigen
B. confined to a specific area
C. a linking or binding molecule
D. a class of compounds that mediate the inflammatory functions of leukocytes

57. _____ lyse
58. _____ memory
59. _____ mitogen
60. _____ morbidity

A. immunologic response to an antigenic stimulus, usually leaves the immune system changed
B. to break apart or dissolve
C. a condition of being diseased
D. a substance that stimulates cell division

61. _____ mortality
62. _____ myalgia
63. _____ natural resistance
64. _____ necrosis

A. death of cells or localized group of cells
B. innate or inborn mechanisms
C. the rate of death or ratio of the number of deaths
D. pain or tenderness in a muscle

65. _____ neoplastic
66. _____ nosocomial
67. _____ oncogenic
68. _____ parenteral

A. new abnormal tissue growth
B. associated with tumor formation
C. situated outside of the oral cavity
D. pertaining to hospital infection

69. _____ pathogen
70. _____ precipitate
71. _____ prime
72. _____ prodromal period

A. initial sign or symptoms of a developing disease or disorder
B. initial sensitization to an antigen
C. solid mass formed from insoluble components
D. disease-causing microorganism or agent

73. _____ prognosis
74. _____ regimen
75. _____ reticulo-endothelial system
76. _____ self-limiting

A. a schedule of treatment
B. forecast of the probable outcome
C. able to resolve in time
D. mononuclear phagocytic system

77. _____ sepsis

78. _____ sequelae

79. _____ stasis

80. _____ symptom

A. a variation in normal body function
B. stoppage of bleeding
C. microbial infection throughout the systemic circulation
D. a disease condition following or occurring as a consequence of another condition or event

81. _____ titer

82. _____ trans

83. _____ venereal route

84. _____ virion

A. the concentration or strength of an antibody expressed as the highest dilution of the serum that produces agglutination
B. a sexually transmitted mode
C. a complete virus particle
D. across, over, through

Appendix C

Chronic Fatigue Syndrome

Chronic fatigue syndrome (CFS) has also been referred to as chronic fatigue immune deficiency syndrome. This disease originated in the eighteenth century. It was previously known as febricula, neurasthenia, or Da Costa's syndrome during the eighteenth, nineteenth, and early twentieth centuries.

ETIOLOGY

At least nine different RNA and DNA viruses have been considered to be associated with CFS, but no convincing evidence supports any currently recognized infectious agent or any other known etiologic agent to CFS.

CFS presents as a heterogeneous disorder possibly involving an interaction of biologic systems: hormonal, neurologic, and immunologic, and potentially psychological dysfunction. In the late 1980s, attention focused on the possibility that CFS was actually an atypical presentation of infectious mononucleosis caused by the Epstein-Barr virus (EBV). Subsequently, many chronically fatigued patients were diagnosed as having chronic EBV disease, EBV syndrome, or chronic infectious mononucleosis. It is important to rule out other conditions associated with chronic fatigue. These conditions include hepatitis, EBV mononucleosis, cytomegalovirus mononucleosis, acquired toxoplasmosis, Lyme disease, hypothyroidism/thyroiditis, collagen vascular disease, and fibromyalgia. Concomitant illnesses include irritable bowel syndrome, depression, and headaches.

It has been proposed that CFS may be caused by an immunologic dysfunction, for example inappropriate production of cytokines, such as interleukin-1 (IL-1), or altered capacity of certain immune functions. Given that CFS may be an illness of immune dysregulation, numerous studies have attempted to identify abnormalities in circulating immune complexes, increased interferon activity, cytokine levels, lymphocyte cell markers, or natural killer (NK) cells. Recently, patients with CFS were shown to exhibit a normal number of NK cells, but these cells had low NK activity. This finding signifies an inability to replenish activated NK cells.

Some of the symptoms of CFS may be due to cytokines produced by this hyperactive immune response to a virus that is still present in the host or that has been eliminated but leaves abnormal immunologic sequelae. These possibilities offer directions for future studies of CFS and therapeutic approaches to this condition. Cytokines are soluble mediators that are released by activated immune cells during infection and inflammation. The possibility that fatigue is mediated by the effects of cytokines on the central nervous system (CNS) is supported by several converging lines of evidence:

- Infusions of cytokines to immunocompromised patients induce flulike symptoms including fatigue and malaise.
- Peripheral and central injection of cytokines to laboratory rodents induce sickness behavior.
- Symptoms of sickness behavior occurring during experimental infections can be abrogated by administration of anticytokine treatments.
- Although many pitfalls in the detection of cytokines still exist, patients afflicted with the chronic fatigue syndrome have been found in some studies to display instances of excessive production of cytokines.

Experimental studies have confirmed that cytokines are interpreted by the brain as internal signals for sickness. Furthermore, there is evidence that sickness motivates reorganization of the organism's priorities in light of this particular threat that is represented by infectious pathogens. The elucidation of the mechanisms that are involved in these effects and, in particular, the role of the cytokines that are produced in the brain in response to peripheral immune stimuli and to stressors should give new insight into the way sickness and recovery processes are organized in the brain.

EPIDEMIOLOGY

The percentage of patients that meet the 1994 Centers for Disease Control and Prevention (CDC) case definition for CFS is considered to be less than 10%. In general, it is estimated that perhaps as many as 1 million persons in the United States have a CFS-like condition.

CFS is associated with these groups:

- It is primarily a disorder of young to middle-age adults, but cases in children have been recognized. It may also occur in elderly people, but coexisting medical conditions may usually rule out its consideration in this population.
- Most series report that CFS is about twice as common in women as in men.
- Few cases have been reported in minorities or among lower socioeconomic groups. However, the incidence in these groups may be underestimated because of their lack of equal access to health care institutions in which CFS is studied.

Cases of suspected CFS have been reported in most industrialized countries. Chronic debilitating fatigue is common in medical outpatients, but CFS is relatively rare. The prevalence of CFS depends heavily on the case definition used.

A molecular epidemiology component of the CDC's CFS research program has been established. The current major laboratory effort focuses on analysis of gene expression in peripheral white blood cells to profile systemic patterns in CFS patients and control subjects, and to identify molecular markers that distinguish CFS patients. This approach uses two complementary gene expression monitoring technologies (high-density filter arrays and glass microarrays and differential display polymerase chain reactions [DD-PCR]). Results should direct attention to pathways detected as abnormal and may also identify different pathologic entities within the syndrome. Preliminary studies of gene expression in cases and control subjects from a study in Atlanta demonstrated that gene expression profiling was feasible on peripheral blood and yielded intriguing results indicating that case gene expression was distinct from control gene expression. The Molecular Epidemiology Program has incorporated gene expression using microarrays and DD-PCR into most of the CFS program studies in which it is possible to collect a peripheral blood sample.

Genetic expression testing, or gene profiling, examines the activity or transcription of genes by quantitatively measuring messenger RNA in cells. Gene expression is altered by many factors, including cell differentiation, metabolic states, and disease status. New techniques allow quantitative analysis of RNA transcripts from thousands of genes at the same time and reveal the pattern of genes that are active at the time of sampling; gene expression patterns characterize disease states. By comparing the gene expression pattern between samples, characteristic differences can be identified. These differences, known as differential gene expression, can point to markers for diagnosis or to metabolic pathways that are altered.

SIGNS AND SYMPTOMS

In 1987 The Division of Viral Disease of the CDC met to establish a formal definition of the complex array of symptoms of CFS. The case definition of the syndrome was devised based on major, minor, and physical criteria, as well as on the exclusion of conditions known to contribute to chronic fatigue states, including tumors, autoimmune diseases, infections, and endocrine disorders. In 1994 the CDC revised its CFS case definition. To meet the definition for CFS, a person must have clinically evaluated, unexplained persistent or relapsing chronic fatigue that is of new or definite onset (i.e., not lifelong), is not the result of ongoing exertion, is not substantially alleviated by rest, and results in substantial reduction in previous levels of occupational, educational, social, or personal activities.

In addition, the person must have at least four of the following symptoms:

- Substantial impairment in short-term memory or concentration
- Sore throat
- Tender lymph nodes
- Muscle pain
- Multijoint pain without swelling or redness
- Headaches of a new type, pattern, or severity
- Unrefreshing sleep
- Postexertional malaise lasting more than 24 hours

Diagnosis rests on fulfillment of the case definition that was revised in 1994. As currently described in the working criteria proposed by the CDC, chronic fatigue may be associated with multiple, distinct, and possibly unique clinical and/or etiopathogenic subsets. Sjögren's syndrome (SS) is a disease of unknown etiology that is characterized by dryness of the mucous membranes and a variety of autoimmune phenomena and conditions. Subjective manifestations of SS such as neurocognitive dysfunction and fatigue have been stressed by some observers. A large number of patients with unrecognized SS-like illness in a clinic specializing in CFS have provoked a suspicion that the relationship between the two is more than casual.

An important feature of the CDC analysis of CFS is the recognition that many people can have unexplained chronic fatigue and may not necessarily fit the case criteria for CFS. In fact, only about 10% of patients meet the present CFS criteria. Such individuals are defined as having idiopathic chronic fatigue. Idiopathic chronic fatigue may represent a different end of the spectrum of a continuum of illness that includes CFS. These diagnostic criteria are now under study to determine their validity. In general, to receive a diagnosis of chronic fatigue syndrome, a patient must satisfy two criteria:

1. Have severe chronic fatigue of 6 months or longer duration with other known medical conditions excluded by clinical diagnosis
2. Concurrently have four or more of the following symptoms: substantial impairment in short-term memory or concentration, sore throat, tender lymph nodes, muscle pain, multijoint pain without swelling or redness, headaches of a new type, pattern or severity, unre-

freshing sleep, and postexertional malaise lasting more than 24 hours.

The symptoms must have persisted or recurred during 6 or more consecutive months of illness and must not have predated the fatigue.

Autonomic Nervous System Involvement

CFS may be an illness mediated by the CNS. Patients with CFS frequently exhibit cognitive deficits in concentration, attention, and short-term memory. These include immunologic abnormalities, indications of pituitary and hypothalamic involvement, abnormal basal plasma levels of certain neurotransmitter metabolites, and cerebral perfusion abnormalities. The symptom pattern of chronic fatigue syndrome may eventually be explainable in terms of CNS dysfunction. Physical or emotional stress, which is reported as a preonset condition in CFS patients, activates the hypothalamic-pituitary-adrenal (HPA) axis, leading to increased release of cortisol and other hormones. Cortisol and corticotrophin-releasing hormone, which are also produced during the activation of the HPA axis, influence the immune system and many other body systems. Recent studies revealed that CFS patients often produce lower levels of cortisol than normal.

Depression

Depression is a theme that predominates in the history of CFS. It is an emotional issue that patients prefer to dismiss because of the personal and societal stigma attached to psychiatric diagnoses. Three studies verified that two thirds or more of patients with CFS meet existing psychiatric criteria for anxiety disorders, dysthymia, or depression. Among patients who develop viral illnesses, a personal history of a psychiatric disorder preceding the infection is a good predictor of the potential for development of a future mood disorder.

LABORATORY EVALUATION

There is no simple laboratory test that can identify CFS; a physician must exclude other possible causes of the symptoms before diagnosing a person with CFS. Recommended screening tests for detecting common exclusionary conditions are:

- Complete blood count
- Erythrocyte sedimentation rate
- Urinalysis
- Blood chemistries (glucose, blood urea nitrogen, creatinine, total protein, albumin and globulin, calcium, phosphorous, alkaline phosphatase, and thyroid stimulating hormone)

A variety of abnormal laboratory findings have been noted in CFS. These abnormalities include atypical lymphocytosis, elevated immunoglobulin G (IgG) levels, a greater incidence of circulating immune complexes, elevated alkaline phosphatase, elevated total cholesterol, and elevated lactic dehydrogenase levels. Also, antinuclear antibodies are detected in some cases. The immunologic abnormalities are in accord with a growing body of evidence suggesting chronic, low-level activation of the immune system in chronic fatigue syndrome.

Immunologic Abnormalities

Cellular Abnormalities

Immunologic tests can demonstrate cellular immunodeficiencies, including disorders of granulocyte function in many cases. One study has reported an elevation in the number of lymphocyte cells expressing activation markers in the most severely ill CFS patients, but this observation has not been supported by other studies. In addition, some studies have observed a trend among CFS patients to have reduced NK cell activity and/or reduced NK cell numbers. However, NK cell assays have yet to be documented as having any value as a diagnostic marker for CFS.

Soluble Mediators and Antibody Abnormalities

Low levels of IgG3- and IgG1-subclass and decreases in the complement system (CH50, C3, C4, Cl-esterase-inhibitor) have been observed. Various reports have suggested that elevated levels of cytokines (e.g., IL-1, IL-2, IL-6, and tumor-necrosis factor) are associated with CFS, but no cytokine has been identified that serves as a useful diagnostic marker for CFS.

The increased occurrence of autoantibodies in CFS patients (especially antinuclear antibodies, circulating immune complexes, and microsomal thyroid antibodies) suggests that CFS is associated with the beginning of manifest autoimmune disease.

Infectious Disease Testing

Increased antibody titers for Epstein-Barr virus (EBV-EA positive, low EBNA-titers) and HHV-6-virus have been noted. Tests for herpes viruses and *Borrelia, Chlamydia, Candida,* or *Amoeba* spp. are positive in some patients.

Chemical Abnormalities

One of the characteristic complaints of patients with chronic fatigue syndrome is the skeletal muscle-related symptom. However, the abnormalities in the skeletal muscle that explain the symptom are not clear. Herein, we show that our patients with CFS had a deficiency of serum acylcarnitine. As carnitine has an important role in energy production and modulation of the intramitochondrial coenzyme A (CoA)/acyl-CoA ratio in the skeletal muscle, this deficiency might induce an energy deficit and/or abnormality of the intramitochondrial condition in the skeletal muscle, thus resulting in general fatigue, myalgia, muscle weakness, and postexertional malaise in patients with CFS. Furthermore, the concentration of serum acylcarnitine in patients with CFS tended to increase to the normal level with the recovery of general fatigue. Therefore the measurement of acylcarnitine would be a useful tool for the diagnosis and assessment of the degree of clinical manifestation in patients with CFS.

Serum angiotensin-converting enzyme (ACE) levels have been found to be elevated in 80% of patients with CFS. The assay of serum ACE is useful as a diagnostic aid in sarcoidosis and may be a useful marker for CFS, especially if a method can be developed to distinguish ACE in CFS from that in sarcoidosis. Sensitivity of ACE for CFS has been demonstrated to be 80%, with 68% specificity in an endemic area. It has been suggested that an increase in ACE may be an early manifestation of CFS; this supports the concept that CFS is a definite disease state.

The ACE level in CFS is affected by freezing and thawing of serum, which causes activation of a fraction of ACE. Furthermore, storage of the serum at refrigerator temperature (4° C) results in loss of this CFS-associated ACE fraction. This suggests that in CFS, either a specific fraction of ACE is released causing the elevated levels, or that an ACE enhancer is produced causing an increase in ACE activity, and that this ACE fraction differs from that appearing in sarcoidosis.

Currently the recommended procedure for studying the ACE activity in blood from patients suspected of having CFS is:

1. Remove serum from a clotted blood sample and store in freezer until assay can be performed.
2. If the result of initial assay is normal, then refreeze serum and repeat assay within 1 week.
3. Store a portion of serum sample at 4° C for subsequent assay in approximately 3 months to test for loss of ACE activity as a last available means to detect an abnormality. A loss of activity with refrigerator storage is unusual and reflects a possible diagnosis of CFS.

Furthermore, variable deficits of vitamins and trace elements have been seen.

DIAGNOSIS

More recent recommendations by the CDC and the International Chronic Fatigue Syndrome Study Group are even more conservative than some previous recommendations. After a thorough history and physical examination, the patient is asked to keep temperature and weight records and a limited amount of laboratory testing is performed.

TREATMENT

Because there is no known cause of CFS, current treatment remains symptomatic. Numerous clinical trials of pharmacologic agents have been conducted, but no definitive therapeutic benefit has been identified.

Tricyclic antidepressants and selective serotonin reuptake inhibitors (SSRIs) are common therapy for patients with CFS. Tricyclic antidepressants have proven to be effective in reducing clinical depression and improving sleep patterns. Some evidence supports the use of the SSRIs fluoxetine (Prozac) and bupropion (Wellbutrin), but placebo-controlled trials of these drugs have not significantly benefited patients with CFS. A recent study of nicotinamide-adenine dinucleotide therapy reported that the therapy decreased the adenosine triphosphate level, which improved muscle atrophy and neuroendocrine abnormalities.

Cognitive behavior therapy is a psychotherapeutic treatment approach. It examines both the patient's cognition and behavior to identify unhealthy coping skills.

The current suggested management includes exercise, optimal diet, appropriate sleep hygiene, low-dose tricyclic antidepressants and/or an SSRI, combined with cognitive-behavior therapy. Alleviating allergy symptoms and stress may decrease the intensity and frequency of exacerbations. Treatment of concomitant disorders (e.g., migraine headaches) may significantly improve a patient's condition.

Multidisciplinary intervention, consisting of medical, psychiatric, behavioral, and psychologic evaluations and therapy, has been demonstrated to be effective at restoring patients to gainful employment. Future advances in technology (e.g., neuroimaging, genotype profiling, and immune assays) may bring greater consistency to scientific research and the possibility of improved therapy for CFS.

BIBLIOGRAPHY

Barker E et al: Immunologic abnormalities associated with chronic fatigue syndrome, *Clin Infect Dis* 18(Suppl 1):S136-141, 1994.

Bates DW et al: A comparison of case definitions of chronic fatigue syndrome, *Clin Infect Dis* 18(Suppl 1):S11-15, 1994.

Bates DW et al: Prevalence of fatigue and chronic fatigue syndrome in a primary care practice, *Arch Intern Med* 153(24):2759-2765, 1993.

Bates DW et al: Clinical laboratory test findings in patients with chronic fatigue syndrome, *Arch Intern Med* 155(1):97-103, 1995.

Bell DS: Chronic fatigue syndrome update. Findings now point to CNS involvement, *Postgrad Med* 96(6):73-76, 79-81, 1994.

Calabrese I et al: Chronic fatigue syndrome, *Am Fam Physician* 45(3):1205-1213, 1992.

Calabrese LH, Davis ME, Wilke WS: Chronic fatigue syndrome and a disorder resembling Sjogren's syndrome: preliminary report, *Clin Infect Dis* 18(Suppl 1):S28-31, 1994.

Dantzer R: Current studies on the neurobiology of chronic fatigue syndrome, *Encephale* 20(3):597-602, 1994.

Fosnocht M. et al: Approach to the patient with fatigue, May 15, 2002, website: http://www.uptodate.com

Fukuda et al: *Ann Intern Med* 121:953-959, 1994.

Garralda ME et al: Childhood chronic fatigue syndrome, *Am J Psychiatry* 158:1161, 2001.

Gluckman JS: Clinical features of chronic fatigue syndrome, May 15, 2002, website: http://www.uptodate.com

Gold D et al: Chronic fatigue, *JAMA* 264(1):48-53, 1990.

Hilgers A, Frank J: Chronic fatigue syndrome: immune dysfunction, role of pathogens and toxic agents and neurological and cardial changes, *Wien Med Wochenschr* 144(16):399-406, 1994.

Johnson SK: Cognitive functioning of patients with chronic fatigue syndrome, *Clin Infect Dis* 18(Suppl 1):S84-85, 1994.

Jones JF: Serologic and immunologic responses in chronic fatigue syndrome with emphasis on the Epstein-Barr virus, *Rev Infect Dis* 13(Suppl 1):S26-S31, 1991.

Kuratsune H et al: Acylcarnitine deficiency in chronic fatigue syndrome, *Clin Infect Dis* 18(Suppl 1):S62-67, 1994.

Levine PH et al: An approach to studies of cancer subsequent to clusters of chronic fatigue syndrome: use of data from the Nevada State Cancer Registry, *Clin Infect Dis* 18(Suppl 1):S49-53, 1994.

Levy JA: Viral studies of chronic fatigue syndrome, *Clin Infect Dis* 18(Suppl 1):S117-120, 1994.

Lieberman J, Bell DS: Serum angiotensin-converting enzyme as a marker for the chronic fatigue-immune dysfunction syndrome: a comparison to serum angiotensin-converting enzyme in sarcoidosis, *Am J Med* 95(10):407-412, 1993.

Ojo-Amaize EA, Conley EJ, Peter JB: Decreased natural killer cell activity is associated with severity of chronic fatigue immune dysfunction syndrome, *Clin Infect Dis* 18(Suppl 1):S157-159, 1994.

Rasmussen AK et al: Chronic fatigue syndrome—a controlled cross-sectional study, *Ugeskr Laeger* 156(46):6836-6840, 1994.

Rasmussen AK et al: Chronic fatigue syndrome—a defined unity? *Ugeskr Laeger* 156(46):6832-6836, 1994.

Reyes Michele et al: Surveillance for chronic fatigue syndrome—four U.S. cities, September 1989 through August 1993, *MMWR* 46(ss-2):1-13, 1997.

Shafran SD: The chronic fatigue syndrome, *Am J Med* 90(6):730-739, 1991.

Taerk G, Gnam W: A psychodynamic view of the chronic fatigue syndrome. The role of object relations in etiology and treatment, *Gen Hosp Psychiatry* 16(5):319-325, 1994.

Timothy C et al: Chronic fatigue syndrome treatment and evaluation, *Am Fam Physician* 65:1083-1090, 1095, 2002.

Tirelli U et al: Immunological abnormalities in patients with chronic fatigue syndrome, *Scand J Immunol* 40(6):601-608, 1994.

Trinidad EE, Ramirez RC: Chronic fatigue syndrome, *Bol Asoc Med P R* 86(7-9):56-61, 1994.

Walsh RD, Cunha BA: The diagnostic approach to chronic fatigue syndrome, *Intern Med* 14(4):48-50, 1993.

Whiting P et al: Interventions for the treatment and management of chronic fatigue syndrome, *JAMA* 286(11):1360, 2001.

Yalcin S et al: Prevalence of human herpesvirus 6 variants A and B in patients with chronic fatigue syndrome, *Microbiol Immunol* 38(7):587-590, 1994.

Appendix D

A Primer on Vaccines

We become immune to microbial antigens through artificial and natural means. Vaccines give us artificially acquired active immunity to a specific disease. Vaccine development is an important focus of research related to acquired immunodeficiency syndrome (AIDS), malaria, and other devastating diseases. In regard to bioterrorism, the goal of the U.S. Food and Drug Administration (FDA) is to foster the development of vaccines. Many products (e.g., vaccines regulated by FDA) could be affected by bioterrorism. Pathogens or pathogen products adapted for biologic warfare include smallpox (variola), anthrax *(Bacillus anthracis),* plague *(Yersinia pestis),* tularemia *(Francisella tularensis),* brucellosis *(Brucella abortus, B. melitensis, B. suis, B. canis),* Q fever *(Coxiella burnetii),* botulinum toxin (produced by *Clostridium botulinum*), and staphylococcal enterotoxin B.

HISTORY AND USE OF VACCINES

Vaccine production is not new. Edward Jenner, an English physician, discovered one of the fundamentals principles of immunization more than 200 hundred years ago. His observations and experiments with smallpox vaccine paved the way for the development of rabies vaccine by Louis Pasteur and many other vaccines (e.g., diphtheria and typhoid fever).

The concept of vaccination or deliberately introducing a potentially harmful microbe into a patient initially met with suspicion and outrage. Vaccines produced today are safer and more protective than those developed in the early days. Children now receive vaccines to numerous diseases (e.g., German measles [rubella]) that were almost unavoidable diseases of childhood in the past. Adults require updates of vaccinations (e.g., tetanus). International travelers frequently require vaccination to endemic diseases in a particular country (e.g., hepatitis A). Health care professionals are now protected against hepatitis B through the use of vaccines. And each year, many adults prepare for winter and the "flu season" by receiving flu vaccine. The use of vaccines has spread to pets and livestock as well (e.g., Lyme disease).

CHARACTERISTICS OF A VACCINE

The purpose of a vaccine is to stimulate active immunity and to create an immune memory so that exposure to the active disease microorganism will stimulate an already primed immune system to fight the disease.

Traditionally prepared vaccines are preparations of inactivated (killed) or live, attenuated (weakened) bacteria or viruses, parts of the microorganisms, or toxoids (inactivated toxins) from the disease-causing agent. Newer synthetic vaccines use subunit vaccines, conjugate vaccines, and naked DNA vaccines.

No vaccine is totally effective nor is it 100% safe. To be approved by the U.S. Food and Drug Administration (FDA) (Tables D-1 and D-2), a vaccine must meet specific requirements. A vaccine must:
- Produce protective immunity with only minimal side effects
- Be immunogenic enough to produce a strong and measurable immune response
- Be stable during its shelf life with the potency remaining at a proper level. Inactivated vaccines are stored in a powdered form and are reconstituted before administration; live, attenuated vaccines require refrigeration.

SMALLPOX VACCINE

Threats of bioterrorism with smallpox as a weapon have launched a high profile discussion of the reintroduction of smallpox into the general U.S. population. Individuals in "high risk" occupations and positions have already begun to be vaccinated.

Category A Agents

Smallpox vaccination was stopped in 1972 after the disease was eradicated in the United States. Smallpox is classified as a Category A agent by the Centers for Disease Control and Prevention. Other category A agents include anthrax, plague, botulism, tularemia, and viral hemorrhagic fevers. These agents are believed to pose the greatest potential threat for adverse public health impact and have a moderate-to-high potential for large-scale dissemination.

Smallpox Vaccine Preparation

Smallpox vaccine, a preventive vaccine, is the only way to prevent smallpox. The vaccine is made from a "live virus" called *vaccinia,* which is another "pox"-type virus related to smallpox but cannot cause smallpox. A "live virus" vaccine, including measles, mumps, rubella, chickenpox and smallpox

TABLE D-1   Available Types of Vaccines, Fall 2002

Traditional Vaccines	Examples of Vaccines
Inactivated vaccines	Hepatitis A, cholera, plague, flu
Live, attenuated vaccines	Measles, rubella, mumps, yellow fever
Toxoids	Tetanus, diphtheria
New and Second-Generation Vaccines	
Conjugate vaccines	*Haemophilus influenzae* type b (Hib)
Subunit vaccines	*Streptococcus pneumoniae,* a type of meningitis, hepatitis B
Recombinant vector vaccines	None licensed
Future Vaccines	
Microspheres, naked DNA	
Edible vaccines	

TABLE D-2   FDA-Approved Vaccines, Fall 2002

Vaccine	Type	Route	Notes
Adenovirus	Live virus	Oral	Available only to US armed forces; no longer being manufactured.
Anthrax	Inactivated bacteria	SC	
BCG	Live bacteria	ID (preferred) or SC	
Cholera	Inactivated bacteria	SC, IM, or ID	
Diphtheria-tetanus	Toxoids	IM	
Diphtheria-tetanus (booster)	Toxoids	IM	
Diphtheria, tetanus, and pertussis (DTP)	Toxoids and inactivated bacteria	IM	
Hepatitis A	Inactivated viral antigen	IM	Recommended only in selected areas
Hepatitis B	Inactivated viral antigen	IM	
Hepatitis B/Hib	Inactivated viral antigen, polysaccharide-protein conjugate	IM	
Hib	Polysaccharide-protein conjugate	IM	
Influenza	Inactivated whole virus, viral components	IM	
Japanese encephalitis	Inactivated virus	SC	
Lyme disease	Inactivated protein	IM	
Measles	Live virus	SC	Still being manufactured?
Meningococcal	Polysaccharide	SC	
MMR	Live viruses	SC	
Measles-Rubella	Live viruses	SC	Still being manufactured?
Mumps	Live virus	SC	Still being manufactured?
Pertussis	Inactivated bacteria	IM	Not sure this is still being manufactured; may be available in Michigan only
Plague	Inactivated bacteria	IM	
Pneumococcal	Polysaccharide	IM or SC	
Polio (IPV)	Inactivated virus	SC	
Polio (OPV)	Live virus	Oral	
Rabies	Inactivated virus	IM or ID	
Rubella	Live virus	SC	Still being manufactured?
Tetanus	Toxoid	IM	
Typhoid	Inactivated bacteria	SC	
Typhoid	Polysaccharide	SC (boosters may be ID)	
Varicella	Live virus	SC	
Yellow Fever	Live virus	SC	

From 2000 Red Book: Report of the Committee on Infectious Diseases, ed 25, Elk Grove Village, Ill, 2000, American Academy of Pediatrics.
SC, Subcutaneous; *ID,* intradermal; *IM,* intramuscular.

vaccines, is a vaccine that contains a "living" virus that is able to give and produce immunity, usually without causing illness. For most people with a healthy immune system, live virus vaccines are safe and effective, but the live virus can be transmitted to other parts of the body or to other people from the unhealed vaccination site.

Vaccine Administration

The vaccine is not injected like other types of vaccines. It is given using a bifurcated (two-pronged) needle that is dipped into the vaccine solution. The needle is used to prick the skin a number of times in a few seconds. It takes about 3 weeks for the site to heal with a scar remaining. The first dose of vaccine offers protection from smallpox for 3 to 5 years, with decreasing immunity thereafter. A repeat vaccination offers longer immunity. Vaccination within 3 days of exposure completely prevents or significantly modifies smallpox in the vast majority of persons. Vaccination 4 to 7 days after exposure likely offers some protection from disease or may modify the severity of the disease.

AIDS VACCINE RESEARCH

In the beginning of 2003, 40 clinical trials using at least 39 different vaccines are ongoing worldwide. But not one vaccine has completed a Phase III trial. The status of HIV vaccines to date is:
1. There are no proven effective therapeutic or preventive HIV vaccines.
2. There is a lack of knowledge related to the ability of a vaccine to induce HIV-specific immune responses that are effective in preventing or treating HIV infection.
3. Therapeutic HIV vaccine research is still in its infancy.

Vaccine Development

The goal in producing HIV vaccines is to destroy HIV or keep the virus in check so that it causes no further damage. An ideal vaccine would stop progressive immunodeficiency and restore the immune system to a healthy state.

The requirements for a preventive HIV vaccine are to generate both humoral and cellular immunity against HIV in the host before exposure to the virus. After initial exposure to HIV, the generation of cellular immune responses against HIV may take a while to develop, which makes neutralizing antibodies against free virus important to reduce the initial spread of the virus in the body.

In the United States research is being based on the use of subunit proteins found in the envelope of HIV. Vaccine research scientists are trying to develop three types of HIV vaccines:
1. Preventive or prophylactic vaccines to protect individuals from HIV infection.
2. Therapeutic vaccines to prevent HIV infected patients from progressing to AIDS.
3. Perinatal vaccines for administration to pregnant HIV-infected women to prevent transmission of HIV to the fetus.

Scientists are hopeful that therapeutic and perinatal administration of vaccine will reach a high level of success.

The challenges associated with HIV vaccine development are:
- A high rate of viral mutation and recombination,
- No clearly defined natural immunity to HIV,
- HIV infects cells that are critical to the immune body defenses, and HIV is transmitted as a free virus and within infected cells.

Problems Associated With HIV Vaccine Development

Problems associated with HIV vaccine development are plagued with the lack of scientific understanding of HIV infection and the complex biology of HIV disease/AIDS. Once inside a host cell, HIV is capable of integrating itself into the genetic material of infected cells. For a vaccine to be effective, it would have to produce a constant state of immune protection, which not only would have to block viral entry to most cells but also would continue to block newly produced viruses over the lifetime of the infected person.

Specific problem areas have been identified by HIV vaccine researchers:
- A lack of knowledge related to the critical components in the body's immune response to HIV infection.
- The high risk of using the entire weakened or inactive HIV in a vaccine.
- The extensive rate of viral mutation as HIV replicates. Strains from different parts of the globe vary by as much as 35% in terms of the proteins that comprise the outer coat of the virus. Even an infected person can experience a change in viral protein by as much as 10% over a period of years. This genetic diversity may require an effective vaccine to be based on multiple viral strain.
- The protective effect of a vaccine may only be for a short period of time, and frequent mandatory booster vaccinations would be impractical and expensive.
- Vaccinated persons could become more susceptible to HIV infection because of vaccine-induced enhancement of infection.
- No vaccine clinical trial to date has demonstrated stimulation of the cellular components of the immune system in the way needed to destroy HIV.
- Animal models have severe limitations, including the possibility of integration of DNA into the human genome from monkeys.
- No research studies have successfully demonstrated which immune responses correlate with protection from HIV infection.

Vaccine research scientists at the Seventh Conference on Retroviruses and Opportunistic Infections held in February 2000 lowered their expectations and will settle for a vaccine that does not completely prevent HIV infection. It is estimated that a vaccine with only 30% effectiveness (compared to the usual 85% to 95% effectiveness of other infectious diseases vaccines) against HIV can begin to eradicate the virus if it is widely administered and accompanied by disease prevention education. Based on this premise, the FDA has indicated that the agency will approve an HIV/AIDS vaccine at this level of efficacy.

Future Expectations

Reasons for optimism about HIV vaccine development include:

- Nonhuman primates vaccinated with products based on HIV or simian immunodeficiency virus (SIM) have shown either complete or partial protection against infection with the wild type virus.
- Successful vaccines have been developed against the feline immunodeficiency virus, also a retrovirus.
- Almost all humans develop some form of immune responses that are protective or that are able to control the viral infection over a long period of time. In fact, some individuals remain disease free for up to 25 years, frequently with undetectable viral load levels.

A VACCINE USED IN LEUKEMIA

The search to develop vaccines for cancer has had a recent breakthrough with the development of a therapeutic vaccine directed at patients with acute myelogenous leukemia (AML). A pilot study to demonstrate the effectiveness and safety of an AML vaccine is underway. The phase I stage of the clinical trial with AML patients is aimed at determining if the PR1 peptide vaccine (a 9 amino acid HLA A2–restricted peptide derived from proteinase 3) can elicit T cell immunity in leukemia patients whose disease had been resistant to treatment.

GLOSSARY

conjugate vaccine Conjugate vaccine is a vaccine in which proteins that are easily recognized by the immune system are linked to the outer coat of the disease-causing microorganism to stimulate an immune response.

naked DNA vaccine Naked DNA vaccine is a vaccine made up of DNA that is not encased or encapsulated. In naked DNA vaccines, genetic material is injected directly into the vaccine recipient.

subunit vaccine Subunit vaccine is a vaccine that uses one or more components of a disease-causing microorganism, instead of the whole microbe, to stimulate an immune response.

toxoids A toxoid is an inactivated toxin, the harmful substance produced by a microbe.

BIBLIOGRAPHY

Advance for Medical Laboratory Professionals: *Clinical clips,* website: www.advanceformlp.com/mtclinical.html, retrieved December 23, 2002.

Bozzette SA et al: A model for smallpox vaccination policy, *N Engl J Med,* website: www.NEJM.org, December 19, 2002.

Centers for Disease Control and Prevention, Smallpox Fact Sheet, website: www.bt.cdc.gov/agent/smallpox, modified December 9, 2002.

Schraeder TL, Campion: Smallpox vaccination—the call to arms, *N Engl J Med* 348:1-2, 2003.

Stine GJ: *AIDS UPDATE 2003,* Prentice Hall, 2003, Upper Saddle River, NJ

Appendix E

Apoptosis

In multicellular organisms homeostasis is maintained through a balance between cell proliferation (mitosis) and physiologic cell death (apoptosis). The term *apoptosis* was coined in a now classic paper by Kerr, Wyllie, and Currie (*Br J Cancer* 26:239) in 1972 as a means of distinguishing a morphologically distinctive form of cell death that was associated with normal physiology.

FACTORS INFLUENCING APOPTOSIS

Apoptosis can be influenced by a wide variety of regulatory stimuli. Cell survival appears to depend on the constant supply of survival signals provided by neighboring cells and the extracellular matrix. Inducers of apoptosis include:

- Cytokines (e.g., tumor necrosis factor family)
- Damage-related inducers (e.g., viral infection, bacterial toxins, oncogenes, tumor suppressors [p53], oxidants, free radicals, and heat shock)
- Therapy-associated agents (e.g., chemotherapeutic drugs, gamma, and ultraviolet radiation)
- Toxins (e.g., ethanol)

APOPTOSIS VERSUS NECROSIS

Apoptotic cell death can be distinguished from necrotic or accidental cell death. Apoptotic cell death is controlled autodigestion of the cells. Apoptosis is characterized by nuclear condensation and fragmentation, cell shrinkage, and elimination of dead cells by phagocytosis. By comparison, necrotic cell death is a pathologic form of cell death resulting from acute cellular injury characterized by rapid cell swelling and lysis.

ALTERATIONS IN APOPTOSIS

During embryonic development excess numbers of developing cells die, and in hormone-responsive tissues (e.g., uterus) cyclical depletion of a particular hormone leads to death. In all of these situations, cell death occurs by the process of apoptosis.

Alterations in cell survival contribute to the pathogenesis of a number of human diseases (e.g., cancer, autoimmune disease, and acquired immunodeficiency syndrome [AIDS]). Certain diseases are associated with the inhibition of apoptosis; other diseases are associated with increased apoptosis.

Diseases associated with inhibition of apoptosis include:
- Cancer (e.g., follicular lymphomas, carcinomas with p53 mutations, and hormone-dependent tumors such as breast, ovarian, and prostate cancer)
- Autoimmune disorders (e.g., systemic lupus erythematosus, immune mediated glomerulonephritis)
- Viral infections (e.g., herpesvirus, adenoviruses)

Diseases associated with increased apoptosis include:
- AIDS
- Neurodegenerative disorders (e.g., Alzheimer's disease, Parkinson's disease)
- Myelodysplastic syndromes (e.g., aplastic anemia)
- Ischemic injury (e.g., myocardial infarction, stroke)
- Toxin-induced liver disease (e.g., alcohol)

LYMPHOCYTES AND APOPTOSIS

Programmed cell death plays a key role in controlling the size of the lymphocyte pool at many stages of lymphocyte maturation and activation. Immature lymphocytes that do not express functional antigen receptors or are not positively selected in the thymus or bone marrow undergo programmed death. If lymphocytes never encounter an antigen after cellular maturation, they die by apoptosis. A fraction of the progeny of antigen-activated lymphocytes also die if they do not receive adequate growth factors or continued stimulation. Susceptibility to apoptosis appears to correlate inversely with fluctuation in the levels of expression of Bcl-2 or Bcl-x$_1$ during lymphocytic maturation and activation. Lymphocytes also can undergo a second form of apoptotic death, activation-induced cell death, resulting from receptor-mediator activation. Activation-induced apoptosis is important for the death of lymphocytes that recognize self-antigens and also plays a role in the induction of tolerance to some foreign antigens.

EVALUATION OF APOPTOSIS

Apoptosis can be measured by light microscopy or electron microscopy. Light microscopy can reveal chromatin condensation, nuclear fragments, invagination of plasma membrane, and formation of apoptotic bodies. In vitro assay can detect the fragmentation of nuclear DNA. The TUNEL assay is a precise assay with terminal end-labeling of broken DNA fragments with labeled nucleotides. The reaction is catalyzed by the enzyme terminal deoxyribonucleotidyl transferase (TdT).

Flow cytometry light scattering can differentiate apoptosis from necrosis.

THE ROLE OF APOPTOSIS IN TREATMENT PROTOCOLS

Treatments designed to specifically alter the apoptotic threshold may have the potential to change the natural progression of some diseases. There are implications of apoptosis for cancer chemotherapy, including the pharmacology of anticancer drugs and opportunities for developing new therapies. Many anticancer drugs (e.g., cisplatin, doxorubicin, vincristine) are associated with induction of apoptosis.

Although there is much to be learned about the molecular pathways leading to apoptotic cell death, our ability to manipulate it could allow therapeutic intervention in major diseases (e.g., cancer, AIDS, autoimmunity, and other diseases).

BIBLIOGRAPHY

Abbas AK, Lichtman AH, Pober JS: *Cellular and molecular immunology,* ed 4, Philadelphia, 2000, WB Saunders.

Vermes IL et al: Impact of apoptosis (programmed cell death) for clinical laboratory sciences, American Association for Clinical Chemistry Annual Meeting Workshop, July, 2000.

Appendix F

Diagnostic Tests in Medical Laboratory Immunology

Acetylcholine Receptor (AcHR) Binding Antibody: Measures antibody to acetylcholine receptors at neuromuscular junctions of skeletal muscle. Useful in the diagnosis of myasthenia gravis. Negative in ocular myasthenia, Eaton-Lambert syndrome, and in generalized myasthenia gravis if treated or inactive.

Acetylcholine Receptor (AcHR) Blocking Antibody: Measures antibody to acetylcholine receptors that block binding of 125_I-(alpha)-bungarotoxin. Found in about one third of patients with myasthenia gravis.

Albumin Index: Measures albumin in cerebrospinal fluid and serum. Elevated values suggest blood-brain barrier damage, as seen in Guillain-Barré syndrome and similar conditions, or possibly a traumatic tap. This test is of value in the interpretation of central nervous system immunoglobulin G (IgG) synthesis rates.

Alpha-1-Antitrypsin: Measures the quantity of alpha-1-antitrypsin, an acute-phase inflammatory reactant, in the blood. A deficiency of this protein is found if the alleles Z and S are present; moderate reduction is exhibited by the MS, and MZ phenotypes are increased in chronic or recurrent anterior uveitis and rheumatoid arthritis. The MZ phenotype is also associated with hepatoma and chronic hepatitis in adults. The ZZ phenotype predisposes an individual to the development of severe, early-onset pulmonary emphysema and to liver disease in infancy and childhood.

Alpha-Fetoprotein: Alpha-fetoprotein (AFP) is normally produced during fetal development by the liver and yolk sac, and in small amounts by the gastrointestinal tract. After birth, serum AFP levels in neonates drop rapidly and by 6 months the blood levels are very low. In pregnant females, AFP levels begin to rise at 12 to 14 weeks and peak during the third trimester. AFP is a valuable tumor marker. When used as a tumor marker, increased levels have been observed in patients with primary hepatocellular carcinoma, nonseminomatous testicular carcinomas, and ovarian carcinomas, as well as in other epithelial tumors, especially those of the gastrointestinal tract. AFP is also increased in some nonmalignant hepatic diseases, such as viral hepatitis and active cirrhosis.

ANA: (see antinuclear antibody)

ANCA: (see antineutrophil cytoplasmic antibody)

Antiadrenal Antibody: Measures antibody to adrenal cortex cells. High antibody titers are characteristic of autoimmune hypoadrenalism in about three fourths of cases but are not found in tuberculous Addison's disease.

Anticentriole Antibody: Measures antibody to the cellular ultrastructures, centrioles. The appearance of these antibodies is unusual but can be demonstrated in systemic sclerosis.

Anticardiolipin Antibody: Measures antibody directed to cardiolipin. The presence of antibody in systemic lupus erythematosus (SLE) is associated with arterial and venous thromboses, and in patients with placental infarcts in early pregnancy with or without SLE. Elevation of anticardiolipin antibody may be predictive of the risk of thrombosis or recurrent spontaneous abortions of early pregnancy.

Anticentromere Antibody: Measures anticentrome (antikinetocore) to chromosomal centromeres. Most patients with *c*alcinosis, *R*aynaud's phenomena, *e*sophageal dysfunction, *s*clerodactyly, *t*elangiectasia (CREST) syndrome demonstrate these antibodies. These antibodies are seen in about one third of patients with Raynaud's disease and approximately 10% of patients with systemic sclerosis.

Anti-DNA Antibody: Measures antibody to double-stranded deoxyribonucleic acid (DNA). Increased amounts (>25% by membrane assay) and decreased quantities of the C4 complement component confirm the diagnosis of systemic lupus erythematosus (SLE). These tests are useful in monitoring the activity and exacerbations of SLE. The absence of anti-DNA is demonstrated in about one fourth of SLE patients; therefore a negative test does not rule out SLE.

Anti DNAase B: High levels of neutralizing antibody to DNase-B are commonly found in patients after a group A streptococcal infection. Because it persists longer than other streptococcal antibodies (2 to 3 months), it is the preferred test in patients with chorea suspected to be due to rheumatic fever. Because it is not influenced by the site of infection, DNase-B antibody is more reliable than the streptolysin O antibody test in providing evidence for streptococcal infection in patients with postimpetigo glomerulonephritis. Elevated titers are strongly suggestive of recent or current infection with group A streptococci. Fourfold increases in titer between acute and convalescent samples taken approximately 2 weeks apart are confirmatory.

Antigliadin Antibodies, IgA, and IgG: Gliadin antibodies are IgG and IgA antibodies against a group of proteins found in the gluten of wheat and rye grains. The enzyme-linked immunosorbent assay test for gliadin antibodies is a reliable screening tool for the evaluation of asymptomatic celiac disease in prepubertal children with short stature. Celiac disease results from an intolerance to dietary gluten, resulting in small intestinal villous atrophy with subsequent malabsorption and malnutrition. In celiac disease, IgG antibodies are more sensitive than IgA antibodies, but IgA antibodies are more specific than IgG antibodies. The level of IgA antibodies decreases with a gluten-free diet. IgA and IgG antibodies rise significantly during gluten challenge, sometimes several months before clinical relapse.

Antiglomerular Basement Membrane Antibody: Measures the amount of antibody to glomerular basement membrane (anti-GBM). High titers are suggestive of Goodpasture's disease or anti-GBM nephritis. The test is useful for monitoring anti-GBM nephritis. Negative results, however, do not rule out Goodpasture's disease.

Antiintrinsic Factor: Measures antibodies to intrinsic factor (IF). The presence of IF-blocking antibodies is diagnostic of pernicious anemia and occurs in about 60% of cases.

Antiislet-Cell Antibody: Measures antibodies to the islet cells of the pancreas. This test is useful as an early marker of beta pancreatic cell destruction.

Anti-Jo Antibody: Anti-Jo-1 antibody is found in patients with pure polymyositis, pure dermatomyositis, or myositis associated with another rheumatic disease or with interstitial lung disease.

Anti-LKM Antibody: Measures antibodies to components of renal and hepatic microsomes. The presence of a high titer is diagnostic of hepatic illness and suggests aggressive disease.

Antimitochondrial Antibody: Measures antibodies to the cellular ultrastructures, mitochondria. A high titer strongly suggests primary biliary cirrhosis (PBC); the absence of mitochondrial antibodies is strong evidence against PBC. Other forms of liver disease frequently exhibit low mitochondrial antibody titers.

Antimyelin Antibody: Measures antibody to components of the myelin sheath of nerves of myelin basic protein. Antibodies to myelin are associated with multiple sclerosis or other neurologic diseases. Myelin antibodies are not detectable in the cerebrospinal fluid of multiple sclerosis patients.

Antimyocardial Antibody: Measures antibody to components of the myocardium. The presence of myocardial antibodies is diagnostic of Dressler's syndrome (cardiac injury) or rheumatic fever.

Antinuclear Antibody: Measures antibody to nuclear antigens. Antinuclear antibodies are found in 99% of patients with untreated systemic lupus erythematosus.

Antineutrophil Antibody: Circulating antibodies to neutrophils can mediate neutropenia in a number of different disorders (e.g., systemic lupus erythematosus, Felty's syndrome, and drug-induced neutropenia). Isoimmune destruction of neutrophils also occurs in febrile transfusion reactions and in isoimmune neonatal neutropenia. Antineutrophil antibodies may include anti-HLA antibodies.

Antineutrophilic Cytoplasmic Antibody: Antineutrophil cytoplasmic antibodies (ANCA) are autoantibodies specific for neutrophil lysosomal enzymes, particularly for proteinase 3 and myeloperoxidase. ANCA antibodies have been subdivided into c-ANCA (cytoplasmic) and p-ANCA (perinuclear). The p-ANCA pattern mimics antinuclear antibodies (ANA). This perinuclear pattern reverts to c-ANCA, however, on formalin-fixed neutrophils. In about 80% of cases, c-ANCA has specificity for proteinase 3 and p-ANCA for myeloperoxidase.

Antiparietal Cell Antibody: Measures antibody to parietal cells (large cells on the margin of the peptic glands of the stomach). The majority (80%) of patients with pernicious anemia have parietal cell antibodies. In the presence of these antibodies, gastric biopsy almost always demonstrates gastritis. Low antibody titers to parietal cells are often found with no clinical evidence of pernicious anemia or atrophic gastritis and are sometimes seen in elderly patients.

Antiplatelet Antibody: Measures immunologically attached IgG on platelets. The presence of platelet antibodies, measured indirectly, is associated with immune thrombocytopenia and systemic lupus erythematosus.

Antiphospholipid Antibody: (see Anticardiolipin Antibodies)

Antireticulin Antibody: Measures antibody to reticulin, an albuminoid or scleroprotein substance present in the connective framework of reticular tissue. The majority (80%) of cases of childhood gluten-sensitive enteropathy demonstrate reticulin antibodies. These antibodies can also be found in dermatitis herpetiformis and adult gluten-sensitive enteropathy and in about one fifth of patients suffering from chronic heroin addiction.

Antirheumatoid Arthritis Nuclear Antigen (Anti-RANA) Antibody: (also called Rheumatoid Arthritis Precipitin-RAP). Measures antibody to a component of the Epstein-Barr virus. Antibody is found in the majority of patients with rheumatoid arthritis and in about 15% of patients with systemic lupus erythematosus. Anti-RANA is not useful in diagnosis or differential diagnosis of arthritis.

Antiribosome Antibody: Measures the presence of antibodies to the cellular organelles, ribosomes. Ribosomal antibodies are found in about 10% of patients with systemic lupus erythematosus.

Antinuclear Ribonucleoprotein (Anti-nRNP) Antibody: Measures an antinuclear antibody (ANA), nuclear ribonucleoprotein. A high titer of this antibody is characteristic of mixed connective tissue disease (MCTD) or undifferentiated connective tissue disease. In MCTD, anti-nRNP is found in the absence of various other ANAs. Low titers of anti-nRNP are seen in about one third of patients with systemic lupus erythematosus and are typically found in association with other ANAs such as anti-DNA or anti-Sm.

Anti-Scl or Anti-Scl-70 Antibody: Measures an antibody to a basic nonhistone nuclear protein. The presence of anti-Scl is diagnostic of systemic sclerosis; however, it is demonstrable in only about one fifth of the patients suffering from systemic sclerosis.

Antiskin (Dermal-Epidermal) Antibody: Measures antibody to the basement membrane area of the skin. Antibodies are present in more than 80% of patients with bullous pemphigoid, but the absence of antibodies does not rule out the disorder.

Antiskin (Interepithelial) Antibody: Measures antibody to intercellular substance of the skin. Antibodies can be detected in most (90%) patients with pemphigus. The absence of demonstrable antibody usually excludes the diagnosis. The presence of antibodies is also useful in evaluating "blistering" disease. A rising antibody titer may indicate an impending relapse of pemphigus; a falling titer is suggestive of effective control of the disease.

Anti-Sm Antibody: Measures Sm (Smith) antibody to acidic nuclear protein. Sm antibody is demonstrated by about one third of patients with systemic lupus erythematosus (SLE). Presence of the antibody confirms the diagnosis of SLE, but the absence of antibody does not exclude the diagnosis.

Antismooth Muscle Antibody: Measures antibody to components of smooth muscle. A high and persistent titer suggests the autoimmune form of chronic active hepatitis. Antismooth muscle antibodies are also seen in viral disorders such as infectious mononucleosis.

Antisperm Antibody: Evaluates the presence of reproductive cell, or sperm, antibodies. Half of vasectomized males and 40% of males and females with fertility problems demonstrate the antibody.

Anti-SS-A (SS-A Precipitin, Anti-Ro) Antibody: Detects the presence of antibody to acidic nucleoprotein of human spleen extract. SS-A precipitins are demonstrable in more than 70% of patients with Sjögren's syndrome-sicca complex and are often found in a subset of these patients at risk for vasculitis. The antibody is also found in one third of patients with systemic lupus erythematosus or Sjögren's rheumatoid arthritis, or the annular variety of subacute cutaneous lupus erythematosus (LE). In neonatal LE, autoantibodies to SS-A, discoid skin lesions, and congenital heart blocks are common.

Anti-SS-B (SS-B Precipitin, Anti-La) Antibody: Detects antibody to acidic nucleoprotein thymus. Anti-SS-B is demonstrated by most patients with Sjögren's syndrome-systemic lupus erythematosus. One half to three fourths of patients with Sjögren's syndrome-sicca complex have the antibody; it is frequently found in a subset of these patients at risk for vasculitis.

Antistriational Antibody: Measures antibody to components of striated muscle. Antibodies to striated muscle may be detected in patients with myasthenia gravis, thymoma, or with penicillamine treatment. Absence of the antibody in patients with myasthenia gravis generally rules out the presence of thymoma.

Antithyroglobulin and Antithyroid Microsome Antibody: Evaluates the presence of antibody to the thyroid components: thyroglobulin, an iodine-containing protein secreted by the thyroid gland and stored within its colloid substance; and thyroid microsomes, particles derived from the endoplasmic reticulum. The presence of microsome antibodies is considered predictive of an elevated thyroid-stimulating hormone (TSH) level. A positive thyroid antibody test and an elevated TSH titer are associated with a risk of hypothyroidism. Absence of both antibodies is strong evidence against autoimmune thyroiditis.

Beta-Glucuronidase: Measures the enzyme activity of the enzyme, beta-glucuronidase, in cerebrospinal fluid. Increased levels of enzyme activity are associated with bacterial or fungal meningitis; extremely elevated enzyme levels are encountered in untreated leptomeningeal (pia or arachnoid) metastases. Treated cases of leptomeningeal carcinoma may demonstrate decreased enzyme levels. Normal enzyme levels are usually seen in primary brain tumors and parenchymal metastases.

Beta-hCG: Human chorionic gonadotropin (hCG) is found in normal concentration during pregnancy. It can also be a valuable aid in the management of cancer patients with trophoblastic tumors, nonseminomatous testicular tumors, and seminomas when used in conjunction with information available from the clinical evaluation and other diagnostic procedures. Increased serum hCG concentrations have also been observed in melanoma, carcinomas of the breast, gastrointestinal tract, lung, and ovaries, and in benign conditions, including cirrhosis, duodenal ulcer, and inflammatory bowel disease.

Beta$_2$-Microglobulin: Measures the quantity of beta$_2$-microglobulin in either serum or cerebrospinal fluid (CSF). Elevated levels of this protein are associated with central nervous system (CNS) involvement in patients suffering from leukemia or lymphoma. Determination of beta$_2$-microglobulin levels in both serum and CSF are of value in the early diagnosis of CNS involvement and in monitoring intrathecal (within the spinal canal) therapy.

C1 Esterase Inhibitor (C1 Inhibitor): Measures the activity and/or concentration of C1 inhibitor in serum. A deficiency of this protein is characteristic of hereditary angioedema. Some patients demonstrate catalytically inactive protein.

C1q: Evaluates the complement component C1q in serum. Decreased levels can be demonstrated in patients suffering from hypocomplementemic urticarial vasculitis, severe combined immunodeficiency, or X-linked hypogammaglobulinemia.

C1q Binding: Measures the binding of immune complexes containing IgG$_1$, IgG$_2$, IgG$_3$, and/or IgM to the complement component C1q. High values of C1q bindings are associated with the presence of circulating immune complexes of the type that interact with the classic pathway of complement activation. This test can be useful as a prognostic tool at diagnosis and during remission of acute myelogenous leukemia.

C2: Measures the second component of complement. An extremely low level of C2 component is suggestive of a lupuslike disease that may be caused by a genetic deficiency associated with HLA-A25, B18, or DR2. Approximately half of the individuals with decreased levels of C2 have autoimmune disease; the other half are apparently normal but have an increased susceptibility to bacterial infection.

C3: Measures the third component of complement. Extremely decreased levels are seen in patients with poststreptococcal glomerulonephritis or inherited (C3) complement deficiency. This component is also decreased in cases of severe liver disease and in patients with systemic lupus erythematosus who have renal disease.

C3b Inhibitor (C3b Inactivator): Measures the C3b component of complement. This component causes low complement C3 levels, the absence of C3PA in serum, and high C3b levels. A deficiency of C3b inhibitor is associated with an increased predisposition to infection.

C3PA (C3 Proactivator, Properdin Factor B): Evaluates the level of the factor B component, which is consumed by activation of the alternative complement pathway. Assessment of C3PA indicates whether a decreased level of

C3 is due to the classic or alternate pathways of complement activation. A decreased level of complement components C3 and C4 demonstrates activation of the classic pathway. Decreased levels of C3 and C3PA with a normal level of C4 is indicative of complement activation via the alternative pathway.

Activation of the classic pathway (sometimes with accompanying alternative pathway activation) is associated with disorders such as immune complex diseases, various forms of vasculitis, and acute glomerulonephritis.

Activation of the alternative pathway is associated with many disorders, including chronic hypocomplementemic glomerulonephritis, diffuse intravascular coagulation, septicemia, subacute bacterial endocarditis, paroxysmal nocturnal hemoglobinuria, and sickle cell anemia.

In systemic lupus erythematosus, both the classic and alternative pathways are activated.

C4a: Measures the level of component C4 of the classic complement activation pathway. A decreased C4 level with elevated anti-DNA and ANA titers confirms the diagnosis of systemic lupus erythematosus (SLE) in a patient. In cases of SLE, the periodic assessment of C4 can be useful in monitoring the progress of the disorder. Patients with extremely low C4 and CH50 levels in the presence of normal levels of the C3 component may be demonstrating the effects of a genetic deficiency of C1 inhibitor or C4.

C4 Allotypes: Evaluate the antigenically distinct forms of C4A and C4B, alleles located on the sixth chromosome in the major histocompatibility complex. Identification of C4 allotypes in conjunction with specific HLA antigens is a marker for disease susceptibility.

C5b (C5b-9): Measures the concentration of the C5 complement component. A genetic deficiency of the C5 component is associated with increased susceptibility to bacterial infection and is expressed as an autoimmune disorder (e.g., systemic lupus erythematosus). In the case of dysfunction of C5 (Leiner's disease), the patient is predisposed to infections of the skin and bowel, and the disease is characterized by eczema. In such a patient the level of C5 is normal, but the C5 component fails to promote phagocytosis.

C6: Measures the level of the C6 complement component. A decreased quantity of C6 predisposes an individual to significant *Neisseria* infections.

C7: Measures the quantity of the C7 complement component. A decreased level of this component is associated with severe bacterial infections caused by *Neisseria* species, Raynaud's phenomenon, sclerodactyly, and telangiectasia.

C8: Measures the level of the C8 complement component. A decreased quantity of this component is associated with systemic lupus erythematosus. A deficiency of C8 makes patients highly susceptible to *Neisseria* infections.

CA 125: CA 125 assay is useful in monitoring the response to therapy for patients with epithelial ovarian cancer. Serial testing for patient CA 125 values should be used in conjunction with other clinical methods for monitoring ovarian cancer. Elevations may be observed in patients with nonmalignant disease. A CA 125 assay result should not be interpreted as absolute evidence of the presence or absence of malignant disease.

CA 15-3: CA 15-3 is used to aid in the management of Stage II and III breast cancer patients. Serial testing for patient CA 15-3 assay values should be used in conjunction with other clinical methods for monitoring breast cancer. Patients with confirmed breast carcinoma frequently have CA 15-3 assay values in the same range as healthy individuals, and elevations may be observed in patients with nonmalignant disease. This assay should not be interpreted as absolute evidence of the presence or absence of malignant disease.

CA 19-9: CA 19-9 is useful in monitoring pancreatic, hepatobiliary, gastric, hepatocellular, and colorectal cancer. The CA 19-9 assay value should not be interpreted as absolute evidence of the presence or absence of malignant disease.

CA 27.29: The CA 27.29 assay is intended for use as an aid in monitoring patients previously treated for stage II or III breast cancer. Serial testing in patients who are clinically free of disease should be used in conjunction with other clinical methods used for the early detection of cancer recurrence. The test is also intended for use as an aid in the management of breast cancer patients with metastatic disease by monitoring the progression or regression of disease in response to treatment. Patients with confirmed breast carcinoma frequently have CA 27.29 levels within the reference interval. Elevated levels of CA 27.29 can be observed in patients with nonmalignant diseases. This assay cannot be interpreted as absolute evidence of the presence or absence of malignant disease and should always be used in conjunction with other diagnostic procedures, including information from the patient's clinical evaluation.

Carcinoembryonic Antigen (CEA): Detects the presence of CEA in cerebrospinal fluid (CSF). An increased level of CEA in CSF is very suggestive of primary or secondary intradural malignancy. The level of CEA may decline with effective therapy.

Ceruloplasmin: Detects the level of the protein ceruloplasmin in blood. Although increased or decreased levels of this protein are associated with a variety of clinical conditions, a severe decreased or complete absence of ceruloplasmin can be demonstrated in most homozygous patients suffering from Wilson's disease. The absence or gross deficiency of ceruloplasmin in heterozygous carriers of the gene responsible for Wilson's disease is rare.

Cold Agglutinins: Evaluate the ability of antibodies to agglutinate group O erythrocytes at 4° C. The presence of an elevated titer of cold-reacting antibodies can cause acrocyanosis or hemolysis. These antibodies can be demonstrated in patients with primary (chronic) or secondary cold agglutinin syndromes caused by bacterial or viral disease such as *Mycoplasma pneumoniae* or Epstein-Barr virus, or neoplasms such as lymphoma or histiocytic lymphoma.

Complement-Activation Products: Measure the protein fragments of C3 and C4 to reflect in vivo or in vitro activation. In vivo activation of complement (e.g., immune complex diseases), or in vitro activation (e.g., complement degradation), causes proteolytic digestion of these components and altered electrophoretic mobility. Assessment of these components is not considered to be of reliable diagnostic value.

Complement Components (C1r, C1s, C2, C3, C4, C5, C6, C7, C8): Assess various components of complement. These components are often elevated in certain inflammatory conditions, acute illnesses such as myocardial infarction, trauma, or some infectious diseases such as typhoid fever. Homozygous component deficiencies predispose an individual to autoimmune diseases such as systemic lupus erythematosus, chronic glomerulonephritis, infections, arthritis, and vasculitis. Determination of complement levels in synovial (joint) fluid is of value. Increased levels may be demonstrated in Reiter's syndrome; decreased levels (relative to plasma concentrations) may be observed in rheumatoid arthritis.

Complement Decay Rate: Assesses the decrease of CH_{50} activity in plasma at 37° C. A rate greater than 50% is consistent with, but not diagnostic of, a C1 esterase inhibitor deficiency.

Conglutinin Solid-Phase (Kg Sp) Assay for Immune Complexes: Measures the quantity of immune complexes binding to the protein, conglutinin. If circulating immune complexes, which are capable of activating the classic or alternative complement pathways, are present, large quantities of conglutinin-binding activity are demonstrated. The majority of circulating immune complexes can be detected by combining the Kg SP, C1q binding, Raji cell, and polyethylene glycol assays.

C-Reactive Protein (CRP): Assesses one of the acute-phase inflammatory proteins, C-reactive protein. This protein is increased in inflammatory conditions.

Cryofibrinogen: Evaluates cold precipitable fibrinogen and other similar plasma proteins. The presence of cryofibrinogen suggests primary or secondary disorders. Secondary disorders include acute and chronic inflammation, lymphoproliferative and connective tissue disorders, necrosis, or tumors.

Cryoglobulins: Detect the presence of cold precipitable immunoglobulins (Igs) in serum. The major types of cryoglobulins and associated conditions include the following:

- Monoclonal IgM, IgG, or IgA without known antibody specificity or monoclonal Bence
- Jones protein associated with disorders such as Raynaud's phenomenon, myeloma, and macroglobulinemia.
- Monoclonal IgM, IgG, or IgA antibodies directed against polyclonal IgG associated with disorders such as Sjögren's disease, lymphoproliferative disorders, purpura, vasculitis, and macroglobulinemia.
- Mixed (usually IgM and IgG) polyclonal Igs associated with disorders such as Sjögren's disease, systemic lupus erythematosus, vasculitis, or purpura.

Diphtheria Antibodies: Measure the quantity of antibody present after the administration of diphtheria toxoid. The absence of antibody after immunization confirms a patient's inability to form new antibody (i.e., abnormal humoral immunity).

Ferritin: Evaluates the concentration of the storage form of iron, ferritin, in serum. In conjunction with abnormalities of erythrocyte (e.g., mean corpuscular volume and mean corpuscular hemoglobin), this assay is useful in establishing the diagnosis of iron deficiency anemia.

Histone Antibody: Histone antibodies are the predominant autoantibody in patients suffering from systemic or drug-induced lupus erythematosus (SLE). Histone autoantibodies have been detected in 18% to 53% of patients with SLE and up to 95% of patients with drug-induced SLE. Patients with idiopathic SLE have a variety of other autoantibodies in addition to histone autoantibodies. Histone antibodies of the IgG class have been shown to be SLE specific, whereas IgM antibodies are found in normal healthy people, as well as in some other non-SLE conditions.

Histone-Reactive Antinuclear Antibody (HRANA): Measures the presence of HRANA. A high titer of HRANA is highly suggestive of drug-induced (e.g., hydralazine) lupus erythematosus. HRANA may occasionally be demonstrated in patients with systemic lupus erythematosus.

HLA-B27: Assesses one of the human leukocyte antigens (HLA) on the surface of lymphocytes. Detection of HLA-B27 is useful in establishing the diagnosis of ankylosing spondylitis (AS). The majority of white patients with AS are antigen positive, and about half of black patients with AS are antigen positive.

HLA-DR: Assesses one of the human leukocyte antigens (HLA) on the surface of lymphocytes. Detection of HLA-DR is useful in predicting a person's susceptibility to disease and in estimating adverse reactions to certain drugs (e.g., hydralazine).

Identification of combinations of HLA alleles at various loci, such as HLA-A, B, C, and DR antigens, together with the inheritance of allotypes of C4 and allelic forms of C2 and properdin factor B (referred to as supratypes), is becoming a useful tool in diagnosing immunoregulatory abnormalities, as well as different types of clinical diseases and susceptibility to infection.

HLA-DR3: Evaluates one of the human leukocyte antigens (HLA) on the surface of lymphocytes. Detection of HLA-DR3 and an elevated titer of thyroid-stimulating hormone is prognostic for forms of Graves' disease that will not respond or will relapse with antithyroid medication.

Immunoglobulins: Measure the total immunoglobulin concentration in the serum. Increased concentration is representative of hyperglobulinemia. A major decrease in concentration, immunodeficiency, causes recurrent infections, atypical arthritis, or persistent diarrhea.

Immunoglobulin A (IgA): Quantitates the concentration of immunoglobulin A (IgA). Normal concentrations rule out agammaglobulinemias in childhood and selective IgA deficiency. Selective deficiencies of IgA are the most common type of immunodeficiency.

Immunoglobulin D (IgD): Quantitates the concentration of immunoglobulin D (IgD). It is found in very low concentrations in serum, and its functional role is not well characterized.

Immunoglobulin E (IgE): Measures immunoglobulin E (IgE). Markedly increased values can be found in patients with immunodeficient states, especially cell-mediated immunodeficiency and atopic eczema; systemic fungal infections such as allergic bronchopulmonary aspergillosis; and invasive parasitic infections.

Immunoglobulin G (IgG): Quantitates the concentration of the immunoglobulin G (IgG). It is the major antibacterial, antifungal, and antiviral antibody. A severe deficiency is manifested by repeated infections.

Immunoglobulin G (IgG) Index: Compares the relative ratio of IgG to albumin in serum and cerebrospinal fluid. If the IgG index is increased (<0.7) and the IgG synthesis rate is increased in a specimen without oligoclonal Igs, the possibility exists that plasma contamination is present because of a leaky blood-brain barrier or a traumatic spinal tap.

Immunoglobulin G (IgG) Rheumatoid Factors: Measure the quantity of IgG antibodies reacting with human IgG. The role of IgG rheumatoid factor is considered of major pathogenic importance in rheumatoid arthritis.

Immunoglobulin G (IgG) Subclasses: Quantitate the subclasses IgG_1, IgG_2, IgG_3, and IgG_4 in serum. Increased levels of IgG$_4$ can be demonstrated by patients with allergies who have normal IgE levels. A deficiency of IgG$_4$ can be associated with severe, recurrent sinopulmonary infections, symptomatic IgA deficiency, and common variable immunodeficiency (with pneumonia and/or bronchiectasis). In addition, elevated IgG$_4$ is found in some highly allergic patients with normal IgE concentrations.

Immunoglobulin G (IgG) Synthesis Rate: Measures the rate of IgG synthesis in cerebrospinal fluid. Elevated rates are associated with demyelinating disease. Conditions associated with increased rates include multiple sclerosis, bacterial meningitis, subacute sclerosing panencephalitis, lupus-related central nervous system involvement, presenile dementia (Alzheimer's disorder), IgG synthesizing neoplasms, syphilis, cryptococcosis, chronic relapsing polyneuropathy, and acute cerebrovascular disease. If the Ig synthesis rate and IgG index are elevated, contamination of the specimen with plasma protein should be suspected.

IgM Antibodies (Antigen Specific): Provide identification of antigen-specific IgM antibodies in the presence of antigen-specific IgG and rheumatoid factor. The separation of IgM and IgG antibodies is important in the serodiagnosis of congenital infections.

IgM Rheumatoid Factors: Measure IgM antibodies to human IgG fixed to latex particles. Elevated levels of rheumatoid factor are associated with rheumatoid arthritis, but such elevations may also be seen in other disorders. Increased levels of rheumatoid factors in combination with high levels of C-reactive protein are predictive of aggressive rheumatoid disease. In the case of a negative rheumatoid factor assay, a patient may be diagnosed through clinical signs and symptoms as suffering from seronegative rheumatoid disease.

Jo-1 Antibody: Detects precipitins to an acidic nuclear protein from calf thymus. Approximately one third of patients with uncomplicated polymyositis and some patients with dermatomyositis demonstrate this antibody.

Ku Antibody: Detects precipitins to an acidic nuclear protein from calf thymus. About one half of patients with overlapping signs and symptoms of scleroderma and polymyositis demonstrate Ku precipitins.

Lyme Disease Testing: Current Centers for Disease Control and Prevention recommendations for the serologic diagnosis of Lyme disease are to screen with a polyvalent enzyme-linked immunosorbent assay test and confirm equivocal and positive results with Western blot. Both IgM and IgG Western blots should be performed on samples less than 4 weeks after appearance of erythema migrans. Only IgG Western blot should be performed on samples greater than 4 weeks after the disease onset. IgM Western blot in the chronic stage is not recommended and does not aid in the diagnosis of neuroborreliosis or chronic Lyme disease. Submit requests for appropriate Western blot testing within 10 days.

Lymphocyte Mitogen Stimulation: Measures the rate of DNA synthesis by isolated lymphocytes. Decreased proliferation and DNA synthesis are diagnostic of a defect in cellular immunity. Cellular immunity is frequently defective in immunodeficiency disorders, infectious diseases, carcinoma, and occasionally in autoimmune disorders.

Lymphocyte Typing: Differentiates and measures (using monoclonal antibodies to identify cell surface markers) the quantities of T cells and B cells in the circulating blood.

Useful in distinguishing T and B cell leukemias and lymphomas. Determination of T cell subsets (helper/inducer, suppressor/cytotoxic) is helpful in monitoring treatment in patients with immunodeficiencies such as HIV infection or transplant recipients.

Myelin Basic Protein: Measures the concentration of myelin basic protein in cerebrospinal fluid. Elevated values indicate extensive and active demyelination of the central nervous system. Disorders in which the level of myelin basic protein can be increased include multiple sclerosis, subacute sclerosing panencephalitis, transverse myelitis, and optic neuritis. Increased values can also be observed in conditions producing damage to nervous tissue but in which demyelination is not the primary process (e.g., radiation or chemotherapy of neoplasms in or near the central nervous system).

Oligoclonal Banding/Multiple Sclerosis: Evaluate the presence of abnormal bands of immunoglobulins (Igs) in cerebrospinal fluid (CSF). Abnormal bands of monoclonal Igs are associated with disorders such as multiple sclerosis (MS), subacute sclerosing panencephalitis, paraprotein disorders, and infections.

Oligoclonal bands are present in the CSF of approximately 90% of MS patients. A patient is considered positive for CSF oligoclonal bands if there are two or more bands in the CSF Ig region that are not present in the serum. To confirm local production of oligoclonal IgG in CSF, a matched serum sample is required. Oligoclonal bands present in CSF, but not in serum, indicate central nervous system production.

Oligoclonal bands and elevated levels of CSF IgG may be present in other disease states, including meningoencephalitis, neurosyphilis, Guillain-Barré syndrome, and meningeal carcinomatosis. Up to 10% of patients with clinically supported MS are negative for oligoclonal bands.

Platelet-Associated IgG (PAIgG): Detects IgG found on the surface of platelets after thorough washing. Elevated levels of PAIgG with inversely proportional platelet counts are found in patients with immune thrombocytopenic purpura. Increased values can also be found in patients suffering from systemic lupus erythematosus.

Platelet Antibody: Evaluates the quantity of platelets with immunologically attached IgG by the use of fluorescein-tagged antihuman immunoglobulin (Ig) specific for the Fc portion IgG. Antibodies can be demonstrated by this indirect test in less than half of patients with immune thrombocytopenia and the majority (82%) of patients with systemic lupus erythematosus.

PM-1 Antibody: Detects antibodies to an acidic nuclear protein from calf thymus. These precipitins are found in the majority (87%) of patients with polymyositis scleroderma. More than half the patients suffering from polymyositis demonstrate the antibody, but the antibody is detected in less than one fifth of patients with dermatomyositis.

Prostate Specific Antigen (PSA): PSA is a laboratory method approved for use as an aid in the detection of prostate cancer when used in conjunction with a digital rectal examination in men age 50 years and older. Serial measurement of PSA can be of value in the prognosis and management of patients with prostate cancer. Elevated PSA concentrations can only suggest the presence of prostate cancer until biopsy is performed. PSA concentrations can also be elevated in benign prostatic hyperplasia or inflammatory conditions of the prostate. PSA is generally not elevated in healthy men or men with nonprostatic carcinoma.

Raji Cell Assay: Measures the binding of immune complexes to complement receptors on a lymphoblastoid cell line, Raji cells.

Rheumatoid Factor (RF): RF may be found in patients with a variety of autoimmune diseases, as well as in up to 10% of apparently healthy individuals. RF assays may be positive in some patients with syphilis, viral infections, chronic liver diseases, sarcoidosis, leprosy, neoplasms, and a variety of other chronic inflammatory conditions. High concentrations of RF are found in patients with rheumatoid arthritis and Sjögren's syndrome. Juvenile onset rheumatoid arthritis is seldom associated with a positive test for RF. The RF test should be used with caution in the diagnosis of rheumatoid arthritis because of the low predictive value of the test for this disease. The percentage of positive RF assays in the normal population increases with age.

Skin Testing: Evaluates delayed hypersensitivity reactivity. The inability to respond to an antigenic challenge strongly suggests that cell-mediated immunity is depressed.

Streptolysin O Antibody (ASO): In the past, the streptolysin O antibody (ASO) test was routinely used to provide serologic evidence of previous group A streptococcal infection in patients suspected of having complications (e.g., acute glomerulonephritis or acute rheumatic fever). Use of the ASO for diagnosis of an acute group A streptococcal infection is rarely indicated today unless the patient has received antibiotics that would render a culture negative.

An ASO performed on serum obtained during the presentation of a nonsuppurative complication that shows a titer two dilutions above the upper limit of normal is evidence for an antecedent streptococcal infection. It is recommended, however, to use a second test (e.g., anti-DNase B) to confirm antecedent infections. Elevated serum ASO titers are found in about 85% of individuals with rheumatic fever. When both ASO and anti-DNase B are used, the result is more than 95%.

Tetanus Antibody: Measures antibody to tetanus toxoid. If a patient has a history of immunization and antibodies are not demonstrable, abnormal humoral immunity is suspected.

Thyroid Peroxidase (TPO) Antibody: The thyroid microsomal antigen has been shown to be the enzyme thyroid peroxidase (TPO).

The measurement of low levels of TPO antibodies in serum can be useful in the assessment of a number of thyroid disorders. More than 90% of patients with autoimmune thyroiditis (Hashimoto's thyroiditis) have thyroglobulin or TPO antibodies. Although the detection of TPO antibodies is not diagnostic, it can aid in predicting the progression of chronic thyroiditis and in further substantiating thyroid disease in patients with nonthyroidal illness.

Antibodies to TPO have also been found in most patients with idiopathic hypothyroidism (85%) and Graves' disease (50%) and less frequently in patients with other thyroid disorders. Low titers may also be found in 5% to 10% of normal individuals.

BIBLIOGRAPHY

ARUP's guide to clinical laboratory testing, Salt Lake City, October 2002, ARUP Laboratories,website: www.arup.com.

Specialty Laboratories Test Menu, Santa Monica, Calif, October 2002, website: www.specialtylabs.com.

Glossary

A   The nucleotide adenine.

abruptio placentae   The premature separation of a normally situated placenta.

acquired   Incurred because of external factors; not inherited.

acquired immunity   (*see* adaptive immunity)

acquired immunodeficiency syndrome (AIDS)   An immune disorder affecting T4 lymphocytes. This disorder is caused by the human immunodeficiency virus (HIV), which was previously called human T-lymphotropic retrovirus (HTLV) or LAV virus.

acquired or secondary immunodeficiency   A defect in the normal immune response caused by external factors or an existing disease or condition.

activated partial thromboplastin time (aPTT)   A coagulation procedure to detect factors that are active in the external mechanism (stage I) of blood coagulation.

active immunity   The form of immunity produced by the body in response to stimulation by a disease-causing organism (naturally acquired active immunity) or by a vaccine (artificially acquired active immunity).

acute   A condition of sudden and short duration.

acute glomerulonephritis   A sudden inflammation of the small convoluted mass of capillaries of the kidney, primarily the capsule.

acute-phase proteins (acute-phase reactants)   A group of glycoproteins associated with nonspecific inflammation of body tissues.

adaptive immunity   The augmentation of body defense mechanisms in response to a specific stimulus, which can cause the elimination of microorganisms and recovery from disease. This response frequently leaves the host with specific memory (acquired resistance), which enables the body to respond effectively if reinfection with the same microorganism occurs.

adenocarcinoma   A malignant new growth derived from glandular tissue or from recognizable glandular structures.

adenopathy   Swelling or enlargement of the lymph nodes.

adrenal medulla   The inner core of the small endocrine gland that rests on top of each kidney.

afferent lymphatic duct   The vessel that carries transparent liquid and antigens into the lymph node.

affinity   Propensity; the bond between a single antigenic determinant and an individual combining site.

agammaglobulinemia   The absence of plasma gammaglobulin because of either a congenital or acquired condition.

agglutination   The clumping or aggregation of particles that have antigens on their surface (e.g., erythrocytes) by antibody molecules that form bridges between the antigenic determinants.

agglutinin   The older term for antibody.

agglutinogen   The older term for antigen.

aggregation   (*see* agglutination)

allele   One or more genes that occur at the same locus on homologous chromosomes.

allergic rhinitis   Inflammation of the mucous membrane of the nose caused by a hypersensitivity reaction to environmental substances such as pollen or mold.

alloantibodies   Immunoglobulins (antibodies) produced in response to exposure of foreign antigens of the same species.

allogenic   Genetically different individuals of the same species.

allograft   A graft of tissue from a genetically different member of the same species (e.g., human kidney).

alopecia   Loss of hair; baldness.

alveolar   The thin-walled chambers of the lungs are referred to as *pulmonary alveoli.*

amniocentesis   The process of removing fluid from the amniotic sac for study (e.g., biochemical analysis).

amplicon   A DNA fragment produced by amplification of a specific DNA sequence.

amplification   A process to produce multiple copies of a specific DNA sequence.

amyloidosis   A condition of intercellular deposition of an abnormal protein with a waxy, translucent appearance in various tissues.

anaerobic metabolism   (Also referred to as the Embden-Meyerhof glycolytic pathway or the TCA cycle.) It is the major, non-oxygen–associated, energy-yielding pathway connected with the breakdown of glucose (glycolysis) in body cells.

anamnestic antibody response   An antibody "memory" response. This secondary type of response occurs on subsequent exposure to a previously encountered and recognized foreign antigen and is characterized by the rapid production of IgG antibodies.

anaphylactic reaction   A severe allergic reaction that can develop in IgA-deficient patients who have developed anti-IgA antibodies.

anaphylactic shock   A severe allergic reaction.

anaphylactoid reaction   A severe reaction to soluble constituents in donor plasma that produces edema.

anaphylatoxins   The complement components, C3a and C5a, which stimulate release by mast cells of their vasoactive amines.

anaphylaxis   An immediate (type I) hypersensitivity reaction characterized by local reactions such as urticaria (hives) and angioedema (redness and swelling) or by systemic reactions in the respiratory tract, cardiovascular system, gastrointestinal tract, and skin.

angioedema   Redness and swelling.

anicteric   Without icterus or lacking a yellow discoloration of the skin and sclera.

anneal   The bonding or hybridization of two complementary nucleic acid strands to one another.

anomalies   Marked deviations from normal.

anorexia nervosa   An eating disorder prevalent in adolescent females.

antenatal   Before birth.

antibodies (antibody)   Specific glycoproteins (immunoglobulins) produced in response to an antigenic challenge. Antibodies can be found in blood plasma and body fluids (e.g., tears, saliva, milk). These serum globulins have a wide range of specificities for different antigens and can bind to and neutralize bacterial toxins or bind to the surfaces of bacteria, viruses, or parasites.

antibody affinity   (*see* affinity)

antibody-dependent cell-mediated cytotoxicity reaction (ADCC)   A cellular activity exhibited by both K cells and phagocytic and nonphagocytic myelogenous-type leukocytes. The target cell in ADCC is coated with a low concentration of IgG antibody.

antibody-mediated immunity   (*see* humoral immunity)

antibody titer   (*see* titer)

anticore window   The period of time in which antigen cannot be detected in the circulating blood, such as in hepatitis B testing.

antigen (immunogen)   A foreign substance that can stimulate the production of antibodies (immune response).

antigenic determinant(s)   The combining site or sites with which antibodies react.

antigenicity   The ability of an antigen to stimulate an immune response.

antineutrophil antibody   An autoantibody divided into either antineutrophil cytoplasmic antibody (c-ANCA) or antibody producing a perinuclear staining of ethanol-fixed neutrophils (p-ANCA).

antistreptolysin O antibody (ASO)   An antibody produced against streptolysin O, a hemolysin produced by streptococci, particularly group A.

aplastic anemia   A deficiency of blood cells such as erythrocytes caused by the lack of cell production (hematopoiesis) in the bone marrow. This form of anemia may result from exposure to toxic chemicals or drugs such as chloramphenicol.

artherosclerotic   (Also referred to as *arteriosclerosis.*) This is a condition of loss of elasticity (hardening) of the walls of the blood vessels (e.g., arteries).

arthralgia   Pain in a joint.

arthritis   Inflammation of a joint.

arthropathy   Joint disease.

aseptic technique   Handling of materials or specimens without the introduction of extraneous microorganisms.

ASO   (*see* antistreptolysin O antibody)

asthma   A respiratory condition characterized by recurrent attacks of dyspnea (difficult or painful breathing) and wheezing caused by spasmodic constriction of the bronchi (larger air passages to or within the lungs).

astrocyte   A nerve cell characterized by fibrous or protoplasmic processes. Collectively these cells are called macroglia or astroglia tissue.

asymptomatic   Exhibiting no symptoms of a disease or disorder.

ataxia   Irregularity of muscular action or faulty muscular coordination.

atopic eczema   Inflammation of the epidermis (skin) characterized by redness, itching, and weeping, which is caused by a hypersensitivity reaction.

atrophy   Wasting or lack of growth of tissues or organs.

autoantibody   An immunoglobulin produced against a self-antigen.

autoimmune hemolytic anemia   A condition of destruction of erythrocytes by antibodies to self-antigens.

autoimmunity   A condition in which the body's own antigenic structures stimulate an immune response and react with self-antigens in a manner similar to the destruction of foreign antigens. This process may cause autoimmune disease.

autologous   A synonym for *self* or part of the same individual.

autonomic nervous system   The branch of the nervous system that functions without conscious control.

autosomal dominant gene   A genetic trait that expresses itself, if present, and is carried on one of the 1 through 22 pairs of (autosomal) chromosomes.

autosomal recessive gene   A genetic trait carried on one of the 1 through 22 pairs of chromosomes that is expressed only if present in a homozygous state.

avascular necrosis   The death of nonvascular cells or tissues.

avidity   The strength with which a multivalent antibody binds to a multivalent antigen.

B cell-growth factor-2   (*see* interleukin-5 [IL-5])

B cell-stimulating factor-2   (*see* interleukin-4 [IL-4])

B cell-stimulating factor-2   (*see* interleukin-6 [IL-6])

B lymphocyte   A lymphocyte subset type that secretes antibody, the humoral element of adaptive immunity.

bacteremia   An infection of the blood caused by bacterial microorganisms.

bare lymphocyte syndrome   An infrequent cause of severe combined immunodeficiency (SCID).

base pair   A nucleotide (either adenine, guanine, cytosine, thymidine, or uracil) and its complementary base on the opposite strand.

Bence Jones (BJ) protein   The abnormal protein frequently found in the urine of patients with multiple myeloma. It precipitates at 50° C, disappears at 100° C, and reappears on cooling to room temperature.

benign   Nonmalignant or noncancerous.

bilirubin   A breakdown product of erythrocyte catabolism. If increased levels of this substance accumulate in the circulation, it will be deposited in lipid-rich tissues such as the brain and will be manifested by the skin and sclera as jaundice/icterus.

blast transformation   The conversion of a B lymphocyte into a plasma cell.

blotting   Transfer or fixation of nucleic acids onto a solid matrix (e.g., nitrocellulose) so that the nucleic acids may be hybridized with a probe.

bond   Physiochemical forces that hold atoms together to form molecules.

bone marrow   The structure that contains hematopoietic (blood-forming) tissues.

Burkitt's lymphoma   An undifferentiated malignant neoplastic disorder of the lymphoid tissues.

bursa of Fabricius   An outgrowth of the cloaca in birds that becomes the site of formation of lymphocytes with B-cell characteristics.

C   The nucleotide, cytosine.

C3   The most abundant and important component of complement that produces a small (C3a) and a large peptide (C3b) when activated.

C5 The complement component split by C3b into C5a and C5b.

C6789 The lytic complement sequence that is activated by C5b and terminates in lysing the cell membrane.

carrier state The asymptomatic condition of harboring an infectious organism. The term may also refer to a heterozygous individual or the carrier of a recessive gene.

catarrhal symptoms An older term used to describe the manifestations of inflammation of the mucous membranes, particularly of the head or throat, with an accompanying discharge.

catecholamines Biologically active amines, including epinephrine and norepinephrine, that have a marked effect on the nervous and cardiovascular systems, metabolic rate and temperature, and smooth muscle.

CD4 The protein receptor on the surface of a target cell to which the gp 120 protein of the HIV viral envelope binds.

cDNA Complementary DNA, produced from mRNA using reverse transcriptase.

cell-mediated immunity The type of immunity dependent on the link between T cells and macrophages.

cellulitis Inflammation within solid tissues, usually loose tissues beneath the skin, that is manifested by redness, pain, swelling (edema), and interference with function.

centromere The constricted portion of a chromosome.

cerebrospinal fluid (CSF) The fluid formed by the choroid plexus in the ventricles of the brain and found within the subarachnoid space, the central canal of the spinal cord, and the four ventricles of the brain.

cerebrovascular accident Stroke.

C$_H$ Constant region of the immunoglobulin heavy chain gene locus.

chancre A lesion that begins as a papule and erodes into a red ulcer. It is the primary wound of syphilis that occurs at the site of entry of the spirochete.

Chédiak-Higashi syndrome A rare inherited autosomal recessive trait characterized by the presence of large granules and inclusion bodies in the cytoplasm of leukocytes.

chemiluminescence Luminescence in which the light emission is caused by the products of a specific chemical reaction.

chemotactic factor (*see* interleukin-8 [IL-8])

chemotaxis The release of substances that attract phagocytic cells as the result of traumatic or microbial damage.

cholestasis The blockage or suppression of the flow of bile.

choreoathetosis A condition characterized by rapid, jerky, involuntary movements or slow, irregular, twisting, snakelike movements seen mostly in the upper extremities (e.g., hands and fingers).

chorioretinitis Inflammation of the choroid (the middle layer) and the retina (the innermost layer) of the eye.

chronic A condition of long duration.

chronic glomerulonephritis An inflammation of long duration of the small convoluted mass of capillaries of the kidney, primarily the capsule.

circulating immune complex An antigen-antibody in the blood flow.

clone Cells descended from the same single cell (daughter cells), all having identical phenotypes and growth characteristics as the original precursor cell.

coagglutination (CoA) This technique is similar to latex agglutination for detecting antigen. Protein A, a uniformly distributed cell wall component of *Staphylococcus aureus*, is able to bind to the Fc region of most IgG isotype antibodies leaving the Fab region free to interact with antigens present in the applied specimens. Visible agglutination of the coated particles indicated an antigen-antibody reaction.

coalesce A fusion of components.

collagen A protein found in skin, tendons, bone, and cartilage.

collagen disease Diseases of the skin, tendons, bone, and cartilage, such as systemic lupus erythematosus and rheumatoid arthritis.

collecting tubule A small duct that receives urine from several renal tubules.

colony-stimulating factors Molecular substances that stimulate hematopoietic progenitor cells to form colonies.

combining site The portion of the Fab molecule that possesses specificity.

common immunocyte Any cell of the lymphoid series that can react with an antigen to produce an antibody or participate in cell-mediated reactions.

common thymocyte Lymphocytes arising in the thymus that precede mature (OKT 10, OKT6 surface antigen) thymocytes in development.

complement A group of proteins (enzymes) present in the blood that can produce inflammatory effects and lysis of cells when activated. Some bacteria activate complement directly, whereas others only do so with the help of antibody. If this cascading sequence of proteins is activated directly, it follows the alternate pathway; if it is activated by antigen-antibody interaction, it follows the classic pathway.

complement cascade The sequential activation of plasma proteins that cause lysis of a cell.

complement fixation This older procedure detects the presence of a specific antigen-antibody reaction by causing the in vitro activation of complement. If complement is not fixed, lysis of the preantibody-coated reagent erythrocytes occurs.

complete antibody An older term for an IgM antibody.

congenital rubella syndrome (*see* rubella syndrome)

conjugate A laboratory substrate prepared by joining two substances, such as fluorescein to an immunoglobulin molecule.

conjugate vaccine A vaccine in which easily recognizable proteins are linked to the outer coat of the disease-causing organism to stimulate an immune response.

convalescence period The time of recovery from conditions such as illness, injury, or surgery.

Coombs' test The older term for the anti-human globulin test.

cooperativity Interaction of specific cellular elements (lymphocytes), cell products (immunoglobulins and cytokines), and nonlymphoid elements.

cortical-hypothalamic-pituitary axis The interrelated association between the outer layer of the brain, the structure located at the base of the cerebrum, and a small endocrine gland.

corticosteroid Any of the hormones produced by the outer layer of the gland located on top of each kidney.

cosmopolitan distribution   Widely distributed.

counterimmunoelectrophoresis (CIE)   A procedure in which oppositely charged antigen and antibody are propelled toward each other by an electrical field. Using this technique, detection of concentrations of antigens and antibodies 10 times smaller than the lowest concentrations measurable by immunodiffusion or double diffusion can be made.

cranial nerve neuritis   An inflammation of any of the nerves that are attached to the brain and pass through the openings of the skull.

C-reactive protein   A nonspecific, acute-phase reactant glycoprotein.

cross-reactivity   A condition in which some of the determinants of an antigen are shared by similar antigenic determinants on the surface of apparently unrelated molecules and a proportion of these antigens interact with the other kind of antigen.

cryoglobulin   An abnormal protein that precipitates at cold temperatures but redissolves at warm temperatures.

cryptogenic cirrhosis   A condition of the liver with an obscure or doubtful cause.

CSF   (*see* colony-stimulating factors)

cutaneous   Refers to the skin (epidermis).

cutaneous T-cell lymphoma   A malignant neoplasm with epidermal manifestations that involves the T subset of lymphocytes.

cytokines   Polypeptide products of activated cells (lymphocytes or macrophages) that control a variety of cellular responses and thereby regulate the immune system.

cytomegalovirus   A herpes-family virus that can cause congenital infections in the newborn and a clinical syndrome resembling infectious mononucleosis.

cytopenia   A severe decrease in hematologic cells.

cytotoxic T cell   A subset type of lymphocyte that can kill other cells infected by viruses, fungi or some types of bacteria, or cells transformed by malignancy.

cytotoxicity   A condition in which macrophages can kill some targets (possibly tumor cells) without phagocytizing them.

Dane particle   The intact, double-shelled hepatitis B virus.

DAT   (*see* direct antiglobulin test)

Davidsohn differential test   The classic laboratory reference test for the diagnosis of infectious mononucleosis.

delta agent   An RNA virus that causes hepatitis but requires the coexistence of hepatitis B infection.

dementia   An irreversible condition of organic loss of mental function.

denaturation   The process of heating and separating two DNA strands.

denatured DNA   Double-stranded helix separates into two single strands. Hydrogen bonds break from heat, pH, nonphysiologic concentration of salts, organic solvents (e.g., alcohol), or detergents.

dendritic cells   The weekly phagocyte Langerhans' cell of the epidermis, and similar, nonphagocytic cells in the lymphoid follicles of the spleen and lymph nodes. These cells may be the main agent of T-cell stimulation, but the precise region of these dendritic cells is not yet certain.

deoxyribonucleic acid (DNA)   The nucleic acid that forms the main structure of the genes.

dermatomyositis   An inflammatory condition included in the collage disorders in which the skin, subcutaneous tissues, and muscles are involved. Necrosis of the muscles is characteristic.

D$_H$ Diversity region of the immunoglobulin heavy-chain gene locus.

diagnosis   Determination of the nature of a disorder or disease.

diapedesis   Ameboid movement of cells.

direct agglutination   A general term in which macroscopic clumping can be observed because particulate reagents are used as an indicator of the presence of an antigen-antibody reaction.

direct antiglobulin test   A test performed to detect the coating of erythrocytes with antibodies.

direct fluorescent antibody   This procedure uses direct detection of antigens using fluorescent labeled antigen-specific antibody.

discoid lupus   The term used to differentiate the benign dermatitis of cutaneous lupus from the cutaneous involvement of systemic lupus erythematosus (SLE).

disease   A pathologic condition characterized by a specific and unique set of signs and symptoms.

disorder   An abnormality of body function.

distal tubules   Ducts in the kidney located farthest from the center of the structure.

DNA amplification   An ultrasensitive polymerase chain reaction technique for the detection of HIV-1 that amplifies minute amounts of viral nucleic acid in the DNA of lymphocytes.

DNA "dot-blot" hybridization   The rapid molecular biology technique used to detect the presence of a specific DNA in a specimen.

domain   The basic unit of an antibody structure. Variations between the domains of different antibody molecules are responsible for differences in antigen binding and in biological function.

dot blot   A technique used to determine whether a particular nucleotide sequence is present in a patient's specimen.

downstream   Toward the 3′ end of a nucleic acid molecule.

dsDNA   Double-stranded DNA.

D^u   Now referred to as weak D, a phenotype of the Rh blood group system.

D^u Rosette Test   A procedure that uses D-positive indicator erythrocytes to form identifiable rosettes around individual D-positive fetal cells that may be in the maternal circulation.

dysplastic   Faulty or abnormal development of body tissue.

dyspnea   Difficulty in breathing.

dysproteinemia   An abnormality of the protein content of the blood.

early antigen (EA)   A "new" antigen expressed by B lymphocytes infected with Epstein-Barr virus in infectious mononucleosis. EA consists of early antigen-diffuse (EA-D), which is found in both the nucleus and cytoplasm of B cells, and early antigen-restricted (EA-R), which is usually found as a mass only in the cytoplasm.

early thymocyte   Immature T cell in the thymus that precedes the common thymocyte in maturational development.

electrophoresis   A method for separating macromolecules on the basis of net electrical charge and size.

ectopic pregnancy   The gestation of a fertilized egg outside of the uterus, most commonly in the fallopian tube.

eczema   An inflammatory condition of the skin (epidermis) characterized by redness, weeping, and itching.

edema (edematous)   Accumulation of fluid in the tissues that produces swelling.

EDTA   Ethylenediamine tetraacetic acid, disodium salt. A common in vitro anticoagulant.

efferent lymphatic duct   The tubule through which semitransparent fluid (lymph) and possible antigens exit the lymph node.

efficacy   The ability of a vaccine to produce the desired clinical effect at the optimal dosage and schedule.

electrophoresis   (*see* serum electrophoresis)

ELISA   (*see* enzyme-linked immunosorbent assay)

eluate   The product of purposely manipulating a red cell suspension to break an antigen-antibody complex, with the subsequent release of the antibody into the surrounding medium.

embryogenesis   The growth and development of a living organism. In humans, this period is from the second to approximately the eighth week of gestation.

encephalopathy   Any degenerative disease of the brain.

endemic   Present at all times, such as the continual existence of a specific microorganism in a population of individuals or in a geographic location.

endocarditis   An inflammation of the inner lining of the heart (endocardium).

endothelial cell   The type of epithelial cell that lines body cavities such as the serous cavities, heart, and blood and lymphatic vessels.

endotoxemia   A condition of having bacterial cell wall heat-stable toxins in the circulation. These toxins are pyrogenic and increase capillary permeability.

end-stage renal disease   An irreversible, pathologic condition of the kidneys.

enterocolitis   An inflammation of the small intestine and colon.

env gene   A gene of a retrovirus such as HIV that encodes for a polyprotein that contains numerous glycosylation sites.

enzyme immunoassay (EIA)   (Also called ELISA.) A general term for quantitative testing of both antigens and antibodies. The method uses color-changed products of enzyme-substrate interaction or inhibition to measure the antigen-antibody reactions.

enzyme-linked immunosorbent assays (ELISA)   A quantitative method of laboratory analysis. Either antigen or antibody can be measured using enzyme-labeled antibody or antigen bound to a solid support. Direct ELISA is a technique for measuring antigen using competition for antibody-binding sites between enzyme-labeled antigen and patient antigen. Indirect ELISA measures antibody concentrations using bound antigen to interact with specimen antibodies.

epidemiology (epidemiologic)   Pertains to the study of infectious disease or conditions in many individuals in the same geographic location at the same time.

epilepsy   A transient disturbance of nervous system function caused by abnormal electrical activity in the brain.

episomal DNA   An accessory, extrachromosomal-replicating genetic element.

epithelial cell   Cell of a type of body tissue that forms the covering of external and internal surfaces or composes a body structure, such as glandular epithelium.

epitope   A single antigenic determinant. It is functionally the portion of an antigen that combines with an antibody paratope (the part of the antibody molecule that makes contact with the antigenic determinant).

Epstein-Barr virus   A human herpes DNA virus found in association with leukocytes and B lymphocytes. It is the causative agent of infectious mononucleosis in Western countries and Burkitt's lymphoma in Africa.

erysipelas   A febrile disease caused by group A streptococci. The disease is manifested by inflammation and redness of the skin and subcutaneous tissues and by fever, vomiting, or headache.

erythema   Redness of the skin caused by inflammation, infection, or injury.

erythematosus   characterized by erythema (*see* erythema).

erythrocyte   The scientific term for a red blood cell.

erythropoiesis   The process of producing red blood cells.

estrogen   The term for the female sex hormones including estradiol, estriol, and estrone.

etiology   A synonym for the study of or the cause(s) of disease.

exchange transfusion   The replacement of an infant's coated erythrocytes with donor blood until a one or two total blood volume transfer is accomplished.

extramedullary hematopoiesis   Production of erythrocytes outside the bone marrow, which can produce enlargement of the liver and spleen.

extravascular destruction   The destruction of an erythrocyte through phagocytosis and digestion by macrophages of the mononuclear-phagocytic system.

extravascular hemolysis   The phagocytizing and catabolizing of erythrocytes by the mononuclear-phagocytic system.

Fab fragments   Two of the three fragments formed if a typical monomeric IgG is digested with a proteolytic enzyme such as papain. These fragments retain the ability to bind antigen and are called the antigen-binding fragments.

Fc portion   The third fragment formed in addition to the two Fab fragments if a typical monomeric IgG is digested with a proteolytic enzyme such as papain. This fragment is relatively homogenous and sometimes crystallizable.

Fc receptor   The portion of an antibody responsible for binding to antibody receptors on cells and the C1q component of complement.

Fd fragment   The fragment consisting of a light chain and half of a heavy chain if the interchain disulfide bonds in the Fab fragment are disrupted.

febrile agglutinin   Antibodies demonstrated in microbial diseases that are manifested by a high fever.

febrile disease   A pathologic process in which an extremely high fever is a characteristic manifestation.

femur   The bone of the leg that extends from the pelvic girdle to the knee (the thigh bone).

fibrin   A meshy protein clot formed by the action of thrombin on fibrinogen.

fibroblast   An immature fiber-producing cell of connective tissue capable of differentiating into a cartilage-forming cell (chondroblast), a collagen-forming cell (collagenoblast), or a bone-forming cell (osteoblast).

fimbriae   Fringed or fingerlike.

floccculation   The clumping together of particles to form visible masses.

flow cytometry   Computerized equipment is used for the separation, classification, and quantitation of particles (e.g., blood cells or antibodies). The technique is based on the passing of a monocellular stream for particles through a beam of laser light. The particles are categorized by size and then analyzed. Monoclonal antibodies can be used for the determination of specific subsets of cells.

Fluorescent antibody (FA) assay   This is a general term used to describe procedures that use the visual detection of fluorescent dyes coupled (conjugated) to antibodies that react with the antigen when present using fluorescent microscopy.

Forssman antibody   A heterophil type of immunoglobulin that is stimulated by one antigen and reacts with an entirely unrelated surface antigen present on cells from different mammalian species. It can be absorbed from human serum by guinea pig kidney cells.

Franklin's disease   A dysproteinemia that is synonymous with gamma heavy-chain disease. This abnormality is characterized by the presence of monoclonal protein composed of the heavy-chain portion of the immunoglobulin molecule.

fulminant   To occur suddenly with great intensity, such as lightninglike flashes of pain.

G   The nucleotide, guanine.

gag gene   A gene of a retrovirus such as HIV that encodes for the major core structural protein.

GALT   (*see* gut-associated lymphoid tissue)

gamma heavy-chain disease   (*see* Franklin's disease)

gastroenteritis   An inflammation of the lining of the stomach and intestine.

genitalia   The female and male reproductive organs and associated external structures such as the penis.

gene cloning   A method for producing quantities of a specific DNA sequence.

genome   The complete set of hereditary factors contained in the haploid set of chromosomes; the complete set of chromosomes contributed by one of the male-female pair.

gestation   The period of development and growth of the unborn in viviparous animals (e.g., humans), from fertilization of the ovum to birth.

giant cell; epithelioid cell   Macrophage-derived cells typically found at sites of chronic inflammation. A giant multinucleated cell is formed by the coalescing of cells into a solid mass, or granuloma.

giardiasis   A parasitic infection associated with the unicellular *Giardia* species.

glial cell   Also known as neuroglial cell. It is the non-nervous or supportive tissue of the brain and spinal cord known to produce minute amounts of CD4 or an alternate receptor molecule, which allows it to be infected with HIV virus.

glomerulonephritis   (*see* acute glomerulonephritis or chronic glomerulonephritis)

glomerulus (pl. glomeruli)   The small structure in the malpighian body of the kidney composed of a cluster of capillary blood vessels in a cluster and enveloped in a thin wall.

goodness of fit   The complementary matching of antigenic determinants and the antigen-binding sites of corresponding antibodies that influences the strength of bonding between antigens and antibodies.

grafting   The transfer of cells or organs from one individual to another or from one site to another in the same individual.

graft-versus-host disease   An intense and frequently fatal immunologic reaction of engrafted cells against the host caused by the infusion of immunocompetent lymphocytes into individuals with impaired immunity.

grand mal seizures   A major epileptic attack with or without loss of consciousness.

granulocyte   A type of leukocytic white blood cell.

granuloma   A macrophage-derived lesion containing sequestered noxious agents such as foreign bodies, some types of bacteria, and others that cannot be eliminated.

granulomatous lesion   A wound composed of granuloma.

Guillain-Barré syndrome   A relatively rare disease of the nerves. Also called acute idiopathic polyneuritis.

gummas   A granuloma that may result from delayed hypersensitivity. It is the soft tumor of the tissues characteristic of the tertiary stage of syphilis.

gut-associated lymphoid tissue (GALT)   The GALT and bone marrow may play a role in the differentiation of stem cells into B lymphocytes; functions as the bursal equivalent in humans.

haptene(s)   Very small molecules that can bind to a larger carrier molecule and behave as an antigen.

helper/inducer subset   (Also referred to as T_4.) A major phenotypic lymphocyte subset of T lymphocytes.

hemagglutination   A laboratory technique for the detection of antibodies that involves the agglutination of red blood cells.

hemagglutination inhibition technique (HAI)   A laboratory technique for detecting antibodies that involves the blocking of agglutination of red blood cells.

hematopoicsis (hematopoietic tissues)   Blood-producing structures of the body such as the liver, spleen, and bone marrow.

hemodynamic shock   A physiologic condition such as decreased blood pressure, resulting from the rapid loss of 15% to 20% or more of blood volume.

hemoflagellate   A protozoan parasite found in the blood and/or body tissues.

hemolysin   A substance such as streptolysin O and streptolysin S produced by most group A strains of streptococci that disrupts the membrane integrity of red blood cells, causing the release of hemoglobin.

hemolysis   The rupturing of the cell membrane (e.g., an erythrocyte), with the subsequent dumping of cytoplasmic contents.

hemolytic anemia   A severe decrease in circulating erythrocytes and associated findings caused by the rupturing of circulating erythrocytes.

hemolytic disease of the newborn   (previously referred to as *erythroblastosis fetalis*). An immunologic incompatibility between mother and fetus that can produce severe or fatal consequences in the unborn or newborn because of destruction of erythrocytes and the accumulation of breakdown products.

hemolyzed   Ruptured erythrocytes.

hemoptysis   Coughing and spitting up of blood as the result of bleeding from any part of the respiratory system.

hemostatic   Stoppage of bleeding.

hepatitis   Inflammation of the liver caused by a virus or other agents such as drugs.

hepatomegaly   Excessive enlargement of the liver.

hepatosplenomegaly   An enlarged liver and spleen.

herpes virus   Any of a large group of DNA viruses such as herpes simplex and varicella.

heterogeneous   Different; not originating in the body.

heterosexual disease   A pathologic condition transmitted between individuals of the opposite sex.

heterozygous   The genetic state of having two dissimilar genes for the same trait.

histamine   An amine produced by the catabolism of histidine, which causes dilation of blood vessels.

histiocyte   A large phagocytic interstitial cell of the mononuclear phagocytic system, a macrophage.

histocompatibility (HLA) antigen   Cell surface protein antigen found on blood and body cells (e.g., leukocytes and platelets) that readily provokes an immune response if transferred into a genetically different (allogenic) individual of the same species.

histone   A simple protein found in combination with acidic substances such as nucleic acids.

Hodgkin's lymphoma or Hodgkin's disease   A major form of malignant lymphoma.

homogeneous   Uniform; the same.

homozygous   In genetics, when the genes for a trait on homologous chromosomes are the same.

HTLV III (human T-lymphotropic retrovirus)   A type of retrovirus also known as LAV or HIV; a causative agent of acquired immunodeficiency syndrome (AIDS).

human B cell lymphotropic virus (HBLV)   A herpesvirus that can interact with human immunodeficiency virus (HIV) in a way that may increase the severity of HIV infection.

human herpes virus 6 (HHV-6)   A herpes virus that can interact with human immunodeficiency virus (HIV) in a way that may increase the severity of HIV infection.

human immunodeficiency virus (HIV)   (Also referred to as human T-lymphotropic virus type III, HTLV-III, LAV, or human immunodeficiency virus [HIV-1].) This virus is a causative agent of acquired immunodeficiency syndrome (AIDS).

human T lymphotropic virus type III   (Also referred to as HTLV-III, LAV, or human immunodeficiency virus.) This virus is a causative agent of acquired immunodeficiency syndrome (AIDS).

humoral   Any fluid or semifluid in the body.

humoral immunity   A form of body defense against foreign substances represented by antibodies and other soluble, extracellular factors in the blood and lymphatic fluid.

hutchinsonian triad   The characteristic manifestation of congenital syphilis. The three major features are notched teeth, interstitial keratitis, and nerve deafness.

hyaluronidase   (Also called spreading factor.) An enzyme that breaks down hyaluronic acid found in connective tissue.

hybridization   Interaction between two single-stranded nucleic acid molecules to form a double-stranded molecule.

hybridoma   Cell lines created in vitro by fusion of two different cell types. A hybridoma is usually formed from a lymphocyte or plasma cells, one of which is a tumor cell.

hydrophilic   Water loving.

hydrophobic   Water hating.

hypercalcemia   A marked increase in ionized calcium in the circulating blood.

hypergammaglobulinemia   An increased gammaglobulin fraction of plasma protein.

hyperkeratosis   A condition of increased growth of the upper layer of the skin (epidermis) or overgrowth of the cornea.

hypersensitivity   An unpleasant or damaging condition of the body tissues caused by antigenic stimulation. Hypersensitivity reactions include allergies such as hay fever.

hyperviscosity   An increase in the thickness (viscosity) of substances such as blood plasma.

hyperviscosity syndrome   A collection of symptoms resulting from increased resistance (viscosity) of the flow of blood in the circulation.

hypervolemia   An increase of total blood volume.

hypogammaglobulinemia   A decrease in the gammaglobulin fraction of plasma protein.

hypoplastic   Defective or incomplete development of a tissue or organ.

hypothalamus   The portion of the brain beneath the thalamus at the base of the cerebrum that forms the floor and part of the walls of the third ventricle.

icterus (icteric)   A synonym for jaundice or the yellow appearance of the skin and mucous membranes because of bilirubin (a product of red cell breakdown) accumulation.

idiopathic   A disorder or disease without an identifiable external cause or self-originated.

idiotype   The antigenic characteristic of the antibody-variable region.

Ig   (*see* immunoglobulin)

iliac nodes   Small rounded structure located in the lower three fifths of the small intestines from the jejunum to the ileocecal valve or in the inguinal region.

immature B cell   The receptor cell that is finally programmed for insertion of specific IgM molecules into the plasma membrane.

immune complex   The noncovalent combination of an antigen with its specific antibody. An immune complex can be small and soluble or large and precipitating, depending on the nature and proportion of the antigen and antibody.

immune deficiency disease   A condition in which a defect exists in the ability to detect antigens and/or to produce antibodies against foreign antigens.

immune status   The ability of a host (an individual) to recognize and respond to foreign (nonself) substances (e.g., antigens).

immune system   The structures (e.g., the bone marrow, thymus, lymph nodes), cells (e.g., macrophages and lymphocytes), and soluble constituents of the circulating blood (e.g., complement) that allow the host to recognize and respond to foreign (nonself) substances such as antigens.

immunity   The process of being protected against foreign antigens.

immunoblot   (*see* Western blot)

immunocompetent   The ability to mount an immune response; a host who is able to recognize a foreign antigen and build specific antigen-directed antibodies. The term specifically refers to lymphocytes that acquire thymus-dependent characteristics, which allow them to function in an immune response.

immunodeficiency   A dysfunction in body defense mechanisms that cause a failure in detection of foreign antigens and production of antibodies against these foreign (nonself) substances.

immunodiffusion   (Also called double diffusion.) A laboratory method for the quantitative study of antibodies (e.g., radial immunodiffusion [RID]) or qualitative identity of antigens (e.g., Ouchterlony technique). This classic technique is used to detect the presence of antibodies and determine their specificity by visualization of "lines of identity" (precipitin lines). These precipitin lines (precipitated antigen-antibody complexes) form where the binding concentrations of antigen and antibody are equivalent. Patient serum diffuses from one well through the gel and reacts with a known specific antigen or antibody that diffuses through the gel from a second well. Double diffusion is a qualitative technique.

immunoelectrophoresis (IEP)   This is a two-step procedure involving the electrophoretic separation of proteins, followed by the linear diffusion of antibodies into the electrophoretic gel from a trough that extends through the length of the gel adjacent to the electrophoretic path. The reactions produce precipitin arcs at positions of equivalence. Visual estimates of concentration can be made.

immunofixation (IFIX)   This is an enhancement of immunoelectrophoresis. Specific antibodies are used to produce sensitive and specific qualitative visual identification of paraproteins by electrophoretic position.

immunofluorescent assay (IFA)   A laboratory method that uses a fluorescent substance in immunologic studies. For example, particular antigens can be identified microscopically in tissues or cells by the binding of a fluorescent (light-emitting) antibody conjugate.

immunogen   A large organic molecule that is either protein or large polysaccharide and rarely, if ever, lipid.

immunogenic   (*see* antigen)

immunoglobulin   A synonym for *antibody*. The term describes all globulins with antibody activity and has replaced the term *gammaglobulin* because not all antibodies have gamma electrophoretic mobility. Immunoglobulins are divided into five classes, with IgG being the most abundant.

immunologic dysfunction   (*see* immune deficiency disease)

immunology   The study of all aspects of body defenses, such as antigens and antibodies, allergy, and hypersensitivity.

immunosuppression   Repressing the normal adaptive immune response with drugs, chemicals, or other means. This process is frequently necessary before organ transplantation or to alter a hypersensitivity reaction.

immunosuppressive agent   Drug, chemical, or other mechanism that prevents the immune system from recognizing and responding to nonself.

impetigo   A skin infection caused by streptococci that begins as a papule.

inactivated toxins   Toxins produced by bacteria and viruses that have been killed and are no longer capable of causing disease.

inactivated vaccine (killed vaccine)   A vaccine made from a whole microorganism (bacteria or virus) whose biological ability to grow or reproduce is ended.

incomplete antibody   An older term that refers to IgG-type antibodies.

indirect fluorescent antibody (IFA)   This procedure is used to detect antibodies to specific antigenic material in the substrate using fluorescent microscopy.

indirect hemagglutination technique   (Also called *passive* hemagglutination technique.) This laboratory method uses erythrocytes passively coated with substances such as extracts of bacterial cells, rickettsiae, pathogenic fungi, protozoa, purified polysaccharides, or proteins for the detection of antibody.

infarction   An area of tissue, such as heart muscle, that undergoes necrosis (tissue breakdown) because of the lack of oxygen from the circulating blood. A condition of oxygen deprivation may be caused by a narrowing of blood vessels (stenosis) or a blockage of the blood circulation in the vessel (occlusion).

infection   A pathogenic condition caused by microorganisms (i.e., viruses or bacteria) that produce injurious effects.

infectious material   Body fluids or excretory products, or nonhuman substances contaminated with body fluids that contain disease-causing microorganisms.

infectious mononucleosis   A benign lymphoproliferative disorder.

inflammation   Tissue reaction to injury caused by physical or chemical agents, including microorganisms. Symptoms include redness, tenderness, pain, and swelling.

inflammatory response   (*see* inflammation)

inguinal adenopathy   Enlarged lymph nodes in the region of the groin.

in situ hybridization   A laboratory technique for demonstrating the presence of HIV-1 in lymphocytes in primary lymph nodes and in peripheral blood from HIV-infected patients.

interferon alpha   Originally called leukocyte interferon. This protein may be an immunosuppressive agent important in controlling the immune response in a negative manner.

interferon beta   Originally called fibroblast interferon or B-cell stimulatory factor-2. This protein has been reclassified as interleukin-6 (IL-6).

interferon beta-2   (*see* interleukin-6 [IL-6])

interleukin-1 (IL-1)   Originally called lymphocyte-activating factor. A cytokine that activates resting T cells as its most prominent biologic activity.

interleukin-2 (IL-2)   Originally called T-cell growth factor. This cytokine is best known for its ability to initiate proliferation or clonal expansion of activated T cells. IL-2 also dramatically enhances the cytolytic activity of a population of natural killer cells (lymphokine-activated killer cells [LAK] against certain tumor cells.

interleukin-3 (IL-3)   Originally called multicolony-stimulating factor (mCSF). This cytokine principally promotes the growth of early hematopoietic cell lines.

interleukin-4 (IL-4) Originally called B cell-stimulating factor-1. This cytokine is a growth factor for the early activation of resting B cells and influences production of certain immunoglobulin synthesis.

interleukin-5 (IL-5) Originally called T-cell replacing factor or B-cell growth factor-2. This cytokine shares many activities with IL-4, but it is not active on early lymphoid cells.

interleukin-6 (IL-6) Originally called interferon beta-2 or B-cell-stimulating factor-2. This cytokine induces secretion of immunoglobulin and is a major factor in induction of the acute-phase reaction.

interleukin-7 (IL-7) Originally called lymphopoietin-1. This cytokine stimulates early B-cell progenitor cells.

interleukin-8 (IL-8) Originally called monocyte-derived neutrophil chemotactic factor. This cytokine is an inflammatory cytokine that is chemotactic for both neutrophils and T cells.

interleukin-9 (IL-9) This cytokine is a potent lymphocyte growth factor.

interleukin-10 This cytokine inhibits cytokine synthesis in various cells.

interleukin-11 This regulator of hematopoiesis-stroma stimulates the production of megakaryocyte and myeloid progenitors; increases the number of Ig-secreting B lymphocytes.

interleukin-12 Enhances the activity of cytotoxic effector T cells; acts as a growth factor for NK/lymphokine-activated killer cells and for activated T cells of both the CD4+ and CD8+ subsets.

interleukin-13 (IL-13) IL-13 possesses many biologic effects similar to IL-4. The major action of IL-13 on macrophages is to inhibit their activation and to antagonize IFN-γ.

interleukin-14 (IL-14) IL-14 acts as a B-cell growth factor (BCGF).

interleukin-15 (IL-15) IL-15 is biologically similar to IL-2. Endogenous IL-15 is a key condition for IFN-γ synthesis.

interleukin-16 (IL-16) IL-16 acts as a T-cell chemoattractant. It takes part in the regulation of many cytokines IL-1, IL-4, IL-6, IL-10, IL-12, IFN-gamma. Histamine and serotonin increase the production of IL-17. Mimics many of the proinflammatory actions of TNF α and β.

interleukin-18 (IL-18) IL-18 acts as a synergist with IL-12 in some of their effects, especially in the induction of IFN gamma production and inhibition of angiogenesis. It stimulates the production of IFN-γ by NK cells and T cells and synergizes with IL-12 in this response.

interleukin-19 (IL-19) The biologic function is similar to IL-10. Regulates the functions of macrophages, suppresses the activities of Th$_1$ and Th$_2$.

interleukin-20 (IL-20) IL-20 plays an important role in skin inflammations.

interleukin-21 (IL-21) IL-21 regulates hematopoiesis and immune response, influences the development of lymphocytes. Similar to IL-2 and IL-15 in antitumor defense system.

interleukin-22 (IL-22) IL-22 is similar to IL-10 but does not prohibit the production of proinflammatory cytokines through monocytes.

interleukin-23 (IL-23) This newly discovered cytokine shares some in vivo functions with IL-12 including the activation of the transcription factor STAT4 (signal transducer and activator of the transcription factor-4).

interleukin-25 (IL-25) This cytokine, also called SF20, is a novel secreted bone marrow stroma-derived growth factor.

interstitial pneumonitis An inflammation situated between or in the interspaces of the lung tissue.

intraperitoneal fetal transfusion (IPT) The administration of blood to a fetus (unborn infant) via the abdominal cavity.

intrarenal obstruction A blockage within the kidney.

intratubular precipitation The formation of a solid mass from soluble substances within the tubules of the kidney.

intrauterine Within the uterus.

intravascular coagulation The formation of a clot within a vessel (i.e., blood vessels of the circulatory system).

intravascular destruction An alternate pathway for erythrocyte breakdown, which normally accounts for less than 10% of red cell destruction.

intravascular hemolysis An alternate pathway of red cell destruction in which the cells are lysed in the vessels of the circulatory system.

intravenous urography The radiologic study of any part of the urinary tract by the administration through a vein of an opaque medium, which is rapidly excreted in the urine.

intrinsic coagulation mechanism The initial stage of blood coagulation that can be activated by antigen-antibody complexes.

intrinsic factor (IF) A substance secreted by the parietal cells of the mucosa in the fundus region of the stomach.

in vitro A term used to designate outside the body (i.e., in the test tube).

in vivo A term used to designate in the living organism.

isoelectric focusing Separation of molecules on the basis of their charge. Each molecule migrates to the point in the pH gradient where it has no net charge.

isoimmune Possessing antibodies to antigens of the same system.

isotype A term that refers to genetic variation within a family of proteins or peptides so that every member of the species will have each isotype of the family represented in its genome (e.g., immunoglobulin classes).

isotypic varion The heavy-chain constant region structure associated with the different classes and subclasses. Isotopic variants are present in all healthy members of a species.

jaundice (*see also* icterus) A yellow appearance of the skin, sclerae, and body excretions.

Kahler's disease An alternate term for multiple myeloma.

Kaposi's sarcoma A rare, malignant, metastasizing disorder chiefly involving the skin. An increased incidence of this malignancy has been observed in patients suffering from acquired immunodeficiency syndrome.

keratinization The development of or conversion into keratin (an extremely tough scleroprotein found in structures such as hair and nails).

kernicterus The deposition of increased bilirubin, a red cell breakdown product, in lipid-rich nervous tissue such as the brain, which can produce mental retardation or death in the newborn. This condition can occur when circulating plasma bilirubin levels reach 20 mg/dL in a full-term infant and at lower levels in a premature infant.

killer T cells   (Also referred to as cytotoxic T cells, cytotoxic lymphocytes, CTLs.) This subset of lymphocytes can kill cancer cells and cells infected with viruses, fungi, or certain bacteria.

kinetochore   A term for the centromere (the constricted area of the chromosome that demarcates the upper and lower arms of the structure).

kinetoplast   A structure that may also be called the micronucleus. It is an accessory body found in many protozoa.

kinin   A small, biologically active peptide.

kinin system   A series of serum peptides sequentially activated to cause vasodilation and increased vascular permeability.

Kleihauer-Betke test   A testing method based on the differences in solubility between adult and fetal hemoglobin. The test is performed on a maternal blood specimen for the detection of fetal-maternal hemorrhage.

Kupffer cell   A phagocytic type of cell that lines the minute blood vessel (sinusoids) of the liver.

lag period   The period of time between a stimulus (i.e., antigenic stimulation), and a reaction (i.e., immunoglobulin response).

LAK   (*see* lymphokine-activated killer cells)

Langerhans' cell   A macrophage found in the skin.

large granular lymphocyte (LGL)   This term can refer synonymously to a NK cell. About 75% of LGLs function as NK cells and appear to account fully for the NK activity in mixed cell populations.

latent   Hidden or inactive.

latent infection   Persistent infections characterized by periods of reactivation of the signs and symptoms of the disease.

latex agglutination   A technique similar to hemagglutination except smaller, antigen-coated latex particles are substituted for erythrocytes for the detection of antibodies. Antibodies can be absorbed into the latex particles by binding to the Fc region of antibodies, leaving the Fab region free to interact with antigens present in the patient specimen.

lattice formation   The establishment of cross-links between sensitized particles such as erythrocytes.

leukocyte   A type of leukocyte that functions in antigen recognition and antibody formation.

leukocyte interferon   (*see* interferon alpha)

leukocytosis   A marked increase in the total circulating white blood cell concentration.

leukopenia   A marked decrease in the total circulating white blood cell concentration.

leukotrine   A term for the newly identified class of compounds that mediate the inflammatory functions of leukocytes. These substances are a collection of metabolites of arachidonic acid, with powerful pharmacologic effects.

ligand   A linking or binding molecules.

light-chain disease (LCD)   A dysproteinemia of the monoclonal gammopathy type. In LCD only kappa or lambda monoclonal light chains, or Bence Jones proteins, are produced.

lipopolysaccharide (LPS)   The major component of some gram-negative bacterial cell walls, which protects them from phagocytosis but activates C3 directly. LPS can also act as a B-cell mitogen.

liposome   A particle of fatlike substance held in suspension in tissues.

live, attenuated vaccine   A vaccine whose biologic activity has not been inactivated, but whose ability to cause disease has been weakened.

localized   Confined to a specific area.

localized inflammatory response   A tissue reaction confined to a specific area. This response is caused by physical or chemical agents, including microorganisms. The manifestations of the response include redness, tenderness, pain, and swelling.

long terminal redundancy (LTR)   A structure that exists at each end of the proviral genome and plays an important role in the control of viral gene expression and the integration of the provirus into the DNA of the host.

LPS   (*see* lipopolysaccharide)

lymphadenopathy   Disease of the lymph nodes.

lymph node   Any of the accumulations of lymphoid tissue organized as definite lymphoid organs along the course of lymphatic vessels.

lymphoblast   The most immature stage of the lymphocyte-type of leukocyte.

lymphocyte   A small white blood cell found in lymph nodes and the circulating blood. Two major populations of lymphocytes are recognized: T and B cells.

lymphocyte-activating factor   (*see* interleukin-1 [IL-1])

lymphocyte recirculation   This process enables lymphocytes to come in contact with processed foreign antigens and to disseminate antigen-sensitized memory cells throughout the lymphoid system.

lymphocytopenia   A severe decrease in the total number of lymphocytes in the peripheral blood.

lymphocytosis   A significant increase in the total number of lymphocytes in the peripheral blood.

lymphokine   (*see* soluble mediator) This soluble protein mediator is released by sensitized lymphocytes on contact with an antigen.

lymphokine-activated killer cells (LAK)   A population of natural killer cells with enhanced cytolytic activity resulting from the addition of IL-2.

lymphoma   Solid, malignant tumor of the lymph nodes and associated tissues or bone marrow.

lymphopoietin-1   (*see* interleukin-7 [IL-7])

lymphoproliferative disorder   A group of diseases characterized by the proliferation of lymphoid tissues and/or lymphocytes.

lymphosarcoma   Malignant neoplastic disorders of the lymphoid tissues, excluding Hodgkin's disease.

lyse   To break apart or dissolve.

lysis   Irreversible leakage of cell contents that occurs after membrane damage.

lysozyme (muramidase)   An enzyme secreted by macrophages that attacks the cell walls of some bacteria.

m-protein   (*see* monoclonal protein)

macroglobulin   A high-molecular-weight protein of the globulin type.

macrophage   A large mononuclear phagocytic cell of the tissues that exists as either a wandering type or a fixed type that lines the capillaries and sinuses of organs such as the bone marrow, spleen, and lymph nodes. This cell phagocytizes, processes, presents antigens to T cells, and is also responsible for removing damaged tissue, cells, bacteria, and others from the host.

macrophage migration inhibitory factor (MIF) A lymphocyte product that is chemotactic for monocytes. Other similar factors stimulate monocyte and macrophage functions.

macular lesion A discolored, unraised spot on the skin.

maculopapular A lesion with both macular and papular characteristics.

malaise A general feeling of tiredness or discomfort.

malignant (malignancy) Cancerous.

manifestation The development of the signs and symptoms of a disease or disorder.

mast cell A large tissue cell with basophilic granules containing vasoactive amines and heparin. When the cell is damaged, the granules release these inflammatory mediators, which increase vascular permeability and allow complement and phagocytic cells to enter damaged tissues from the circulating blood.

mature B cell Concerned with synthesis of circulating antibodies.

mediastinum The tissues and organs such as the heart, trachea, esophagus, and lymph nodes that separate the sternum in the front (ventral side) from the vertebral column in the back (dorsal side) of the body.

megakaryocytic thrombocytopenic purpura A severe deficiency of the cells (thrombocytes/platelets) related to blood clotting that causes large, purple discolorations of the skin.

melanocyte A cell that produces melanin (the dark pigment normally found in structures such as the hair, eyes, and skin). It can also occur abnormally in certain tumors, melanomas.

memory The immunologic response to an antigenic stimulus that usually leaves the immune system changed.

memory cell Also called a memory B cell. These cells are lymphocytes that recall prior antigen exposure.

meningoencephalitis An inflammation of the brain and its membranous covering (the meninges).

meningovascular A term that refers to the blood vessels of the covering of the brain and spinal cord (meninges).

mesothelium A type of epithelium, originally derived from the mesoderm lining the primitive embryonic body cavity, that becomes the serous membrane of body surfaces, such as the peritoneum (the membrane viscera and lining of the abdominal cavity, except the kidneys), the pleura (the membrane covering the lungs), the walls of the thoracic cavity (the chest and diaphragm), and pericardium (the sac enclosing the heart).

microencephaly Abnormally small brain.

microglia The phagocytic cells of the brain, thought to be derived from incoming blood monocytes.

microplate A compact plate of rigid or flexible plastic with multiple wells.

MIF (*see* macrophage migration inhibitory factor)

microspheres Tiny, microscopic spheres that can carry vaccines or drugs and can pass easily through the body's tissues.

mitogen A substance that stimulates cell division (mitosis).

mobility The ability of specific and nonspecific cells of the immune system to circulate.

monoclonal antibody Purified immunoglobulins produced by cells cloned from a single fusion-type hybridoma cell. Monoclonal antibodies are directed against antigens derived from a single cell line.

monoclonal gammopathy A dysproteinemia in which a single type of immunoglobulin is increased. This immunoglobulin is secreted by a single clone of plasma cells.

monoclonal protein (M protein, paraprotein) A protein characterized by a narrow peak or a localized band on electrophoresis, by a thickened bowed arc on immunoelectrophoresis, and by a localized band on immunofixation.

monocyte A type of leukocyte found in the peripheral blood.

monocytic Refers to the leukocyte type, monocytes.

monokine A soluble protein mediator.

mononuclear cell Cell types including the monocytes, promyelocytes, myelocytes, and blasts.

mononuclear-phagocyte system Formerly called the reticuloendothelial system (RES). This system is the body defense system and is composed of macrophages and a network of specialized cells of the spleen, thymus, and other lymphoid tissues.

monovalent An antigen with only one antigenic determinant.

morbidity A condition of being diseased; the ratio of sick to healthy persons or the number of cases of a specific illness in a designated population.

mortality The rate of death or ratio of the number of deaths to living individuals in a designated population.

multicolony-stimulating factor (mCSF) (*see* interleukin-3 [IL-3])

multiple myeloma A malignant disorder of plasma cells also known as plasma cell myeloma or Kahler's disease.

multipotential stem cell (MSC) Precursor cells in the bone marrow capable of differentiating into various blood cell (hematopoietic) types.

murine hybridoma The fusion product of a malignant and normal cell that produces large quantities of monoclonal antibodies.

myalgia Pain or tenderness in the muscles.

myelitis An inflammation of the spinal cord or bone marrow.

myeloma cell Plasma cells derived from malignant tumor strains.

myeloma clone A group of neoplastic cells that are descendants of a single, neoplastic cell.

myeloma kidney Abnormalities of the kidney associated with the neoplastic disorder multiple myeloma.

myelomatosis A term for multiple myeloma.

myeloperoxidase An important enzyme in the process of phagocytosis.

myocarditis An inflammation of the cardiac muscle tissue.

myosin One of the two main contractile proteins found in muscles.

naked DNA vaccine Vaccine made up of deoxyribonucleic acid that is not encased or encapsulated.

nasopharyngeal carcinoma A malignancy involving the nose and throat.

natural killer cell (NK cells, previously called *null cells*) A population of effector lymphocytes that produces such mediators as interferon and interleukin-2.

natural resistance Innate or inborn.

necrosis The death of cells or a localized group of cells.

necrotizing vasculitis An inflammation of a vessel such as a blood vessel that results in tissue destruction.

neonatal septicemia A systemic disease caused by pathogenic microorganisms or their toxins in the blood of an infant up to 4 weeks old.

neonate An infant up to 4 weeks old.

neoplasm Any new and abnormal tissue such as a tumor.

neoplastic Refers to new, abnormal tissue growth.

nephelometry A laboratory assay method based on the measurement of the turbidity of particles in suspension. A nephelometer can be used for assays such as quantitating immunoglobulin concentrations in serum.

nephritis An inflammation of the kidney.

nephritogenic An agent or microorganism capable of causing an inflammation of the kidney.

nephropathy Any inflammatory, degenerative, or sclerotic disease of the kidneys.

nephrosis A condition of the kidney, particularly tubular degeneration, without the signs and symptoms of inflammation.

nephrotic syndrome A disorder of the kidneys characterized by a decreased concentration of albumin in the circulating blood, marked edema (swelling), increased protein in the urine (proteinuria), and increased susceptibility to infection.

nephrotoxic An agent such as a specific toxin that is destructive to kidney cells.

neurologic sequelae Morbid nervous system signs and symptoms that follow or are caused by a disease.

neurotoxic cytokine A substance able to destroy nervous tissue.

neutralization This procedure is similar to complement fixation but can be used only when the antibody being measured is directed against a hemolysin (a bacterial toxin capable of directly lysing red blood cells).

neutropenia A marked decrease in the neutrophil-type of leukocyte.

neutrophil A granulocyte-containing type of leukocyte.

NK cell (*see* natural killer cell)

non-Hodgkin's lymphoma A condition of solid, malignant tumors of the lymph nodes and associated tissues or bone marrow that is not of the Hodgkin's type.

nonself A term covering microorganisms as well as cells, organs, and other materials from a different animal or individual. The term is not generally applied to food or drugs, although they are sometimes involved in immunity.

nonsymptomatic An abnormal condition such as an infectious disease that does not manifest the signs and symptoms of the disorder.

normal flora Microorganisms that normally inhabit areas of the body such as the skin, mucous membranes, and intestinal tract.

normocytic, normochromic anemia A deficiency of erythrocytes; however, the erythrocytes present in the circulation are of normal size and color.

Northern blot This molecular biology technique is similar to the Southern blot technique, except that messenger-RNA (m-RNA) from the specimen is separated and blotted. If specific RNA is present, the radiolabel can be detected.

nosocomial Pertaining to a hospital. For example, a nosocomial infection is a hospital-acquired infection.

null cell (*see* natural killer cells)

oligonucleotide probe A string of nucleotides used to detect the presence of a complementary nucleic acid sequence.

oncogene A transforming gene of cellular origin contained in retroviruses and associated with acute leukemias.

oncogenic Associated with tumor formation.

oocyst The encysted form of a fertilized gamete occurring in certain sporozoa; an immature ovum.

opportunistic infection A microbial disease that infects a debilitated host.

opsonization When the complement component C3b is attached to a particle, it promotes the adherence of phagocytic cells because of the C3 receptors. Antibody, if present, augments this by binding to Fc receptors.

oropharynx The part of the throat between the soft palate and the upper edge of the epiglottis.

osteoclast A giant, multinucleated cell formed in the bone marrow of growing bones. This cell is associated with reabsorption and removal of unwanted tissue.

osteomyelitis An inflammation of bone/bone marrow.

osteonecrosis The accelerated destruction of bone tissue.

osteoporosis Increased porosity of bone that causes softening and thinning of the bone.

otitis media Inflammation of the middle ear.

pancreatitis An inflammation of the structure, with endocrine and exocrine functions located behind the stomach, between the spleen, and duodenum.

papule A small, solid, elevated lesion of the skin.

paraprotein (*see* M protein or monoclonal protein)

parenchymal Refers to the functional constituents of an organ as opposed to the framework (stroma).

parenteral Situation outside of the alimentary (oral) canal. Parenteral medications, for example, can be administered subcutaneously (beneath the skin), intramuscularly, or intravenously.

parotid gland The largest of the three salivary glands located near the ear.

paroxysmal cold hemoglobinuria (PCH) A form of destruction of erythrocytes (red blood cells) caused by an IgG protein that reacts with the erythrocytes in colder parts of the body and subsequently causes complement components to irreversibly bind to erythrocytes. It is commonly seen as an acute transient condition secondary to viral infection.

paroxysmal nocturnal hemoglobinuria (PNH) A disorder in which the patient's erythrocytes act as a complement activator. The activation of complement results in excessive lysis of the patient's erythrocytes.

passive hemagglutination technique (*see* indirect hemagglutination technique)

pathogen A disease-causing microorganism or agent.

pathogenesis The origin of disease.

pathogenic (pathogenicity) The disease-producing potential of a microorganism.

perforation A hole or break in the wall or membrane of an organ or body structure.

periarteritis nodosa An inflammation of the layers of small and medium-sized arteries. This condition is manifested by a variety of systemic signs and symptoms, including febrile manifestations.

pericarditis An inflammation of the serous membrane lining of the sac surrounding the heart and the origins of the great blood vessels.

perinatal Preceding, during, or after birth.

perineal region The external region between the vulva and anus in the female or between the scrotum and anus in the male.

peritonitis An inflammation of the serous membrane covering the intestines and abdominal organs (viscera) and the abdominal cavity.

pernicious anemia An erythrocytic disorder associated with defective vitamin B_{12} uptake.

petechiae Small, purple hemorrhagic spots on the skin or mucous membranes.

PG (*see* prostaglandins)

phagocyte Any cell capable of engulfing and destroying foreign particles such as bacteria.

phagocytosis A form of endocytosis. This important body defense mechanism is the process in which specialized cells engulf and destroy foreign particles such as microorganisms or damaged cells. Macrophages and segmented neutrophils (PMNs) are the most important phagocytic cells.

phagolysosome A vacuole (secondary lysosome) formed by the fusion of a phagosome and a primary lysome(s) in which microorganisms are killed and digested.

phagosome A membrane-bound vesicle in a phagocyte containing the phagocytized material.

pharyngitis An inflammation of the throat.

pharynx The throat.

phototherapy The use of ultraviolet light to accelerate the breakdown of bilirubin that has abnormally accumulated in the skin.

phytohemagglutinin A specific substance, a lectin, that is derived from plants and has the ability to agglutinate erythrocytes.

plasma The straw-colored fluid component of blood in circulating or anticoagulated blood.

plasma cell A few mature plasma cells can be found in the bone marrow, but they are not normally seen in the circulating blood.

plasma cell myeloma (*see* multiple myeloma)

plasmacytoid Plasma cell-like.

plasmacytoid lymphocyte A cell that resembles a plasma cell.

plasmin A proteolytic enzyme with the ability to dissolve formed fibrin clots.

plasminogen The inactive precursor to plasmin, which is converted to plasmin by the action of substances such as urokinase.

platelet factor-3 An important factor associated with blood thrombocytes (platelets).

pleura The membrane covering the lungs, the walls of the thoracic cavity (chest), and diaphragm.

pleuritis An inflammation of the serous membrane lining, the pleura.

pluripotent (*see* multipotential stem cells)

PMN (*see* polymorphonuclear leukocyte)

Pneumocystis carinii A protozoa that causes interstitial plasma cell pneumonia. This microorganism is frequently observed as an opportunistic pathogen in patients with acquired immunodeficiency syndrome (AIDS).

pol gene A gene of a retrovirus such as HIV that encodes for reverse transcriptase, endonuclease, and proteases activities.

polyarthritis Inflammation of several joints.

polyclonal gammopathy A dysproteinemia in which the products of a number of different cell types are demonstrated.

polyendocrinopathies A disease condition that involves several endocrine glands.

polymerase chain reaction (PCR) This molecular biology technique uses amplification of low levels of specific DNA sequences in a sample to reach the threshold of detection. The reaction products are hybridized to a radioactively labeled DNA segment complementary to a short sequence of the amplified DNA. After electrophoresis, the radiolabeled product of specific size is detected by autoradiography.

polymorphonuclear leukocyte A short-lived scavenger blood cell whose granules contain powerful bactericidal enzymes.

polymyositis Inflammation of several muscles at the same time. This condition is manifested by a number of signs and symptoms including pain, edema, deformity, and sleep disturbance.

polyneuropathy A disease involving several nerves.

polyserositis A condition of general inflammation of serous membrane with effusion (the escape of fluid). The inflammation is progressive and especially prevalent in the upper abdominal cavity.

posterior cervical In the back (dorsal surface) and associated with the vertebral bone of the neck.

postnatal After birth.

postoccipital lobe The back portion (lobe) of the cerebral hemisphere that is shaped like a three-sided pyramid.

postpartum A term referring to after birth.

potency The strength of a substance.

pre-B cell An early, rapidly dividing mature B-cell precursor.

precipitate The formation of a solid mass from previously soluble components. An alternate definition is to occur suddenly or unexpectedly.

prenatal A term that refers to before birth.

presentation of antigens The activity associated with the conveying of an altered antigenic molecule to T and B cells by macrophages. This process is necessary for most adaptive responses.

prime To give an initial sensitization to antigen.

primary antibody response An immunologic (IgM antibody) response that occurs after a foreign antigen challenge.

primary biliary cirrhosis Cirrhosis (interstitial inflammation of an organ) of the liver caused by chronic retention of bile. The causative agent (etiology) is unknown in the primary form of the disorder.

primary immunodeficiency Dysfunction in an immune organ such as the thymus.

primary immunoglobulin deficiency A genetically determined disorder associated with certain diseases.

primary lymphoid tissue or organ The bone marrow and thymus gland are classified as primary or central lymphoid tissues.

primitive stem cell The early form of uncommitted, multipotential blood cells that replicate themselves and generate more differentiated daughter cells.

procainamide A drug that functions as a cardiac depressant used in the treatment of cardiac arrhythmias.

prodromal period (prodrome, prodromal)   The earliest or initial sign or symptom of a developing disease or disorder. For example, the prodromal period of an infectious disease manifested by rash would be the space of time between the earliest symptoms and the appearance of the rash or fever.

prognosis   A forecast of the probable outcome of a condition, disorder, or disease.

progressive systemic sclerosis (PSS)   A disorder of loss of tissue elasticity throughout the body that advances in severity over time.

prophylaxis   A synonym for prevention.

prostaglandin   A prostaglandin is a pharmacologically active derivative or arachidonic acid. Prostaglandins are naturally occurring unsaturated fatty acids that stimulate and suppress the effects of many inflammatory processes and stimulate the contraction of uterine and other smooth muscle tissues. Different prostaglandins are capable of modulating cell mobility and immune responses.

prostration   A condition of extreme exhaustion (lack of strength or energy).

proteinuria   Protein (albumin) in the urine.

proteolysis   The breaking apart of a protein molecule.

proteolytic enzyme   A substance able to break apart a protein molecule.

prothrombin time (PT)   A blood coagulation test that assesses the process of clotting beginning with the formation of factor X.

protocol   The steps usually followed in a situation such as laboratory testing or patient treatment.

proximal humeri   The end portion of the upper bone of the arm nearest the center of the body (shoulder).

prozone phenomenon   A possible cause of false-negative antigen-antibody reactions caused by an excessive amount of antibody.

psychoneuroimmunology   The relationship between the mind and the body that combines research in basic science with psychologic and psychosocial factors.

psychosocial factors   Related to both psychologic and social factors.

PT   (*see* prothrombin time)

purpura   An extensive area of red or dark purple discoloration of the skin.

pyelonephritis   An inflammation of the kidney and pelvis region of the kidney (the funnel-shaped expansion of the upper end of the ureter into which the renal calices open).

pyoderma   Any purulent (pus-producing) skin disease.

pyrogenic   Microorganisms that cause the production of pus.

pyroglobulin   An abnormal (IgM) globulin that precipitates on heating to $50°$ or $60°$ C but does not redissolve on cooling or intensified heating as do typical Bence Jones pyroglobulins.

radial immunodiffusion (RID)   A quantitative variation of immunodiffusion. The diameter of the precipitin ring formed from evenly distributed antigen (or antibody) and its counterpart from the test sample diffuses into agar gel from a single well, resulting in a circular ring of precipitin around the sample well. The diameter of the precipitin ring is proportional to the concentration of specific antibody (or antigen) present in the test specimen. A comparison to known standards allows for quantitation of the test specimen.

Radioallergosorbent test (RAST)   This procedure detects the presence of IgE (and IgG) antibodies to allergens.

radioimmunoassay (RIA)   A laboratory technique involving the use of radioactive substances to evaluate immunoglobulins. Traditional RIA is done with specific antibodies in liquid solution. Solid-phase RIA uses antibody bound to solid support (e.g., tubes, glass beads).

Raynaud's phenomenon (Raynaud's disease)   A condition of episodic constriction of small arteries of the extremities (usually fingers or toes) induced by cold temperatures or emotional stress that would not affect an unafflicted person. The signs and symptoms of the condition include two forms: a pale appearance and numb feeling followed by redness and tingling or a swollen, red, and painful condition. Heat relieves the condition if the stimulus was cold-induced.

reagin   An antibody-like protein that binds to a test antigen such as cardiolipid-lecithin-coated cholesterol particles in the venereal disease research laboratory (VDRL) serologic method of testing for syphilis; or an old term for IgE with a specificity for allergens.

reagin antibodies   Nontreponemal antibodies produced by a patient infected with *Treponemal pallidum* against components of their own or other mammalian cells.

reanneal   To reassemble or recombine two nucleic acid strands.

recessive   The term used to describe a gene that is not expressed unless it is in the homozygous form.

receptor   A cell surface molecule that binds specifically to particular proteins or peptides in the fluid phase.

recirculation   In reference to lymphocytes, mostly T cells, which pass from the circulating blood through the lymphatic system back to the circulating blood.

recombinant DNA technology   (Also referred to as recombinant genetic engineering.) The technique in which genetic material from one organism is inserted into a foreign cell or another organism in order to mass-produce the protein encoded by the inserted genes.

recombinant vector vaccine   A vaccine that combines a vector, a harmless bacterium or virus used to transport an antigen into the body to stimulate protective immunity, and an antigen or immunogen from an organism other than the vector.

refractory anemia   A form of anemia (decreased erythrocytes in the circulation) resistant to ordinary treatment.

regimen   A schedule of treatment.

regional adenopathy   Swelling or enlargement of the lymph nodes in a certain area or areas of the body.

relative lymphocytosis   An increase of lymphocytes in the circulating blood in relationship to the total number of leukocytes in the circulation.

renal impairment   Dysfunction of the kidneys.

renal insufficiency   Inadequate functioning of the kidneys.

replicability   The ability of specific and nonspecific cells of the immune system to produce daughter cells.

restriction endonuclease   Bacterial enzyme that recognizes short sequences of DNA and cleaves the DNA near this restriction site; each enzyme is named after the bacteria from which it has been isolated.

reticuloendothelial system   (*see* mononuclear phagocytic system)

retinal hemorrhage   Extreme bleeding from the inner layer (the retina) into the fluid-filled interior of the eye.

retinitis   An inflammation of the inner layer (the retina) of the eye.

retroauricular   Behind the protruding portion of the external ear that surrounds the opening (auricle).

retrovirus   A type of virus that carries a single, positive-stranded RNA and uses a special enzyme, reverse transcriptase, to convert viral RNA into DNA.

reverse passive hemagglutination   A laboratory method that uses erythrocytes as an indicator cell to observe the absence of agglutination in the presence of antibodies.

reverse transcriptase   An enzyme found in the single, positive-stranded RNA core of a retrovirus.

Reye's syndrome   An acute and frequently fatal childhood disease that may follow a variety of common viral infections within several hours or days. The signs and symptoms of disease include persistent vomiting followed by delirium caused by edema of the brain, hypoglycemia, dysfunction of the liver, convulsions, and coma.

rheumatic fever   A disease caused by the toxins produced by group A beta streptococci.

Rh factor   This blood group antigen, named for the rhesus monkey, was originally identified because an antibody agglutinated the erythrocytes of all rhesus monkeys and 85% of humans. The antibody was later discovered to be the Landsteiner-Wiener antibody, which is dissimilar from the Rh antibody.

rhinorrhea   Watery discharge from the nose.

rouleaux (rouleaux formation)   Pseudoagglutination or the false clumping of erythrocytes when the cells are suspended in their own serum. This phenomenon is caused by an abnormal protein in the serum, plasma expanders (e.g., dextran), or Wharton's jelly from cord blood samples. Rouleaux formation appears as rolls resembling stacks of coins on microscopic examination.

rubella   The viral cause of measles.

rubella syndrome   A number of congenital anomalies such as mental retardation and cardiovascular defects caused by the rubella virus.

scarlet fever   An acute infectious disease caused by group A streptococcus. The rash and other signs and symptoms are caused by the erythema-producing toxin produced by the streptococci.

sclerodactyly   A chronic disorder characterized by progressive fibrosis of the fingers and toes.

scleroderma   A progressive fibrosis beginning with the skin.

sebum   The oily secretion of the sebaceous glands whose ducts open into the hair follicles.

secondary immunoglobulin deficiency   An acquired disorder associated with certain diseases.

secondary lymphoid tissue or secondary lymphoid organs   The secondary tissues include the lymph nodes, spleen, and Peyer's patches in the intestine.

self-limiting   Confined, able to resolve in time.

senescence   The process of growing old.

sensitivity   The frequency of positive EIA results obtained in the testing of a population of individuals who are truly positive for antibody (e.g., anti-HIV).

sensitization   Physical attachment of antibody molecules to antigens on the erythrocytic membrane.

sepsis   Microbial infection throughout the systemic circulation.

septic arthritis   An inflammation of the joints caused by the presence of pathogenic microorganisms.

septicemia   The presence of pathogenic microorganisms in the blood.

sequelae   A disease condition occurring after or as a consequence of another condition or event.

seroconversion   The development of a demonstrable antibody response to a disease or vaccine.

seroepidemiologic   The evidence of antibodies to a disease in a defined population.

seronegative   The lack of evidence of an antibody to a disease.

serositis   An inflammation of the membrane consisting of mesothelium, a thin layer of connective tissue, having lines enclosing the body cavities.

serum   Straw-colored fluid present after blood clots.

serum electrophoresis   A technique for separating ionic molecules, principally proteins, into five fractions on a medium such as paper or cellulose acetate. The separation is based on the rate of migration based on size and ionic charge of these individual components in an electrical field. The components can be visualized by staining and quantitated using a densitometer.

serum sickness   A hypersensitivity reaction occurring after a single, large injection of serum from an animal of another species.

sex-linked   A genetic trait associated with the X chromosome.

sialic acid   Found on red blood cell membranes; produces a negative surrounding charge.

sickle cell anemia   An inherited form of anemia caused by a genetically defective hemoglobin.

sIg   (*see* surface immunoglobulin)

silent carrier   A carrier of a disease who manifests no clinically obvious symptoms or signs.

single-strand conformational polymorphism   A technique used to detect subtle differences in nucleotide sequences; typically used to compare sequences from two or more individuals to determine whether or not they are identical or if a mutation has occurred.

sinusitis   An inflammation of the cavity in a bone, such as in the paranasal sinuses.

sinusoid   A specialized capillary found in locations such as the bone marrow, spleen, and liver through which blood passes to reach the veins, allowing the lining macrophages to remove damaged or antibody-coated cells.

Sjögren's syndrome   An autoimmune disorder manifested by enlargement of the parotid glands, chronic polyarthritis, and dryness of the conjunctiva, throat, and mouth.

SLE   (*see* systemic lupus erythematosus)

solid-phase assay   A laboratory method in which one of the reactants is bound to surface.

soluble mediator   (Also called lymphokine.) A substance secreted by monocytes, lymphocytes, or neutrophils that provides the mechanism of cell-to-cell communication. Important lymphokines include migration inhibitory factor (MIF), interleukin-2 (T-cell growth factor), chemotactic factors, and interleukin-1.

somnolence   A condition of prolonged drowsiness or a state resembling a trance.

sor gene   A gene of a retrovirus such as HIV. The product of the small, open-reading frame is a protein that induces antibody production in the natural course of infection.

Southern blot analysis   A molecular biology laboratory technique used in DNA analysis. DNA from a patient specimen is denatured, treated with enzymes to produce DNA fragments; then the single-stranded DNA fragments are separated by electrophoresis. These fragments are further treated, and radiolabeling is introduced. The resulting DNA with the radiolabel is then, if present, detected by autoradiography. This technique has many applications including studying the HIV-1 sequence in peripheral blood cells and tissues such as lymph nodes, liver, and kidney.

specificity   1. The ability of a particular antibody to combine with one antigen instead of another based on the fact that the binding sites of antibodies directed against determinants of one antigen are not complementary to determinants of another dissimilar antigen. 2. The proportion of negative EIA test results obtained in the population of individuals who actually lack the antibody in question (e.g., anti-HIV).

spirochete   A type of bacteria with a twisted or spiral appearance when viewed microscopically.

spleen   A large, glandlike organ located in the upper left quadrant of abdomen under the ribs. The spleen is the body's largest reservoir of mononuclear-phagocytic cells.

splenomegaly   A markedly enlarged spleen.

stasis   Stoppage of bleeding.

steric hindrance   Mutual blocking of dissimilar antibodies with the same binding constant, directed against antigenic determinants located in close proximity on a cell's surface.

streptokinase   An enzyme that dissolves clots by converting plasminogen to plasmin.

subclinical infection   An early or mild form of a disease without visible signs.

substrate   A substance on which another substance such as an enzyme acts.

supernatant   Fluid above the solid portion (e.g., cells in a centrifuged or sedimented specimen).

suppressor/cytotoxic   (Also referred to as T8.) A major phenotypic lymphocyte subset of T lymphocytes.

supraglottic larynx   The area above the true vocal cords.

surface immunoglobulin (sIg)   Immunoglobulin, at first cytoplasmic and later surface bound, is the key feature of B cells, through which they recognize specific antigens.

surrogate testing   Procedures performed in place of specific tests for an infectious agent such as non-A, non-B hepatitis.

susceptibility   Having little resistance, such as resistance to infectious disease.

symptom   An indication of a disorder or disease, or a variation in normal body function.

symptomatic   A deviation from usual function or appearance.

syncytia   Giant, multinucleated groups or masses of cells.

syndrome   A collection of symptoms that occur together.

synergistic   The action of two or more agents that frequently produces a much greater effect than the expected sum of the individual agents.

systemic   Throughout the body.

systemic circulation   Blood circulation throughout the body.

systemic lupus erythematosus (SLE)   An autoimmune disorder expressed as a group of multisymptom disorders that can affect practically every organ of the body.

systemic sclerosis   Loss of tissue elasticity of vessels such as blood vessels throughout the whole body.

T cell   (*see* T lymphocyte)

T-cell growth factor   (*see* interleukin-2 [IL-2])

T-cell replacing factor   (*see* interleukin-5 [IL-5])

T lymphocyte or T cell   The cells responsible for the cellular immune response and involved in the regulation of antibody reactions.

Tabes dorsalis   A slowly progressive degeneration of the nervous system caused by syphilis. In untreated patients this condition may appear from 5 to 20 years after the initial infection with *Treponema pallidum*.

tachycardia   An abnormally fast heart rate.

tart cell   When a blood preparation is microscopically examined for the presence of cells associated with systemic lupus erythematosus (SLE), tart cells may be seen. Tart cells usually represent monocytes that have phagocytized another whole cell or nucleus, often a lymphocyte. These cell formations can be mistaken for the classic LE cell connected with SLE.

TdT   (*see* terminal deoxynucleotidyl transferase)

telangiectasia   A vascular lesion formed by the dilation of a group of capillaries and occasionally of terminal arteries.

terminal deoxynucleotidyl transferase (TdT)   An intracellular DNA polymerase found mainly in cortical, and therefore young thymocytes. These cells are lost from the thymus after corticosteroid treatment.

thrombocytopenia   A severe deficiency of circulating blood platelets (thrombocytes).

thrombophlebitis   An inflammation of a vein that develops before the formation of a thrombus (clot).

thrombosis   A condition of formation of a blood clot or thrombus.

thrombus   A clot.

thymoma   A tumor derived from the epithelial or lymphoid elements of the thymus.

thymosin   (Also called thymic hormone.) A humoral factor secreted by the thymus that promotes the growth of peripheral lymphoid tissue.

thymus   A primary or central lymphoid tissue responsible for processes of lymphocytes into the T type of cell. This ductless, glandlike structure is located beneath the sternum (breastbone).

titer   The concentration or strength of an antibody expressed as the highest dilution of the serum that produces agglutination (e.g., 1:4, 1:8).

TNF   (*see* tumor necrosis factor)

toxic shock syndrome   A serious and potentially fatal disorder caused by toxins produced by *Staphylococcus aureus*.

Toxoplasma gondii   A protozoal microorganism that can be transmitted from an infected mother to an unborn infant. The disease can result in encephalomyelitis.

trans   A prefix meaning across, over, or through.

transaminase (ALT/SGPT)   A surrogate test for non-A, non-B hepatitis.

transforming-growth factors   Cytokines identified as products of virally transformed cells. These molecules can induce phenotypic transformation in non-neoplastic cells.

transplacental hemorrhage The entrance of fetal blood cells into the maternal circulation.

treponemes *(Treponema)* A genus of spirochetes.

tubular cell injury Damage to cells of the renal tubules.

tumor necrosis factor A cytokine that can destroy tumor cells.

ubiquitous Existing everywhere.

ulcerative lesion An open sore.

unilateral blindness The lack of vision in one eye.

Universal Blood and Body Fluid Precautions Specific regulations and practices, such as wearing gloves, that conform to current state and federal requirements. These precautions assume that *all* specimens (e.g., blood) have the potential for transmitting disease.

urticaria Hives.

vaccination A method of stimulating the adaptive immune response and generating memory and acquired resistance without suffering disease. A form of artificial active-acquired immunity.

vaccine A suspension of killed or attenuated (inactivated) infectious agents administered to establish resistance to the disease.

variable region The antigen-binding portion of an immunoglobulin molecule.

variable lymphocyte A type of white blood cell that lacks the characteristics of a normal lymphocyte.

varicella A term for chickenpox.

varicosity A condition of having distended veins.

vasculitis An inflammation of a vessel such as a blood vessel.

vasoamine Vasoactive amines (e.g., histamine, 5-hydroxytryptamine), produced by mast cells, basophils, and platelets and causing increased capillary permeability.

vector A bacterium or virus that does not cause disease in humans and is used in genetically engineered vaccines.

venereal route A sexually transmitted mode of infection.

viral capsid antigen (VCA) A "new" antigen expressed by B lymphocytes infected with Epstein-Barr virus in infectious mononucleosis.

viremia A systemic (blood) infection caused by a virus.

virion A complete virus particle.

virulence The degree of pathogenicity or ability to cause disease of a microorganism.

Waldenström's primary macroglobulinemia (Waldenström's macroglobulinemia) A neoplastic proliferation of the lymphocyte-plasma cell system.

Wasserman test The first diagnostic serologic test for syphilis; no longer in use.

Western blot A molecular biology technique similar to the Northern blot and Southern blot procedures. This procedure is used to detect antibodies to specific epitopes of electrophoretically separated subspecies of antigens. Western blot is often used to confirm the specificity of antibodies detected by an ELISA screening procedure.

Index

NOTE: Page numbers followed by f indicate figures; t tables; b boxes.